THE CIRCULATING PLATELET

Edited by SHIRLEY A. JOHNSON

Thrombosis Research Laboratory
Veterans Administration Hospital
and
Department of Physiology
Georgetown University School of Medicine
Washington, D. C.

1971

ACADEMIC PRESS   New York and London

ACADEMIC PRESS, INC.
111 Fifth Avenue, New York, New York 10003

United Kingdom Edition published by
ACADEMIC PRESS, INC. (LONDON) LTD.
Berkeley Square House, London W1X 6BA

LIBRARY OF CONGRESS CATALOG CARD NUMBER: 72- 127686

PRINTED IN THE UNITED STATES OF AMERICA

CONTENTS

v

4.   Energy Metabolism

Rudolf Gross and Wolfgang Schneider

5.   Membrane Glycoproteins of Blood Platelets

G. A. Jamieson and D. S. Pepper

6.   Platelet Proteins

Ralph L. Nachman

7.   Thrombosthenin

Ernst F. Lüscher and M. Bettex-Galland

8. Functions of Platelet Membranes

Aaron J. Marcus, Lenore B. Safier, and Harris L. Ullman

9. Platelet Aggregation

Louis M. Aledort

10. Endothelial Supporting Function of Platelets

Shirley A. Johnson

11. Role of Platelets in Blood Clotting

Walter H. Seegers

12. Platelets in Hemostasis and Thrombosis

Shirley A. Johnson

13. Role of Platelets in Fibrinolysis

Hau C. Kwaan

14. Immunological Reactions Involving Platelets

Roger M. Des Prez and Samuel R. Marney, Jr.

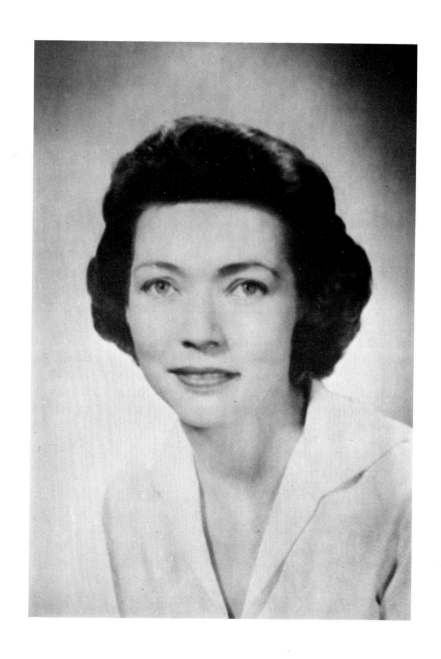

SHIRLEY A. JOHNSON

(April 15, 1922–September 11, 1970)

Our great American, Thomas Jefferson, gave much attention to criteria whereby he estimated the strength of the mind. He listed four qualities in the order of their importance: (1) good humor, (2) integrity, (3) industry, and (4) science. These characteristics can be cultivated. Paying attention to our goals becomes most profitable when they are accurately established. In our Memorial Service, I was interested in utilizing to the utmost the mind qualities exemplified by Shirley Johnson Greenwalt. In each individual these live and work and grow.

Evidently an imprint of basic value was brought from the Canadian prairie provinces of Saskatchewan and Alberta where she was born and lived. Moral soundness, honesty, and uprightness were further nurtured in Victoria College (B. A., 1945) and the Graduate School (Ph.D., 1949) of the University of Toronto. Character builds itself in the stream of life. With Shirley Johnson the commonplace affairs generally proved to be viewed in a special way. Every moment is, of course, new, fresh, and bright, and the one who takes notice of this is soon noticed. On the occasion of her becoming a citizen of the United States of America the oath was administered in just another room by an official. This time, however, the witnesses knew they were especially selected. They appeared in finest dress, and further meaning was added by having a special luncheon after the conferring of citizenship. In her home a dinner or breakfast was prefaced by a short prayer in the finest religious tradition. An ordinary reprint of my Harvey Lecture was presented to me under a special cover before a small group of students, and thus was elevated to extraordinary status. About ten years ago, she and Tibor J. Greenwalt were married. The wedding and the modest reception which followed were attended by only a few, but were very special to all. The marriage was great news for the little world-family of hematologists. Frequently I pass the small church in Grosse Pointe Farms, Michigan, where the ceremony took place, and repeatedly it pleases me that this adventure was such a great success.

For the presentation of a scientific paper by Shirley Johnson a manuscript was first perfected and then read. The remarks, which carried clearly, were synchronized precisely with the projection of lantern slides. These were prepared with meticulous care. With color added, the meaning was easy to grasp. The quality of the presentation was a supplement to the excellence of the work itself. Presentations were made at congresses in Paris, Sydney, Moscow, Istanbul, Vienna, Munich, London, and many another city. These left impressions which generated respect for experimental work in the United States, and especially for women in science. This demonstrated that "all virtue and goodness tend to make men powerful in the world; but they who aim at the power have not the virtue" (Newman's law).

Since Jefferson assigned a high rating to good humor or good-naturedness, I feel I must introduce another attitude. When Shirley switched from home economics studies to science technology, it was observed in her characteristic fashion: "There is more to life than cooking cabbage." Consider another incident. Organizing the International Symposium on Platelets at the Henry Ford Hospital was a laborious extracurricular task, but the work was all completed efficiently and, as usual, everything was in good order. The symposium was scheduled to begin on a Friday morning in January. About Thursday noon, or exactly when airplanes from near and far distances were expected to land with participants, a snowstorm started and made safe landing at Detroit impossible for several hours. It was observed good-naturedly that "the timing of the storm was certainly very accurate." On another occasion, there was a heated discussion at a meeting. It was regarded as serious because "even Doctor Jones got very peppery."

The first position after graduation was at Kirksville, Missouri, where the main effort was devoted to instruction. In 1951, research was begun at Wayne State University. She was living with her brother and family in Detroit at the time, and came to the department where I was chairman saying she wanted to work in physiology. It was our first meeting. On such short notice it was not possible to provide for funds. There were only prospects, but this did not stop Doctor Johnson. She began to work on a volunteer basis. This was an unusual beginning for someone destined to rise to the top ranks. Years later, the University presented her with one of its centennial medals. This was in recognition of outstanding scholarship and loyal support of the ideals and programs of the University.

The work at Wayne State University was begun with enthusiasm and continued at a high level of productivity later at the Henry Ford Hospital

(1956–1960), then at Milwaukee County Hospital, the Veterans Administration Hospital, and Marquette University in Milwaukee where Doctor Greenwalt lived. When he became Medical Director, Blood Program, American National Red Cross in Washington, D.C., Doctor Johnson became Chief of the Thrombosis Research Laboratory of the Veterans Administration Hospital and held appointments in physiology at George Washington University and Georgetown University. At each place there was the difficult task of finding funds and help and arranging the laboratory.

The first experiments at Wayne State University were with blood platelets and the blood coagulation mechanisms. Quite soon platelets were obtained in large quantities from bovine plasma, and the substance(s) required to correct the procoagulant power of hemophilia B plasma was found in serum. When oral anticoagulants were being used, this substance could not be found in serum, and its metabolic synthesis was considered to be vitamin K dependent. A theory was advanced to account for the inactivity of the antihemophilic globulin in serum. Activity was recovered by ether extraction. Antifibrinolysin activity was found in platelets. Plasma antithrombin activities were differentiated. Her studies on functional aberration of platelets in clinical states became well known. There was a study of the defects in the blood coagulation mechanisms in polycythemia vera. The morphological location of platelet factor 3 was studied, as well as the suppression of its activity in uremia, in macroglobulinemia, and by dextran. The endothelial supporting function of platelet factor 3 was demonstrated, and this concept was enlarged. This observation was at the level of basic physiology. During the course of histological studies on blood clots, Doctor Johnson prepared herself to do ultrastructural work. The electron microscope was applied to the study of the physiology of hemostasis. The difficult technology was mastered in a short time. A careful analysis was made of a sequence of events in the physiology of hemostasis. A correlation included observations on ultrastructural forms, ADP formation, thrombin formation, fibrin formation, hemostasis, and clot retraction. I quote a summary from a review:

> The main function of platelets, the maintenance of hemostasis, depends on three of their properties, the endothelial supporting function of platelets, the ability to form hemostatic plugs and to release lipoprotein material (platelet factor 3). When the number of circulating platelets is reduced the capillary endothelium becomes weakened as platelets are not available to enter the endothelial cytoplasm to support it and the capillary wall ruptures when exposed to minor trauma. The bleeding through the ruptured vessel wall is arrested by formation of a clump of platelets forming a hemostatic plug. Damage to the vessel wall initiates both the coagulation mechanisms and degradation of adenosine triphosphate. The products of each of these reactions, namely, thrombin and ade-

nosine diphosphate, bring about aggregation of platelets to form the hemostatic plug. These are the platelet functions performed following a transfusion of platelets into a thrombocytopenic recipient. The platelets remaining in the circulation and which are counted in platelet survival studies are those in excess of immediate need of the recipient.

During a time span of less than two decades, Doctor Johnson's name appeared on almost 100 contributions in journals and books. All of these are having their impact. Along with this, three important symposia were programmed. Five books were produced under her leadership and planning. One was coauthored by Tibor J. Greenwalt, while the others contained chapters by various authors. The titles are impressive and sustain the original interest in platelets: (1) "Blood Platelets," (2) "Coagulation and Transfusion in Clinical Medicine," (3) "Physiology of Hemostasis and Thrombosis," (4) "Dynamics of Thrombus Formation and Dissolution," and (5) "The Circulating Platelet."

Such is the nature of an inspiring mind that lives on with good humor, integrity, industry, and science. I quote: "It is not the mere cry of moralists, and flourish of rhetoricians; but it is noble to seek truth, and it is beautiful to find it. It is the ancient feeling of the human heart—that knowledge is better than riches; and it is deeply and sacredly true!" (Sydney Smith).

From my studies in integrative physiology, I learned that I am always gaining. Loss is only apparent. This is a truth which prevails, even if an event is incomprehensible. It is like the problem of evil, which is solved by seeing that it is good not understood. So, under trying conditions, *I remind myself to appreciate all there is*, and proceed in a life-affirming manner.

WALTER H. SEEGERS
Washington, D.C.

LIST OF CONTRIBUTORS

Numbers in parentheses indicate the pages on which the authors' contributions begin.

LOUIS M. ALEDORT (259), Department of Medicine, Mount Sinai School of Medicine, New York, New York

M. BETTEX-GALLAND (225), Department of Anatomy, University of Berne, Berne, Switzerland

E. J. WALTER BOWIE (473), Department of Clinical Pathology and Internal Medicine, Mayo Clinic, and Mayo Graduate School of Medicine, Rochester, Minnesota

ROGER M. DES PREZ (415), Vanderbilt University Medical School, and Veterans Administration Hospital, Nashville, Tennessee

SHIRLEY EBBE (19), St. Elizabeth's Hospital, and Tufts School of Medicine, Boston, Massachusetts

RUDOLF GROSS (123), Medizinische Universitätsklinik, Köln, Germany

G. A. JAMIESON (189), The American National Red Cross, Blood Research Laboratory, Bethesda, Maryland

SHIRLEY A. JOHNSON (183, 355),* Thrombosis Research Laboratory, Veterans Administration Hospital, and Department of Physiology, Georgetown University School of Medicine, Washington, D.C.

HAU C. KWAAN (395), Department of Medicine, Northwestern University Medical School, and Hematology Section, Veterans Administration Research Hospital, Chicago, Illinois

* Deceased.

ERNST F. LÜSCHER (225), Theodor Kocher Institute, University of Berne, Berne, Switzerland

AARON J. MARCUS (241), Hematology Section, New York Veterans Administration Hospital, and Department of Medicine, Cornell University Medical College, New York, New York.

SAMUEL R. MARNEY, JR. (415), Vanderbilt University Medical School, and Veterans Administration Hospital, Nashville, Tennessee

RALPH L. NACHMAN (207), Cornell University Medical College, Division of Hematology and Department of Medicine, New York Hospital, New York, New York

CHARLES A. OWEN, JR. (473), Department of Clinical Pathology and Biochemistry, Mayo Clinic, and Mayo Graduate School of Medicine, Rochester, Minnesota

D. S. PEPPER (189), Blood Transfusion Service, Regional Blood Transfusion Centre, Royal Infirmary, Edinburgh, Scotland

SEYMOUR PERRY (541), National Cancer Institute, Bethesda, Maryland

JOHN W. REBUCK (1), Division of Laboratory Hematology, The Henry Ford Hospital, Detroit, Michigan

LENORE B. SAFIER (241), Hematology Section, New York Veterans Administration Hospital, and Department of Medicine, Cornell University Medical College, New York, New York

WOLFGANG SCHNEIDER (123), Medizinische Universitätsklinik, Homburg, Saar, Germany

WALTER H. SEEGERS (20), Department of Physiology and Pharmacology, Wayne State University School of Medicine, Detroit, Michigan

HARRIS L. ULLMAN (241), Hematology Section, New York Veterans Administration Hospital, and Department of Medicine, Cornell University Medical College, New York, New York

JAMES G. WHITE (45), Department of Pediatrics, University of Minnesota School of Medicine, Minneapolis, Minnesota

RONALD A. YANKEE (541), Leukemia Service Medicine Branch, National Cancer Institute, Bethesda, Maryland

PREFACE

In 1951, the first United States Government funds designated for research into the biochemistry and physiology of platelets became available. The possibility of atomic warfare created a very practical need for the technical knowledge required for successful transfusion of platelets into thrombocytopenic recipients. It is clear from the type of research which resulted that the members of the scientific community responsible for awarding these funds appreciated that practical advances depend on basic knowledge in biochemistry and physiology.

Interdisciplinary backgrounds and tools were focused on this subject, and extraordinary productivity has resulted in the last two decades. Such productivity would only come from a scientific body possessed of health and excitement. As Sir Kenneth Clark has stated "that civilisation ... requires confidence—confidence in the society in which one lives, belief in its philosophy, belief in its laws, and confidence in one's own mental powers" ("Civilisation," Harper and Row, New York, 1969). While scientific achievement is not equated with civilization, it is a part of it.

Although all the contributors submitted comprehensive outlines to the editor before the chapters were written, some repetition of the subject matter has occurred. In each case there is no repetition of point of view so it seemed best to leave the chapter contents unchanged. For the reader interested in these subjects it will be invaluable to read about the same topic from several different vantage points.

The information contained herein has almost all been obtained during the past twenty years, and, I think, represents one of the milestones in expansion of biological knowledge. The success of "The Circulating Platelet" belongs to the contributors, all of whom are authorities in the area they have written about. Their enthusiasm has made organization of this work a pleasure.

SHIRLEY A. JOHNSON

THE CIRCULATING PLATELET

1

HISTORICAL PERSPECTIVES AND THE BLOOD PLATELETS

JOHN W. REBUCK

I. THE DISCOVERY OF BLOOD PLATELETS

> That is the Oxford, strong to charm us yet:
> Eternal in her beauty and her past.
>
> *Lionel Johnson**

From this "weathered cloister and worn court" Robb-Smith (1967) has amassed such an array of early Victorian scientific manuscripts as to illumine past perspectives and still leave something more to motivate our

* From *Oxford* written in 1890 and published in *Ireland and Other Poems*.

present-day electronic approach to the twenty-first century. The biologist, unlike the poet, is still confined to the regions circumscribed by his tools and methods. Blood platelets, increasingly more important as determinants of therapeutic life-span, demand, however, exact knowledge of their milieu before they can be studied, indeed, before they can be discovered.

A. Discovery Leading to Function

Before platelets were discovered then Hewson (1773) must necessarily devise the first anticoagulants, which were neutral salts such as sodium sulfate, and discover that hemolysis could be prevented with serum as a diluent. Only then and with the introduction of the achromatic objective to overcome the chromatic aberrations in the compound microscope could Gulliver (cf. Gerber, 1842) describe minute spherules in the blood which were 2.5 mμ in diameter and which then transformed to granulated particles in a few hours. Unfortunately in a later paper as related by Robb-Smith, Gulliver rejected the concept of a relationship between his minute spherules and fibrin formation. The second English discoverer of the platelets, William Addison (1842), observed the beginning of fibrin formation in association with minute bodies in the blood; his drawing (his Fig. 1) illustrates a platelet–fibrin clot. Quite fairly Robb-Smith cites the observations of platelets by the two Germans Simon (1842) and Zimmerman (1846) in the very same period. In 1850, T. W. Jones had induced fibrin thrombi by trauma to the vessel wall in the web of a frog's foot (1851); his Fig. 2 is an excellent drawing of an experimental thrombus but there is little evidence that he envisioned the role of the previously described blood particulate elements as important in its formation. Similarly Virchow (1858), who coined the term fibrinogen which he believed was converted into the fibrin clot, rejected Zimmerman's observation of small colorless bodies, refractile and with well-defined outlines as formed elements of anticoagulated blood. Virchow described the center of the thrombus as composed of fibrin and a faintly granular substance, but having rejected the identity of the platelets, missed the significance of the central fibrin-related granular substance.

In 1865 Schultze devised a warm stage and was able to observe the coalescence of platelets into granular masses, a finding of inestimable importance concerning platelet aggregation. Osler (1874) was able to extend this work by finding that there was no tendency for individual platelets to stick together within the blood vessels of the rat's connective tissue but if blood were removed from the animal, the granular masses formed at once. Furthermore, pseudopodia as "two, three, or even more tail-like processes of extreme delicacy" were described for the first time as a property of the platelets and depicted in his Fig. 5k. In confirming platelet aggregation Osler furthermore observed process formation at the periphery of the platelet masses, but he concluded that nothing could be said of the nature of these bodies or of their origin. He was certain that they did not arise from disintegration of white blood cells as had been previously postulated. However, Osler had entered into the literature this observation: "In specimens examined without any reagents the filaments of fibrin adhere to the (platelets)."

In the previous year two French observers (Ranvier, 1873; Vulpian, 1873) noted, respectively, that fibrin formed in relation to granules in the blood and that such corpuscular blood elements adhered promptly to glass and had a definite relationship to the clotting of blood. A finding supported by the first photomicrographs of these forms by Norris (1882) who was active in photomicrography from 1877 to 1880 (cf. Robb-Smith, 1967). The stage was now set for the discovery of the function of these elements. At this point in time it was now certain that platelets were not artifacts, that they were particulate elements of the normal blood and in some way they were related to coagulation and thrombosis, and that they deserved a name.

B. Platelet Function

Repeating Jones' experiments on the damaged vessel wall, Bizzozero (1882) of Turin observed that adhesion of platelets to the damaged area was the first stage in the formation of a thrombus and better than anybody before him displayed the role of platelets in coagulation (cf. his Figs. 1–14). Furthermore, he was able to separate platelets from the blood and reinfuse them for the first time and after removal of platelets from the circulation of an animal determine that it took 4 or 5 days before normal numbers repopulated the blood. Just before this, the great French hematologist Hayem (1878) had established the identity of the platelets, had counted them, and was elucidating their morphology and functions. But where Hayem clung tenaciously to the concept that platelets as "hematoblasts" were concerned as well with red cell development, Bizzozero did not believe them related to either leukocytes or erythrocytes although, of course, their origin was still unknown; it was Bizzozero who finally gave the platelets their name. Both Hayem and Bizzozero were discerning enough to note that in submammalian species the particulate element of the blood associated with hemostasis, thrombus formation, and fibrin deposition was nucleated. It was indeed Bizzozero (1882) who described such forms in the frog as "nucleated platelets." A separate section below will be devoted to the comparative biology of such thrombocytes as they came to be called.

From such beginnings the knowledge of platelet function proceeded swiftly and continually to the time of this writing. By 1886, Eberth and Schimmelbusch had extended Bizzozero's work to the point that "viscous metamorphosis" was introduced as their term for the structural and physiological changes in platelets by which they stuck to each other and foreign surfaces. Much later Wright and Minot (1917) unfortunately used the same term "viscous metamorphosis" for a later stage following platelet aggregation in which they observed a glassy optical transformation in the platelet masses. At present ultrastructural studies tend to follow the original designation for the earliest of platelet aggregates but extend the term to cover the later changes as well.

Krauss (1883) and Denys (1887) found that in certain patients afflicted with purpura these very platelets were reduced in number. Hayem (1896) confirmed their finding of the thrombocytopenic state in purpura and in this experiment of nature correctly related the paucity of platelets to the inability of the clot to retract. Wright (1906, 1910), almost unnoticed, by employing his own version of the polychrome stain to platelets, depicted azurophilic granules within the platelet itself. But a long, agonizing period in platelet history then began marked by important yet only meager gleanings of platelet functional studies, while little by little the extension of Wright's discovery of the megakaryocyte as the source of platelets yielded their exact structural nature. Equally important, the plasma coagulation factors had to be painstakingly identified one by one before the exact role of the platelet in relation to its environment could begin to emerge. Before these two goals had been achieved, the platelet was well into the mid-twentieth century.

The first electron microscopy in hematology (Wolpers and Ruska, 1939) confirmed irrevocably Osler's observations on the pseudopodial processes of platelets in shed blood. An interesting note was the observation that hypotonicity led not to platelet disintegration but merely to the formation of a single, extremely long, pointed process. Gurevitch and his fellow workers (1958) confirmed this single, swordlike protrusion produced by increasingly hypotonic saline environment and Ulutin and his associates (1963) took advantage of this normal property of the platelet to devise an ultrastructural platelet osmotic resistance test with the sword form as the normal endpoint.

The additional magnification of the electron microscope enabled Bessis (1948, 1950) and Bessis and Burstein (1949) to establish four structural states of the platelet: (1) discoidal or round; (2) dendritic; (3) transitional; and (4) expanded or spread. Rebuck and his co-workers (1960, 1961) devised an ultrastructural platelet differential based on the chronology of transformation and established the now generally accepted transformational changes as comprising: (1) circulating or round forms; (2) dendritic or pseudopodial stages leading to; (3) platelet aggregation or early viscous metamorphosis (VM); (4) intermediate or transitional stage; and (5) expanded or spread forms. Customarily the last two stages take place within the platelet aggregate. Zucker and Borrelli (1964) further noted that the circulating or discoidal form became irregularly spherical with beginning transformation.

The granular content (azurophilic granules) of the platelet first depicted by Wright (1906, 1910) was called the chromomere, and by 1942 Fonio began the search for the anatomical location of the rich source of lipid substances in platelets which could markedly accelerate the clotting of blood, a search which culminated in the work of Johnson et al. (1959) in assigning this function to the common dense granules of the platelet hyaloplasm. Recently, White and Krivit (1966) further revealed that within the platelet these common granules themselves undergo transformation into lameller particles with the configuration of lipid micelles and that such platelet micelles are released through the platelet cell membrane prior to aggregation. This was the structural pinpointing of the platelet phosphatides which had first been implicated by the work of Chargaff et al. in 1936.

With these concepts only beginning to unfold, Braunsteiner et al. (1953) perceived that ultrastructural platelet disease was marked, on the one hand, by failure of normal pseudopodial process formation termed "thrombocytoasthenia" linked to poor clot retraction, and, on the other, to excessive platelet spreading termed "thrombocytopathy" (Braunsteiner and Pakesch, 1956) soon linked to an abnormal platelet retention of its dense plateletfactor 3 containing granules (Rebuck et al., 1960; Johnson et al., 1961).

The observation by Born (1956) that platelets contained large amounts of ATP and that its degradation was concurrent with transformational events, especially pseudopodial extrusion during clotting, suggested that platelet ADP was the cause of platelet aggregation by thrombin. Ollegaard (1951, 1961) found that an extract from erythrocytes would increase platelet stickiness and aggregation. The material increasing platelet adhesiveness was later defined as the nucleotide adenosine diphosphate (ADP) (Hellem, 1960; Gaarder et al., 1961). It was under the influence of ADP that structural changes and disk–sphere transformation with pseudopodial projections were found to be concurrent with increased stickiness followed by aggregation (Hovig, 1962; Rodman et al., 1963; Zucker and Borrelli, 1964).

Platelet microtubules (Haydon and Taylor, 1965; Behnke, 1965) in the platelet discoid shape are concentrated in a circumferential band to support the circulating configuration (White, 1967). With ADP the microtubular system is redistributed to form a thick band about the dense granules concentrated in the central portions of the now irregularly sphered platelet (White, 1968).

Of teleological importance were the early observations of Achard and Aynaud (1908; Aynaud, 1911) that chilling of platelets, such as occurs with extravastion of blood, led to platelet changes comparable to those produced by coagulation or hemostasis. White and Krivit (1967) determined the ultrastructural basis for this decisive cold-dependent platelet transformation as one of reversible randomization of the above mentioned normal discoid supporting microtubular bands. As the threshold of molecular structure is approached, a further filamentous substructure of the marginal microtubular band has been discovered (Behnke and Zelander, 1966).

Of equal importance has been the delineation of a larger serpentine tubular system which opens at and is continuous with the platelet surface membrane and winds into the depths of the platelet serving as a conduit for the passage of material from the external environment into the platelet hyaloplasm as well as channels of egress for hyaloplasmic constuents, such as the common dense granules and recently described very dense granules (amines) (Behnke, 1967; White, 1968a).

One of the more startling discoveries concerning platelet structure was the realization (Behnke, 1968) that the platelet surface was not the disorderly arranged surface of broken megakaryocytic cell body that such a platelet origin might have conferred but instead was a highly ordered, trilaminar structure composed of an external coat of sulfated acid mucopolysaccharide surmounting a unit membrane contiguous to a submembranous portion, all containing the openings of the larger canalicular channel system. In other words, a complete cell membrane had been disclosed!

It is this outer coat which changes rapidly for adhesion to the severed small vessels to form the platelet plug of hemostasis as first depicted in man by Monto (1955), to attach the platelet to collagen (Hughes and Lapiere, 1964) and to allow the endothelial supporting function as postulated by Downey (1938) to emerge as platelet–endothelial intercellular transfer (Johnson et al., 1964).

It is beyond the scope of this chapter to trace the historical development of the individual platelet factors (in arabic numerals) and the role of platelet–fibrin relationships within and external to the platelet. Most that is known will be found in the reviews listed below.

Some idea of the complexity of the current status of our understanding of platelet structure and function and its relationship to hemostasis and blood clotting can be obtained by the consideration of the relatively few reviews of these subjects before 1960: Frank (1925); Bunting (1928); Rosenthal (1938); Tocantins (1938); Fonio and Schwender (1942); and Rebuck (1947). In comparison, the last decade affords the future student of platelet history the works of Johnson *et al.* (1961), Bowie *et al.* (1965), Johnson and Greenwalt (1965), Marcus and Zucker (1965), Johnson and Seegers (1967), Kowalski and Niewiarowski (1967), Haanen *et al.* (1968), Jensen and Killmann (1968), Schulz (1968), Johnson and Guest (1969), Maupin (1969), Johnson (1971), and Brinkhous (1971).

II. COMPARATIVE HEMATOLOGY

Deprived of the urgency of arresting hemorrhage in the human patient or the urgency of preventing circulatory occlusion by thrombosis in the human patient, study of the comparative biology of the platelets or their nucleated representative, the thrombocyte, nevertheless progressed.

A. Invertebrates

Recognition of platelet precursors in invertebrates has been complicated by the similarities in appearance of leukocytic amebocytes merely filling in the gaps to repair inflicted wounds and thrombocytes functioning to form plugs of a coagulative nature to prevent fluid loss. Cuenot (1906) observed that removal of a small piece of sea urchin led to plugging of the hole with three kinds of amebocytes comprising a plasmodium. Next Tait (1908) pointed out that if the main antennal vessel of the sand flea was amputated, blood flowed out until sticky clumps of cells, first seen only at the edge of the cut vessel, finally were massed to close the opening. Individual cells in the clump were then transformed into a granular mass. Florkin (1960) described an island of coagulation surrounding certain crustacean blood cells. Finally evidence was obtained that hemocytes of the American lobster contributed to the formation of fibrin clots. Stewart *et al.* (1966) prepared protein extracts from the hemocytes of this species which promoted clotting of its plasma. More recently Bang (1970) observed two stages in the repair of the cut antennal vessel of the hermit crab. At first there was sticking of the blood cells to the cut tissue. Second, the mass contracted to seal off the wound. Cellular outlines disappeared, spikes protruded from individual cells at the edge of the mass, and the seal became tight. Ultrastructurally this was accompanied by the appearance of microtubules which were interwoven between interdigital pseudopodial processes. Warren (1965) describes "explosive" corpuscles of certain crustaceans which explode in plasma with coagulation occurring in their immediate vicinity long before it takes place away from them.

B. Vertebrates

Vertebrate studies next focused on the structural appearances and makeup of the cells involved in the coagulative process. In the least complex of the vertebrates, the hagfish, Jordan (1938) has both described and depicted the thrombocyte as a cell transformed from a more primitive lymphoid hemoblast. The thrombocyte, oval or irregular in shape, as stained with Wright's stain shows a coarsely reticulated nuclear pattern with a slightly grooved nuclear outline. Its pale blue cytoplasm containing fine red-purple granules is very cohesive and is capable of shedding cytoplasmic bits as "plastids." The granules were capable to a slight extent of mediating fibrin formation in the thrombus. In the lamprey hemocytoblasts which enter the venous blood channels transform into thrombocytes.

In the *Dipnoi*, represented by the lungfish, thrombocytes possess meager bipolar azurophilic granules but the thrombocytes themselves exhibit considerable ameboid activity. Among the *Ganoids* the bowfin thrombocytes which are small and frequently adherent to each other have large clear vacuoles at both poles of lymphocyte-like nucleus in addition to meager azurophilic granules. In skates and the dogfish shark (*Elasmobranchs*) the thrombocytes are characterized by their hemoblast origin and fine, reddish granulation aggregated in the perinuclear area. In bony fishes (*Teleosts*) the specific granulation of the thrombocytes is only rarely demonstrable although the blood of the bony fishes is said to coagulate more rapidly than that of the cartilaginous fishes. In the latter it is interesting that Reznikoff and Reznikoff (1934) were able to produce a decrease in thrombocytes by interperitoneal injections of turpentine in the dogfish. Although Warren (1965) notes that erythrocyte formation and thrombocyte formation are closely associated in the lower vertebrates as they are in higher forms, it is interesting that Walvig (1958) has been able to describe and illustrate thrombocytes in the antarctic icefish, notorious for its lack of erythrocytes.

The large thrombocytes of *Triturus* of the *Amphibia* are oval cells with a central lymphocyte-like nucleus whose cytoplasm has a bright red granular component with Wright's stain as well as a delicate hyaline extragranular layer. The thrombocytes are motile and phagocytic for a black granular pigment more marked after starvation. A most exciting attribute is the ability of the salamander's thrombocytes to project long pseudopods capable of segmentation into cytoplasmic compartments called "plastids" comparable to megakaryocytic thrombocytopoiesis in mammals. Giant thrombocytes are formed after splenectomy in Triturus when thrombocytopoiesis is shifted from the spleen to the circulation. Wright (1906, 1910) was aware of a similar cytoplasmic shedding of plastids or platelets from the blood thrombocytes of *Batrachoseps* and mentions this observation in his classic papers on the origin of platelets from megakaryocytes in man. Emmel (1925) observed that usually such striking cytoplasmic segmentation and shedding of thrombocytic cytoplasm was marked in lungless species of the *Urodela* in which it occurred in 5 of 11 species investigated. Mitoses were observed in young thrombocytes in the blood of salamanders (Jordan, 1938). By lowering the environmental pressure on the blood, Gordon (1935) was able to observe increased numbers of thrombocytes in *Necturus*.

In the *Anurans*, as evidenced by the leopard frog, the thrombocytes continue to be formed intravascularly from lymphocytes. As noted above in the *Cyclostomes* and *Urodela* the cytoplasm of these thrombocytes projects pseudopodial processes which undergo segmentation resulting in granular plastids seemingly homologous with the platelets of mammals. Furthermore, the thrombocytes here are ameboid and phagocytic. With supravital staining there are a relatively small number of neutral red staining granules and smaller globules.

Moving to the reptiles, Alder and Huber (1923) described thrombocytes in both *Lacerta* and *Tarentola* with the thrombocytes together with the hemocytoblasts comprising from 72–73% of all nonerythrocytic forms in the blood, while in *Emys* thrombocytes alone were 25%. In the box turtle, Jordan (1938) found thrombocytes to be oval or spindle-shaped, devoid of granules, and with a cytoplasm apparently homogeneous. They are only slightly differentiated small lymphocytes but have a tendency to fuse into large clumps. In lizards the thrombocytes such as those of *Chamaeleon* are again sharply fusiform or oval, but small, lilac-colored granules are found in their blue cytoplasm.

Lucas and Jamroz (1961) devoted a considerable portion of their atlas of avian hematology to description and illustration of the avian thrombocytes which are small, intermediate, and large in size, oval in outline, and contain specific, minute conspicuous granules.

Progressing to the marsupials among the mammals (Jordan, 1938) a decided change is noted, for, instead of the slightly modified lymphoid cell or lymphocyte as the intravascular source of a nucleated thrombocyte, the spleen of the oppossum contains very large cells, megakaryocytes, with dark large polymorphous nuclei and abundant cell bodies. The pseudopodia from such red granule-containing megakaryocytic cytoplasm project into the splenic sinuses and are compartmentalized to form free platelets, the nonnucleated particulate forms of mammalian blood with thromboplastic activity.

III. MEGAKARYOCYTES AND THE ORIGIN OF PLATELETS

A. Megakaryocytic Function

Megakaryocytes were first observed in the marrow by Robin (1849) although their function as a source of platelets was not elucidated until 1906 by Wright. Indeed the blood-forming function of the marrow was not known until the almost simultaneous observations of Neumann and Bizzozero in 1865. By 1872, Kölliker had described the multinucleated osteoclast as one of the marrow giant cells and in 1890 Howell was able to differentiate the normally giant polymorphonuclear marrow cell which he designated as "megakaryocyte" from the previously described osteoclast.

Wright (1906, 1910) who discovered the megakaryocytic function of platelet formation, described the process in the marrow as follows:

> All of the blood platelets are detached portions or fragments of the cytoplasm of the megakaryocytes, which are in such relation to the blood channels in the marrow that detached portions of their cytoplasm are quickly carried by the blood current into the circulation. The breaking up of the cytoplasm into the platelets... takes place in various ways but usually by pinching off of small rounded projections or pseudopods from the cell body...

Wright further described granular masses, the size of the future platelets, sharply marked off by zones of hyaline cytoplasm in the tips of the pseudopods and observed that the line of cleavage was through the hyaline zones. Downey (1913) soon confirmed Wright's description of the platelet-forming megakaryocytes by a similar structural analysis with the light microscope. Direct observations of megakaryocyte formation of platelets were made decades later by Bessis (1959) and Pulvertaft (1959) in oxygen depleted cell cultures. Bessis further was able to make cinematomicrographic records of the actual process (Bessis, 1959). There remained only the ultrastructural evidence afforded by Weiss (1965e,c) that pseudopodial platelet formation by the megakaryocyte into the adjacent marrow sinus was indeed functional by reason of ultrastructural changes in megakaryocytic pseudopods lying in the marrow of a rat with induced phenylhydrazine hemolytic anemia, in which the megakaryocytic cytoplasm showed changes identical with those that platelets show in clots.

Earlier O. P. Jones (1960) had produced ultrastructural evidence that the Golgi complex of the megakaryocyte-concentrated products for the formation of the future platelet granules within vesicles budded off from the edges of its doubled membrane-bounded lamellae. Yamada (1957) in his classic description of the fine structure of platelet formation had wisely chosen the noncommital term "demarcation membranes" to outline the liberation of platelets by extension of these demarcation membranes through the marginal zone of the cell to insert into the plasma membrane of the megakaryocyte and only then to be followed by separation of the paired demarcation membranes.

A mode of platelet formation, alternate to the pseudopodial form, was first observed by Sabin (1923) in her supravital studies in which platelets were set free by simultaneous disintegration of large portions of the entire megakaryocytic cell body. These observations have been confirmed by Pisciotta et al. (1953) using phase microscopy and by Reisner (1959) in his living megakaryocytic preparations.

As soon as the role played by megakaryocytes in platelet formation was made clear, then the cytogenesis of their earliest form, the megakaryoblast was traced to the hemocytoblast (marrow stem cell, myeloblast) by Ferrata and Negreiros-Rinaldi (1915). Katzenstein (1926) and Koerner (1926) found an alternate reticuloendothelial origin for the megakaryocytic series: an heteroplastic derivation invoked after cataclysmic destruction of the myeloblastic pool (Liebow et al., 1949). A hitherto unrecognizable stem cell, intermediate between the myeloblast and the megakaryoblast, yet committed to megakaryocyte formation has been required by the kinetics of megakaryocytopoiesis as delineated by Ebbe (1968) and her colleagues (Ebbe et al., 1968a,b). Frey (1928) distinguished between the platelet-forming megakaryocytes and a mature but reserve form to complete the series.

B. Life-Span Kinetics

The best evidence for the time required for transformation of the stem cell precursor through the various megakaryocytic maturational stages until platelet formation can be effected is the 9–11-day period evidenced by the patient of Schulman and his associates (1960). This patient was shown to be deficient in a thrombopoietic factor supplied by the administration of fresh, stored, or fresh–frozen plasma which brought about maturation of her marrow megakaryocytes in the time stated. A similar 10-day megakaryocytic cycle was obtained in a single human by the radiolabel observations of Cronkite and his fellow workers (1961).

Odell and Jackson (1968), after microspectrophotometric measurement of the DNA content of rat megakaryocytes with concurrent Feulgen staining, demonstrated that megakaryocytes in that species undergo synchronous replication of their DNA by a factor of 2 up to $32N$. In man, analyses of multipolar mitoses (Rebuck et al., 1971) have yielded a similar maximum polyploidy of $32N$ for normals which was not exceeded even in megakaryocytic leukemia.

Platelet depletion in the peripheral blood can be replenished then in three ways: (1) by the aforementioned conversion of pluripotential stem cells to a stem cell pool decided for megakaryocyte formation leading to (2) hyperplasia of the entire megakaryocytic series; and (3) by maximal, maintained polyploidy resulting in individual macromegakaryocytes (Harker, 1966).

Monstrous or giant abnormal platelets are detached from the megakaryocytic cell body in two conditions: (1) chronic myelogenous (granulocytic) leukemia as first described by Naegeli (1914) and Oelhafen (1914); and (2) agnogenic myeloid metaplasia (Downey and Nordland, 1939).

C. Megakaryocytic Dysfunction

Immunologic thrombocytopenic purpura first described by Werlhof in 1735 (cf. Werlhof, 1775) as "morbus maculosus hemorrhagicus" was marked by depression of platelet numbers by Krauss (1883) and Denys (1887). Furthermore Hayem (1896) was able to ascribe the poor clot retraction exhibited by the blood of such patients to their concurrent thrombocytopenia. As early as 1911, Le Sourd and Pagniez induced experimental thrombocytopenia by injections of antiplatelet antibodies. By 1925, Frank had worked out the paradox of increased megakaryocytic numbers in the marrow of this patient group and coupled it with the apparent inability of the megakaryocytes to produce platelets. In 1951 the classic work of Harrington and his associates had unravelled the immunologic etiology of the disease.

Bunting (1909) began the experimental manipulation of the megakaryocytic series by bringing about profound thrombocytopenia with turpentine and saponin, a depression followed by megakaryocytic hyperplasia and thrombocytosis, a similar immunologic induction was cited above (Le Sourd and Pagniez, 1911). By 1916 Selling had associated disappearance of marrow megakaryocytes with benzol poisoning and had started the long list of megakaryocytotoxic agents known today.

In deficiencies of vitamin B_{12} Gaspar (1926) and O. P. Jones (1936) were able to relate the characteristic thrombocytopenia to profoundly altered marrow megakaryocytes which were not only diminished in number but were marked by nuclear structural changes of hypersegmentation, multinucleation, and immaturity of chromatin pattern. It was inevitable that limited overgrowths of the megakaryocytic–platelet system would be described, the "primary thrombocythemias" (Epstein and Goedal, 1934; Akazaki and Hamaguchi, 1939). The uncontrolled leukemic manifestations centered on the same system (Dubinskaja, 1928).

Of great interest is the concept of precocious megakaryocytic activation to thromboplastic activity before platelet formation, and precluding thrombocytopoiesis. As early as 1906 Le Sourd and Pagniez had demonstrated that clot retraction could be specially induced by megakaryocyte-rich fractions of the marrow. Weiss (1965) had ultrastructural evidence of *in situ* megakaryocytic thromboplastic activity, while Goodall (1968) linked myelofibrosis to peculiar aggregations of fibrin around degenerating megakaryocytes which formed complexes obstructing the microcirculation of the marrow.

Exposure of platelets to temperatures above 40°C results in severe and irreversible structural and functional changes (Macfarlane, 1938, Budtz-Olsen, 1951). Similarly in heat stroke in man there is an almost specific injury of the megakaryocytic series. Severe nuclear pyknosis, karyorrhexis, and disintegration of megakaryocytic nuclei were produced within 6 hours after exposure to temperatures above 106°C (Malamud *et al.*, 1946).

The recognition of diseases affecting megakaryocytopoiesis has increased in relation to the vast store of ultrastructural and functional information increasingly available to us. Little by little with knowledge of their mechanisms will come the ability to withstand them.

IV. PROJECTION

From the historical perspective at least one projection, if not warranted, at least seems required. When one considers that megakaryocytic filamentous pseudopodial projections are a necessary prelude to platelet formation

(Thiëry and Bessis, 1956) and that the megakaryocytic plasma membrane is identical to the exquisitely elaborated trilaminar plasma membrane of the platelet (Behnke, 1969), then it is reasonable to conclude that the demarcation membranes of the megakaryocyte are merely cytoplasmic membrane invaginations whose task of platelet envelopment is simplified to invagination across the mere breadth of the filamentous pseudopod. In other words, the platelet is truly a nonnucleated corpuscle encrusted completely with its assigned portion of megakaryocyte surface, as truly a functioning independent corpuscle as the erythrocyte. Yet, where nature has chosen to produce the erythrocytes through a combination of differentiational stages coupled with a series of daughter cells each undergoing multiplicative mitoses to produce the enormous clone of red blood corpuscles, almost unnoticed until the present, she has similarly produced a host of just as individualized platelet corpuscles by nuclear polyploidy and cytoplasmic hoarding until that ripe moment when surface membrane invagination is facilitated by filamentous cytoplasmic projection.

REFERENCES

Achard, C., and Aynaud, M. (1908). *C. R. Soc. Biol.* **65**, 57.
Addison, W. (1842). *London med. gaz.* [N.S.] **30**, 144.
Akazaki, K., and Hamaguchi, I. (1939). *Beitr. Pathol. Anat. Allg. Pathol.* **103**, 95.
Alder, A., and Huber, E. (1923). *Folia Haematol. (Leipzig)* **29**, 1.
Aynaud, M. (1911). *Ann. Inst. Pasteur, Paris* **25**, 56.
Bang, F. B. (1970). *J. Reticuloendothel. Soc.* **7**, 161.
Behnke, O. (1965). *J. Ultrastruct. Res.* **13**, 469.
Behnke, O. (1967). *Anat. Rec.* **151**, 121.
Behnke, O. (1968). *J. Ultrastruct. Res.* **24**, 51.
Behnke, O. (1969). *J. Ulstrastruct. Res.* **26**, 111.
Behnke, O., and Zelander, T. (1966). *Exp. Cell Res.* **43**, 236.
Bessis, M. (1948). *C. R. Soc. Biol.* **142**, 1948.
Bessis, M. (1950). *Blood* **5**, 1803.
Bessis, M. (1959). Cited by Rebuck *et al.* (1970).
Bessis, M., and Burstein, M. (1949). *Hematology* **3**, 48.
Bizzozero, G. (1882). *Virchows Arch. Pathol. Anat. Physiol.* **90**, 261.
Born, G. V. R. (1956). *J. Physiol. (London)* **133**, 61P.
Bowie, E. J., Thompson, J. H., and Owen, C. A., Jr. (1965). *Mayo Clin. Proc.* **40**, 625.
Braunsteiner, H., and Pakesch, F. (1956). *Blood* **11**, 965.
Braunsteiner, H., Fellinger, K., and Pakesch, F. (1953). *Klin. Wochenschr.* **31**, 21.
Brinkhous, K., ed. (1971). "The Platelets." Williams & Wilkins, Baltimore, Maryland.
Budtz-Olsen, O. E. (1951). "Clot Retraction." Blackwell, Oxford.
Bunting, C. H. (1909). *J. Exp. Med.* **11**, 415.

Bunting, C. H. (1928). *In* "Special Cytology" (E. V. Cowdry, ed.). pp. 417–424. Harper (Hoeber), New York.

Chargaff, E., Bancroft, F. W., and Stanley-Brown, M. (1936). *J. Biol. Chem.* **116**, 237.

Cronkite, E. P., Bond, V. P., Fliedner, T. M., Paglia, D. A., and Adamik, E. R. (1961). "Blood Platelets" (S. A. Johnson *et al.*, eds.), p. 595. Little, Brown, Boston, Massachusetts.

Cuenot, L. (1906). *C. R. Soc. Biol.* **60**, 880–882.

Denys, J. (1887). *Cellule* **3**, 445.

Downey, H. (1913). *Folia Haematol.* (*Leipzig*) **15**, 25.

Downey, H. (1938). Hematology Lectures. University of Minnesota.

Downey, H., and Nordland, M. (1939). *Folia Haematol.* (*Leipzig*) **62**, 1.

Dubinskaja, B. (1928). *Virchows Arch. Pathol. Anat. Physiol.* **270**, 192.

Ebbe, S. (1968). *In* "Blood Platelets" (K. G. Jensen and S. A. Killmann, eds.), Williams & Wilkins, Baltimore, Maryland.

Ebbe, S., Stohlman, F., Jr., Donovan, J., and Overcash, J. (1968a). *Blood* **32**, 787.

Ebbe, S., Stohlman, F., Jr., Overcash, J., Donovan, J., and Howard, D. (1968b). *Blood* **32**, 383.

Eberth, J. C., and Schimmelbusch, C. (1886). *Virchows Arch. Pathol. Anat. Physiol.* **103**, 39.

Emmel, V. E. (1925). *Amer. J. Anat.* **35**, 31.

Epstein, E., and Goedel, A. (1934). *Virchons Arch. Pathol. Anat. Physiol.* **292**, 233.

Ferrata, A., and Negreiros-Rinaldi (1915). *Folia med.* **1**, 65.

Florkin, M. (1960). *In* "The Physiology of Crustacea" (T. H. Waterman, ed.), Vol. I, Chapter 4 Academic Press, New York.

Fonio, A., and Schwender, J. (1942). "Die Thrombozyten des Menschlichen Blutes." Huber, Bern.

Frank, E. (1925). "Die haemorrhagischen Diathesan in die Krankheiten des Blutes und der blutbildenden Organe" (A. Schittenhelm, ed.), p. 289. Springer, Berlin.

Frey, H. C. (1928). *Frankfurt. Z. Pathol.* **36**, 419.

Gaarder, A., Jansen, J., LaLand S., Hellem, A. J., and Owren, P. A. (1961). *Nature* (*London*) **192**, 531.

Gaspar, S. (1926). *Frankfurt. Z. Pathol.* **34**, 460.

Gerber, F. (1842). "Elements of General and Minute anatomy of Man and the Mammals" (added notes and appendix comprising researches on the anatomy of the blood, chyle, etc.). G. Gulliver, London.

Goodall, H. B. (1968). "Symposium on Myeloproliferative Disorders of Animals and Man," Program, p. 47. Batelle Northwest Inst., Richland, Washington.

Gordon, A. (1935). *Proc. Soc. Exp. Biol. Med.* **32**, 820.

Gurevitch, J., Nelken, D., and Danon, D. (1958). *Blood* **13**, 773.

Haanen, C., and Jurgens, J. (1968). "Platelets in Haemostasis." Karger, Basel.

Harker, L. A. (1966). *Blood* **28**, 1014.

Harrington, W. J., Minnich, V., Hollingsworth, J. W., and Moore, C. V. (1951). *J. Lab. Clin. Med.* **38**, 1.

Haydon, G. B., and Taylor, A. D. (1965). *J. Cell Biol.* **26**, 673.

Hayem, G. (1878). *Arch. Physiol. Norm. Pathol.* **5**, 692.

Hayem, G. (1896). *C.R. Acad. Sci.* **123**, 894.

Hellem, A. J. (1960). *Scand. J. Clin. Lab. Invest.* **12**, Suppl. 51.

Hewson, W. (1773). "The Works" (edited with an introduction and notes by G. Gulliver). Sydenham Soc., London, 1841.

Hovig, T. (1962). *Thromb. Diath. Haemorrh.* **8**, 455.

Howell, W. H. (1890). *J. Morphol.* **4**, 117.

Hughes, J., and Lapiere, C. M. (1964). *Thromb. Diath. Haemorrh.* **11**, 327.

Jensen, K. G., and Killmann, S. A., eds. (1968). "Blood Platelets." Williams & Wilkins, Baltimore, Maryland.

Johnson, S. A. (1971). *In* "The Platelets" (K. Brinkhous, ed.). Williams & Wilkins, Baltimore, Maryland.

Johnson, S. A., and Greenwalt, T. J. (1965). "Coagulation and Transfusion in Clinical Medicine," esp. pp. 65–66. Little, Brown, Boston, Massachusetts.

Johnson, S. A., and Guest, M. M., eds. (1969). "Dynamics of Thrombus Formation and Dissolution." Lippincott, Philadelphia, Pennsylvania.

Johnson, S. A., and Seegers, W. H., eds. (1967). "Physiology of Hemostasis and Thrombosis." Thomas, Springfield, Illinois.

Johnson, S. A., Sturrock, R. M., and Rebuck, J. W. (1959). *In* "Blood Clotting Factors" (E. Deutsch, ed.) Pergamon Press, Oxford.

Johnson, S. A., Monto, R. W., Rebuck, J. W., and Horn, R. C., Jr., eds. (1961). "Blood Platelets." Little, Brown, Boston, Massachusetts.

Johnson, S. A., Balboa, R. S., Dessel, B. H., Siegesmund, K. A., and Greenwalt, T. J. (1964). *Exp. Mol. Pathol.* **3**, 115.

Jones, O. P. (1936). *Proc. Soc. Exp. Biol. Med.* **34**, 694.

Jones, O. P. (1960). *Anat. Rec.* **138**, 105.

Jones, T. W. (1851). *Guy's Hosp. Rep.* [2] **7**, 1.

Jordan, H. E. (1938). *In* "Handbook of Hematology" (H. Downey, ed.), Vol. 2, pp. 703–862. Harper (Hoeber), New York.

Katzsenstein, W. F. (1926). *Z. Gesamte Exp. Med.* **48**, 607.

Koerner, K. (1926). *Virchons Arch. Pathol. Anat. Physiol.* **259**, 617.

Kölliker, A. (1872). "Sitzung am Marz 2." *Phys. Med. Ges.*, Wurzburg.

Kowalski, E., and Niewiarowski, S., eds. (1967). "Biochemistry of Blood Platelets." Academic Press, New York.

Krauss, E. (1883). Inaugural Dissertation, Heidelberg.

Le Sourd, L., and Pagniez, P. (1906). *C. R. Soc. Biol.* **61**, 109.

Le Sourd, L., and Pagniez, P. (1911). *J. Physiol. Pathol. Gen.* **13**, 56.

Liebow, A., Warren, S., and De Coursey E. (1949). *Amer. J. Pathol.* **25**, 853.

Lucas, A. M., and Jamroz, C. J. (1961). "Atlas of Avian Hermatology," Agr. Monogr. 25. U.S. Dept. of Agriculture, Washington, D.C.

Macfarlane, R. G. (1938). M. D. Thesis, University of London.

Malamud, N., Haymaker, W., and Custer, R. P. (1946). *Mil. Surg.* **99**, 397.

Marcus, A. J., and Zucker, M. B. (1965). "The Physiology of the Blood Platelets." Grune & Stratton, New York.

Maupin, B. (1969). "Blood Platelets of Man and Animals." Pergamon Press, Oxford.

Monto, R. W. (1955). *Fed. Proc., Fed. Amer. Soc. Exp. Biol.* **14**, 413.

Naegeli, O. (1914). *Verh. Deut. Ges. Pathol.* **17**, 550.

Odell, T. T., and Jackson, C. W. (1968). *Blood* **32**, 102.

Oelhafen, H. (1914). *Folia Haematol. (Leipzig)* **18**, 171.

Ollegaard, E. (1951). *Acta Haematol.* **6**, 220.

Ollegaard, E. (1961). *Thromb. Diath. Haemorrh.* **6**, 86.

Osler, W. (1874). *Proc. Roy. Soc., London* **22**, 391.

Pisciotta, A. V., Stefanini, M., and Dameshek, W. (1953). *Blood* **8**, 703.

Pulvertaft, R. J. V. (1959). Cited by E. Ponder in Rebuck *et al.* (1970).

Ranvier, L. A. (1873). *C. R. Soc. Biol.* **5**, 46.

Rebuck, J. W. (1947). *J. Lab. Clin. Med.* **32**, 660.

Rebuck, J. W., Riddle, J. M., Johnson, S. A., Monto, R. W., and Sturrock, R. M. (1960). *Henry Ford Hosp. Med. Bull.* **8**, 273.

Rebuck, J. W., Riddle, J. M., Brown, M. G., Johnson, S. A., and Monto, R. W. (1961). *In* "The Blood Platelets" (S. A. Johnson *et al.*, eds.). Little, Brown, Boston, Massachusetts.

Rebuck, J. W., Boyd, C. B., and Monto, R. W. (1971). *In* "The Platelets" (K. Brinkhous, ed.), William & Wilkins, Baltimore, Maryland.

Reisner, E. H. (1959). Cited in Rebuck *et al.* (1970).

Reznikoff, P., and Reznikoff, D. G. (1934). *Biol. Bull.* **66**, 115.

Robb-Smith, A. H. T. (1967). *Brit. J. Haematol.* **13**, 618.

Robin, C. (1849). *Gaz. Med.* **4**, 992.

Rodman, N. F., Mason, R. G., and Brinkhous, K. (1963). *Fed. Proc., Fed. Amer. Soc. Exp. Biol.* **22**, 1356.

Rosenthal, N. (1938). *In* "Handbook of Hematology" (H. Downey, ed.), Vol. I, pp. 447–496. Harper (Hoeber), New York.

Sabin, F. R. (1923). *Bull. Johns Hopkins Hosp.* **34**, 277.

Schulman, I., Pierce, M., Lukens, A., and Currinmbhoy, Z. (1960). *Blood* **16**, 943.

Schultze, M. (1865). *Arch. Mikrosk. Anat.* **1**, 1.

Schultz, H. (1968). "Thrombocyten und Thrombose im Elektronen Mikroskopischen Bild." Springer, Berlin.

Selling, L. (1916). *Johns Hopkins Hosp. Rep.* **17**, 83.

Simon, J. F. (1842). "Physiologische und pathologische Anthropochemie mit Berucksichtigung der eigentlichen Zoochemie." Berlin.

Stewart, J. E., Dingle, J. R., and Odense, P. H. (1966). *Can. J. Biochem.* **44**, 1447–1459.

Tait, J. (1908). *Quart. J. Exp. Physiol.* **1**, 247.

Thiëry, J. P., and Bessis, M. (1956). *Rev. Hematol.* **11**, 162–174.

Tocantins, L. M. (1938). *Medicine (Baltimore)* **17**, 175.

Ulutin, O. N., Riddle, J. M., and Rebuck, J. W. (1963). *New Instanbul Contrib. Clin. Sci.* **6**, 142.

Virchow, R. (1858). "Die Cellularpathologie in Begründung auf physiologische und pathologische Gewebelehre." Hirschwald, Berlin.

Vulpian, E. F. A. (1873), *C.R. Soc. Biol.* **5**, 49.

Walvig, F. (1958). *Nytt. Mag. Zool.* **6**, 11–120.

Warren, A. (1965). "Comparative Hematology." Grune & Stratton, New York.

Weiss, L. (1950). *Anat. Rec.* **151**, 433.

Weiss, L. (1965). *J. Morphol.* **117**, 467.

Werlhof, P. G. (1775). "Opera medica," Coll. et auxit. J. E. Wichmann. Hanover, Helwingrorum.

White, J. G. (1968a). *Amer. J. Pathol.* **53**, 791.

White, J. G. (1968b). *Blood* **31**, 604.

White, J. G., and Krivit, W. (1966). *Blood* **27**, 167.

White, J. G., and Krivit, W. (1967). *Blood* **30**, 625.

Wolpers, C., and Ruska, H. (1939). *Klin. Wocenschr.* **18**, 1077.

Wright, J. H. (1906) "Origin and Nature of the Blood Plates." Boston, Massachu-
  setts.
Wright, J. H. (1910). *J. Morphol.* **21**, 263.
Wright, J. H., and Minot, G. R. (1917). *J. Exp. Med.* **26**, 295.
Yamada, E. (1957). *Acta Anat.* **29**, 267.
Zimmerman, G. (1846). *Rust's Mag. gesamte Heilk.* **65**, 410.
Zucker, M. B., and Borrelli, J. (1964). *Fed. Proc., Fed. Amer. Soc. Exp. Biol.* **23**, 299.

2

_____

ORIGIN, PRODUCTION, AND
LIFE-SPAN OF BLOOD PLATELETS*

SHIRLEY EBBE

When the concentration of circulating blood platelets is too low or too high, spontaneous hemorrhage may occur. Thrombocytopenia is the more common clinical disorder, and Gaydos *et al.* (1962) made an effort to

* Supported in part by grant AM-08263 and Research Career Development Award 1-K3 AM-8634 from the National Institute of Arthritis and Metabolic Diseases, by a Research Grant from the American Cancer Society (Massachusetts Division), Inc., and Grant No. T-505 from the American Cancer Society, Inc.

determine if there was a critical minimum level of platelets necessary to maintain hemostasis in man. Their results indicate that platelet concentrations of 20,000–50,000/mm^3 are adequate to prevent grossly visible hemorrhage, suggesting that the normal amounts of 150,000–450,000/mm^3 (Brecher and Cronkite, 1950) are far in excess of the number required. However, in human beings there probably is not a critical minimum value for platelet concentration that would apply to all, because as Cronkite (1966) has emphasized, there may not always be a close correlation between the platelet count and bleeding tendency. He related the bleeding tendency, in part, to rapidity of onset of thrombocytopenia, but the status of the vascular system and the rest of the coagulation mechanism also appear to influence the degree and type of hemorrhage in thrombocytopenic patients. The number of circulating platelets as measured in peripheral venous blood is determined by three factors: rate of production; distribution; and rate of destruction. This chapter will present some aspects of these determinants of platelet quantity in the normal steady state and adjustments which may occur in states of perturbed thrombocytopoiesis.

I. PLATELET PRODUCTION

It is generally agreed that platelets are produced by megakaryocytes (Wright, 1906). The origin of the megakaryocytes, however, is not so clear. The compartment of recognizable megakaryocytes is a nonproliferating compartment which is maintained by continuous influx from precursor compartments (Feinendegen et al., 1962). Consequently, the proliferative capacity of the thrombocytopoietic system is in the precursor compartments which are not recognizable by morphological criteria. An evaluation of megakaryocytopoiesis must, therefore, include a consideration of these precursor compartments as well as the population of recognizable megakaryocytes.

A. Origin of Megakaryocytes

1. PLURIPOTENTIAL STEM CELL

Hematopoietic cells produced in the bone marrow consist of cells of the megakaryocytic, granulocytic, and erythrocytic systems. Comparison of the differentiated, and, hence, recognizable, components of the three systems reveals differences in kinetic behavior as well as in morphology. However, consideration of the complete cell systems reveals several similarities. Some of these similarities are shown in Fig. 1.

Clinical observations of myeloproliferative disorders (Dameshek, 1951) showed the tendency for all three hematopoietic cell lines to be affected, suggesting that the basic disorder was at the level of a common precursor cell. Demonstration of the Philadelphia chromosome in granulocytic, erythroid, and polyploid mitoses in bone marrows of patients with chronic granulocytic leukemia gave further support to this notion (Whang *et al.*,

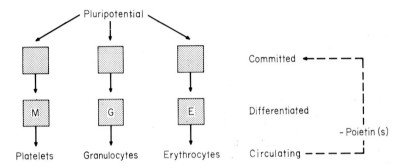

FIG. 1. A model for hematopoiesis which indicates that the compartments of mega-karyocytes (M), granulocytic precursors (G), and erythroid cells (E) arise from separate committed, but unrecognizable, precursor pools. The committed stem cells, in turn, all derive from the pluripotential stem cell. Each committed compartment appears to be a site of action of the respective-poietin which may develop in response to cytopenia.

1963; Tough *et al.*, 1963), and Killmann (1968) has more recently proposed that acute leukemia may also be a disorder at the level of a common stem cell.

In experimental animals, transplantation of hematopoietic tissue to irradiated and/or genetically receptive recipients has permitted more direct study of the pluripotential stem cell compartment. When normal mouse bone marrow cells are transplanted to irradiated mice, splenic colonies of hematopoietic cells form in the recipients, and a single colony may contain all three types of hematopoietic cells (Till and McCulloch, 1961). Each colony appears to arise from one (Becker *et al.*, 1963) or two (Lewis *et al.*, 1967) transplanted progenitor cells which must, therefore, be hematopoietic precursor cells with the potential to differentiate along more than one cell line (the pluripotential stem cell or colony forming unit or CFU). A common origin of granulocytes and erythroid cells has been further documented by the demonstration of the same marker chromosomes in granulocytic and erythroid cells of splenic colonies (Wu *et al.*, 1967) as well as by a reciprocal relationship between proliferative capacities of the two compartments (Harris *et al.*, 1966; Hellman and Grate, 1967).

Megakaryocytic differentiation from the same common stem cell may be surmised from the formation of rat platelets in irradiated mice transplanted with rat marrow (L. H. Smith *et al.*, 1957) and by the appearance of megakaryocytes, either as mixed or pure colonies, in the spleens of irradiated mice transplanted with syngeneic mouse hematopoietic cells (Till and McCulloch, 1961; Lewis and Trobaugh, 1964; Brecher *et al.*, 1967; Davis *et al.*, 1968). In the normal steady state, the transplantable colony forming unit is not actively replicating and appears, rather, to be in a state of prolonged cell cycle or no cell cycle (W. W. Smith *et al.*, 1962; Fliedner *et al.*, 1964; Becker *et al.*, 1965; Morse *et al.*, 1970).

2. COMMITTED STEM CELL

Stohlman *et al.* (1964) believed that the pluripotential stem cell was a common precursor, but that it did not feed directly into the differentiated compartments. Instead, they proposed that there was a more differentiated immediate precursor for each cell line, the committed stem cell. Subsequent observations have tended to substantiate this hypothesis. For erythropoiesis, the stem cell which responds to erythropoietin appears to be different from the pluripotential colony forming unit (Till *et al.*, 1967; Kubanek *et al.*, 1968; Rencricca *et al.*, 1969; Morse *et al.*, 1970). Recent studies suggest that the granulocytic compartment also may be maintained, in part, by a committed stem cell which, in turn, may be responsive to a stimulus initiated by neutropenia (Morley and Stohlman, 1970; Rickard *et al.*, 1970).

For the megakaryocytic compartment, it is clear that there are morphologically unrecognizable precursors interposed between the pluripotential stem cell and recognizable megakaryocytes. After an injection of tritiated thymidine (^{3}HTdR) in man (Cronkite *et al.*, 1960), rats (Feinendegen *et al.*, 1962; Ebbe and Stohlman, 1965), or rabbits (Cooney and Smith, 1965), there is a steady influx of labeled cells into the compartment of recognizable cells. This indicates that the immediate precursor, unlike the pluripotential stem cell, spends a large proportion of time in active DNA synthesis. Figure 2 presents a model for megakaryocytopoiesis which has been derived from a number of observations made in the normal steady state and in conditions of perturbed thrombocytopoiesis. The differentiated compartment is composed of three morphological types (Bessis, 1956) which we have designated stages I, II, and III (Ebbe and Stohlamn, 1965); the labeling pattern with tritiated thymidine confirms the morphological impression that they are successive stages of maturation (Ebbe and Stohlman, 1965) as does their sequential disappearance after irradiation (Simpson, 1959).

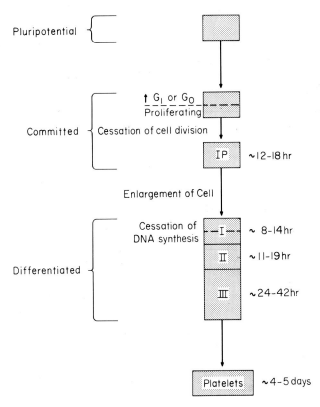

FIG. 2. A model for megakaryocytopoiesis in the rat. IP is the immediate precursor compartment.

Megakaryocytes are polyploid cells, and, since DNA content of individual cells corresponds to $2^x N$ quantities, polyploidy appears to be achieved by synchronous nuclear replication without cell division (Garcia, 1964; Odell et al., 1965). The most immature recognizable megakaryocytes consist of cells of all ploidy values (Odell and Jackson, 1968), as would be anticipated from the fact that the more mature megakaryocytes do not incorporate tritiated thymidine. The stage I compartment matures rapidly, and only a small proportion ($\sim$25%) is in DNA synthesis at any one time; consequently, it seems likely that some degree of polyploidy is achieved at the precursor cell level. Odell et al. (1968) calculated generation times and DNA synthetic periods for immature megakaryocytes from the labeling of mitotic figures by tritiated thymidine and concluded that this compartment of morphologically homogeneous cells consists of two parts. The first, which consists of less than half of the cells, is capable of DNA synthesis, and the second is not. Odell and Jackson (1970) believe that, in the rat, most cells enter the pool of recognizable megakaryocytes as $8N$ cells, some stay in the endoreduplicating fraction for one or two cell cycles before maturing further while others mature without further DNA synthesis. An alternative explanation would be that those stage I cells which incorporate tritiated thymidine are, in fact, cells of the immediate precursor compartment that differentiated during their own DNA synthetic period (Ebbe and Stohlman, 1965). The stage I megakaryocytes which synthesize DNA in the rat are initially heavily labeled by a single injection of tritiated thymidine. For the next 12–18 hours, there is an influx of cells which are equally heavily labeled from the immediate precursor compartment. Then the intensity of the label drops to about half the initial value, probably signifying the influx of the first wave of cells which have undergone cell divison. For this reason, the average time spent in the immediate precursor compartment, which is envisioned as primarily a compartment of nuclear replication, is estimated to be 12–18 hours in the rat. From the time at which the platelet counts of mice fall after sublethal irradiation, it has also been estimated that the immediate precursor compartment is as radioresistant as the differentiated megakaryocytes and has a maturation time of about a day (Ebbe, 1970a).

There are few data from which one can derive information about the earlier megakaryocytic precursors. Because of the rapid turnover of megakaryocytes and their need for constant replacement, it seems reasonable to propose that cellular proliferation occurs before the cells mature to the level of nuclear replication without cell division. Nakamura *et al.* (1969) reported that the thrombocytopoietic response of mice to irradiation could be modified by preirradiation production of immunothrombocytopenia. Recent observations indicate that the population of precursor cells which is responsive to the thrombocytopoietic stimulus of acute peripheral platelet depletion is, in part, resistant to sublethal doses of X-radiation (Ebbe and Stohlman, 1970). This suggests that there are megakaryocytic precursors which may be radioresistant by virtue of being in a state of prolonged cell cycle (prolonged G_1) or no cell cycle (G_0), but the possibility of a direct effect of a thrombopoietin on the pluripotential stem cell can not be discarded with available data. In this regard, the megakaryocytic system may again be compared to erythropoiesis. Stohlman *et al.* (1955) demonstrated that anemia or hypoxia stimulated erythropoiesis in sublethally irradiated animals, and this effect was found to be due to the humoral factor, erythro-poietin (EP) (Stohlman and Brecher, 1956). Recent observations (Morse *et al.*, 1970) show that, while the erythropoietin-responsive stem cell is in cycle, it normally has a prolonged G_1 and, hence, might be expected to have a degree of resistance to small doses of radiation. A direct effect of erythropoietin on the pluripotential stem cell has not been demonstrable (Kubanek *et al.*, 1968; Rencricca *et al.*, 1969).

B. Recognizable Megakaryocytes

In the compartment of recognizable megakaryocytes, a portion of stage I megakaryocytes retains the ability to synthesize DNA, and this ability has been shown to be limited to cells which have a single, nonsegmented nucleus (deLeval and Paulus, 1969). The appearance of multiple nuclei in more mature megakaryocytes, therefore, must result from a process of nuclear segmentation (Bessis, 1956) rather than from repeated endomitotic nuclear division as previously proposed (Japa, 1943).

Maturation of recognizable megakaryocytes is associated with cyto-plasmic growth and differentiation as well as with nuclear segmentation. Fully mature megakaryocytes (stage III) are, on the average, about twice the size of their stage I precursors (Ebbe *et al.*, 1968a). Final cell size and cytoplasmic volume may, in part, be determined by the degree of polyp-loidy (Paulus, 1967; Harker, 1968; Odell and Jackson, 1970). In conjunction with growth, megakaryocytic cytoplasm develops granules and an extensive network of tubules which eventually subdivide the cytoplasm into platelet units (Yamada, 1957; Behnke, 1968). Behnke (1969) has shown that the final step of release of platelets is preceded by formation of extensions of megakaryocyte cytoplasm between other cells or into sinusoids.

II. REGULATION OF PLATELET PRODUCTION

A. Response to Thrombocytopenia

There is a considerable amount of evidence that megakaryocytopoiesis is stimulated by thrombocytopenia. Acute platelet depletion in experimental animals is generally followed by a reactive thrombocytosis and evidence of accelerated platelet production (Craddock *et al.*, 1955; Matter *et al.*, 1960; Odell *et al.*, 1962; Ebbe *et al.*, 1968a). An increased rate of differentiation of precursors into the megakaryocytic compartment and an increased number of megakaryocytes in response to thrombocytopenia were described in the early studies (Craddock *et al.*, 1955; Witte, 1955; Odell *et al.*, 1962). Matter *et al.* (1960) did not believe that the increase in numbers of mega-karyocytes was sufficient to account for the increase in platelet production which they observed and suggested that an alteration in cytoplasmic production was more important. Witte's finding (1955) of giant forms of mega-karyocytes also suggested that cytoplasmic mass might increase out of proportion to the numbers of megakaryocytes. In his studies, however, the possibility that the giant forms resulted from an action of a potent antiplatelet serum rather than from the thrombocytopenia itself could not be ruled out. Harker (1968) has reported that the sizes of individual mega-karyocytes are increased in rats in which thrombocytopenia is maintained for 4 days by thrombocytopheresis, suggesting that the macrocytosis occurs in response to thrombocytopenia. At the same time, he found a moderate increase in megakaryocyte numbers. With prolongation of the thrombo-cytopenia for 10 days, megakaryocyte size did not increase further, but their numbers did.

In the rat subjected to acute platelet depletion, there is a lag period of 2 days before the production rate of platelets increases (Matter *et al.*, 1960; Odell *et al.*, 1962; Ebbe *et al.*, 1968a). During this time, changes in mega-karyocytopoiesis occur which lead to maximal changes in stage III, platelet-producing megakaryocytes 2 days after induction of thrombocytopenia, the time at which platelet production increases. Megakaryocyte size remains normal for the first 9 hours, and maturation rate is normal for the first 24 hours. One day after induction of thrombocytopenia, macrocytosis is present in young megakaryocytes and becomes maximal in stage III at 48 hours. The rate of differentiation and maturation of megakaryocytes is accelerated during the second postthrombocytopenic day (Ebbe *et al.*, 1968a,b), during which time there is also an increase in numbers of mega-karyocytes and in mitotic index of the young forms (Odell *et al.*, 1969). These findings seem to indicate that the stimulatory effect of thrombocyto-penia acts primarily at the level of precursor cells to increase their size, maturation rate, and number. However, thrombopoietin, like the other -poietins (Stohlman *et al.*, 1964; Patt *et al.*, 1957), may also affect the differ-entiated cells, since the maturation rate of recognizable megakaryocytes becomes accelerated.

It is well known that nonspecific thrombocytosis may occur in response to tissue damage, and it is not clear if this occurs as a result of activation of the same feed-back mechanism which responds to thrombocytopenia or by a different mechanism. Consequently, before the alterations in mega-karyocytopoiesis, which occur in response to platelet depletion which, in turn, was induced by a surgical procedure (e.g., exchange transfusion) can be ascribed to the thrombocytopenia alone, it must be shown that the procedure itself did not produce the alterations. Harker (1968) found that sham operated rats had no changes in megakaryocyte size or number. Ebbe et al. (1968a) were unable to attribute the macromegakaryocytosis seen after thrombocytopheresis to the procedure, but megakaryocyte maturation was somewhat accelerated in sham operated controls (Ebbe et al., 1968b).

B. Response to Thrombocytosis

There is also evidence that an elevated platelet count may lead to sup-pression of megakaryocytopoiesis and platelet production (Cronkite, 1957; Cronkite et al., 1960; Odell et al., 1967; Harker, 1968; Evatt and Levin, 1969). Odell et al. (1967) found that sustained transfusion-induced thrombo-cytosis in rats resulted in a decrease of megakaryocyte numbers and in reduction of platelet production as measured by incorporation of ^{35}S-Na$_2$SO$_4$. Suppression of platelet production by thrombocytosis has also been demonstrated by a decrease in incorporation of ^{75}Se-selenomethi-onine (Evatt and Levin, 1969). Harker (1968) also found a decrease in megakaryocyte numbers and, in addition, diminution in their sizes. After a single platelet transfusion, however, Cronkite et al. (1960) did not observe a decrease in megakaryocyte numbers, and we (Ebbe et al., 1966c) did not see an alteration in maturation rate with sustained thrombocytosis of moderate degree. Microcytosis of megakaryocytes after a single platelet transfusion is also less reproducible than is the macrocytosis which may be induced by only a moderate degree of thrombocytopenia (Ebbe, 1970b). From these observations it appears that the megakaryocytic system may be more sensitive to stimulation than to suppression.

C. Thrombopoietin

The mechanism by which the message that peripheral platelets are low or high is fed back to the bone marrow has not been elucidated. Recently, new techniques have been used to evaluate the thrombopoietic effect of plasma from thrombocytopenic animals, the pitfalls of older assay tech-niques having been pointed out by Abildgaard and Simone (1967). Transfusions of plasma from animals with thrombocytopenia have been reported to increase the incorporation of ^{35}S-Na$_2$SO$_4$ (Harker, 1969) or ^{75}Se-seleno-methionine (Evatt and Levin, 1969) into the platelets of recipients in which thrombocytopoiesis was suppressed by transfusion-induced thrombocytosis. Harker (1969) has reported that plasma from rats with transfusion-induced thrombocytosis had less effect than normal plasma in stimulating incorporation of ^{35}S into platelets of recipient animals. Evatt and Levin (1969) have emphasized that the degree of incorporation of isotopically labeled substances into platelets may be more a measure of the mass of platelets produced than their number. Considering the fact that newly-formed platelets may be larger than those which have aged in the circulation (see section III, B), estimation of the mass of platelets produced may be a more sensitive measure of thrombocytopoiesis than determination of only their number.

The stimulus for elaboration of a thrombopoietin is not clear, and it has been suggested that it may depend more on the total body content of platelets than upon their concentration in the blood (deGabriele and Penington, 1967b; Aster, 1967). DeGabriele and Penington (1967a) have suggested the interesting possibility that the concentration of thrombopoietin may be controlled by absorption or inactivation by platelets.

III. PLATELET DESTRUCTION

A. Use of Platelet Transfusions

Studies of platelet kinetics have accelerated and proliferated since the development of a practical method for the preparation and transfusion of platelet concentrates (Dillard *et al.*, 1951). The subsequent demonstration of a technique for labeling of these cells with ^{51}Cr-sodium chromate *in vitro* (Aas and Gardner, 1958) also provided an important tool to evaluate platelet turnover. With the use of platelet transfusions it was possible to elucidate the true nature of the postirradiation hemorrhagic state (Cronkite *et al.*, 1952; Woods *et al.*, 1953). Additional valuable information of the pathogenesis of human diseases and platelet immunology has accumulated as a result of observations of the survival of transfused platelets, and the techniques for preparing platelet concentrates have improved to the point that administration of platelet transfusions to thrombocytopenic patients has become routine. Gardner and Cohen (1966) considered the various methods available for determination of platelet life-span in the nonthrombocytopenic subject and concluded that irregular labeling or reutilization of the isotopic label made most procedures unsatisfactory except for labeling with ^{51}Cr. However, critical analysis of even this method for estimating the rate of platelet destruction may lead to the conclusion expressed by Cronkite (1966) that "the ideal method for performing such studies has not been described." Consequently, interpretation of the data with regard to platelet turnover in the normal steady state should be done with caution. At this point it may be of value to discuss some of the considerations which lead to these conclusions.

B. Platelet Aging

It has been clearly demonstrated that for platelet transfusions to correct the hemostatic defect of thrombocytopenic recipients, the transfused platelets must be capable of recirculation after transfusion (Hjort et al., 1959; Jackson et al., 1959). The converse, that all platelets which circulate are hemostatically effective has not been clearly demonstrated. The observations of Shulman et al. (1968), in fact, suggest that older platelets may continue to circulate after they have lost their maximum effectiveness to prevent capillary hemorrhage. Other observations also indicate that circulating platelets are not homogeneous with regard to size, density, metabolism, or hemostatic function and that the differences may be related to cell age. Newly-formed platelets have been shown to be both larger than those which have aged in the circulation and more dense (Detwiler et al., 1962; McDonald et al., 1964; Minter and Ingram, 1967; Booyse et al., 1968). Young platelets also have the capacity for protein synthesis (Shulman et al., 1968; Booyse et al., 1968; Steiner and Baldini, 1969; Karpatkin, 1969a), and cell-free extracts containing messenger RNA capable of synthesizing contractile protein have been prepared from platelets (Booyse and Rafelson, 1967; Steiner, 1969). Thus, it would appear that young platelets, like young red cells, may be released into the circulation while still containing RNA and, hence, still capable of protein synthesis. Ingram and Coopersmith (1969) have recently reported that these young cells may be recognized morphologically after staining by a technique which demonstrates reticulocytes.

Shulman et al. (1968) determined bleeding times to measure the hemostatic effectiveness of platelets in vivo, and their findings suggested that only those platelets which were synthesizing protein and, hence, were newly-formed were hemostatically effective. Other observations have indicated that young platelets may have greater clot retracting ability (Detwiler et al., 1962), more facility to adhere to collagen (Hirsh et al., 1968), more tendency to aggregate with ADP (Manucci and Sharp, 1967; Karpatkin, 1969b), and more tendency to aggregate and release ADP and platelet factor 4 under appropriate stimulation (Karpatkin, 1969b) than the older platelets in the circulation. Melchinger and Nemerson (1967) and Manucci and Sharp (1967) were unable to relate the adhesiveness of platelets to glass beads to their size. However, Kagnoff (1969) found that recovery of platelet adhesiveness preceded the increase in platelet count during recovery from radiation-induced thrombocytopenia in dogs which suggests that this property of platelets may also be more prominent in newly-formed platelets. These findings all suggest that circulating platelets are heterogeneous and that there may be a gradual age-related loss of hemostatic effectiveness. They have also been found to be nonhomogeneous with regard to sensitivity to osmotic shock. Webber and Firkin (1965) found two morphological populations by electron microscopy after exposure to osmotic stress, and Karpatkin (1969a) found that the large and heavy (young) platelet had greater resistance to osmotic shock than did the small and light (old) cells. Other metabolic differences between young and old platelets have also been described (Karpatkin, 1969a; Okuma *et al.*, 1969).

In the past, many of the investigators who determined platelet survival from the rate at which platelets labeled with a radioactive isotope were removed from the circulation attempted to extrapolate the mode of platelet destruction from the shape of the platelet survival curve. It was believed that the shape of the curve would indicate if platelets were removed from the circulation in predominantly a random fashion due to utilization or if their destruction was dependent in larger part on cell death due to senescence. Conclusions in this regard were not unanimous, and the differences have recently been summarized (Ebbe, 1968). In addition to the methodological problems which were previously emphasized, the functional heterogeneity of the platelet population may complicate an analysis of survival curves. Shulman *et al.* (1968) estimated that platelets become hemostatically ineffective after circulating for more than two days of their 8–10 day survival; hence, only 20–25% of circulating platelets may be fully functional. This may mean that only this fraction is maximally susceptible to destruction by randomly occurring processes and the rest are functionally effete particles which continue to circulate until some intracellular change determines that they should be phagocytosed by the reticuloendothelial system (Aster, 1969). These considerations seem to agree with the model proposed by Davey (1966) from data obtained with ^{51}Cr-labeled platelets in which human platelets have a predetermined life-span of 7–13 days upon which is superimposed the random removal of 10–20% per day.

C. Methodology

1. PLATELET TRANSFUSIONS

Additional factors which make platelet survival data difficult to interpret with regard to platelet kinetics in the normal, nonthrombocytopenic steady state are related to methodology. In those techniques involving concentration, labeling, and transfusion of platelets, it is questionable that any provide an *ex vivo* environment which is truly physiological and, therefore, does not alter the platelet. Probably the least damaging to the platelets is that technique in which platelets are labeled *in vivo* with ^{32}P-orthophosphate and transfused as whole blood (Adelson *et al.*, 1957). However, this method has only limited applicability to human beings as the platelet donors must be patients with myeloproliferative disorders receiving therapeutic doses of ^{32}P (Adelson *et al.*, 1957; Kissmeyer-Nielsen and Madsen, 1961), and the platelets from some such patients have been shown to have an intrinsic defect affecting survival (Lander and Davey, 1964). In small animals, the yield of transfused platelets in the recipient's circulation may be difficult to determine, probably because of the large volume of labeled blood which must be transfused to achieve satisfactory levels of platelet radioactivity (Ebbe *et al.*, 1965).

Early transfusions of ^{51}Cr-labeled platelets or unlabeled platelets were prepared from blood anticoagulated with EDTA (Dillard *et al.*, 1951; Aas and Gardner, 1958). However, this anticoagulant damages platelets as shown by sphering, swelling, and ultrastructural changes (Zucker and Borrelli, 1954; Bull and Zucker, 1965; White, 1968). The survival curves showed initial sequestration of a large proportion of transfused platelets (Aas and Gardner, 1958), and the maximum yield in the recipient's circulation was only about 30% of infused platelet-bound radioactivity (Baldini *et al.*, 1960). The use of ACD as an anticoagulant resulted in higher yields of transfused platelets (Kissmeyer-Nielsen and Madsen, 1961). Aster and Jandl (1964) found that acidified ACD could be used to prepare platelet concentrates for labeling and transfusion and that, when this was done, the initial sequestration did not occur. Also, platelets in ACD do not show the swelling which was seen with EDTA (Bull and Zucker, 1965).

The cold temperatures which have generally been used for preparation of platelet concentrates have also been shown to produce reversible changes such as sphering (Zucker and Borrelli, 1954), swelling (Bull and Zucker, 1965; Salzman *et al.*, 1969), and ultrastructural changes (Behnke, 1967; White and Krivit, 1967). With regard to determination of optimum temperature for *ex vivo* processing of platelets, it is of interest that platelets maintained at 37°C show preservation of apparently normal volume (Bull and Zucker, 1965; Salzman *et al.*, 1969) and ultrastructure (Behnke, 1967; White and Krivit, 1967), but reduced viability when transfused (Abrahamsen, 1968; Murphy and Gardner, 1969). The optimum temperature for preservation of platelet viability has been empirically determined to be room temperature (Abrahamsen, 1968; Murphy and Gardner, 1969); however, changes in platelet volume and ultrastructure have been demonstrated at room temperature (Bull and Zucker, 1965; Behnke, 1967). Thus, not all factors which appear to be noxious or beneficial to the platelet when judged by one parameter may appear to have the same influence when judged by another. This is further illustrated by the effects of ADP. The addition of ADP to platelets *in vitro* produces not only aggregation but also swelling (Bull and Zucker, 1965; Salzman *et al.*, 1969) and reversible ultrastructural changes which differ from those seen with cold or EDTA (White, 1968). In spite of this, Flatow *et al.* (1966) found that platelet concentrates prepared with the addition of ADP to platelet-rich plasma (PRP) were nearly as effective as transfusions of platelet-rich plasma in recirculating after transfusion to thrombocytopenic recipients and better than concentrates prepared by other techniques.

Over the years, methodology for preparing and administering platelet concentrates has improved greatly. The purpose of this resumé was to emphasize the uncertainties which still exist, and the consequent dangers from trying to derive absolutely quantitative data with regard to platelet turnover *in situ* from the rate and pattern of destruction of transfused platelets. Discrepancies resulting when platelet production was calculated from destruction rate of isotopically labeled platelets and platelet count have been summarized (Ebbe, 1968). It is clear that none of the available transfusion techniques preserve all of the facets of platelet structure and viability to equal degrees. Some changes may be reversed when the platelets are transfused back into a physiological environment. Mustard *et al.* (1966) discussed a model for platelet destruction in which multiple, reversible insults may be required before eventual destruction occurs. In light of this model, the reversible changes in platelets which may be incurred during preparation for transfusion might represent insults which would eventuate in alteration of their pattern of destruction from that which would have occurred had they remained for their entire life-span within the physiological milieu of the circulation.

2. LABELING WITH DIISOPROPYLFLUOROPHOSPHATE

To avoid the problems with transfusion of platelets, platelet kinetics have been studied by determination of platelet-bound radioactivity after injection of a radioisotopically labeled compound which labels platelets *in situ*. Diisopropylfluorophosphate (DFP) labeled with ^{32}P (Leeksma and Cohen, 1956) or tritium (^{3}H) (Adelson *et al.*, 1965) has been used for this purpose. The initial observations with diisopropylfluorophosphate (Leeksma and Cohen, 1956) suggested that this substance might be the ideal platelet label in that it appeared to irreversibly bind to circulating platelets without labeling megakaryocytes or being reutilized. However, subsequent evaluation has not verified this promise. Labeling of megakaryocytes *in vivo* by radioactive diisopropylfluorophosphate has been reported to be demonstrable by autoradiographic methods (Mustard *et al.*, 1964; Bithell *et al.*, 1967) but other investigators have found that it was not detectable (Kurth *et al.*, 1961; Ebbe *et al.*, 1966a; Cooney *et al.*, 1968). Zucker *et al.* (1961) followed platelet and red cell radioactivity from diisopropylfluorophosphate which had been injected preoperatively in patients undergoing surgery and transfusions with banked blood. They found that specific activity of circulating platelets fell less than that of the red cells as a result of this partial exchange of labeled blood with the nonradioactive transfused blood. From this they concluded that there are noncirculating depots of platelets which label with diisopropylfluorophosphate and proposed the megakaryocytes as a possible location. We have recently analyzed data obtained from labeling of rat platelets with diisopropylfluorophosphate during the phase of recovery from acute platelet depletion induced by exchange transfusion with platelet-poor homologous blood (Ebbe *et al.*, 1970). These observations showed that circulating platelet-bound radioactivity fell more slowly than normal when platelets were labeled 1–2 days after platelet depletion. This could not be attributed to longer survival of the cohorts of young platelets which were labeled. Rather, persistence of high levels of circulating platelet-bound radioactivity corresponded in time to the acceleration of platelet production which occurred in response to thrombocytopenia and appeared to be best explained by production of labeled platelets from megakaryocytes. Thus, labeling of megakaryocytes with consequent delivery of labeled platelets into the circulation probably influences the platelet "survival' curves and may account, in part, for their longer duration and different shape when labeling with diisopropylfluorophosphate *in situ* is compared with survival of transfused platelets (Ebbe *et al.*, 1966b; Bithell *et al.*, 1967; Ginsburg and Aster, 1969). Use of diisopropylfluorophosphate to quantify platelet turnover is further complicated by reutilization of ^{32}P and its appearance in platelet lipids as it disappears from platelet proteins (Mizuno *et al.*, 1959; Cooney *et al.*, 1968).

3. LABELING OF MEGAKARYOCYTE CYTOPLASM

Another approach to determination of platelet life-span has been to measure platelet radioactivity after administration of a radioactive compound which does not label circulating platelets directly but, rather, becomes incorporated into them by way of the megakaryocytes. After a single administration, platelet radioactivity gradually increases then declines; the time between the points of half maximum radioactivity on the ascending and descending curves gives an estimate of the platelet life in the circulation. Radioactive sodium sulfate has been used in rats (Odell *et al.*, 1955) and man (Vodopick and Kniseley, 1963), and ^{75}Se-selenomethionine has been used in dogs (Cohen *et al.*, 1965), man (Cohen *et al.*, 1965; Najean *et al.*, 1969), and rabbits (Evatt and Levin, 1969). Daily injections of ^{35}S-Na$_2$SO$_4$ have been used in man (Odell and Anderson, 1959; Vodopick and Kniseley, 1963), rats (Odell and Anderson, 1959), and mice (Odell and McDonald, 1961). With this technique, circulating platelet-bound radioactivity gradually increases and platelet life-span can be estimated from the time at which the curve of platelet radioactivity forms a plateau, because this is the time at which all unlabeled platelets have been replaced by labeled platelets.

D. Platelet Life-Span

A large number of studies have been reported in which platelet survival has been estimated by transfusion of labeled or unlabeled platelets, by labeling of circulating platelets *in situ*, or by labeling of platelets within the megakaryocyte cytoplasm. Some of them have been cited, and some of the pitfalls in interpreting the data have been enumerated. However, these studies provide estimates of the duration of time that platelets stay in the peripheral circulation, and these may be summarized as follows: man ~7–14 days; dogs ~7–8 days; calves ~10 days; rabbits ~2–5 days; rats ~4–5 days; and mice ~4 days.

IV. DISTRIBUTION OF PLATELETS

After their release from the bone marrow, platelets apparently do not enter a pool in which they are evenly distributed throughout the circulation, and the spleen appears to be the major area in which platelet concentration exceeds that of peripheral blood. Penny *et al.* (1966) determined the splenic platelet content by perfusion of surgically removed human spleens. They found that the platelet pool size was disproportionately greater than the blood contained, indicating that platelets are concentrated by the spleen. The size of the pool appeared to be dependent on splenic size only. Aster (1966) found that splenic blood had higher concentrations of platelets than did the peripheral blood. He also administered ^{51}Cr-labeled platelet concentrates to normal, asplenic, and hypersplenic people and determined yield of transfused platelets, surface radioactivity over the splenic area and the effect of epinephrine on platelet count, circulating platelet-bound radioactivity and surface activity. His findings indicate that about one-third of the total platelet mass is concentrated in a normal spleen, and that this portion may be increased when the spleen is enlarged. The platelets concentrated in the spleen appeared to be freely exchangeable with those in the peripheral circulation.

There is general agreement that the action of the spleen in influencing the peripheral platelet count is due, in large measure, to its capacity to concentrate platelets (Bosch, 1965; Aster, 1966; Davey, 1966; deGabriele and Penington, 1967b; Aster, 1967). In these studies, the influence of the spleen on the maximum yield of transfused, ^{51}Cr-labeled platelets was observed, and it was found that this value, for the most part, was determined by spleen size, and that the largest proportion of transfused platelets recirculated in the peripheral blood in asplenic individuals. Technical differences or differences in the way results were expressed probably account for the failure of other investigators to demonstrate the splenic pool (Hjort and Paputchis, 1960; Cohen *et al.*, 1961).

The size of the splenic platelet pool has been estimated to be about one-third of the total platelet mass in man (Aster, 1966) and 12% (Aster, 1967) or 40% (Heyssel *et al.*, 1967) in rats. These values were derived from determinations of the proportion of transfused, labeled platelets which apparently entered the splenic pool. Aster (1967) also estimated the splenic pool to contain 10–15% of the total platelet mass from the rate at which platelet-bound ^{51}Cr was removed from the circulation of rats by exchange transfusion. In the rat, we have done serial platelet counts during the course of exchange transfusions with platelet-poor homologous blood. The effectiveness of the procedure in replacing the animal's own blood with transfused blood was evaluated with ^{51}Cr-labeled red cells, and it was found that replacement of ^{51}Cr-labeled red cells by unlabeled red cells corresponded to calculations based on the animal's weight, a blood volume of 6% of body weight, and the volume of blood exchanged. Comparison of serial platelet counts with calculated effectiveness of exchange transfusion with platelet-poor blood suggested that the platelet count fell slightly less than expected from the amount of blood exchanged in intact animals. In splenectomized rats, there was a closer correlation. To further compare the sizes of the red cell and platelet pools, four intact and four splenectomized rats were exchange transfused with nonradioactive, platelet-poor homologous blood 1 or 2 days after their red cell compartment had been labeled with ^{51}Cr-labeled red cells. A comparison of the rate of fall of platelet counts and red cell radioactivity is shown in Fig. 3. If the red cell and platelet pools were

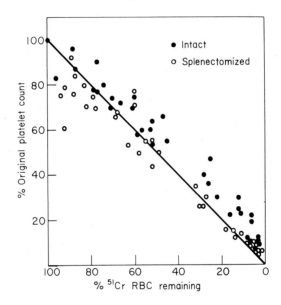

Fig. 3. Decrease in platelet count and circulating radioactivity during exchange transfusion of rats with platelet-poor, nonradioactive blood after labeling of their red cell compartments with ^{51}Cr-red cells. The points are from 4 intact and 4 splenectomized rats. If red cell and platelet compartments were equal in size, the points should be evenly distributed about the straight line.

of equal size, the values should have been evenly distributed about the line. There is little difference between intact and splenectomized rats, but there appears to be a closer correlation between sizes of red cell and platelet pools in the splenectomized rats. In intact rats, platelets were removed from the circulation somewhat more slowly than red cells, thus, further suggesting that there is a small splenic platelet pool in rats. However,

Matter *et al.* (1960) found no evidence of reserve stores of platelets in the rat during the course of platelet depletion by exchange transfusion. The small size of the splenic pool in this species may make its detection in the normal animal almost impossible, considering the errors in the techniques involved.

Matter *et al.* (1960) also found that the rate of increase of platelet counts after acute platelet depletion was the same in normal and asplenic rats, and our results (Fig. 4) confirm this finding. In human beings, however,

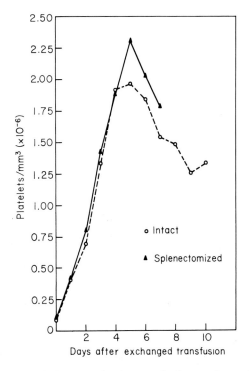

FIG. 4. Platelet counts in intact and splenectomized rats after exchange transfusion with platelet-poor blood to platelet levels of ~7–8% of pretreatment values. Each point is the average of 2–10 intact or 4–6 splenectomized rats.

Shulman *et al.* (1968) found that regeneration of circulating platelets occurred more promptly after thrombocytopheresis in asplenic than in normal individuals. This finding tended to confirm their other observations which indicated that the spleen retains newly formed platelets in a non-exchangeable pool for about 2 days. The inability to demonstrate a difference between intact and asplenic rats may be due to a species difference with regard to splenic trapping of newly-formed platelets or to the brevity of the sequestration period in the rat which has a more rapid turnover of platelets than does man. In rabbits, as in man, platelet adhesiveness is increased after splenectomy suggesting that the more adhesive platelets may normally be sequestered in the spleen (McBride and Wright, 1968).

In summary, the model for distribution and fate of human blood platelets shown in Fig. 5 seems to be appropriate from the data which are currently available. Platelets appear to undergo an aging process after they are released from megakaryocytes, and their age appears to determine, in part, their distribution, their hemostatic effectiveness, and, hence, perhaps, their susceptibility to utilization. Aster's observations (1969) indicate that the bulk of senescent platelets are destroyed in the reticuloendothelial system of the spleen, liver, and bone marrow.

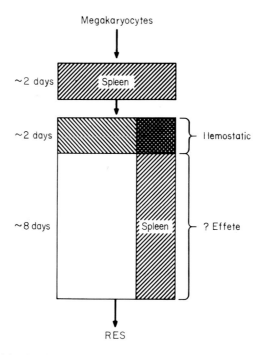

FIG. 5. Model for distribution of platelets in man. The nonexchangeable splenic pool of newly-formed platelets and the possibility that platelets are hemostatically ineffective after more than 2 days in the circulation are based on the observations of Shulman *et al.* (1968). In addition to the nonexchangeable pool, about one-third of the total mass of circulating platelets appears to be sequestered in the spleen. After about 10 days in the circulation and exchangeable splenic pool, platelets are destroyed by the reticuloendothelial system (RES).

V. SUMMARY

The thrombocytopoietic system consists of unrecognizable precursor, or stem, cells in addition to recognizable megakaryocytes of several stages of maturation. This system appears to be subject to homeostatic control which is regulated, in part, by the number of peripheral platelets. This control mechanism exerts its effects, in large measure, by action at the stem cell level. However, little is known about the nature of the feed-back mechanism(s). The distribution and hemostatic effectiveness of platelets may be determined, in part, by their age, but techniques which are currently available do not permit precise determination of platelet turnover, pattern of distribution, or mode of destruction.

REFERENCES

Aas, K. A., and Gardner, F. H. (1958). *J. Clin. Invest.* **37**, 1257.

Abildgaard, C. F., and Simone, J. V. (1967). *Semin. Hematol.* **4**, 424.

Abrahamsen, A. F. (1968). *Scand. J. Haematol.* **5**, 53.

Adelson, E., Rheingold, J. J., and Crosby, W. H. (1957). *J. Lab. Clin. Med.* **50**, 570.

Adelson, E., Kaufman, R. M., Berdeguez, C., Lear, A. A., and Rheingold, J. J. (1965). *Blood* **26**, 744.

Aster, R. H. (1966). *J. Clin. Invest.* **45**, 645.

Aster, R. H. (1967). *J. Lab. Clin. Med.* **70**, 736.

Aster, R. H. (1969). *Blood* **34**, 117.

Aster, R. H., and Jandl, J. H. (1964). *J. Clin. Invest.* **43**, 843.

Baldini, M., Costea, N., and Dameshek, W. (1960). *Blood* **16**, 1669.

Becker, A. J., McCulloch, E. A., and Till, J. E. (1963). *Nature (London)* **197**, 452.

Becker, A. J., McCulloch, E. A., Siminovitch, L., and Till, J. E. (1965). *Blood* **26**, 296.

Behnke, O. (1967). *Vox Sang.* **13**, 502.

Behnke, O. (1968). *J. Ultrastruct. Res.* **24**, 412.

Behnke, O. (1969). *J. Ultrastruct. Res.* **26**, 111.

Bessis, M. (1956). "Cytology of the Blood and Blood-forming Organs." Grune & Stratton, New York.

Bithell, T. C., Athens, J. W., Cartwright, G. E., and Wintrobe, M. M. (1967). *Blood* **29**, 354.

Booyse, F., and Rafelson, M. E., Jr. (1967). *Blood* **30**, 553.

Booyse, F. M., Hoveke, T. P., and Rafelson, M. E., Jr. (1968). *Fed. Proc., Fed. Amer. Soc. Exp. Biol.* **27**, 569.

Bosch, L. J. (1965). "Studies on Platelet Transfusion in Man." Wolters, Groningen.

Brecher, G., and Cronkite, E. P. (1950). *J. Appl. Physiol.* **3**, 365.

Brecher, G., Smith, W. W., Wilson, S., and Fred, S. (1967). *Radiat. Res.* **30**, 600.

Bull, B. S., and Zucker, M. B. (1965). *Proc. Soc. Exp. Biol. Med.* **120**, 296.

Cohen, P., Gardner, F. H., and Barnett, G. O. (1961). *N. Engl. J. Med.* **264**, 1294.

Cohen, P., Cooley, M. H., and Gardner, F. H. (1965). *J. Clin. Invest.* **44**, 1036.

Cooney, D. P., and Smith, B. A. (1965). *Brit. J. Haematol.* **11**, 484.

Cooney, D. P., Smith, B. A., and Fawley, D. E. (1968). *Blood* **31**, 791.

Craddock, C. G., Jr., Adams, W. S., Perry, S., and Lawrence, J. S. (1955). *J. Lab. Clin. Med.* **45**, 906.

Cronkite, E. P. (1957). *Brookhaven Symp. Biol.* **10**, 96.

Cronkite, E. P. (1966). *Transfusion (Philadelphia)* **6**, 18.

Cronkite, E. P., Jacobs, G. J., Brecher, G., and Dillard, G. (1952). *Amer. J. Roentgenol. Radium Ther.* **67**, 796.

Cronkite, E. P., Bond, V. P., Fliedner, T. M., Paglia, D. A., and Adamik, E. R. (1960). *In* "Blood Platelets" (S. A. Johnson *et al.*, eds.), p. 595. Little, Brown, Boston, Massachusetts.

Dameshek, W. (1951). *Blood* **6**, 372.

Davey, M. G. (1966). "The Survival and Destruction of Human Platelets." Karger, Basel.

Davis, M. L., Upton, A. C., Cosgrove, G. E., and Satterfield, L. C. (1968). *Proc. Soc. Exp. Biol. Med.* **128**, 1149.

deGabriele, G., and Penington, D. G. (1967a). *Brit. J. Haematol.* **13**, 210.

de Gabriele, G., and Penington, D. G. (1967b). *Brit. J. Haematol.* **13**, 384.

deLeval, M., and Paulus, J. M. (1969). *Blood* **34**, 529.

Detwiler, T. C., Odell, T. T., Jr., and McDonald, T. P. (1962). *Amer. J. Physiol.* **203**, 107.

Dillard, G. H. L., Brecher, G., and Cronkite, E. P. (1951). *Proc. Soc. Exp. Biol. Med.* **78**, 796.

Ebbe, S. (1968). *Ser. Haematol.* **1** (2), 65.

Ebbe, S. (1970a). *In* "The Platelet." Williams & Wilkins, Baltimore, Maryland (in press).

Ebbe, S. (1970b). *In* "Regulation of Hematopoiesis" (A. S. Gordon, ed.), p. 1587. Appleton, New York.

Ebbe, S., and Stohlman, F., Jr. (1965). *Blood* **26**, 20.

Ebbe, S., and Stohlman, F., Jr. (1970). *Blood* **35**, 783.

Ebbe, S., Baldini, M., and Donovan, J. (1965). *Blood* **25**, 548.

Ebbe, S., Stohlman, F., Jr., Donovan, J., and Howard, D. (1966a). *J. Lab. Clin. Med.* **68**, 233.

Ebbe, S., Stohlman, F., Jr., Donovan, J., and Howard, D. (1966b). *J. Lab. Clin. Med.* **68**, 813.

Ebbe, S., Stohlman, F., Jr., Donovan, J., and Howard, D. (1966c). *Proc. Soc. Exp. Biol. Med.* **122**, 1053.

Ebbe, S., Stohlman, F., Jr., Overcash, J., Donovan, J., and Howard, D. (1968a). *Blood* **32**, 383.

Ebbe, S., Stohlman, F., Jr., Donovan, J., and Overcash, J. (1968b). *Blood* **32**, 787.

Ebbe, S., Sapienza, P., Duffy, P., and Stohlman, F., Jr. (1970). *Blood* **35**, 613.

Evatt, B. L., and Levin, J. (1969). *J. Clin. Invest.* **48**, 1615.

Feinendegen, I. E., Odartchenko, N., Cottier, H., and Bond, V. P. (1962). *Proc. Soc. Exp. Biol. Med.* **111**, 177.

Flatow, F. A., Levin, R. H., and Freireich, E. J. (1966). *Transfusion (Philadelphia)* **6**, 205.

Fliedner, T. M., Thomas, E. D., Meyer, L. M., and Cronkite, E. P. (1964). *Ann. N. Y. Acad. Sci.* **114**, 510.

Garcia, A. M. (1964). *J. Cell Biol.* **20**, 342.

Gardner, F. H., and Cohen, P. (1966). *Transfusion (Philadelphia)* **6**, 23.

Gaydos, L. A., Freireich, E. J., and Mantel, N. (1962). *N. Engl. J. Med.* **266**, 905.

Ginsburg, A. D., and Aster, R. H. (1969). *Clin. Res.* **17**, 325.

Harker, L. A. (1968). *J. Clin. Invest.* **47**, 458.

Harker, L. A. (1969). *J. Clin. Invest.* **48**, 35a.

Harris, P. F., Harris, R. S., and Kugler, J. H. (1966). *Brit. J. Haematol.* **12**, 419.

Hellman, S., and Grate, H. E. (1967). *Nature (London)* **216**, 65.

Heyssel, R. M., Silver, L. J., Wasson, M., and Brill, A. B. (1967). *Blood* **29**, 341.

Hirsh, J., Glynn, M. F., and Mustard, J. F. (1968). *J. Clin. Invest.* **47**, 466.

Hjort, P. F., and Paputchis, H. (1960). *Blood* **15**, 45.

Hjort, P. F., Perman, V., and Cronkite, E. P. (1959). *Proc. Soc. Exp. Biol. Med.* **102**, 31.

Ingram, M., and Coopersmith, A. (1969). *Brit. J. Haematol.* **17**, 225.

Jackson, D. P., Sorensen, D. K., Cronkite, E. P., Bond, V. P., and Fliedner, T. M. (1959). *J. Clin. Invest.* **38**, 1689.

Japa, J. (1943). *Brit. J. Exp. Pathol.* **24**, 73.

Kagnoff, M. F. (1969). *Int. J. Radiat. Biol.* **15**, 587.

Karpatkin, S. (1969a). *J. Clin. Invest.* **48**, 1073.

Karpatkin, S. (1969b). *J. Clin. Invest.* **48**, 1083.

Killmann, S. (1968). *Ser. Haematol.* **1** (3), 103.

Kissmeyer-Nielsen, F., and Madsen, C. B. (1961). *J. Clin. Pathol.* **14**, 630.

Kubanek, B., Tyler, W. S., Ferrari, L., Porcellini, A., Howard, D., and Stohlman, F., Jr. (1968). *Proc. Soc. Exp. Biol. Med.* **127**, 770

Kurth, D., Athens, J. W., Cronkite, E. P., Cartwright, G. E., and Wintrobe, M. M. (1961). *Proc. Soc. Exp. Biol. Med.* **107**, 422.

Lander, H., and Davey, M. G. (1964). *Australas. Ann. Med.* **13**, 207.

Leeksma, C. H. W., and Cohen, J. A. (1956). *J. Clin. Invest.* **35**, 964.

Lewis, J. P., and Trobaugh, F. E., Jr. (1964). *Nature* **204**, 589.

Lewis, J. P., O'Grady, L. F., Passovoy, M., Simmons, J., and Trobaugh, F. E., Jr. (1967). *Exp. Hematol.* **13**, 15.

McBride, J. A., and Wright, H. P. (1968). *Brit. J. Haematol.* **15**, 297.

McDonald, T. P., Odell, T. T., Jr., and Gosslee, D. G. (1964). *Proc. Soc. Exp. Biol. Med.* **115**, 684.

Mannucci, P. M., and Sharp, A. A. (1967). *Brit. J. Haematol.* **13**, 604.

Matter, M., Hartmann, J. R., Kautz, J., DeMarsh, Q. B., and Finch, F. A. (1960). *Blood* **15**, 174.

Melchinger, D., and Nemerson, Y. (1967). *J. Appl. Physiol.* **22**, 197.

Minter, N., and Ingram, M. (1967). *Blood* **30**, 551.

Mizuno, N. S., Perman, V., Bates, F. W., Sautter, J. H., and Schultze, M. O. (1959). *Blood* **14**, 708.

Morley, A., and Stohlman, F., Jr. (1970). *Blood* **35**, 312.

Morse, B. S., Rencricca, N. J., and Stohlman, F., Jr. (1970). *Blood* **35**, 761.

Murphy, S., and Gardner, F. H. (1969). *N. Engl. J. Med.* **280**, 1094.

Mustard, J. F., Murphy, E. A., Robinson, G. A., Rowsell, H. C., Ozge, A., and Crookston, J. H. (1964). *Thromb. Diath. Haemorrh.* Suppl. 13, 245.

Mustard, J. F., Rowsell, H. C., and Murphy, E. A. (1966). *Brit. J. Haematol.* **12**, 1.

Najean, Y., Ardaillou, N., and Dresch, C. (1969). *Annu. Rev. Med.* **20**, 47.

Nakamura, W., Kojima, E., Minamisawa, H., Kankura, T., Kobayashi, S., and Eto, H. (1969). *In* "Comparative Cellular and Species Radiosensitivity" (V. P. Bond and T. Sugahara, eds.), p. 202. Igaku Shoin Ltd., Tokyo.

Odell, T. T., Jr., and Anderson, B. (1959). *In* "The Kinetics of Cellular Proliferation" (F. Stohlman, Jr., ed.), p. 278. Grune & Stratton, New York.

Odell, T. T., Jr., and Jackson, C. W. (1968). *Blood* **32**, 102.

Odell, T. T., Jr., and Jackson, C. W. (1970). *In* "Hemopoietic Cellular Proliferation" (F. Stohlman, Jr., ed.). p. 278. Grune & Stratton, New York.

Odell, T. T., Jr., and McDonald, T. P. (1961). *Proc. Soc. Exp. Biol. Med.* **106**, 107.

Odell, T. T., Jr., Tausche, F. G., and Gude, W. W. (1955). *Amer. J. Physiol.* **180**, 491.

Odell, T. T., Jr., McDonald, T. P., and Asano, M. (1962). *Acta Haematol.* **27**, 171.

Odell, T. T., Jr., Jackson, C. W., and Gosslee, D. G. (1965). *Proc. Soc. Exp. Biol. Med.* **119**, 1194.

Odell, T. T., Jr., Jackson, C. W., and Reiter, R. S. (1967). *Acta Haematol.* **38**, 34.

Odell, T. T., Jr., Jackson, C. W., and Reiter, R. S. (1968). *Exp. Cell Res.* **53**, 321.

Odell, T. T., Jr., Jackson, C. W., Friday, T. J., and Charsha, D. E. (1969). *Brit. J. Haematol.* **17**, 91.

Okuma, M., Steiner, M., and Baldini, M. (1969). *Blood* **34**, 712.

Patt, H. M., Maloney, M. A., and Jackson, E. M. (1957). *Amer. J. Physiol.* **188**, 585.

Paulus, J. (1967). *Blood* **29**, 407.

Penny, R., Rozenberg, M. C., and Firkin, B. G. (1966). *Blood* **27**, 1.

Rencricca, N. J., Rizzoli, V., Howard, D., Duffy, P., and Stohlman, F., Jr. (1969). *Blood* **34**, 836.

Rickard, K. A., Shadduck, R. K., Morley, A., and Stohlman, F., Jr. (1970). *In* "Hemopoietic Cellular Proliferation" (F. Stohlman, Jr., ed.), p. 238. Grune & Stratton, New York.

Salzman, E. W., Ashford, T. P., Chambers, D. A., Neri, L. L., and Dempster, A. P. (1969). *Amer. J. Physiol.* **217**, 1330.

Shulman, N. R., Watkins, S. P., Jr., Itscoitz, S. B., and Students, A. B. (1968). *Trans. Assoc. Amer. Physicians* **81**, 302.

Simpson, S. M. (1959). *Int. J. Radiat. Biol.* **2**, 181.

Smith, L. H., Makinodan, T., and Congdon, C. C. (1957). *Cancer Res.* **17**, 367.

Smith, W. W., Brecher, G., Stohlman, F., Jr., and Cornfield, J. (1962). *Radiat. Res.* **16**, 201.

Steiner, M. (1969). *Blood* **34**, 526.

Steiner, M., and Baldini, M. (1969). *Blood* **33**, 628.

Stohlman, F., Jr., and Brecher, G. (1956). *Proc. Soc. Exp. Biol. Med.* **91**, 1.

Stohlman, F., Jr., Cronkite, E. P., and Brecher, G. (1955). *Proc. Soc. Exp. Biol. Med.* **88**, 402.

Stohlman, F., Jr., Lucarelli, G., Howard, D., Morse, B., and Leventhal, B. (1964). *Medicine (Baltimore)* **43**, 651.

Till, J. E., and McCulloch, E. A. (1961). *Radiat. Res.* **14**, 213.

Till, J. E., Siminovitch, L., and McCulloch, E. A. (1967). *Blood* **29**, 102.

Tough, I. M., Jacobs, P. A., Court Brown, W. M., Baikie, A. G., and Williamson, E. R. D. (1963). *Lancet* **1**, 844.

Vodopick, H. A., and Kniseley, R. M. (1963). *J. Lab. Clin. Med.* **62**, 109.

Webber, A. J., and Firkin, B. G. (1965). *Nature (London)* **205**, 1332.

Whang, J., Frei, E., III, Tjio, J. H., Carbone, P. P., and Brecher, G. (1963). *Blood* **22**, 664.

White, J. G. (1968). *Blood* **31**, 604.

White, J. G., and Krivit, W. (1967). *Blood* **30**. 625.

Witte, S. (1955). *Acta Haematol.* **14**, 215.
Woods, M. C., Gamble, F. N., Furth, J., and Bigelow, R. R. (1953). *Blood* **8**, 545.
Wright, J. H. (1906). *Boston Med. Surg. J.* **154**, 643.
Wu, A. M., Till, J. E., Siminovitch, L., and McCulloch, E. A. (1967). *J. Cell. Physiol.* **69**, 177.
Yamada, E. (1957). *Acta Anat.* **29**, 267.
Zucker, M. B., and Borrelli, J. (1954). *Blood* **9**, 602.
Zucker, M. B., Ley, A. B., and Mayer, K. (1961). *J. Lab. Clin. Med.* **58**, 405.

3

PLATELET MORPHOLOGY*

JAMES G. WHITE

* Supported by grants from the USPHS # HE-11880, AI-05153, and CA-08832, Cardiovascular Clinical Research Program Project, and the Life Insurance Medical Research Fund.

I. INTRODUCTION

The evolution of knowledge concerning blood platelets and their role in hemostasis and thrombosis followed closely the development of and improvements in microscopic methods (Tocantins, 1948; David-Ferreira, 1964; Robb-Smith, 1967; Schulz, 1968). Early studies depended almost entirely on crude optical instruments for viewing hemostatic processes *in vivo* and *in vitro*. Despite technical problems and the limited resolution of optical systems, nearly all major facets of platelet function were recognized before the turn of the century (Donne, 1842; Jones, 1851; Osler, 1874; Bizzozero, 1882; Hayem, 1882; Eberth and Schimmelbusch, 1886; le Sourd and Pagniez, 1906; Aynaud, 1911; Wright and Minot, 1917). Drawings appearing in early publications demonstrate clearly the processes of adhesion, aggregation, platelet–fibrin interaction, hemostatic plug formation, and clot retraction. The discoid form of unaltered platelets, the shape changes occuring during the hemostatic reaction, the apparent fusion of aggregated platelets to seal sites of vascular injury, and the availability of some substance or substances from platelets important in clot formation were also recognized. Controversy normal to the development of scientific knowledge obscured the importance of these findings, but in retrospect most of the early observations appear to agree quite closely with current concepts of platelet physiology. Recent reviews have examined the historical contributions made by morphologists, and the reader is urged to consult these references for detailed information on a fascinating era of platelet research (David-Ferreira, 1964; Quick, 1966; Robb-Smith, 1967; Schulz, 1968).

The lack of adequate instruments, problems encountered in studying platelets, and emphasis on other areas of medical investigation contributed to a long pause in the first half of this century during which little was added to the understanding of blood platelets. At the onset of World War II a renewed interest in platelet physiology and the pathogenesis of thrombotic disease developed. Many factors contributed to this interest, including improvements in microscopic techniques (Sharp, 1961). The electron microscope and its application to the study of platelets had an important influence during this era (David-Fereira, 1964; Robb-Smith, 1967; Schulz, 1968; Wolpers and Ruska, 1939). Although the initial efforts left much to be desired, they indicated more clearly than the light microscope the intimate relationship between platelet structure and function (Wolpers and Ruska, 1939; Burstein and Bessis, 1948; De Robertis *et al.*, 1953; Bloom, 1954; Braunsteiner, 1961). The development of thin sectioning techniques added a new dimension to platelet evaluation (Bernhard and Leplus, 1955). Many new concepts evolved from the study of platelet ultrastructure, and the information helped greatly in the development of our current state of knowledge.

Improvements in methods used to prepare platelets for study in the electron microscope and the application of cytochemical, histochemical, biochemical, and immunochemical techniques which could be combined with ultrastructural study have had an important impact on the investigation of blood platelets in recent years. The current status of morphology is far removed from the separate science it was considered a few years ago. Today the emphasis is on structural physiology, rather than on morphology per se. As a result it has been possible to bring chemical, physiologic, and structural concepts into a cohesive framework which markedly improves understanding of basic mechanisms involved in normal and abnormal platelet function. This chapter will be concerned primarily with structural features of platelets. When possible the functional significance will be stressed and reference made to more detailed descriptions of platelet structural physiology (Marcus and Zucker, 1965; Johnson and Seegers, 1967; Brinkhous, 1967; Kowalski and Niewiarowski, 1967; Hagen *et al.*, 1968; Jensen and Killmann, 1968; Michal and Firkin, 1969).

II. GENERAL FEATURES OF PLATELET MORPHOLOGY

Blood platelets viewed in the light or phase contrast microscopes offered a deceptively simple appearance. The cells resembled small bits of protoplasm containing a variable number of granules dispersed in clear fluid and enclosed by a plasma membrane. When the platelets were smeared on slides before observation, the interaction with glass caused the cell surface to spread out in a transparent mantle, and granules to be condensed together in the cell centers. The separation of cell sap from formed organelles on glass slides or during hemostatic reactions led to their separate designations as the hyalomere and granulomere, respectively. These terms served a useful purpose in providing a basic nomenclature of platelet anatomy for workers throughout the world. "Fusion of platelets" and "viscous meta-morphosis" were of similar value in creating an acceptable visual image of the dynamic morphological changes of platelets during hemostatic function.

However, the simple terminology derived from early microscopic studies has for the most part outlived its usefulness. Electron microscopic investigations (Figs. 1, 2, 3, 4) have shown that platelets are far more complex than

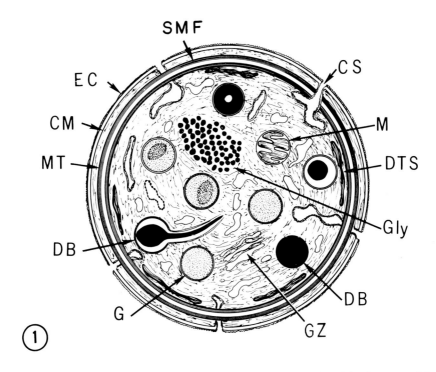

FIGS. 1 and 2. The anatomy of normal human platelets sectioned in the equatorial plane. Figure 1 is a diagramatic representation summarizing observations made on many cells similar to the example shown in Fig. 2. In the text platelet anatomy is organized in three functional divisions, including the *peripheral zone*, the *sol–gel zone*, and the *organelle zone*. Structural elements of the peripheral zone include the exterior coat (EC), the unit membrane (CM), and a submembrane area containing submembrane filaments (SMF). Submembrane filaments (SMF) are also included with the circumferential band had been conceived when the nomenclature was originated. The "plasma membrane" of platelets is not merely a barrier separating cell contents from the surrounding milieu. "Hyaloplasm" suggests a clear watery matrix, but the internal substance of the platelet is not a solution, nor is it clear. "Granulomere" suggests homogeneity of organelles, but the platelet contains several kinds of formed structures with different functions. Unfortunately the old

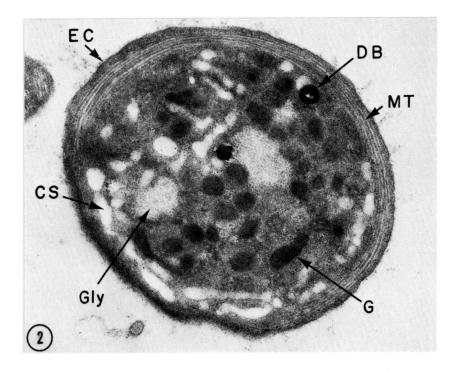

of microtubules (MT) and microfilaments as the three major fiber systems constituting the matrix of the sol–gel zone. Granules (G), dense bodies (DB), and mitochondria (M) are the formed organelle zone. Three systems of channels are present in the platelet substance, including the open canalicular system (CS) continuous with the cell surface the dense tubular system (DTS) associated with the circumferential band of microtubules and a Golgi zone (GZ) found in about 10% of platelets. Glycogen particles (Gly) are usually concentrate in masses in the matrix. Figure 2, 24,900×.

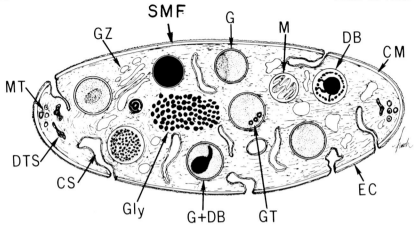

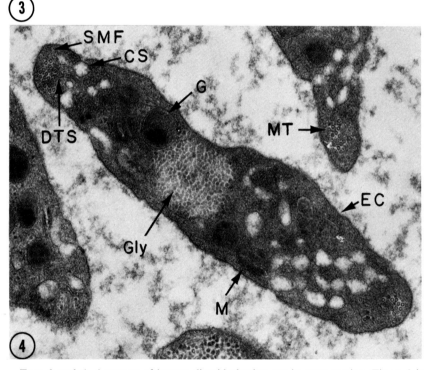

FIGS. 3 and 4. Anatomy of human discoid platelets cut in cross section. Figure 3 is a diagramatic sketch based on study of many cells, and Fig. 4 is a thin section of a human platelet. The symbols are the same as those in the first two illustrations. Various forms of dense bodies are indicated in Figs. 1 and 3 including the dense body found in the substance of a granule (G + DB). Tubular structures (GT) resembling microtubules are often seen in platelet granules. Figure 4, 45,800×.

terminology was perpetuated into the era of electron microscopic study, but it is difficult to understand why it has persisted to the present day. There are many reasons why the lexicon of terms used to describe the anatomy of platelets should be updated. Although platelets are unique in many respects, they have many structural features which are identical or very similar to almost all living cells (Grette, 1962; Born *et al.*, 1965; White, 1967a; Stormorken, 1969). The development of a nomenclature, cognizant of the similarities rather than the differences, would facilitate comparisons between platelets and other cell types.

An attempt to develop a more appropriate terminology has begun (White, 1970a,b,c). The suggested revision is based on the concept that anatomical zones of the platelet are related to specific functions. Correlation of physical and functional zones permits a more dynamic concept of structural elements and their role in platelet physiology and pathology. The *peripheral zone* is involved in adhesion and aggregation, the *sol–gel zone* in cytoskeletal support and contraction, and the *organelle zone* in storage and secretion.

III. THE PERIPHERAL ZONE

The interface between platelets and plasma was believed to be the lipo-protein-rich unit membrane for many years. Recent studies, however, have indicated that the trilaminar surface is covered by a thick exterior coat (Stehbens and Biscoe, 1967; White and Krivit, 1967b; Behnke, 1967, 1968a). Furthermore, the area immediately under the unit membrane has unique structural features which suggest it is specially adapted for interaction with the cell wall. These findings have led us to consider the wall of the platelet as a unique area best referred to as the *peripheral zone*.

A. The Exterior Coat

The outermost layer of the platelet peripheral zone is the exterior coat. When osmic acid was used as the only fixative this layer was not visible (Rodman *et al.*, 1962). Double fixation in glutaraldehyde and osmic acid preserved a coarse, whispy substance on platelets (Figs. 2, 4), but the best methods for demonstrating coat material are by negative staining and cytochemistry (Fig. 5) (B. J. Bull, 1966; Behnke, 1967, 1968a; Nakao and

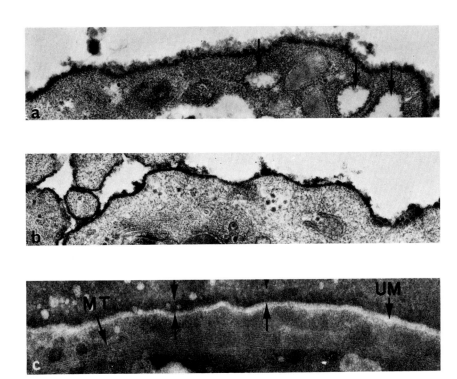

Fig. 5. The exterior coat of the platelet peripheral zone. Coat material is visible as a coarse film covering osmium–glutaraldehyde-fixed platelets (Figs. 2 and 4), but is demonstrated more clearly by cytochemical techniques. (a) This platelet is from a sample of citrate platelet-rich plasma exposed to horse radish peroxidase (HRP) prior to fixation. Electron dense particles of horse radish peroxidase are embedded in the exterior coat covering the surface of the cell and lining the channel system (↑). (b) Platelet from sample exposed to ruthenium red during fixation. The agent is embedded in the exterior coat. (c) Whole mounted, spread platelet stained with phosphotungstic acid. A microtubule (MT) composed of parallel subfilaments is evident near the unit membrane (UM) which is electron transparent. The exterior coat (↯) stained by phosphotungstic acid is twice as thick as the unit membrane. (d) Exterior coat substance of surface and channel (↑)

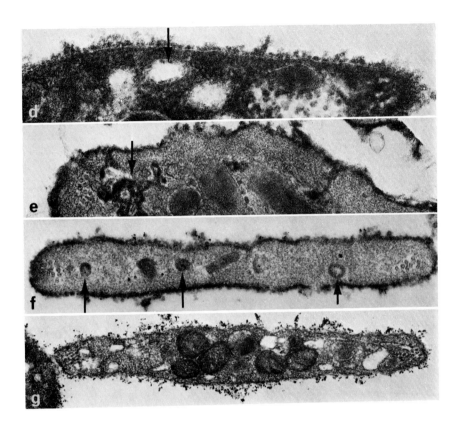

precipitated by alcian blue during fixation. (e) Lanthanum nitrate combined with fixative solutions is embedded in the coat substance of the surface and channel system (↑). (f) This platelet was vitally stained with horse radish peroxidase and thorium dioxide for 30 minutes prior to fixation. The particles of thorium dioxide tend to rest on the surface of horse radish peroxidase embedded in the coat substance (↑). (g) Platelet from sample of citrate platelet-rich plasma fixed in glutaraldehyde and exposed to thorotrast at pH 1.8 before fixation in osmic acid. Platelets are heavily coated with thorium dioxide, indicating the presence of acidic carbohydrate groups in the exterior coat capable of binding divalent cation.

Angrist, 1968; White and Krivit, 1967b; White, 1968a). Experiments designed to localize sites of ATPase in platelets resulted in demonstration of the exterior coat when reaction product in the form of lead phosphate deposited in a layer outside the unit membrane (White and Krivit, 1965; White, 1970a). Evaluation of platelets by the negative stain whole-mount method defined the coat as a dense layer 150–200 Å in thickness (B. J. Bull, 1966; White, 1968a, 1970a). Ferritin conjugated antifibrinogen antibody, colloidal iron, horse radish peroxidase, lanthanum nitrate, ruthenium red, thorium dioxide, modified silver methenamine, and surface staining of sections with phosphotungstic acid have revealed the rich content of acidic mucopolysaccharides and glycoprotein in the platelet exterior coat, and its tendency to bind proteins and cations (Behnke, 1967, 1968a; White *et al.*, 1965; White, 1970a,d; Rambourg and Leblond, 1967). Some evidence suggested that exterior coat substance was a labile component of the peripheral zone (B. J. Bull, 1966), but more recent studies indicate that the coat remains on platelets throughout aggregation and viscous metamorphosis (White, 1970d).

Efforts to demonstrate the exterior coat by cytochemical methods have confirmed that the platelet surface exposed to plasma is far more extensive than had been considered (Behnke, 1967, 1968a; White, 1968b). A number of tortuous channels randomly dispersed in the interior of the platelet are stained in the same manner as the outside surface. These findings and others have shown that platelets contain an open channel system continuous with the cell surface through which plasma can penetrate into the cell interior. The surface area of the open channel system markedly increases the total area of the platelet available for stimulation by agents which trigger the hemostatic reaction.

The origin of the exterior coat on platelets has not been determined. Early studies suggested that platelet surfaces derived from cytomembranes within the substance of the megakaryocyte (Paulus, 1967). Behnke, however, has demonstrated that demarcation membranes are formed by invaginations of the megakaryocyte surface (Behnke, 1968b, 1969). This finding suggests that coat material must reach the outside surface of the developing megakaryocyte in order to provide the characteristics which distinguish the platelet. The mechanism involved is unknown, but may involve *in situ* synthesis or a process whereby granules formed in megakaryocyte cytoplasm are transferred to the channels which drive into the cell during demarcation.

Clarification of the source of the exterior coat is important because defects in the process of formation may lead to specific disorders of circulating platelets.

B. The Unit Membrane

The trilaminar membrane of the platelet peripheral zone is morphologically indistinguishable from unit membranes enclosing other blood and tissue cells. Its role in homeostasis of platelets, therefore, is most likely similar to the function of other plasma membranes (Weiss and Mayhew, 1967). Despite the absence of distinguishing physical characteristics, however, the platelet unit membrane is considered to be of critical importance in the physiology of hemostasis (Marcus, 1969). During platelet aggregation and transformation the cells provide an essential substance for acceleration of blood coagulation. This substance, often referred to as platelet factor 3, is believed to reside in the lipoprotein-rich unit membrane (Marcus et al., 1966). The mechanism by which the membrane becomes exposed to serve as a catalytic surface for plasma proteins is not known. Several possibilities have been suggested, including disintegration or disruption of the platelet surface, stripping of coat substance covering the unit membrane, or reorientation of molecular constituents in the unit membrane during shape change and aggregation (Marcus et al., 1966; B. J. Bull, 1966; Marcus, 1969). None of these explanations appears adequate, however. For example, shape changes identical to those occurring during aggregation and viscous metamorphosis can be induced by EDTA, chilling, vincristine, and aggregating agents without causing availability of platelet factor 3 (White and Krivit, 1967c; White, 1968c,d,e). Adhesion of platelets during the initial, completely reversible first wave of aggregation does not cause platelet factor 3 to become available. The coat substance covering the unit membrane can be stained by ruthenium red or other cytochemical agents at any time during aggregation and viscous metamorphosis, and vital stains attached to platelets before aggregation remain on the cells throughout transformation (White, 1970d). Vital and passive electron stains are excluded from the interior substance of the platelet during transformation, though they are known to enter the cytoplasm of damaged cells. These findings argue against some of the theories proposed to explain the availability of unit membrane lipoprotein, but by no means prove that the cell wall is not the origin of platelet factor 3. Other explanations may resolve this difficult problem for only minute amounts of lipoprotein are required to stimulate clotting (Marcus, 1969). Focal injury or changes in the coat substance and unit membrane currently beyond the resolution of the electron microscope may ultimately prove to be the mechanism underlying availability of platelet factor 3.

Until such a mechanism can be defined, however, it is reasonable to continue searching for platelet factor 3 in some locus other than the cell wall of the platelet. Since stripping of coat substance, damage or disruption of the cell wall, and disintegration are not required for platelet factor 3 availability, and shape change, swelling, and adhesion can occur without exposing lipoprotein, it may be possible that the substance comes from inside the cell (White and Krivit, 1966). Investigations of other chemical substances secreted by platelets during aggregation and viscous metamorphosis have shown that they are released in parallel from intracellular storage sites (Grette, 1962). The release reaction is a physiological process dependent on energy metabolism and the contractile mechanism of the platelet (Grette, 1962; Karpatkin, 1967; Lüscher, 1967). Secretion or release of endogenous chemical constituents occurs when the contractile mechanism is triggered with sufficient force to empty storage organelles into the open channel system (White, 1968a, 1970d). Aggregation and contraction of the platelet mass facilitates discharge of components, and the time course of their secretion parallels the availability of platelet factor 3 (Hardisty and Hutton, 1966). The storage organelles containing the products of the release reaction originate from granules (White, 1968f), and granules are known to have the same lipoproteins as platelet membranes (Marcus et al., 1966). It seems possible, therefore, that platelet factor 3 may become available through the platelet release reaction.

C. The Submembrane Area

The area lying just under the unit membrane of the platelet surface has special characteristics which impel its inclusion with other structural components of the peripheral zone. It has been evident for some time that organelles inside the matrix of unaltered platelets never contact the cell wall. The nature of the special barrier under the cell surface has been obscure. Recently the submembrane area has been shown to contain a relatively regular system of filamentous elements (White, 1969a) (Fig. 6). The submembrane filaments are obscured by the dense matrix of the sol–gel zone, but can be seen peripheral to the circumferential band of microtubules in discoid cells. Treatment with aspirin or sodium salicylate causes submembrane filaments to be more prominent, and chemical or osmotic shock render them visible as a distinct system under the unit membrane (White 1968g; Zucker-Franklin, 1968). Submembrane filaments are physically similar to microfilaments and subfilaments of microtubules (White, 1968h) It is by no means certain that they represent a different protein species. There is evidence which suggests that all fibrous systems in the platelet interior are composed of similar subunits, and that the state of polymeriza-

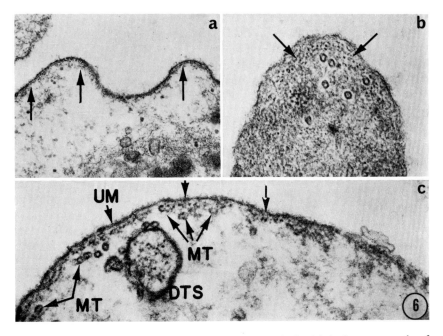

FIG. 6. Platelet submembrane filaments. The example in (a) is from a sample of chemically shocked platelets. Thin filaments (↑) cut in cross section or lying in the plane of section form a network under the unit membrane. The platelet in (b) is from citrate platelet-rich plasma treated with aspirin, which ·.so makes the SMF more prominent (↑). A chemically shocked platelet in (c) reveals SMF (↑) under the unit membrane (UM), microtubules (MT) in various stages of disassembly, and a' residual channel of the DTS containing filaments similar to SMF, microfilaments and subfilaments of microtubules. a, 29,000 × ; b, 74,500 × ; c, 81,000 ×.

tion varies with location in the cell and with stages in platelet transformation (White, 1968d,h; Lüscher and Bettex-Galland, 1968). The close association of submembrane filaments with the cell surface is the only distinguishing feature of this system, and the reason why it is considered part of the peripheral zone. Functionally, the submembrane filaments may cooperate with circumferential microtubules to maintain platelet discoid shape, play a role in the extrusion and stabilization of pseudopods, and interact with other elements of the platelet contractile mechanism to effectuate viscous metamorphosis and clot retraction.

IV. THE SOL–GEL ZONE

Light and phase contrast microscopic studies revealed the presence of organelles inside blood platelets, but the transparency of the matrix prevented recognition of other structural components. The formed bodies were felt to be dispersed in a fluid suspension or salt solution, the clarity of which suggested the term hyaloplasm. Although it is now apparent that the internal environment of platelets is made up of many structural elements, the idea that these components are in solution or suspension remains prevalent. A similar concept governs the thinking about the state of hemoglobin inside intact erythrocytes, even though Ponder some years ago suggested that the cytoplasm of the red cell had a consistency close to that of molten metal (Itano, 1953).

When thin sections of platelets were examined in the electron microscope the internal matrix appeared to consist of an irregular meshwork of fibrous material in which formed organelles were imbedded (Schulz, 1968). It was suggested that the matrix was an artifact created by precipitation of protein from solution during fixation. To some extent this concept was correct. However, the asymetric shape of platelets and separation of granules from one another visible in the light microscope should have suggested that the hyaloplasm must be extremely viscous. Since high internal viscosity results to a large extent from molecular interaction, it was predictable that protein polymers would be present in platelet hyaloplasm.

The introduction of glutaraldehyde fixation at 37°C prior to treatment with osmic acid at low temperature revealed that the matrix of the platelet was a dense mat of fibrous elements (Haydon and Taylor, 1965; Behnke, 1965, 1966; Bessis and Breton-Gorius, 1965; Silver, 1965; Sandborn et al., 1966; Sixma and Molenaar, 1966). At first these elements were thought to be artifacts of fixation, but studies by the negative stain whole-mount method revealed that fibers of various types were present in unfixed platelets (B. J. Bull, 1966; White, 1968h). Subsequent investigations have shown that changes in the state of polymerization and movement of the fibrous components of the matrix are intimately related to support of platelet discoid shape and to internal contraction (While and Krivit, 1967a; White,

1968a,d). Since it is clear that the matrix inside platelets resembles a gel, it seems appropriate to focus on this characteristic by renaming the hyaloplasm the *sol–gel zone*.

A. Microtubules

At least three systems of fibers are present in the matrix of the platelet, including *submembrane filaments, microtubules,* and *microfilaments*. Submembrane filaments were discussed with the peripheral zone of the platelet. The most prominent of the three systems is the circumferential band of microtubules (Figs. 2, 4, 7). Cross sections of fixed platelets reveal microtubules as a group of 8–24 circular profiles, each approximately 250 Å in diameter, at the polar ends of the lentiform cell. When platelets are sectioned in the equatorial plane, the bundle of tubules is apparent just under the cell wall along its greatest circumference. Circumferential tubules are

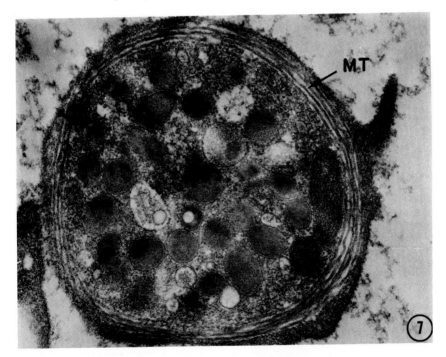

FIG. 7. Platelet microtubules. The circumferential band of microtubules (MT) lying under the cell surface forms a complete circle in this platelet. Complete annular bundles of microtubules are common in spread whole-mount preparations, but are rarely observed in thin section. 35,600×.

always slightly separated from each other, though small bridges between tubules can occasionally be identified. Although the bundle lies close to the cell wall it never appears to contact it. The space between the tubules and the surface is often occupied by submembrane filaments cut in cross section.

Study of circumferential band microtubules by the negative stain whole-mount method revealed their substructural characteristics (Behnke and Zelander, 1966, 1967; White, 1968h). Each tubule is in itself a fibrous system. When fully spread, the tubules consists of 12–15 subfilaments (Figs. 8, 9). The subfilaments lie in parallel association with a center to center spacing of approximately 70 Å. Individual subfilaments appear to be approximately

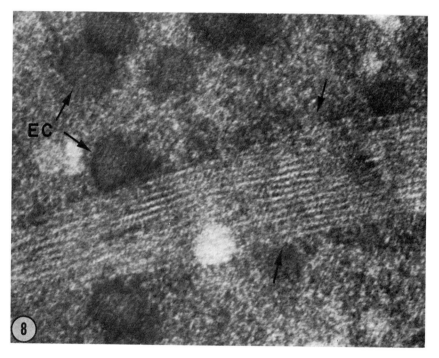

FIG. 8. Platelet microtubules. The substructure of the platelet microtubule is evident in this example of a spread whole mount stained with phosphotungstic acid. Each tubule is composed of 12–15 subfilaments in parallel association. The subfilaments resemble twisted ropes composed of globular subunits. Globular subunits of adjacent subfilaments are not in exact parallel register, and the asymmetry results in a periodic pattern (↑) cutting diagonally across the long axis of the spread tubule. The findings indicate the platelet microtubules are helical complexes of helical subfilaments. Dark particles adjacent to the microtubule are fragments of exterior coat (EC) stained by phosphotungstic acid. 365,600 ×.

35 Å in diameter when in parallel association, and to consist of globular subunits stacked in an offset manner to yield a helical twist. Globular subunits of adjacent subfilaments are not in exact parallel register. As a result a diagonal periodic pattern is evident across the long axis of the spread tubules. This finding suggests that the intact tubule has a helical conformation, as well as each of its subfilaments. At points where spread

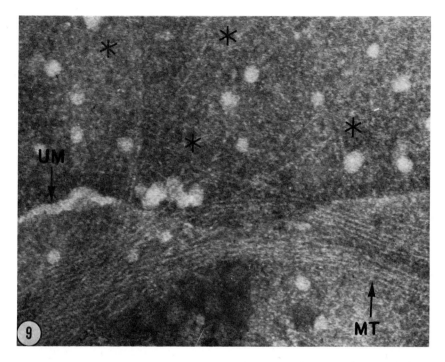

FIG. 9. Platelet microtubules (MT). The microtubules (↑) near the surface (UM) of this platelet were fractured during preparation of the whole mount. Individual subfilaments (*) remain intact as they spread out from the site of fracture. Subfilaments, therefore, appear more stable than the microtubule itself. The individual subfilaments are indistinguishable from microfilaments which fill the sol–gel matrix. 284,200×.

tubules are broken, individual subfilaments can be seen spreading out from the fracture (Fig. 9). This finding suggested that subfilaments are more stable than the microtubule, and the polymerization of subfilaments may precede their parallel association into the tubule form. In addition the subfilaments escaping from fractured tubules appear to be approximately 50 Å in diameter, and are indistinguishable from microfilaments which fill the matrix of the platelet.

Behnke and Zelander originally described the substructure of platelet microtubules, and made several important observations which bear on their function (1966, 1967). They noted that the circumferential bundle appeared to consist of a single tubule coiled on itself. Further, they found that the coiled tubule tended to expand or straighten when freed from the confines of the surface membrane. This fascinating observation indicated that the band of microtubules of intact platelets would tend to impose an externally directed force on the inside of the cell wall, causing it to assume the configuration of the annular bundle. This finding will have important implications when we consider the fate of the circumferential band during the platelet transformation induced by aggregating agents.

The circumferential band of microtubules appears to serve a cytoskeletal supportive function in unaltered cells. Its location in the equatorial plane suggested this possibility, and the supportive function has been confirmed

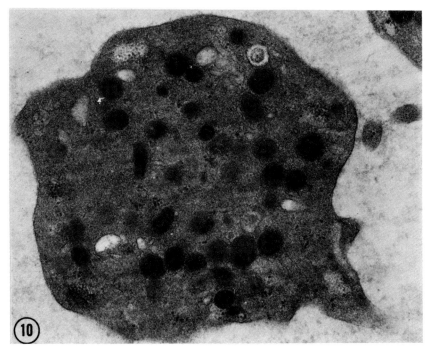

FIG. 10. Platelet microtubules. Platelet from sample of citrate platelet-rich plasma chilled to 4°C for 10 minutes before fixation. Microtubules are disassembled completely by cold, but the loss of disk shape and increase in platelet volume associated with their disappearance are not accompanied by central movement of organelles. The granules and other formed elements in this platelet are as far apart or more separated then in unaltered discoid cells (see Figs. 2, 4, and 7). 33,200×.

in several ways. Platelets are well known to lose their disk shape and become swollen and irregular in contour when exposed to low temperature for brief periods of time (Aynaud, 1911; Zucker and Borrelli, 1954) (Fig. 10). Restoration of the disk form occurs if the cells are returned to 37°C for about 1 hour. The loss of disk shape induced by chilling is associated with complete disappearance of the circumferential tubules, and recovery with restoration of the circumferential band in its usual position under the cell wall (White and Krivit, 1967c). These findings suggest that the band of tubules is involved in maintaining the discoid shape of the cell. Colchicine and vincristine also cause disassembly of platelet microtubules and loss of discoid form (White, 1968e). Observations made during disassembly suggested that bonds between subfilaments were affected, permitting the filamentous elements to separate and tubules to dilate. Swelling of adjacent tubules appeared to result in formation of a compact honeycomb-like

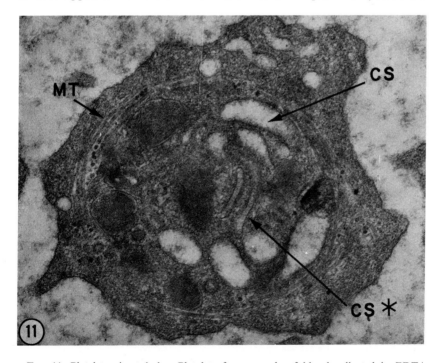

FIG. 11. Platelet microtubules. Platelets from sample of blood collected in EDTA anticoagulant and maintained at 37°C. The swelling and changes in surface contour produced by the chelating agent have not altered the circumferential band of microtubules (MT) in this cell. Organelles within the annular bundle remain randomly distributed. Some channels of the canalicular system are swollen (CS) while others became narrow (CS*) after exposure to EDTA. 41,500×.

inclusion in many platelets (White, 1968i). A similar inclusion referred
to as a crystal has been found in leukocytes and other cells after treatment
with vincristine (Bensch and Malawista, 1969). An important feature of
alkaloid treated platelets and chilled cells was that despite removal of the
band of microtubules, loss of disk shape, and swelling, the organelles
inbedded in the matrix remained as far apart or more separated than had
been observed in unaltered cells.

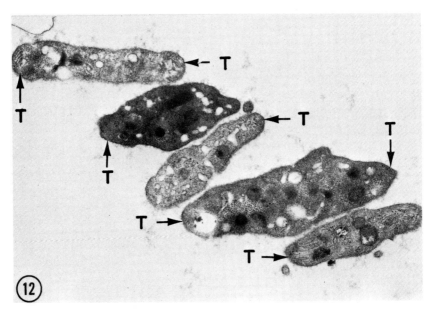

FIG. 12. Platelet microtubules. A sample of citrate platelet-rich plasma exposed to
epinephrine and fixed immediately after onset of the first wave of aggregation during
observation on the platelet aggregometer. Platelets become sticky and adhere to one
another without changing shape when exposed to epinephrine or norepinephrine. The
microtubules (T) in clumped platelets retain their peripheral location and organelles
remain randomly distributed. 12,900×.

Experiments with EDTA answered another question about microtubules
(White, 1968c). Platelets separated from blood collected in EDTA anticoagulant and maintained at 37°C lose their disk form and became spiny
spheres (Fig. 11). The changes in surface contour under these conditions
were not associated with disappearance or alteration in the circumferential
band of microtubules until the cells had been damaged by incubation for
long periods. Granules within the band remained separated until swelling
of the channel system resulted in their transfer to canaliculi. Thus changes

in platelet surface contour and swelling induced by the chelating agent could occur without internal shift, expansion, or loss of the band of microtubules.

All of these experiments were designed to clarify the nature of the internal reorganization in platelets when the cells are combined with aggregating agents (Figs. 12–28). After platelets are exposed to collagen, thrombin,

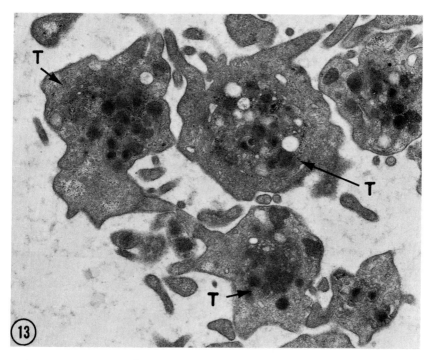

Fig. 13. Platelet microtubules. Sample of citrate platelet-rich plasma aggregated by ADP and fixed just prior to onset of the second wave of clumping as the process was recorded on the platelet aggregometer. The cells have lost their disk shape, developed multiple surface projections or pseudopods, and formed loose aggregates. Organelles are grouped in the center of the altered cells, but are not fused. Circumferential bundles of microtubules (T) are reduced in circumference and displaced toward the cell centers where they encircle the clumped organelles. 13,500×.

ADP, serotonin, epinephrine, or norepinephrine the cells lose their discoid shape and become irregular with multiple pseudopods. Changes in surface contour are accompanied by movement of granules toward the cell center where they are closely encircled by the centrally displaced circumferential band of microtubules and microfilaments (White and Krivit, 1967c; White,

1968a,d, 1969b, 1970a–d) (Figs. 16–20). The extent of internal transformation varies from platelet to platelet. In some cells the process is advanced with organelles in close apposition, while in others the only manifestation is an irregularity in surface contour. The more platelets manifesting internal transformation and the more advanced the internal changes in single cells the more likely the process is to go on to irreversible aggregation. If internal

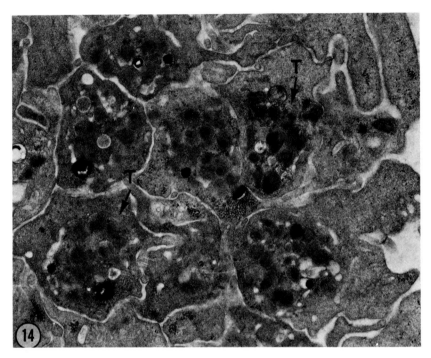

FIG. 14. Platelet microtubules (T). Sample of citrate platelet-rich plasma exposed to epinephrine and fixed early in the second wave of aggregation. The changes which develop in epinephrine aggregated platelets just prior to the release reaction are identical to those found in cells clumped by ADP, serotonin, and thrombin prior to onset of the second phase of aggregation. 14,500×.

reorganization is limited in extent and involves few platelets, the process is completely reversible. Aggregates disperse and platelets recover their unaltered discoid shape with randomly dispersed organelles and circumferential band of microtubules located under the cell surface. The physical changes can precede, accompany, or follow adhesion of platelets, or develop without aggregation. However, far advanced internal reorganization in a significant number of platelets invariably precedes or is apparent at the time of the release reaction no matter which agent is used. Even unphysiologic agents, such as kaolin particles and heat, trigger the same internal reaction in platelets as the usual chemical aggregating substances (White, 1968j) (Figs. 19, 20).

The central displacement and reduction in circumference of the annular bundle of microtubules is an intriguing feature of the platelet transformation.

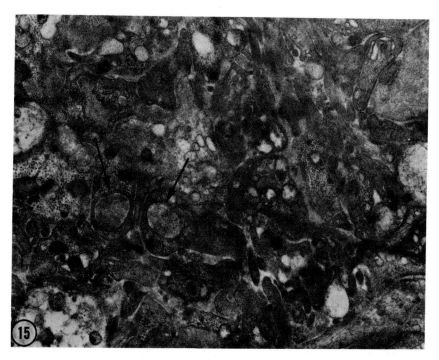

FIG. 15. Platelet microtubules. Late second wave changes in epinephrine aggregated platelets. Centrally clumped masses of granules have fused (↑). The platelet aggregate has contracted resulting in the crushed appearance of the cells. Microtubules are prominent in pseudopods at this stage of viscous metamorphosis but are not clearly visible at this magnification. 16,100 ×.

Shape changes induced by several aggregating agents are known to be accompanied by an increase in cell volume (B. S. Bull and Zucker, 1965). If the circumferential band of microtubules is under tension to expand as Behnke and Zelander suggest (Behnke and Zelander, 1966, 1967), then an increase in the circumference of the annular bundle should accompany platelet swelling. This does occur in some platelets swollen by exposure to hypotonic conditions (White, 1968h), but is never apparent in platelets

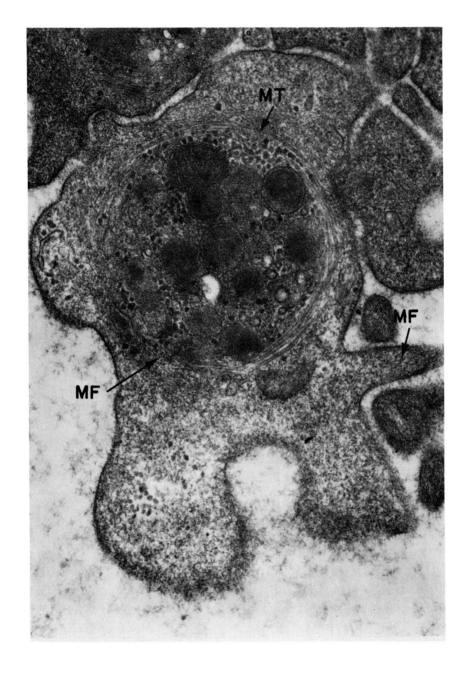

aggregated by agents which cause the volume increase. The possibility that water leaking into platelets during physiological swelling caused dilution of the gel and passive collapse toward the cell center was also considered. However, chilling which produces shape change and swelling does not cause organelles to move together in platelet centers. The granules are usually farther apart in platelets exposed to low temperature than in unaltered cells (White and Krivit, 1967a). Since microtubules are removed from chilled platelets, it was important to determine if the presence of the annular bundle in swollen platelets might favor passive central collapse of the gel. EDTA had been shown to produce the shape change and swelling caused by aggregating agents. When EDTA platelets were examined, the increase in volume and alteration in surface contour were apparent, but the band of microtubules was undisturbed and granules remained separated. These findings support the concept that central movement and reduction in circumference of the annular band of tubules in platelets exposed to aggregating agents is an active process. In fact it appears that the bundle of microtubules is involved in a centripitally oriented wave of contraction forcing platelet organelles into close apposition and ultimate fusion in the cell centers.

It was not certain, however, whether the microtubules were contracting, were part of a contractile mechanism, or were acted upon by a contractile system (White, 1968d). To solve this problem platelets were treated with colchicine, vincristine, or velban to remove microtubules and then studied for their contractile activity. Initial studies demonstrated that removal of microtubules by chemical dissection did not impair the capacity of the cells

---

Fig. 16. Platelet microtubules. The platelet shown in this illustration is part of an ADP-induced aggregate. Internal transformation is far advanced in this cell. Organelles are clumped together and fusion may be in progress. The circumferential band of microtubules (MT) has been reduced in circumference, and together with microfilaments (MF) forms a tight web encircling the mass of organelles. Pseudopods are swollen, revealing the presence of microfilaments. Amorphous or fine fibrillary material separates the unit membranes of adjacent platelets in the aggregate. The changes in this cell are typical, but the variability in degree or extent of internal transformation from cell to cell in the aggregate is great. However, the alterations always precede or accompany the platelet release reaction. The more cells manifesting the change at the end of the first phase of clumping, the more likely the process will be to continue into an irreversible second wave of aggregation. 53,900×.

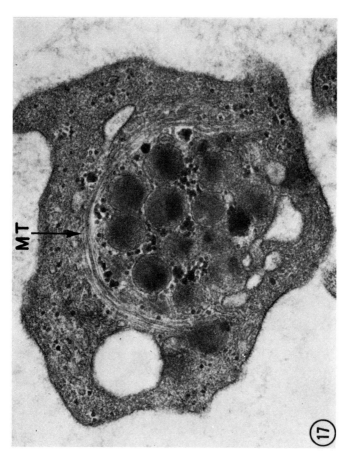

FIG. 17. Platelet microtubules. Platelet from sample of citrate platelet-rich plasma exposed to thrombin and fixed during the first wave of aggregation. Alterations in this cell are similar to but not as advanced as in the platelet shown in the previous illustration. The circumferential band of microtubules (MT) closely encircles the centrally clumped organelles. 43,100×.

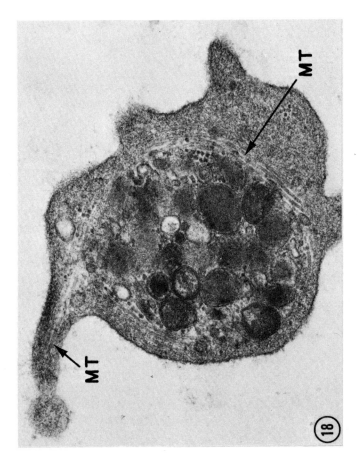

Fig. 18. Platelet microtubules. The cell in this illustration was obtained during the first wave of aggregation induced by serotonin. The similarity to thrombin and ADP induced changes is apparent. Microtubules (MT) form a tight band around centrally clumped organelles and extend into a pseudopod. This type of observation has suggested that microtubules do not necessarily contract, but interact with the contractile mechanism which decreases the circumference of the circle much as a watch spring is tightened. 37,300 ×.

to retract clots (White, 1968e). This finding eliminated the concept that intact microtubules were required for platelet contractile function. However, clot retraction is a gross measure of contractile function, and another set of experiments was designed to evaluate the role of microtubules in the platelet release reaction. Dissected platelets were compared with untreated cells from the same sample of citrate platelet-rich plasma as to their ability to

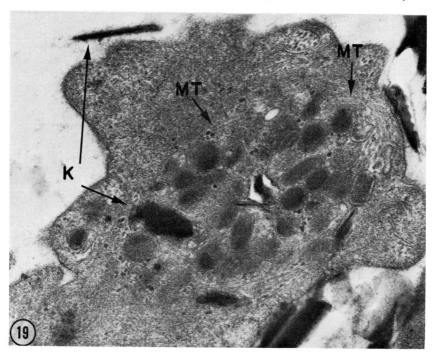

FIG. 19. Platelet microtubules. Platelet from sample of citrate platelet-rich plasma incubated with kaolin. Kaolin particles (K) have been ingested by the cell, and internal changes similar to those which develop after exposure to chemical aggregating agents have occurred. Phagocytosis of collagen particles also triggers internal reorganization. However, platelets take up many small particles such as thorium dioxide, ferritin, colloidal gold, horse radish peroxidase, and lanthanum nitrate which do not trigger internal contraction, though they can cause degranulation. The size of ingested particles as well as their nature influence the platelet response. MT, microtubules. 33,200 ×.

develop a double wave of aggregation after exposure to identical concentrations of ADP and epinephrine on the platelet aggregometer (White, 1969b). Comparable samples were also examined in the electron microscope. The samples of vincristine treated platelets developed a single wave of clumping, whereas untreated cells reacted with a biphasic response. In the electron microscope normal aggregated platelets had undergone internal reorganization, but the organelles in treated cells were widely dispersed. Since the second wave of aggregation is dependent on the release of endogenous chemical constituents, it was apparent that removal of microtubules had affected the secretory capacity of the treated platelets. Furthermore the release reaction is directly related to the contractile function of platelets.

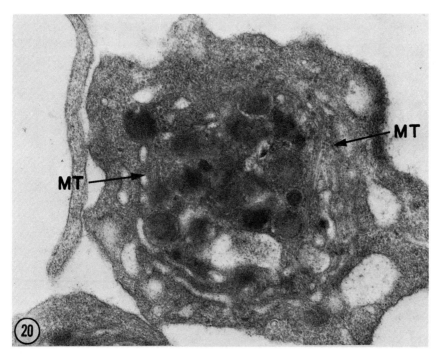

FIG. 20. Platelet microtubules. This platelet is from a sample of citrate platelet-rich plasma warmed to 45°C for 15 minutes. Heat triggers platelet internal contraction just as it stimulates muscle contraction and contraction of actomyosin gels. Internal transformation is similar to changes which develop when the cells are exposed to physiological aggregating agents. However, the surface of the cells is altered by heat. They do not respond to ADP and are incapable of retracting clots. MT, microtubules. 37,300×.

Therefore, it was concluded that removal of the circumferential band of microtubules impaired the centripetal internal wave of contraction and the release reaction necessary for the second wave of platelet aggregation.

The investigations described above have suggested that one principal function of circumferential microtubules is to orient the wave of contraction which results in extrusion of endogenous platelet products. Tubules may not contract upon themselves, but their intimate association with contractile filaments, and semirigid state permit them to orient the web of contractile elements so that contraction has direction. Why should the platelet, a secretory cell markedly similar to cells of endocrine tissue, have such a specialized means for releasing chemical substances? The answer to this question can only be speculated upon. Yet platelets in circulating blood

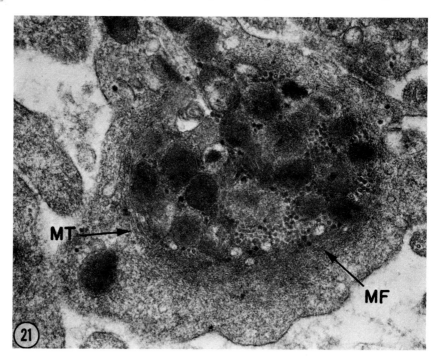

Fig. 21. Platelet microtubules. Platelet from citrate platelet-rich plasma exposed to thrombin and fixed early in the second wave of aggregation. Microtubules (MT) are still evident in the ring surrounding centrally clumped organelles, but most of the fibers are microfilaments (MF). Most granules remain discrete but some appear to have fused. 38,200×.

are constantly exposed to chemical agents known to cause cell transformation and the release reaction. Platelets must be exquisitely sensitive to these agents in order to exercise their hemostatic function, but overreaction in the circulating blood could result in catastrophic thromboembolism. The unusual nature of platelet internal transformation probably acts as a protective mechanism, as well as means of accomplishing secretory function. Platelets respond in a graded fashion proportional to the nature of the stimulating agent, its concentration, and individual sensitivity of the cell. This capacity has been emphasized previously as a contraction–relaxation cycle in the primary response of platelets to aggregating agents (White, 1968k). Thus the contractile system of the platelet may be organized specifically to afford protection to the host as well as rapid response in event of vascular injury.

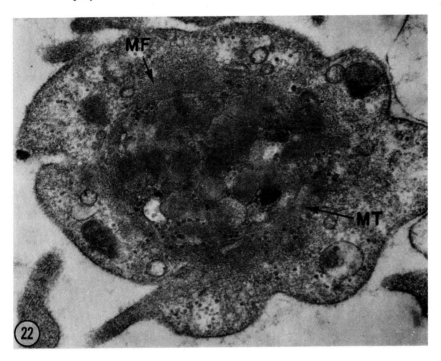

FIG. 22. Platelet microtubules. Collagen-induced platelet internal transformation. The changes are essentially identical to those produced by thrombin in the platelet shown in the previous illustration. Microtubules (MT) in the web of fibers have been largely replaced by microfilaments (MF) which extend into pseudopods. 41,500×.

The function of the circumferential band of microtubules appears to be completed when centrally clumped granules undergo fusion during the second wave of platelet aggregation (Figs. 21, 26). When fusion has occurred, the internal changes are no longer reversible. The ring of tubules surrounding the fused granules breaks down into component subfilaments which are physically identical to microfilaments. As contraction of the mass of aggregated platelets continues new microtubules appear in the pseudopods (Figs. 27, 28). Some of these tubules may originate from the annular bundle, while others appear to result from compression of parallel micro-filaments in elongated pseudopods as the cell mass contracts. The function of microtubules which appear during viscous metamorphosis is not known. They are not essential for clot retraction (White, 1968e).

The precise relationship of microtubules to the contractile mechanism of platelets is still under investigation. Puszkin and Aledort have recently

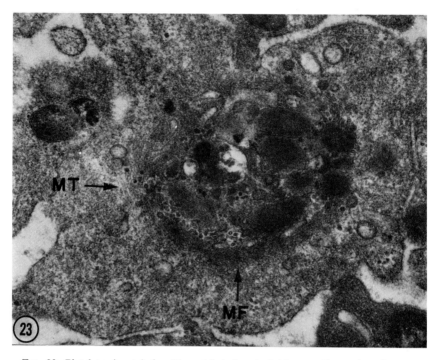

FIG. 23. Platelet microtubules. Thrombin-induced platelet transformation after onset of the second wave of aggregation. Fusion of centrally clumped granules is in progress. A ring of microfilaments (MF) and a few residual microtubules (MT) surround the mass of organelles. 33,200×.

isolated a colchicine binding protein from platelets with actinlike properties (1969). Their findings suggest that platelet microtubules are the storage form of the actin component of thrombosthenin, and subunits interact with thrombosthenin M at the colchicine binding site. Lüscher has come to a similar conclusion regarding the actinlike properties of the subunits making up platelet microtubules (Lüscher and Bettex-Galland, 1968). These views are entirely compatible with the evidence compiled from electron micro-scopic studies.

B. Microfilaments

Microfilaments constitute the third system of fibers in the platelet sol–gel zone (Bessis and Breton-Gorius, 1965; Behnke, 1966; Sixma and Molenaar, 1966). They appear more numerous than other polymers, and are so concentrated in the matrix of unaltered platelets that they cannot be resolved in thin sections. However, they can be identified readily in whole-mounts

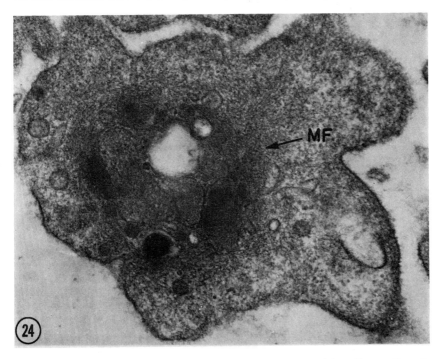

FIG. 24. Platelet microtubules. Platelet from sample aggregated by collagen. Granule fusion is nearly complete, and only microfilaments (MF) are apparent in the enclosing ring of fibers. 45,650×.

of spread platelets and in thin sections of platelet pseudopods (Zucker-Franklin *et al.*, 1967; Zucker-Franklin, 1969; B. J. Bull, 1966) (Figs. 28, 29, 30). The state of microfilaments in unaltered platelets is not yet clear. Subunit proteins of microfilaments may exist primarily in a pregel resembling the viscous state of hemoglobin molecules in intact red blood cells. Polymerization into filaments may be a constant, or alternating process, or may occur only as a result of stimulation during the hemostatic reaction of platelets. Whichever the case may be it is apparent that the organization of the platelet internal matrix is governed by the balance of sol–gel trans-formation. While many other components may be dissolved in the sol–gel zone, microfilaments appear to be the primary structural constituents.

Studies in this laboratory have emphasized the similarity of microfila-ments, submembrane filaments, and subfilaments of microtubules. All are composed of globular subunits stacked end-to-end in a slightly offset manner yielding a helically twisted structure. The platelet filaments are

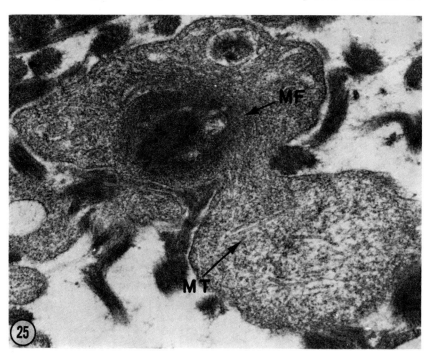

FIG. 25. Platelet microtubules. Platelet from sample of recalcified citrate platelet-rich plasma fixed early in clot retraction. Centrally clumped granules have fused within a ring of microfilaments (MF). Microtubules (MT) are prominent in pseudopods at this stage of transformation. Fibrin strands are apparent in the surrounding plasma. 41,500×.

approximately 50 Å in diameter and resemble actin-like filaments found in other cells, particularily muscle (Zucker-Franklin et al., 1967; Zucker-Franklin, 1969). Extracts of platelet contractile protein contain masses of filamentous structures strikingly similar to microfilaments, subfilaments of microtubules, and submembrane filaments. These findings suggest that filaments of the platelet are structural elements of the contractile mechanism. However, platelet thrombosthenin consists of a myosin moiety as well as actin-like filaments. The nature of the myosin component, thrombosthenin M, remains obscure (Lüscher and Bettex-Galland, 1968). Identification of this protein, its structural analogue, and localization in platelets will help to solve the remaining mysteries of platelet contraction.

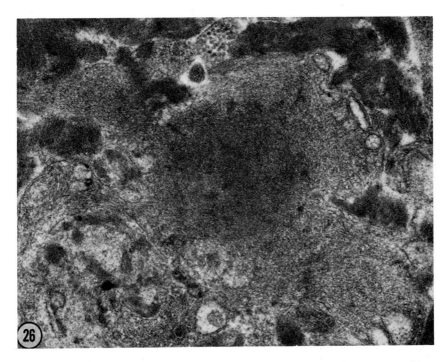

Fig. 26. Platelet microtubules. Late clot retraction. Fused granules form an amorphous mass in this cell. Microfilaments are incorporated into the condensed mass and spread from it throughout the platelet. Microtubules are no longer present in the central regions of contracted platelets at this stage of clot retraction. 38,240×.

V. THE ORGANELLE ZONE

A large number of formed organelles and particles are imbedded in the sol–gel matrix of the platelet. Particulate elements are mainly glycogen (Figs. 2 and 4). The glycogen is usually concentrated in a single large mass, but individual particles are often seen throughout the cell. Glycogen particles have a characteristic morphology at high magnification, and should not be mistaken for ribosomes (White, 1967a). Recognition of the platelet's capacity to synthesize protein (Booyse and Rafelson, 1968; Warshaw et al.,

1967) caused some confusion about the nature of the small particles, but at the present time there is no evidence that ribosomes or ribosomal aggregates are present in the platelet substance. This observation does not negate the evidence that platelets can synthesize large proteins, but suggests that the mechanism may not involve the pathways found in other cells.

The formed organelles of the platelet consist of numerous granules, a few dense bodies, and occassional mitochondria.

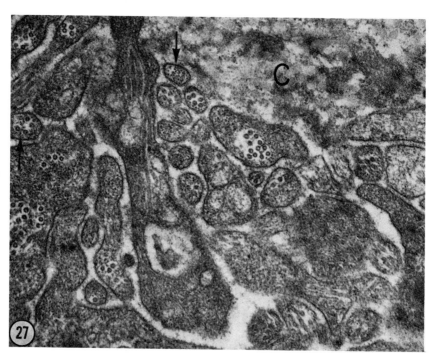

FIG. 27. Platelet microtubules. Collagen (C) induced platelet aggregate. The prominance of microtubules and their close relationship to microfilaments in pseudopods are evident in this example. Arrows (↑) indicate areas in which tubules appear to be forming from or disassembling into microfilaments. 41,500×.

A. Granules

Granules are the most numerous of the formed organelles in the platelet (Figs. 2 and 4). The structures vary in size and shape, but are generally believed to constitute a single species. Each granule is approximately 0.2–0.3 μ in diameter, and enclosed by a unit membrane similar to the plasma membrane of the peripheral zone. Two zones of differing electron opacity are evident in the coarse matrix of the granule. Rodman (1967) observed a membrane separating the dark zone from the less opaque area, but this appears to be quite rare. The basis for compartmentalization is not known, but it suggests that chemical constituents of the granules are physically segregated. Some granules do not appear to have two zones of differing density. The apparent uniformity of substructure in these organelles may be due to the plane of section, but the possibility that they represent a

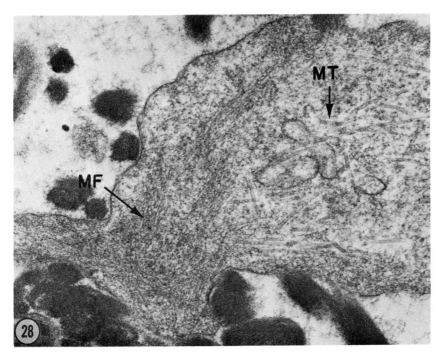

Fig. 28. Platelet microtubules. Swollen pseudopod at periphery of platelet aggregate in retracted clot. The interdigitation of microtubules (MT) and microfilaments (MF) is apparent. 37,350×.

different population must also be considered. Tubular elements resembling microtubules are found frequently in the matrix of normal platelet granules (White, 1968l) (Fig. 31). The basis for their occurrence inside the organelles is unknown.

Biochemical studies have shown that granules are rich in phospholipids, and contain hydrolytic enzymes similar to those found in lysosomes (Marcus et al., 1966). Other studies have suggested that granules are storage sites for platelet fibrinogen, thrombosthenin, serotonin, catecholamines, glyco-

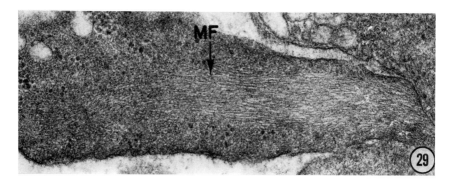

FIG. 29. Platelet microfilaments. The microfilaments (MF) are difficult to resolve in unaltered platelets. They are prominent in pseudopods, however, after platelet transformation, and often form parallel masses. 49,800×.

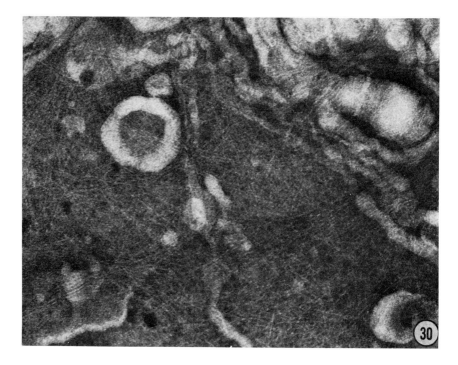

FIG. 30. Platelet microfilaments. Negatively stained whole mount of spread platelet. The matrix of the cell is filled with an irregular meshwork of microfilaments. The 50 Å fibers are indistinguishable from the subfilaments of microtubules and submembrane filaments. 272,000×.

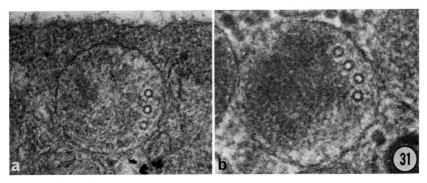

FIG. 31. Platelet granules. The examples shown in (a) and (b) reveal circular profiles in their matrix resembling cross sections of microtubules. Tubular elements are common in platelet granules, but their function is unknown. a, 111,700×; b, 125,000×.

proteins, and a nonmetabolic pool of ATP and ADP (Born *et al.*, 1958; Wurzel *et al.*, 1965; Baker *et al.*, 1959; Da Prada *et al.*, 1967; Holmsen *et al.*, 1969; Day *et al.*, 1969; E. Weber *et al.*, 1968). Recently cytochemical investigations have suggested that mucopolysaccharides are also constituents of platelet granules (Rambourg and Leblond, 1967; Spicer *et al.*, 1969; White, 1970a). It is difficult to understand how so many different chemical constituents can be stored in a single population of organelles. Siegel and Lüscher (Siegel and Lüscher, 1967) have suggested that hydrolytic enzymes are stored in a light fraction which sediments more slowly in sucrose than the granules, but the recent studies of Day *et al.* (1969) again emphasize the location of hydrolytic enzymes in the granule fraction.

B. Dense Bodies

A few of the organelles present in thin sections of glutaraldehyde–osmium fixed human platelets are extremely opaque to the electron beam (Tranzer *et al.*, 1966). Because of their opacity they are referred to as dense bodies (Fig. 2). The number of dense bodies in platelets from different mamalian species varies with the content of serotonin in the cells. Platelets with abundant 5-HT have many dense bodies, whereas human platelets with a low content of the amine are considered to have few opaque organelles (Figs. 32 and 33). Reserpine or tyramine treatment *in vivo* or *in vitro* depletes platelet serotonin and dissolves the dense bodies. Depleted platelets incubated with 5-HT *in vitro* recover their content of serotonin and reform opaque organelles. Biochemical studies on dense bodies isolated by density gradient centrifugation also reveal their high content of serotonin, and 5-HT has been localized in the dense bodies by ultrastructural autoradiography (Solatunturi and Paasonen, 1966; Bak *et al.*, 1967; Da Prada *et al.*, 1967; Davis and White, 1968). Additional investigations have shown that dense bodies contain ATP, ADP, and catecholamines; a lamellar substructure

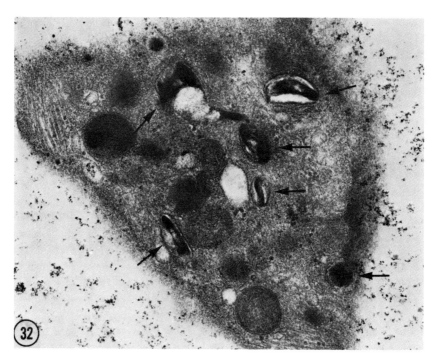

FIG. 32. Dense bodies. The opaque organelles are storage sites for serotonin and other products of the platelet release reaction. Animal platelets rich in serotonin contain many dense bodies, but the organelles are considered rare components of human platelets which transport less of the amine. However, this has not been our experience. The cell shown in this illustration is from human citrate platelet-rich plasma incubated with thorium dioxide before fixation. Six dense bodies (↑) are present in the matrix of the cell. Thorium dioxide is often transferred from the channel system to intact granules, but rarely appears in dense bodies. This finding suggests that the opaque organelles are not formed in the channel system. 41,500 ×.

observed in some investigations suggested that they might contain phospholipid (B. J. Bull, 1966). The results of the various investigations suggest that dense bodies are storage organelles for most if not all of the endogenous products secreted by platelets during the release reaction (Holmsen *et al.*, 1969).

The electron opacity of platelet-dense bodies was initially related to their avidity for osmic acid (Tranzer *et al.*, 1966). Glutaraldehyde and serotonin in test tube experiments were found to form a complex resembling a Schiff base which precipitated added osmic acid. The reaction of glutaraldehyde-fixed platelet dense bodies with osmic acid appeared to follow the reaction suggested by *in vitro* experiments, and the opacity of the organelles was believed to result from a heavy deposit of osmium. A similar interpretation

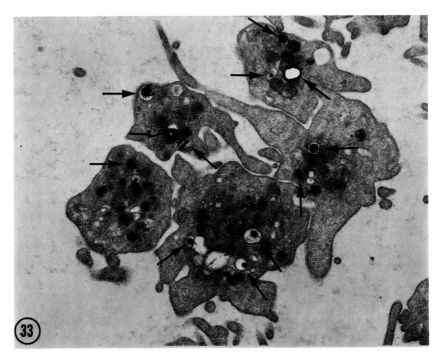

FIG. 33. Dense bodies. ADP-induced aggregate of human platelets fixed during the first wave. Twelve dense bodies (↑) are apparent in the five cells. This number of opaque organelles almost equals a previously reported value of 16 dense bodies per 2000 human platelets in thin section. 12,900 ×.

was made when dense bodies were preserved in glutaraldehyde-fixed platelets after a second fixation in potassium dichromate (Wood, 1965). Deposit of metallic oxydizing fixatives in dense bodies after glutaraldehyde fixation was considered to be a specific cytochemical test for platelet serotonin (Etcheverry and Zieher, 1968).

However, there were several points which argued against this interpretation. Although platelets fixed in osmic acid alone rarely contained dense

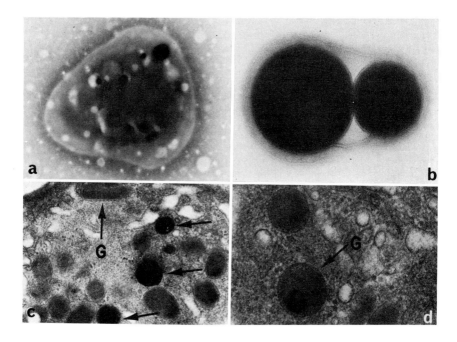

Fig. 34. Dense bodies. The cell in (a) is a whole-mounted platelet from citrate platelet-rich plasma which has not been fixed or stained. Seven dense bodies are apparent in the substance of the cell. The organelles do not require metallic oxidizing fixatives or stains to make them visible for they are inherently electron opaque. Other organelles in whole-mounted platelets are electron transparent. It is for this reason that the opaque organelles are referred to as dense bodies. (b) Reveals two dense bodies confined within the same unit membrane. The cell was fixed in glutaraldehyde but not osmic acid. Platelets are nearly invisible when fixed in glutaraldehyde alone and sections examined without post-staining. However, dense bodies retain their inherent opacity. Several stages of dense body formation (↑) are apparent in (c). A granule with an opaque nucleoid and periodic

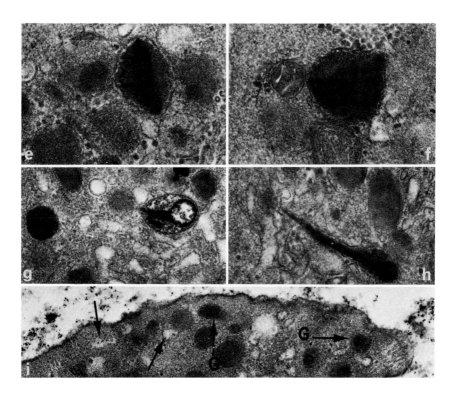

banding of the less dense zone is also present. (d) Demonstrates a granule containing a zone whose opacity is identical to that of serotonin storage organelles. (e) and (f) show more advanced stages in transformation of granules to dense bodies. One of the dense bodies in (g) is completely opaque while a second contains a signet ring with a tail. (h) illustrates a long tailed dense body whose head is associated with granule substance inside the surrounding membrane. The platelet in (i) was incubated with horse radish peroxidase and thorium dioxide before fixation. Both are present on the cell surface and in the open channel system (↑). Only thorium dioxide, however, is transferred from channels to granules (G).

bodies, on occasion they could be found (Davis and White, 1968). The reason for their preservation in some osmic acid-fixed platelets was poorly understood at the time, but is was apparent that glutaraldehyde was not absolutely essential. More important, however, was the observation that platelet dense bodies were inherently electron opaque (White, 1968a, 1969c). When platelets were spread on grid surfaces by the whole-mount method, the dense bodies could be identified readily (Fig. 34). No fixation nor surface staining with phosphotungstic acid was required. Also sections of platelets fixed in glutaraldehyde alone and imbedded in water soluble methacrylate without postfixation in osmic acid or dichromate, and without staining of sections with uranyl acetate and lead citrate also contained opaque organelles (Fig. 34). These experiments established that platelet dense bodies were inherently opaque, and did not require metallic oxydizing fixatives for visualization.

The basis for the inherent opacity of platelet dense bodies has not been specifically defined, but several steps have been taken toward a solution. Various experiments have shown that the opacity is not due to a content of protein, lipid, fibrinogen, or serotonin per se. It is the uptake of serotonin which results in the development of electron density, suggesting that something carried into the organelle with 5-HT must be responsible. Kerby and Taylor had shown that chelation and plasma were important for the uptake of serotonin by platelets (Kerby and Taylor, 1961). This suggested that 5-HT might be transferred across the platelet membrane as a metal chelate, and subsequent concentration of cation could result in complexes of sufficient mass to prevent transmission of electrons. The sedimentation of dense bodies in gradient density also suggested that these organelles have a greater mass than platelet granules (Da Prada et al., 1967). On the basis of these observations and certain principles of electron optics, it was suggested that calcium was most likely responsible for the inherent opacity of dense bodies. However, the possibility that other cations might contribute or be principally involved was not ruled out.

Since the products contained in dense bodies are extruded during the platelet release reaction, it seemed reasonable to consider those ions which appear in plasma during platelet secretion as contributors to opacity. The two ions released by platelets after exposure to aggregating agents are calcium and potassium (Holmsen et al., 1969). Both are derived from nonmetabolic pools in the platelet, and neither is exchangeable with ions outside the cells. Calcium is again of a special interest because of its particular association with platelet lipids (Wallach et al., 1958).

Spicer et al. (1969) have shown recently that platelet dense bodies can be preserved by osmic acid when the fixative is combined with buffered potassium pyrophosphate or pyroantimonate. The results also suggested specific localization of precipitable cation in dense bodies, though the nature of the cation could not be defined. Additional studies have shown that potassium phosphate has a protective effect on platelet dense bodies. Therefore, phosphate, pyrophosphate and pyroantimonate appear to react with cations in platelet dense bodies in some manner which preserves them, or at least prevents their extraction during dehydration and imbedding. The precise nature of the cation remains to be determined.

The development of dense bodies in human platelets appears to involve a relationship between granules and the system of open channels which communicates with the plasma (White, 1968m). Observations on normal platelet samples have revealed multiple stages in the transformation of granules to opaque organelles (White, 1968f) (Fig. 34). The darker zone in the platelet granule appears primarily involved in development of opacity. Dissolution of the light zone may result in the contracted appearance of dense substance within a vacuole presented by most platelet dense bodies. On occassion, however, the entire contents of the organelle appear electron opaque, and a few dense bodies are observed with long, taillike extensions.

The fact that only a few of the platelet granules become electron opaque suggested that a special route must exist for the transfer of serotonin to selected organelles. The only pathway which seemed appropriate for this purpose was the open canalicular system (White and Krivit, 1967b). When thorium dioxide was incubated with platelets *in vitro*, the dense particles entered the open channels without causing platelet transformation (White, 1968m). Some of the thorium particles were transferred from the channels to apparently intact platelet granules. These findings have since been confirmed *in vivo* (Vegge *et al.*, 1968). Recent investigations with two electron dense tracers used simultaneously have demonstrated the selectivity of this process (White, 1970d) (Fig. 34). When thorium dioxide and horse radish peroxidase were added to citrate platelet-rich plasma, both entered the channel system of platelets. However, only thorium particles were transferred to the granules, while horse radish peroxidase was restricted to the exterior coat lining channels and covering the peripheral zone. These findings suggested that the open canalicular system may serve as a major route for uptake and transfer of plasma borne substances to selected platelet granules.

The question arose as to what characteristic of granules might favor the uptake and concentration of cations. Recently Spicer *et al.* demonstrated the fine structural localization of acid mucosubstances in the nucleoid (dense zone) of platelet granules with a dialyzed iron method specific for acidic mucopolysaccharides (Spicer et al., 1969). Polyanionic acidic muco-substances have an affinity for cations, and localization in the zone primarily involved in development of opacity associated with granule conversion to dense bodies may indicate a role in cation deposition. We have used a surface staining technique with phosphotungstic acid and rutherium red staining after platelet degranulation to obtain cytochemical localization of acidic mucopolysaccharides (White, 1970a). The results confirm the presence of these substances in platelet granules, but in contrast to the findings of Spicer et al. the staining reaction appears to involve the entire organelle, rather than a selected region of the substructure (Fig. 35). Preliminary investigations on isolated platelet granules by biochemical techniques also indicate the presence of acidic mucopolysaccharides in these organelles (White, 1970e). Mucopolysaccharides in platelet granules may function as a trap for cations, serve as a matrix separating enzymes and other chemical constituents, and provide a source of mucosubstance for renewal of the exterior coat of the platelet surface.

C. Mitochondria

Platelet mitochondria are few in number and structurally simple. Yet, they contribute significantly to the energy metabolism of the cell (Marcus and Zucker, 1965). Blockade of anaerobic glycolysis does not cause a drop in the level of platelet ATP, nor does it inhibit normal platelet function. Thus mitochondria can alone support platelet energy requirements. ATP has been localized in mitochondria at the fine structural level. Biochemical studies have defined the presence of typical mitochondrial enzymes in isolated fractions and suggested the presence of monamine oxidase activity in these organelles (Solatunturi and Paasonen, 1966). During platelet hemostatic reactions the mitochondria become more dense, suggesting a change in energy state. Intoxication of platelets by drugs often results in formation of electron dense aggregates inside mitochondria. The deposits are commonly found in mitochondria of other tissues, and their significance is uncertain. Incubation of sections on drops of hydrogen peroxide removes the mitochondrial deposits, suggesting that they are complexes of osmic acid with metallic ions or salts. Calcium has been considered a principle component of these deposits in mitochondria, but the point is still in dispute. Pyroantimonate precipitates have been identified in platelet mitochondria, but the cation responsible for precipitation is unknown (Spicer et al., 1969).

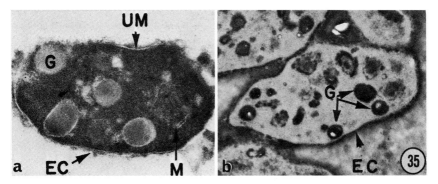

Fig. 35. The platelet (a) was fixed in glutaraldehyde alone and embedded in water soluble methacrylate. Sections were stained with uranyl acetate and lead citrate. Granules (G) take up less stain than mitochondria (M), the sol–gel matrix and the exterior coat (EC). Unit membranes (UM) are not stained. The cells in (b) were fixed and embedded in a similar manner. In this case sections were stained on drops of phosphotungstic acid at a pH of 1.5. Pease has shown that this stain is specific for acidic carbohydrates of mucopolysaccharides under these conditions. Glycogen is also stained, but the stores of this material are removed by alkaline lead whereas the reactive substance in granules, channels and the exterior coat is not.

VI. MEMBRANE SYSTEMS

A. Golgi Apparatus

The open canalicular system which constitutes the major group of specialized membranes in the platelet was discussed above under the peripheral zone. It is physically part of the cell wall, structurally identical to it, and appears to function in a similar manner. A second membrane system consists of stacks of flattened saccules. It occurs in approximately 10% of platelets and is structurally identical to a Golgi apparatus (Fig. 36). Platelet Golgi zones are probably derived from the parent megakaryocyte. There is no available evidence to indicate functional activity of this system in the circulating cell.

B. Dense Tubular System

The third specialized group of membranes in the platelet is the dense tubular system (Behnke, 1967). Channels of this system are closely associated with the circumferential band of microtubules (Fig. 4). A few irregular membranes enclosing material with an opacity similar to the sol–gel

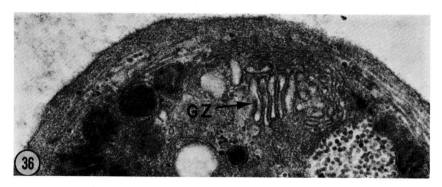

Fig. 36. Golgi zone (GZ). Platelet from sample of citrate platelet-rich plasma containing a stack of flattened saccules. This structure is similar to the Golgi apparatus found in megakaryocytes. Its function in circulating platelets is unknown. 33,200×.

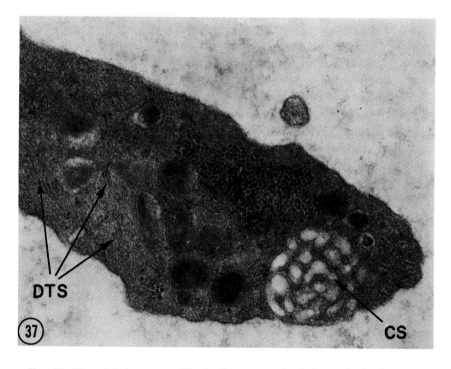

Fig. 37. Dense tubular system. Platelet from a sample of citrate platelet-rich plasma exposed to a high concentration of acetylsalicylic acid. Aspirin at high concentration produced changes in platelet microtubules, microfilaments, and channel systems. The canalicular system (CS) is contracted to one side of the cell and channels of the dense tubular system (DTS) are dispersed in the sol–gel matrix. 21,500×.

zone can usually be identified just under the circular profiles of circumferential microtubules in cross sections of platelets. Behnke (1967) and
Hovig (1968) have indicated that channels of the dense tubular system can
be found distributed randomly in sol–gel cytoplasm, but are difficult to
identify because of their content of similarily opaque material. In our experience dense tubular channels are quite rare except in association with
the band of microtubules. However, when microtubules are removed by
chemical dissection with vincristine, the channels of the dense tubular
system spread randomly throughout the platelet substance (White, 1968i).
Exposure of platelets to high concentrations of aspirin and sodium salicylate
can also cause marked changes in circumferential microtubules, and result
in dispersal of the dense channel system (White, 1968g) (Figs. 37 and 38).
The chemical injury causes slight expansion of the irregular channels, and
fine filaments can be identified within their matrix. Chemical shock causes
marked dilitation of the channels, and under these conditions filaments
identical to microfilaments, submembrane filaments, and subfilaments of

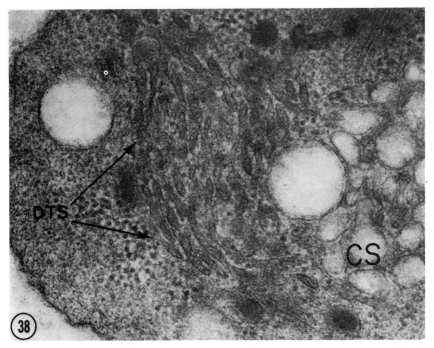

FIG. 38. Dense tubular system. Proliferation of the dense tubular system (DTS) and
separation from the canalicular system (CS) are evident in this aspirin damaged platelet.
Fine filaments are present in the dense substance forming the matrix of DTS channels.
89,500×.

microtubules can be found inside them (White, 1969a) (Fig. 6). In addition microtubules are closely associated with the residual channels of the swollen dense tubular system (Figs. 6 and 39). These findings have suggested that the dense tubular system may be involved in elaboration of filaments for platelet fibrous systems and may serve as a template for organization of the circumferential band of microtubules.

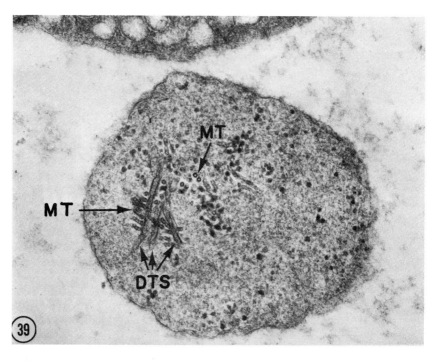

FIG. 39. Dense tubular system. An aspirin injured platelet revealing an association between channels of the DTS and microtubules (MT). A similar close association between the DTS and microtubules is shown in a chemically shocked cell in Fig. 6. The nature of this relationship is not yet known. 33,200 ×.

VII. UNUSUAL FEATURES OF PLATELET MORPHOLOGY

A. Large Platelets

Many aberrations of platelet structure have been reported in the past and some are considered characteristic of certain diseases (Schulz *et al.*, 1958; Jean *et al.*, 1963). However, most anomalies appear to be variations of normal platelet structure occurring more frequently in certain conditions (Hovig, 1968). Giant platelets, for example, are found in high frequency in patients with idiopathic thrombocytopenia (Karpatkin, 1969). The large cells are a reflection of rapid discharge of platelets from the bone marrow, and an increased rate of platelet destruction or removal from the circulation. Entirely similar giant platelets, however, are frequently observed in the buffy coat layer from centrifuged samples of blood from most normal individuals

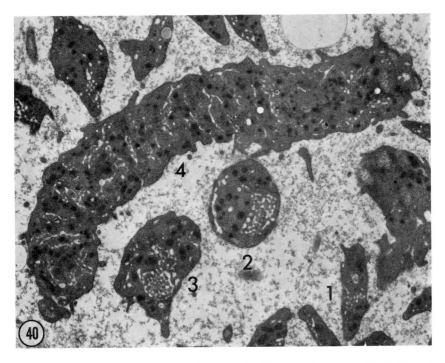

Fig. 40. Unusual platelets. The cells shown in this example are from the buffy coat of normal human blood. When buffy coat layers are fixed *in situ* the upper portion usually contains large platelets. Platelet number (1) is a normal sized cell. Numbers (2) and (3) are somewhat larger. The fourth cell is a giant platelet. The appearance suggests that it is an incompletely demarcated fragment of magakaryocyte cytoplasm. 16,100×.

(Fig. 40). The massive cells appear to be large fragments of incompletely segmented megakaryocyte cytoplasm rather than discrete platelets. It is probable that demarcation and separation into smaller units is completed in the circulation. In patients with the May-Hegglin anomaly, however, giant platelets appear to persist (Wassmuth *et al.*, 1963). The abnormality is not associated with bleeding symptoms. Other disorders characterized

by large platelets in circulating blood have been described, and the giant
cells appear to function poorly (Bernard and Soulier, 1948). Thus far the
only structural difference between giant and normal sized platelets is the
incomplete state of formation of a circumferential bundle of microtubules
in the large cells. Observations on megakaryocytes and the giant cells in
circulating blood have indicated that the annular bundle is formed after
platelets reach the circulation. Whether failure of segmentation or incomplete formation of the circumferential band of tubules are related to presist-
ence of giant forms in abnormal states remains to be determined.

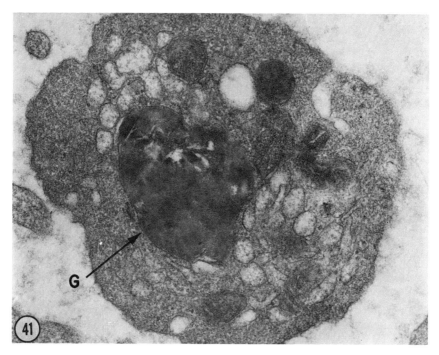

Fig. 41. Unusual organelles. The platelet in this illustration is from a patient with
polycythemia and thrombocythemia. Giant granules (G) were frequently observed in his
platelets. 39,700×.

B. Small Platelets

Recently small platelets have been reported to be a characteristic feature
of the Wiskott-Aldrich syndrome (Grottum et al., 1969). In addition to
their small size, Wiskott-Aldrich platelets have decreased numbers of
granules and dense bodies, a prominent dense tubular system, metabolic

abnormalities, poor function, and short life-span. Some of the reported defects can be induced in normal platelets by incubation with high concentrations of aspirin, but this finding has no relevance to the origin of the abnormalities in platelets of patients with Wiskott-Aldrich syndrome.

C. Granule Abnormalities

Abnormalities in granules have frequently been observed in patients with bleeding disorders due to defective platelet function (Jean *et al.*, 1963; Caen *et al.*, 1966). Decreased numbers, increased frequency of unusual shapes, and presence of giant granules have been reported in platelets from individuals with various hemorrhagic disorders. However, large granules and organelles with unusual shapes are so frequently encountered in normal platelets that they are unlikely to be a causative factor in bleeding syndromes (Figs. 41 and 42). A recent investigation of platelets from patients with

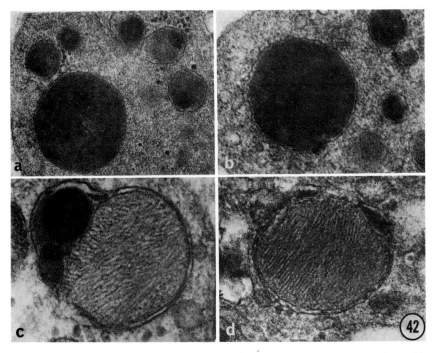

Fig. 42. Unusual organelles. The giant platelet granule in (a) is from a patient with thrombasthenia. A similar giant organelle in (b) is present in a normal platelet. The granules shown in (c) and (d) are from patients with carcinoid syndrome. Some features of these organelles have suggested that they result from cytoplasmic sequestration.

carcinoid syndrome revealed a number of abnormalities including the presence of unusual granules in a significant number of cells (White and Davis, 1969) (Fig. 42). Granule aberrations found in this disorder do not appear to be associated with defective platelet function.

D. Other Structural Variations

In addition to previously described anomalies of platelet structure, there are other variations which occur infrequently (Figs. 43 and 44). They include

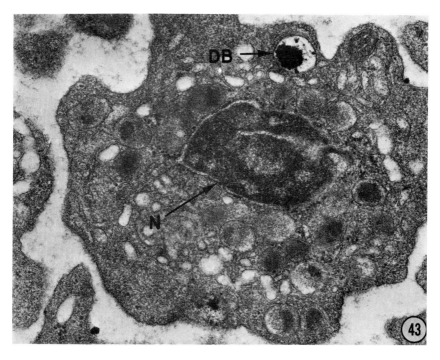

FIG. 43. Unusual organelles. A platelet from normal human blood which contains a mass resembling a nucleus (N). The sample of citrate platelet-rich plasma was chilled before fixation, but the dense body (DB) and granules indicate the cell is a platelet. We have collected seven examples of this type from normal blood. 41,500×.

platelet centrioles, nuclear remnants, and inclusions resembling crystals. Platelets with these variations from normal are so rare that they do not require speculation as to their origin. However, all of them have been found in normal human blood.

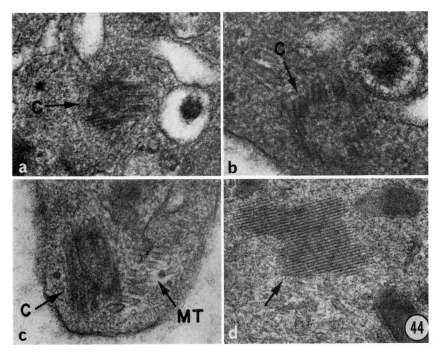

FIG. 44. Unusual organelles. Centrioles (C) are rare in human platelets, but three examples are shown in (a, b, and c). The complex is closely associated with the circumferential microtubules (MT) in (c). All were observed in platelets from normal blood. The crystalline structure in (d) was found in a platelet stored in culture media for 3 days. Similar structures are found in platelets of citrate platelet-rich plasma kept at 37°C for 24 hours. Aspirin in high concentration induces changes in microtubules which result in crystals similar to the one shown in this illustration. Whether all such crystals arise from microtubules is not certain.

VIII. STRUCTURAL PHYSIOLOGY

Redefinition of platelet anatomical features and division into three zones was done for two reasons. The first was to permit comparisons between platelets and other cells, tissues and organ systems which have much in common with the hemostatic cell. A second purpose was to permit direct correlations to be drawn between platelet structure and function. There are three basic mechanisms which appear fundamental to the functional activity of blood platelets in hemostasis. They are adhesion, contraction, and secretion. In a sense the three terms chosen to describe basic mechanisms represent an oversimplification. Adhesion, for example, is not identical to aggregation, for it can occur in the presence of EDTA, whereas platelet-to-platelet clumping requires calcium (Hellem, 1968). However, both adhesion and aggregation imply the development of platelet stickiness, and the basic mechanism involved in this event is still unknown. The purpose of this description of structural physiology is to focus attention on the platelet reaction and anatomical components involved. Therefore, the term adhesion is used to imply development of stickiness and interaction

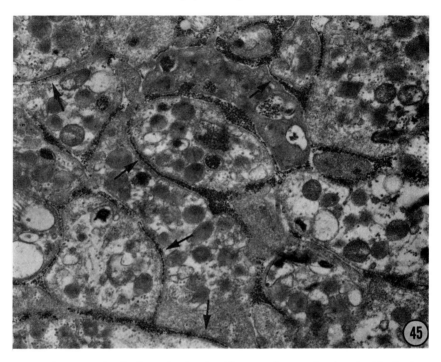

FIG. 45. Zone of adhesion. Platelets in this example were incubated with thorium dioxide before aggregation with ADP. The electron dense particles are compressed between adjacent cell surfaces. Cross sections (↑) indicate that the layers of thorium dioxide are separated from unit membranes by clear spaces. 16,100×.

with other surfaces regardless of their nature. The choice made here should not be confused with the semantics used by others to stress differences between adhesion and aggregation (Spaet and Zucker, 1964).

Aside from the words themselves, the selection of three basic mechanisms to describe platelet function is not an oversimplification. Platelets must adhere to sites of vascular injury and to each other in order to form a hemostatic plug. Secretion is necessary to increase the mass of platelets forming the plug, since the initial coat of adherent cells is inadequate for this purpose. Contractile physiology dominates the hemostatic reaction from its inception. The contractile mechanism protects the cell from over response to minimal stimuli, effectuates the secretion of endogenous chemical constituents, seals the loose mass of aggregated platelets into a hemostatic plug, and retracts the platelet–fibrin meshwork necessary to control bleeding from larger wounds.

The peripheral zone of the platelet is involved primarily in the process of adhesion, the sol–gel zone in contraction and the organelle zone in secretion. Adhesion, contraction, and secretion are separable, but not entirely independent phenomena. Platelets can become sticky and adhere to one another without contracting or releasing endogenous constituents. They can swell and contract to a limited extent without secreting or becoming sticky. Secretion, however, is entirely dependent on contraction, and unless the release reaction occurs, secondary aggregation does not take place. It is the interaction of adhesion, contraction, and secretion, however, which should be stressed. The separation of these mechanisms helps us to understand the nature of the process, but hemostasis results when all three operate efficiently and together. Recent reports have discussed the sequential aspects of platelet transformation in detail (White and Krivit, 1967c; White, 1968a,d,j,k; 1969b,d; 1970a–f) (Figs. 12–28). A few of the principal phenomena will be discussed here.

A. Adhesion

The precise physical and chemical changes involved in the conversion of platelets from a nonsticky to a sticky state are still unclear. A similar problem from the anatomical point of view is the site adhesion takes place. Thin sections of osmic acid-fixed platelet aggregates revealed that surface membranes of adjacent cells did not fuse during viscous metamorphosis (Hovig, 1962). Instead unit membranes on adjacent cells remained separated by an interval of 200–400 Å. Spaces between the aggregated cells appeared structureless until improved methods of fixation and new cytochemical techniques revealed a thick exterior coat covering the platelet peripheral zone (Stehbens and Biscoe, 1967). Fixation of platelet clumps from the first and second waves of aggregation in solutions containing either ruthenium red or lanthanum nitrate revealed that coat material stained specifically by the dense agents remained on the platelet surfaces throughout viscous metamorphosis, and filled the intercellular space (White, 1970d). Experiments in which horse radish peroxidase was added to platelet-rich plasma

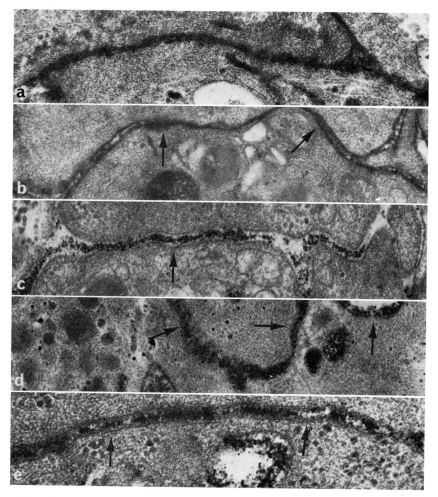

Fig. 46. Zone of adhesion. The platelet aggregates in (a) and (b) were fixed in solutions containing lanthanum nitrate and ruthenium red, respectively. Both stains are embedded in the exterior coats covering adjacent cells. As a result the zone of adhesion is difficult to define because the stain often forms a confluent layer between the cells (↑). In (c), thorium dioxide particles appear to be supported on the surface of exterior coats separating adjacent cells. The appearance suggests that coat substance is intact on aggregated cells, and that adhesion must occur at the periphery of the exterior coat. Platelets forming the aggregate in (d) were incubated in horse radish peroxidase and thorium dioxide before exposure to aggregating agent. In (e) the cells were preincubated in thorium dioxid and fixed in solutions containing ruthenium red after aggregation. Particles of thorium dioxide are supported on layers of horse radish peroxidase embedded in exterior coats of adjacent cells in (d) and on exterior coats stained by ruthenium red in (e). These results have defined the zone of adhesion between platelets at the extreme periphery of exterior coats covering adjacent cells in the aggregates.

before the platelets were aggregated and fixed for study in the electron microscope gave exactly the same results. These findings indicated that exterior coats of blood platelets served as the zone of adhesion between aggregated cells. However, the stains were embedded in exterior coats down to the unit membranes, and often filled the interval between adjacent cells. The precise site of attachment of surface coats could not be clearly defined within the continuous layer of cytochemical reaction product.

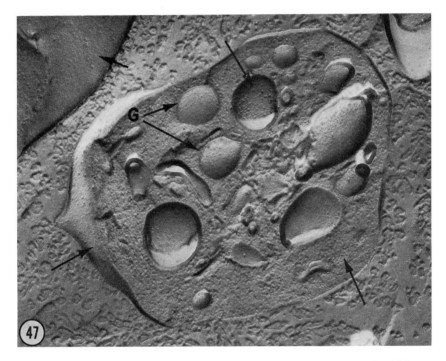

FIG. 47. Zone of adhesion. Platelets in this illustration are from a sample which was frozen, fractured, etched, and shadowed with platinum and carbon. The direction of shadowing is indicated at the lower right. This replica reveals closely packed small particles in the platelet matrix. Slightly larger particles are present in scooped out or projecting granules (G), and on the surfaces of the platelets (↑). Recent studies have shown that the particles are not in the exterior coat. The plane of fracture splits the two layers of the unit membrane. Particles are either on the outside of the inner layer or on the inside of the outer lamellae. 37,350 ×.

Experiments utilizing thorium dioxide as a vital stain helped to resolve this problem (White, 1970d) (Fig. 45). When platelets were incubated with thorium dioxide before aggregation and fixation, the electron dense particles were distributed in a different manner than horse radish peroxidase, lanthanum nitrate, and ruthenium red (Fig. 46). The dense particles were supported on the surface of the exterior coat rather than embedded in it. In platelet aggregates the thorium dioxide formed a thin line between exterior coats. The absence of coat material between unit membranes and the layer of thorotrast suggested that the appearance might be due to extraction or shrinkage during dehydration and embedding. However, when thorium dioxide and horse radish peroxidase were incubated simultaneously with

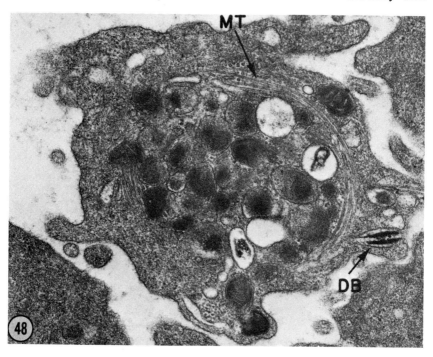

Fɪɢ. 48. Secretion. Platelet from sample aggregated by ADP. Internal changes including central movement of granules and circumferential microtubules (MT) are apparent. A dense body (BD) lies outside the band of tubules in close proximity to the cell surface. The shift of some dense bodies toward the platelet surface while other organelles are concentrated in the cell center has suggested that opaque organelles may be selectively extruded. 29,800×.

platelets before aggregation, or aggregates of platelets pretreated with thorium dioxide and fixed in solutions containing ruthenium red were examined it was apparent that material had not been extracted. Exterior coats on adjacent aggregated platelets were intact and the zone of adhesion between them was clearly defined by the thin layer of thorium dioxide particles overlying the passive or vital electron stain.

The various approaches have suggested that stickiness develops at the most peripheral area of the platelet exterior coat. Components deeper in the coat substance or the unit membrane do not appear to be involved because they are removed from the zone of adhesion by a distance of 150–200 Å. It is possible, however, that the exterior coat is not arranged in layers, but in subunits. In this case chemical components of the unit membrane could project into plasma from between the mosaic of coat subunits.

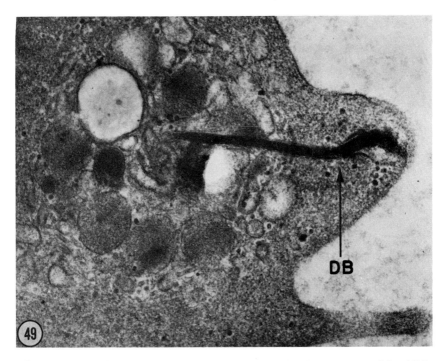

Fig. 49. Secretion. The platelet in this example has also been aggregated by ADP. A dense body (DB) extends from the mass of centrally clumped organelles to the cell periphery. Similar dense bodies with long tails are found occasionally in unaltered platelets, but are more commonly seen in after exposure of the cells to aggregating agents. 49,800×.

Yet, the distances involved are remarkable, and at the present time it seems more reasonable to focus on substances in the outside layer of the exterior coat which might be involved in the development of stickiness.

The physical structure and chemical composition of the extreme periphery of platelets has been extremely difficult to get at. Since platelets are "sponges" surrounded by an "atmosphere plasmatique" (Roskam, 1923), it

is difficult to know where plasma ends and the platelet begins. It was anticipated that other microscopic methods which view the exterior of cells directly
would give the needed information. The limiting resolution of scanning
electron microscopes (150–200 Å), however, is not sufficient to provide
details of molecular organization. Freeze-fracture and etching of platelets
followed by replication appeared to be an excellent means of getting at the
structure of the exterior coat without sacrificing the resolution of the transmission electron microscope (Ruska and Schulz, 1968). Indeed, particulate
subunits are visible on the surface of platelets prepared in this manner.
However, recent work with this method has shown that freeze-fracturing
splits the two layers of unit membranes. As a result the particles observed
on replicas are on the outer surface of the inner half of the unit membrane,
or on the inner surface of the outer half. Thus advanced optical techniques
are still too limited in capacity to provide the details of structure necessary
to define the organization of the platelet exterior coat (Fig. 47).

B. Contraction

The physical units and reasons for considering them to be basic elements
of the platelet contractile system were discussed in the section on the
platelet sol–gel zone. Contractile elements, however, are merely the force
generating components of a far more complex system involving one or
more trigger mechanisms, energy metabolism, calcium activation, and
relaxing factor activity. Understanding of various components involved
in the contractile system and the mode of their interaction is quite limited,
and considerable effort will be required to solve the problems.

In muscle systems the calcium necessary for activation of the contractile
protein, actomyosin, is localized in fenestrated channels referred to as the
sarcoplasmic reticulum (Porter, 1961). The calcium is kept out of the sarcoplasm by an ATP hydrolyzing enzyme associated with the membranous
channels (Nagai et al., 1960; A. Weber, 1966). When nerve depolarization
inactivates the ATPase which acts as a calcium extrusion pump, divalent
cations enter the sarcoplasm, activate the ATPase of actomyosin, and
contraction ensues. Recovery of the calcium pumping ATPase activity of
sarcoplasmic reticulum results in extrusion of calcium ions into the channels
and relaxation of the contractile elements.

There are many different types of muscle and muscle systems in mammals
and nonmammalian species, and primitive motile systems in all organisms
capable of directed self movement (Allen and Kamiya, 1964). The sequestration of calcium necessary for activation of the contractile elements appears

basic in most, if not all, of these contractile systems. It seemed reasonable
that the platelet, which for all practical purposes is a muscle cell (White,
1967b), should also have a calcium repository separate from the contractile
elements in the sol–gel zone. Examination of platelets for a morphological
counterpart to the sarcoplasmic reticulum focused attention on the cell
wall, the tortuous channels of the open canalicular system, and the dense
tubular system. The channels of the open canalicular system resemble the

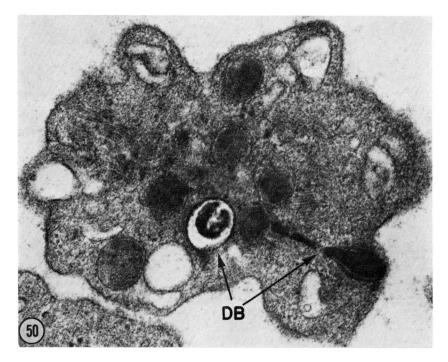

FIG. 50. Secretion. Thrombin-induced platelet transformation. One of the dense
bodies (DB) in this cell is shifted toward the surface of the cell. The tendency of some
dense bodies to move to the cell wall during internal reorganization suggests that they
may be related to the channel system. Such a relationship may facilitate discharge of
dense bodies or their products. 43,100×.

fenestrated channels of sarcoplasmic reticulum, and the surface of smooth
muscle cells is believed to be involved in the process of calcium flux necessary
for contraction (A. Weber, 1966). A material with characteristics of mucopolysaccharide is present in the sarcoplasmic reticulum, and this substance
binds thorium dioxide particles at low pH, suggesting a role in calcium
storage (Philpott and Goldstein, 1967). A magnesium-stimulated calcium

extrusion pump has been demonstrated in the membranes of the channels by biochemical and cytochemical techniques (Ohnashi and Ebashi, 1963). All of these features of the sarcoplasmic reticulum have been identified in the exterior coat covering the cell wall and lining the open channel system of platelets by identical methods (White, 1970a).

Some years ago Grette described a relaxing factor associated with cell free extracts of blood platelets which appeared identical to the relaxing

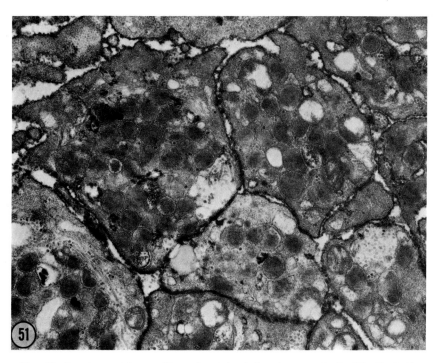

Fig. 51. Secretory pathway. The epinephrine-induced aggregate in this illustration was fixed in solutions containing lanthanum nitrate. Electron dense stain penetrates between the surfaces of adjacent clumped cells but does not enter the sol–gel zone except in channels of the open canalicular system. 16,700×.

factor found in muscle cells (Grette, 1963). More recent investigations of muscle relaxing factor have shown that this activity is related to the magnesium stimulated calcium extrusion pump ATPase associated with the membranes of the sarcoplasmic reticulum (A. Weber, 1966). Since cytochemical and biochemical studies had indicated that an ATPase similar to that associated with the sarcoplasmic reticulum was present in the exterior coat of platelets, it seemed worthwhile to reexamine the relaxing factor described by Grette. The experiments of Statland *et al.* (1969) demonstrated that the supernatant fraction studied by Grette could not have been free of membranes. A membrane fraction from platelets purified by gradient density centrifugation was found to take up calcium ions at the same rate as sarcotubular vesicles from muscle, and to be inhibited by the same agents which prevented uptake in the muscle relaxing factor system including ADP and amytal. The findings of the various investigations indicate that channels of the canalicular system and the cell wall of platelets serve as a sarcoplasmic reticulum excluding calcium from the sol–gel zone until the contractile mechanism is triggered.

The nature of the trigger mechanism is unknown. Many agents can initiate platelet contraction, suggesting that there are a number of different mechanisms involved. Yet the response of the platelets is ultimately the same no matter which agent stimulates the process. Therefore, all agents or mechanisms must affect one key step. On the basis of studies on muscle contraction and adrenal secretion this final common pathway may involve calcium flux. It is not calcium ion transport from plasma, though this may be important in late stages of secondary aggregation, viscous metamorphosis, and clot retraction, but movement of calcium from the platelet sarcoplasmic reticulum into the sol–gel zone. Experiments with atropine and local anesthetics on platelet contraction suggest that calcium flux is involved, but direct measurements have not been made (Aledort and Niemetz, 1968; White, 1969d).

C. Secretion

The capacity of blood platelets to secrete was recognized in early studies before 1900. Hayem (1878) and Bizzozero (1882) both suggested that platelets probably released a factor which was necessary for clot formation. It was Grette's investigation, however, which established the secretory capacity of the hemostatic cell (Grette, 1962). During study of the thrombin catalyzed reactions of platelets, he found that a number of endogenous chemical substances became available simultaneously from the cells during viscous metamorphosis. Grette referred to this secretory process as the platelet release reaction and his findings suggested that a contractile mechanism triggered by calcium ions caused the release reaction.

Subsequent studies by many investigators have shown that all other chemical and physical agents capable of inducing platelet viscous metamorphosis also trigger the release reaction (Holmsen *et al.*, 1969). The endogenous products secreted in parallel during the release reaction initiated by various agents are the same, varying only in amount and rate at which they become available.

Grette chose the term release reaction specifically because the secretory process differed from simple cell lysis. Yet platelet injury, damage, disruption, and disintegration are still cited as mechanisms in the current literature. Holmsen, Day, and Stormorken in a series of studies have shown clearly that the release reaction is not associated with extrusion of chemical sub-

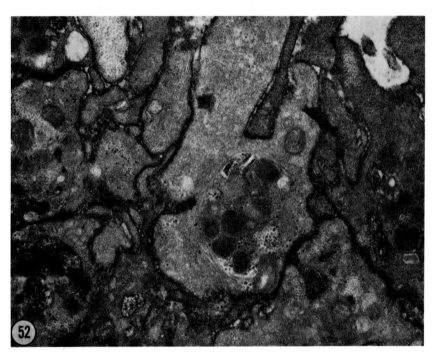

FIG. 52. Secretory pathway. Thrombin-induced aggregate fixed during second wave in solutions containing ruthenium red. The dense stain is embedded in exterior coats of all cells, even those deeply located in large platelet lumps. 25,800×.

stances which would suggest injury (Holmsen *et al.*, 1969). Thus the altered permeability and swelling of platelets which develop immediately after exposure to some aggregating agents are not signs of damage or impending disintegration. They represent characteristic features of the platelet physiological response, and are completely reversible. The fact that platelet ions and chemical constituents do not leak out of swollen platelets also indicates that altered permeability is a controlled phenomenon, not a manifestation of cell damage. These findings and others underline the integrity of the platelet, and emphasize the physiologic character of the platelet release reaction.

Products of the platelet release reaction include the adenine nucleotides, ATP and ADP, serotonin, catecholamines, potassium, calcium, platelet factor 3 and 4, hydrolytic enzymes, mucopolysaccharides, amino acids, and fibrinogen (Holmsen et al., 1969). Biochemical and cytochemical studies have shown that nearly all, if not all, of these substances are constituents of organelles in the platelet sol–gel zone. The adenine nucleotides, potassium, and calcium, might be confused with stores of these substances elsewhere in the platelet, but investigations have shown that the potassium, calcium and adenine nucleotides released during secretion are either nonexchange-able with plasma constituents or exist in nonmetabolic compartments (Buckingham and Maynert, 1964; Holmsen et al., 1969). Not all of the products listed appear simultaneously in the plasma. Adenine nucleotides, serotonin, catecholamines, and cations are released quickly by all agents. The extrusion of other substances takes longer or requires the action of collagen or thrombin for transfer to plasma. Rates of appearance of some components of the release reaction have not been measured.

The heterogeneity of the release reaction suggests that some components are more easily extruded than others, or that various products of the release reaction are localized in different subcellular organelles. There are two storage organelles in the platelet, the granule and the dense body. During conversion of granules to dense bodies, serotonin, catacholamines, adenine nucleotides, and cations became concentrated in the opaque organelles. The process of granule transformation appears to involve a close association with channels from which the plasma borne substances are transferred to the developing dense bodies. Granule matrix is often dissolved as the dense substance is deposited. The granules are lysosomes, and the process of uptake may cause activation of enzymes in the organelle, liquification of the matrix, and transfer of same constituents to the channel system as serotonin is carried in. Long, tail-like processes extending into the channel system from some dense bodies suggest that a direct relationship between granules and canaliculi may exist for a time during transformation, and occasionally sealing off may be incomplete. The proposed sequence is attractive because it explains the selective conversion of a few granules to dense bodies, the opportunity for loss of some chemical components during uptake of others, differences in chemical composition of dense bodies and granules, and the close relationship of dense bodies and channels which appears to facilitate discharge during the release reaction (Figs. 48, 49 and 50). Thus the existence of two types of storage organelles with different chemical components contributes to the heterogeneity of the release reaction, and the special relationship of dense bodies to channels may explain why these organelles or their products are first to appear during secretion (White, 1970a,b,c).

A second problem contributing to the differential character of release is the varying rate at which components coming from granules appear in the

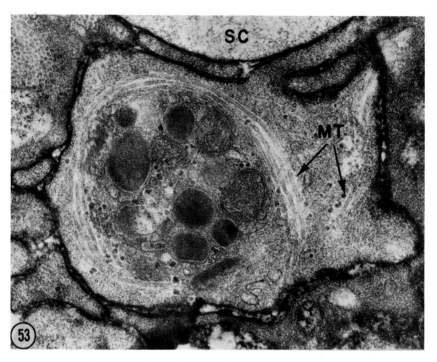

FIG. 53. Secretory pathway. Platelets aggregated by ADP and fixed in solutions containing ruthenium red. Typical internal changes are evident in this cell. Organelles are clumped in the platelet center and encircled by microtubules (MT) which also extend into a pseudopod. Despite the alterations, the stain is excluded. Even the swollen cell (SC) does not permit the entry of ruthenium which is known to penetrate into damaged cells. 43,900×.

plasma. Certain of the hydrolytic enzymes, for example, appear in plasma within 1 minute while acid phosphatase remains with the platelets until the cells are damaged in late viscous metamorphosis. Platelet factor 3 also remains with the aggregated cells, although some unsedimentable platelet factor 3 does appear in plasma (Horowitz and Popayoanou, 1968). The explanation for differential release from the same organelle or organelles is not known. However, acid phosphatase is known to be more tightly linked to lysosomes than other hydrolases, and its release from platelet subcellular particles *in vitro* is difficult (Marcus *et al.*, 1966). This finding suggests that differential release from the same organelle might depend on the chemical nature, structural binding, or location of the substance. Enzymes associated with the matrix of organelles might easily dissolve and be secreted when lysosome labilization occurs, but constituents bound to the granule membrane would tend to remain with the platelet mass.

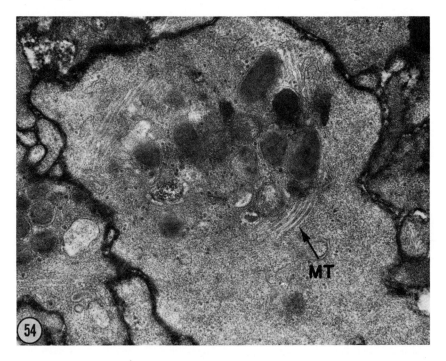

Fig. 54. Secretory pathway. Platelet from sample prepared in the same manner as the cells in the previous illustration. The failure of ruthenium red to enter platelets swollen by aggregating agents indicates that the increase in cell volume is not a manifestation of cell damage. MT, microtubules. 33,200×.

Investigations of the platelet release reaction have revealed several basic principles which should be emphasized. First, secretion is a fundamental characteristic of the platelet physiological response to all agents capable of causing viscous metamorphosis, and release is essential for the second wave of aggregation when the biphasic response of platelets is studied by nephelometry. Second, the release reaction is a physiological process. It does not result from injury, damage, or disintegration of the cells. Third, secretion results from stimulation of the platelet contractile mechanism, and the extent of release is dependent on the degree of completion of the contractile process. Fourth, all of the endogenous chemical products of secretion are confined to storage organelles inside the cells. Transfer of these organelles or their products to the plasma is the process of secretion.

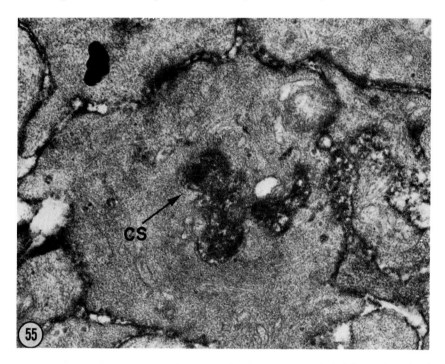

FIG. 55. Secretory pathway. Although ruthenium red is excluded from the sol–gel matrix, it does enter aggregated platelets. The stain penetrates and fills swollen channels of the open canalicular system (CS). 49,800×.

The principles governing platelet secretion lead to an inevitable conclusion about the mechanism involved. If damage is not a factor, then a special route must exist whereby the storage organelles or their products can leave the intracellular compartment and reach the surrounding plasma. A search for the platelet secretory pathway has indicated that the open canalicular system serves this purpose (White, 1970d). Platelet aggregates induced by several agents were fixed before or after the onset of the second wave of aggregation in solutions containing electron dense traces (Figs. 51–56). Ruthenium red and lanthanum nitrate form small molecular aggregates in colloidal suspension which readily penetrate between fixed cells separated by gaps of 10–18 Å. The agents enter the cytoplasm of damaged cells but not cells fixed in an undamaged condition.

Ruthenium red and lanthanum nitrate rarely penetrated into the sol–gel matrix of platelets fixed in the first or second waves of aggregation. Both compounds stained exterior coats of clumped platelets, including cells

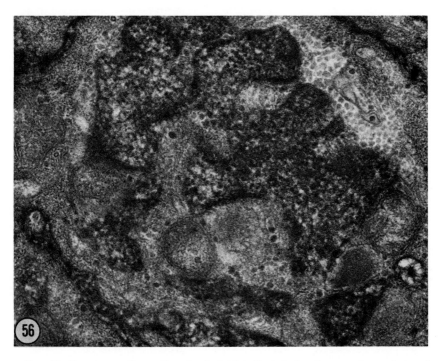

FIG. 56. Secretory pathway. Sample of platelets fixed during the second wave induced by ADP. Swollen channels of the canalicular system have largely replaced the area usually occupied by granules. The granular material can be found in the channels, and it stains positively with ruthenium red. These findings suggest that the open canalicular system serves as a major route for discharge of the products of the platelet release reaction. 59,600×.

deep in the aggregates. The dense stains also entered the open canalicular system of peripheral and deeply located platelets from aggregates fixed before or after the platelet release reaction. Granules deposited in the channel systems during the second wave of aggregation were stained by ruthenium red.

The capacity of the electron dense stain to penetrate between surfaces of aggregated cells into open channel systems of deeply located platelets in aggregates from the first or second wave indicates patency of this route during the release reaction. Staining of granule substance in channel systems by ruthenium red reveals that organelles are transferred to the channels and that granule material reacts with the stain considered specific for mucopolysaccharide. Exclusion of dense stains from the sol–gel matrix throughout both waves of aggregation indicates that cell damage is not a factor in physiologic platelet transformation. All of these findings support the conclusion that the open channel system serves as a conduit for extrusion of the products of secretion during the platelet release reaction.

IX. CONCLUSIONS

Relationships between structure and function have been emphasized in this description of platelet morphology. Platelet anatomy has been organized into zones which correlate with the three basic mechanisms of functional activity. New terms were selected for some features of platelet anatomy to facilitate this correlation and permit comparisons between the structural physiology of platelets and other types of cells. Biochemical, physiological, cytochemical, and autoradiographic experiments have clarified many of the relationships between platelet structure and function and have permitted precise localization of chemical substances important in platelet physiology.

The working hypotheses underlying the experimental approach has been that platelets are muscle cells, not merely in the sense that they are involved in processes resembling contraction, or contain substantial amounts of a protein similar to muscle actomyosin, but that contractile physiology dominates the platelet reaction. Assigning preeminence to the contractile mechanism does not detract from the importance of adhesion and secretion in platelet function. It merely serves to focus attention on the single feature which appears to govern the unique response of platelets. Contractile elements are believed by some workers to be responsible for adhesion and aggregation (Booyse and Raphelson, 1969), though localization of contractile protein in the exterior coat covering the peripheral zone has not been definitely established. We have focused on centripetal internal reorganization as a manifestation of contraction occurring inside platelets. Evidence gathered from the study of seven aggregating agents, the influence of inhibitors, and the effects of chemical dissection have consistently shown that internal transformation is an essential prelude to release, and that both secretion and central movement of organelles are dependent on an internal wave of contraction. The capacity of the cells to undergo partial internal reorganization without secreting, and to recover completely suggested a contraction–relaxation cycle in the primary response of platelets. Further consideration of this feature of the reaction to minimal stimuli has indicated that it serves as a protective mechanism preventing overreaction of circulating platelets. Secretion is entirely dependent on the platelet contractile mechanism; when contraction is blocked, the release reaction does not occur. Sealing of loose platelet aggregates into hemostatic plugs and clot retraction are known to be directly related to platelet contractile capacity. Thus contractile activity is manifested at every stage of the platelet hemostatic response. Skeletal muscle differs from smooth muscle, and both have features not found in primitive contractile systems. The contractile mechanism of the platelet also has certain characteristics which distinguish it from other types of muscle. Yet the basic comparison has been substantiated in many ways, and by focusing on platelet contractile physiology it may be possible to elucidate the basic mechanism of hemostasis.

REFERENCES

Aledort, L. M., and Niemetz, J. (1968). *Proc. Soc. Exp. Biol. Med.* **128**, 658.
Allen, R. D., and Kamiya, N., eds. (1964). "Primitive Motile Systems in Cell Biology." Academic Press, New York.
Aynaud, M. (1911). *Ann. Inst. Pasteur, Paris* **25**, 56.
Bak, I. J., Hassler, R., May, P., and Westerman, E. (1967). *Life Sci.* **6**, 1133.
Baker, R. V., Blaschko, H., and Born, G. V. R. (1959). *J. Physiol. (London)* **149**, 55P.
Behnke, O. (1965). *J. Ultrastruct. Res.* **13**, 469.
Behnke, O. (1966). *Scand. J. Haematol.* **3**, 136.
Behnke, O. (1967). *Anat. Rec.* **158**, 121.
Behnke, O. (1968a). *J. Ultrastruct. Res.* **24**, 51.
Behnke, O. (1968b). *J. Ultrastruct. Res.* **24**, 412.
Behnke, O. (1969). *J. Ultrastruct. Res.* **26**, 111.
Behnke, O., and Zelander, T. (1966). *Exp. Cell Res.* **43**, 236.
Behnke, O., and Zelander, T. (1967). *J. Ultrastruct. Res.* **19**, 147.
Bensch, K. G., and Malawista, S. E. (1969). *J. Cell Biol.* **40**, 95.
Bernard, J., and Soulier, J. P. (1948). *Sem. Hop.* **24**, 217.
Bernhard, W., and Leplus, R. (1955). *Schweiz. Med. Wochenschr.* **85**, 897.
Bessis, M., and Breton-Gorius, J. (1965). *Nouv. Rev. Fr. Hematol.* **5**, 657.
Bizzozero, G. (1882). *Virchows Arch. Pathol. Anat. Physiol.* **90**, 261.
Bloom, G. (1954). *Z. Zellforsch. Mikrosk. Anat.* **40**, 222.
Booyse, F. M., and Rafelson, M. E. (1968). *Biochim. Biophys. Acta* **166**, 689.
Booyse, F. M., and Rafelson, M. E. (1969). *In* "Dynamics of Thrombus Formation and Dissolution" (S. A. Johnson and M. M. Guest, eds.), pp. 149–171. Lippincott, Philadelphia, Pennsylvania.
Born, G. V. R., Ingram, G. I. C., and Stacey, R. S. (1958). *Brit. J. Pharmacol. Chemother.* **13**, 62.

Born, G. V. R., Haslam, J., Goldman, M., and Lowe, R. D. (1965). *Nature (London)* **205**, 678.

Braunsteiner, H. (1961). *In* "Blood Platelets" (S. A. Johnson *et al.*, eds.), pp. 617–628. Little, Brown, Boston, Massachusetts.

Brinkhous, K. M., ed. (1967). "Platelets: Their Role in Hemostasis and Thrombosis." Schattaner, Stuttgart.

Buckingham, S., and Maynert, E. W. (1964). *J. Pharmacol. Exp. Ther.* **143**, 332.

Bull, B. J. (1966). *Blood* **28**, 901.

Bull, B. J., and Zucker, M. B. (1965). *Proc. Soc. Exp. Biol. Med.* **120**, 296.

Burstein, M., and Bessis, M. (1948). *Rev. Hematol.* **3**, 69.

Caen, J. P., Castaldi, P. A., Leclerc, J. C., Inceman, S., Larrieu, M. J., Probst, M., and Bernard, J. (1966). *Amer. J. Med.* **41**, 4.

Da Prada, M., Pletcher, A., Tranzer, J. P., and Knuchel, H. (1967). *Nature (London)* **216**, 1315.

David-Ferreira, J. F. (1964). *Int. Rev. Cytol.* **17**, 99.

Davis, R. B., and White, J. G. (1968). *Brit. J. Haematol.* **15**, 93.

Day, H. J., Holmsen, H., and Hovig, T. (1969). *Scand. J. Haematol.* Suppl. 7, 1–35.

De Robertis, E., Paysero, P., and Reissig, M. (1953). *Blood* **8**, 587.

Donne, A. (1842). *C. R. Acad. Sci.* **14**, 366.

Eberth, J. C., and Schimmelbusch, C. (1886). *Virchows Arch. Pathol. Anat. Physiol.* **103**, 39.

Etcheverry, G. J., and Zieher, L. M. (1968). *J. Histochem. Cytochem.* **16**, 162.

Grette, K. (1962). *Acta Physiol. Scand.* **56**, Suppl. 195, 1–93.

Grette, K. (1963). *Nature (London)*, **198**, 488.

Grottum, K. A., Hovig, T., Holmsen, H., Abrahamsen, A. F., Jeremic, M., and Seip, M. (1969). *Brit. J. Haematol.* **17**, 373.

Hagen, E., Wechsler, W., and Zilliken, F. (1968). *Exp. Biol. Med.* **3**, 1–240.

Hardisty, R. M., and Hutton, R. A. (1966). *Brit. J. Haematol.* **12**, 764.

Haydon, G. B., and Taylor, A. D. (1965). *J. Cell Biol.* **26**, 673.

Hayem, G. (1878). *C. R. Acad. Sci.* **95**, 18.

Hellem, A. J. (1968). *Ser. Haematol.* **1**, 99–145.

Holmsen, H., Day, H. J., and Stormorken, H. (1969). *Scand. J. Haematol.* Suppl. 8, 1–26.

Horowitz, H. I., and Papayoanou, M. F. (1968). *Thromb. Diath. Haemmorrh.* **19**, 18.

Hovig, T. (1962). *Thromb. Diath. Haemorrh.* **8**, 455.

Hovig, T. (1968). *In* "Blood Platelets" (K. G. Jensen and S. A. Killmann, eds.), pp. 1–64. Williams & Wilkins, Baltimore, Maryland.

Itano, H. A. (1953). *Arch. Biochem.* **47**, 148.

Jean, G., Racine, L., Gautier, A., and Marx, R. (1963). *Thromb. Diath. Haemorrh.* **10**, 42.

Jensen, K. G., and Killmann, S. A., eds. (1968). "Blood Platelets." Williams & Wilkins, Baltimore, Maryland.

Johnson, S. A., and Seegers, W. H., eds. (1967). "The Physiology of Hemostasis and Thrombosis." Thomas, Springfield, Illinois.

Jones, T. V. (1851). *Guy's Hosp. Rep.* [2] **7**, 1–100.

Karpatkin, S. (1967). *J. Clin. Invest.* **46**, 409.

Karpatkin, S. (1969). *J. Clin. Invest.* **48**, 1073.

Kerby, G. P., and Taylor, S. M. (1961). *J. Clin. Invest.* **40**, 44.

Kowalski, E., and Niewiarowski, S., eds. (1967). "Biochemistry of Blood Platelets." Academic Press, New York.

le Sourd, L., and Pagniez, P. (1906). *C. R. Acad. Sci.* **142**, 1562.

Lüscher, E. F. (1967). *Brit. J. Haematol.* **13**, 1.

Lüscher, E. F., and Bettex-Galland, M. (1968). *In* "Metabolism and Membrane Permeability of Erythrocytes and Thrombocytes" (E. Deutsch, E. Gerlach, and K. Moser, eds.), pp. 247–253. Thieme, Stuttgart.

Marcus, A. J. (1969). *N. Engl. J. Med.* **280**, 1213, 1278, and 1330.

Marcus, A. J., and Zucker, M. B. (1965). "The Physiology of Blood Platelets." Grune & Stratton, New York.

Marcus, A. J., Zucker-Franklin, D., Safier, L. B., and Ullman, H. (1966). *J. Clin. Invest.* **45**, 14.

Michal, F., and Firkin, B. G. (1969). *Annu. Rev. Pharmacol.* **9**, 95.

Nagai, T., Makinose, M., and Hasselbach, W. (1960). *Biochim. Biophys. Acta* **43**, 223.

Nakao, K., and Angrist, A. A. (1968). *Nature (London)* **217**, 960.

Ohnashi, T., and Ebashi, S. (1963). *J. Biochem. (Tokyo)* **54**, 506.

Osler, W. (1874). *Proc. Roy. Soc., London* **22**, 391.

Paulus, J. M. (1967). *Blood* **29**, 407.

Philpott, C. W., and Goldstein (1967). *Science* **155**, 1019.

Porter, K. R. (1961). *J. Biochem. Biophys. Acta* **39**, 93.

Puszkin, E., and Aledort, L. M. (1969). *Abst. 4th Conf. Blood Platelets, 1969*, Oak Ridge, Tennessee, p. 12.

Quick, A. J. (1966). "Hemorrhagic Diseases and Thrombosis." Lea & Febiger, Philadelphia, Pennsylvania.

Rambourg, A., and Leblond, C. P. (1967). *J. Cell Biol.* **32**, 27.

Robb-Smith, A. H. T. (1967). *Brit. J. Haematol.* **13**, 618.

Rodman, N. F. (1967). *In* "Platelets: Their Role in Hemostasis and Thrombosis" (K. M. Brinkhous, ed.), p. 9. Schattaner, Stuttgart.

Rodman, N. F., Mason, R. G., McDevitt, N. B., and Brinkhous, K. M. (1962). *Amer. J. Pathol.* **40**, 271.

Roskam, J. (1923). *Arch. Int. Physiol.* **20**, 241.

Ruska, C., and Schulz, H. (1968). *Klin. Wochenschr.* **46**, 689.

Sandborn, E. B., Le Buis, J., and Bois, P. (1966). *Blood* **27**, 247.

Schulz, H. (1968). "Thrombocyten und Thrombose im elektronenmikroskopischen Bild." Springer, Berlin.

Schulz, H., Jurgens, R., and Heipler, E. (1958). *Thromb. Diath. Haemorrh.* **2**, 300.

Sharp, A. A. (1961). *In* "Blood Platelets" (S. A. Johnson *et al.*, eds.), pp. 67–88. Little, Brown, Boston, Massachusetts.

Siegel, A., and Lüscher, E. F. (1967). *Nature (London)* **215**, 745.

Silver, M. D. (1965). *Z. Zellforsch. Mikrosk. Anat.* **68**, 474.

Sixma, J. J., and Molenaar, I. (1966). *Thromb. Diath. Haemorrh.* **16**, 153.

Solatunturi, E., and Passonen, M. K. (1966). *Ann. Med. Exp. Biol. Fenn.* Suppl. 14, 427.

Spaet, T. H., and Zucker, M. B. (1964). *Amer. J. Physiol.* **206**, 1267.

Spicer, S. S., Greene, W. B., and Hardin, J. H. (1969). *J. Histochem. Cytochem.* **17**, 781.

Statland, B. E., Heagan, B. M., and White, J. G. (1969). *Nature (London)* **223**, 521.

Stehbens, W. E., and Biscoe, T. J. (1967). *Amer. J. Pathol.* **50**, 210.

Stormorken, H. (1969). *Scand. J. Haematol.* **6**, Suppl. 9, 1–24.

Tocantins, L. M. (1948). *Blood* **3**, 1073.

Tranzer, J. P., Da Prada, M., and Pletcher, A. (1966). *Nature (London)* **212**, 1574.

Vegge, T., Monn, E., and Hjort, P. F. (1968). *Thromb. Diath. Haemorrh.* **20**, 354.

Wallach, D. F. H., Surgenor, D. M., and Steele, B. B. (1958). *Blood* **13**, 589.

Warshaw, A. L., Laster, L., and Shulman, N. R. (1967). *J. Biol. Chem.* **242**, 2094.

Wassmuth, D. R., Hamilton, H. E., and Sheets, R. F. (1963). *J. Amer. Med. Ass.* **183**, 737.

Weber, A. (1966). *Curr. Top. Bioenerg.* **1**, 203.

Weber, E., Morgenstern, E., and Walter, E. (1968). *In* "Metabolism and Membrane, Permeability of Erythrocytes and Thrombocytes" (E. Deutsch, E. Gerlach, and K. Moser, eds.), pp. 259–265. Thieme, Stuttgart.

Weiss, L., and Mayhew, E. (1967). *N. Engl. J. Med.* **276**, 1354.

White, J. G. (1967a). *In* "Physiology of Hemastasis and Thrombosis" (S. A. Johnson and W. H. Seegers, eds.), p. 248. Thomas, Springfield, Illinois.

White, J. G. (1967b). *Blood* **30**, 539.

White, J. G. (1968a). *Scand. J. Haematol.* **4**, 371.

White, J. G. (1968b). *Amer. J. Pathol.* **53**, 791.

White, J. G. (1968c). *Scand. J. Haematol.* **5**, 241.

White, J. G. (1968d). *Blood* **31**, 604.

White, J. G. (1968e). *Amer. J. Phatol.* **53**, 281.

White, J. G. (1968f). *Amer. J. Pathol.* **53**, 791.

White, J. G. (1968g). *J. Cell Biol.* **39**, 141A.

White, J. G. (1968h). *Blood* **32**, 638.

White, J. G. (1968i). *Amer. J. Pathol.* **53**, 447.

White, J. G. (1968j). *Blood* **32**, 324.

White, J. G. (1968k). *Abstr., 12th Int. Congr. Int. Soc. Hematol.* 1968, New York, p. 196.

White, J. G. (1968l). *Blood* **32**, 148.

White, J. G. (1968m). *Amer. J. Pathol.* **53**, 567.

White, J. G. (1969a). *Amer. J. Pathol.* **56**, 267.

White, J. G. (1969b). *Amer. J. Pathol.* **54**, 467.

White, J. G. (1969c). *Blood* **33**, 598.

White, J. G. (1969d). *Scand. J. Haematol.* **6**, 236.

White, J. G. (1970a). *In* "The Platelet" (F. K. Mostofii ed.). Williams & Wilkins, Baltimore, Maryland (in press).

White, J. G. (1970b). *In* "Principles of Hematology." McGraw-Hill, Baltimore, Maryland (in press).

White, J. G. (1970c). *In* "Proceedings of the Eighteenth Wayne State Symposium on Blood" (in press).

White, J. G. (1970d). *Amer. J. Pathol.* **58**, 31.

White, J. G. (1970e). *Fed. Proc., Fed. Amer. Suc. Exp. Biol.* **29**, 623.

White, J. G. (1970f). *Scand. J. Haematol.* **7**, 145.

White, J. G., and Davis, R. B. (1969). *Amer. J. Pathol.* **56**, 519.

White, J. G., and Krivit, W. (1965). *Blood* **26**, 554.

White, J. G., and Krivit, W. (1966). *Blood* **27**, 167.

White, J. G., and Krivit, W. (1967a). *Blood* **30**, 625.

White, J. G., and Krivit, W. (1967b). *J. Lab. Clin. Med.* **49**, 60.

White, J. G., and Krivit, W. (1967c). *In* "Platelets: Their Role in Hemostasis and Thrombosis" (K. M. Brinkhous, ed.), p. 29. Schattaner, Stuttgart.

White, J. G., Krivit, W., and Vernier, R. L. (1965). *Blood* **25**, 241.

Wolpers, C., and Ruska, H. (1939). *Klin. Wochenschr.* **18**, 1077.

Wood, J. G. (1965). *Tex. Rep. Biol. Med.* **23**, 828.

Wright, J. H., and Minot, G. R. (1917). *J. Exp. Med.* **26**, 395.

Wurzel, M., Marcus, A. J., and Zweifach, B. W. (1965). *Proc. Soc. Exp. Biol. Med.* **118**, 468.

Zucker, M. B., and Borrelli, J. (1954). *Blood* **9**, 602.

Zucker-Franklin, D. (1968). *J. Clin. Invest.* **47**, 106A.

Zucker-Franklin, D. (1969). *J. Clin. Invest.* **48**, 165.

Zucker-Franklin, D., Nachman, R., and Marcus, A. J. (1967). *Science* **157**, 945.

4

ENERGY METABOLISM

RUDOLF GROSS and WOLFGANG SCHNEIDER

I. INTRODUCTION

Biological Importance of Biochemical Investigations of Blood Cells

Considering the multiplicity of the individual cellular features, detailed investigations of entirely different cells in lower and higher organisms have yielded an amazing degree of conformance in the morphological structure of the respective cell organelles. But it has also been shown, that these cellular constituents, after separation by appropriate measures, equally show an analogous chemicometabolic organization. The *conformity of the structural elements* in terms of molecular biology actually is so pronounced that it allows discussion of defined metabolic phases without having to refer right away to one specific cell. Cellular metabolism thus is based on an overall organizational plan (Pette, 1965) that is based on the similarity of morphological and functional structures of the living cell and displays only a very limited number of variants. This conformity in the morphologicometabolic cellular structure makes it possible to study specific intracellular reaction mechanisms, e.g., in easily accessible cells and to transfer the results to corresponding metabolic processes which take place in other cells. Individual cells, such as microorganisms, ascites tumor cells, or blood cells, lend themselves particularly well to this purpose, since there is no need to break down cellular assemblies. But in addition, the cell systems occurring in the blood offer yet another outstanding advantage: Due to their loss of certain cell organelles they are *increasingly simplified metabolic systems* which range from leukocytes via platelets and reticulocytes to erythrocytes. They thus provide clear and distinct conditions for investigating the remaining metabolic regulations as mutual coordination in the metabolism of the cell organelles also proceeds along identical principles which maintain the constancy of the chemical composition of the entire cell per se, while still ensuring the sequence of varying catabolic and biosynthetic reactions enabling cellular function (for a review, refer to Krause, 1969).

In the case of blood cells it is thus possible to assess the significance of certain metabolic pathways by comparing the retained functional possibilities of a cell system having lost specific cell organelles with another cell system where they are still present. Due to the absence of numerous regulatory mechanisms in *erythrocytes*, these lend themselves exceedingly well to an investigation of metabolic control of glycolysis. In this respect *thrombocytes* and *leukocytes* also show principal agreement. However, they differ from erythrocytes by their mitochondrial content, and thus by additional capacities for synthesis, e.g., protein synthesis, fat metabolism, and gluconeogenesis. In view of these capacities for synthesis, however, the energy metabolism which renders them possible acquires increased significance. By way of its energy demands and by maintaining compartmentized ionic and metabolic gradients the mitochondrial metabolism thus regulates metabolic functions not only within its own domain, but becomes effective beyond this within the entire cell (Lehninger, 1964; Chance, 1965; Rasmussen, 1966). In view of these relationships, it is not surprising that the thrombocyte metabolism bears much more resemblance to leukocyte metabolism than to erythrocyte metabolism (Seitz, 1965).

While leukocytes, by the presence of a nucleus and genetic and epigenetic regulatory mechanisms thus rendered possible, prove to be of particular interest in connection with lymphocytes, increasing importance has attached in recent years to thrombocytes, quite particularly in view of the fact that despite the loss of a nucleus they still contain mitochondria. By this singular quality which is rather uncommon in nature—disregarding a transient stage of erythrocyte maturation—thrombocytes can be regarded as the examples par excellence of a metabolic coordinating system between different cellular compartments which are *separated by membranes*. Since lack of a nucleus and of epigenetic regulatory mechanisms, which are possible in nucleated cells, is associated with the nearly complete absence of the protein synthesis which makes particularly stringent demands on the energy metabolism, thrombocytes offer highly distinct conditions for investigating such regulatory mechanisms. It thus appears that the unknown mechanism which retains the functional capacity of thrombocytes has to be sought in the maintenance and coordination of *metabolic compartmentation*. On the other hand, their physiological function within the hemostatic mechanism, i.e., adhesion, aggregation, and subsequent destruction with a concurrent release of factors involved in the blood clotting mechanisms—but quite particularly the slow release of chemically bound energy for retraction and the well organized sequence of such platelet functions essential for effective hemostasis—seems to be caused by a stepwise breakdown of metabolic compartmentation. The chronological sequence in the failing function of defined metabolic segments is in turn conditioned by the sensitivity of the subunits of the cell organelles to the metabolic alterations occurring during hemostasis and their concomitants. Apart from intravital functions, as for instance the possible maintenance of vascular integrity, thrombocytes thus are biologically predetermined for destruction which proceeds in the form of an *organized breakdown of their metabolic compartments*.

The above aspects on the regulation of cellular function are novel in our knowledge of thrombocytes and will be in the foreground of the present review of experimental findings available on platelet metabolism.

II. ENERGY METABOLISM OF THROMBOCYTES

Due to the presence of additional intracellular membranes, the thrombocyte, in contrast to mature erythrocytes, shows several *metabolic compartments with independent regulatory mechanisms* and accordingly varying electrolyte and metabolite gradients. For the energy metabolism of the platelets the cytoplasmic and the mitochondrial compartments are of particular significance; it is assumed that, as the hemostatic mechanism proceeds, additional cellular compartments might become effective involving, for instance, the liberation reaction (Grette, 1962; Mills *et al.*,

1968), or the lysosomal compartment which is concerned with the observed degradation processes (Kowalski *et al.*, 1967). Despite certain autonomic functions, the cytoplasmic and the mitochondrial metabolic compartments are subject to *interaction and mutual coordination* in that, because of the pure carbohydrate metabolism in platelets (Waller *et al.*, 1959), glycolysis within the cytoplasmic compartment provides the carbon chains for the oxidative energy production and as substrates for mitochondrial or mito-chondrial-cytoplasmic (glycogen) syntheses. The glycolytic flow rate is in turn controlled in most instances by allosteric reaction mechanisms which on their part are initiated by phosphorylation products of the oxidative energy metabolism (for a review, refer to Krause, 1969). In the present contribution the cytoplasmic and the mitochondrial metabolic pathways are reviewed separately for the sake of clarity and to bring out charac-teristic features of the individual regulatory mechanisms. However, such presentation will of necessity entail certain overlappings and repetitions which cannot be completely avoided.

A. Cytoplasmic Functions

1. GLYCOLYSIS

Anaerobic glycolysis is the principal metabolic pathway in erythrocytes. Generation of ATP by substrates phosphorylation apparently is sufficient to maintain concentration gradients at the erythrocyte membrane, and thus a certain energy potential (Cooley and Cohen, 1967a). Further stabilization of the membrane during the transition from the reticulocyte to the mature erythrocyte stage is an alleviating factor (Rapoport, 1968a). Since the erythrocyte accordingly shows a particularly simple energy metabolism in which the pentose–phosphate shunt is of only minor significance and where glycogen formation and glyconeogenesis are even virtually absent, erythrocytes are of particular advantage for the study of regulatory functions involved in glycolysis (for reviews, see Rapoport, 1968b; Deutsch *et al.*, 1968).

By contrast, the metabolic system in thrombocytes is appreciably more complicated. It is certain that this is due in part to the pronounced reactivity of the platelet membrane (a review has been presented by Born, 1968) which governs all further platelet functions. But the metabolic system is primarily dependent on the presence of mitochondria which is essential for a series of syntheses, such as glyconeogenesis (Schneider and Schumacher, 1969) or lipid synthesis (Majerus *et al.*, 1969), functions which are not being mastered by the erythrocyte. Since these syntheses originate from either pyruvate or its derivative, acetyl-CoA, it is not surprising that a pronounced glycolytic metabolism may also be demonstrated in thrombocytes (Waller et al., 1959; Bettex-Galland and Lüscher, 1960; Chernyak, 1965; Karpatkin and Siskind, 1967; Karpatkin and Langer, 1968). According to Karpatkin and Langer (1968), the *glycolytic flow rate* demonstrable in thrombocytes is considered to be 13 times that of human erythrocytes, and 4.7 times that of skeletal muscle (Keitt, 1966; Beatty et al., 1966). From a comparison with erythrocytes, it seems probable that this active glycolytic metabolism is decisively influenced by the requirements of synthesis. For a considerable period of time there was frequent speculation whether this metabolic system might be causally correlated with the high ATP content in thrombocytes by way of substrate phosphorylation. The relatively low platelet respiration seemed to be in support of this theory; it was found by Waller et al. (1959) that only 20% of the glucose consumed is metabolized to CO_2 and water. However, when considering the lower effectivity of the glycolytic energy yield, which is not more than 2 moles of ATP per mole glucose consumed against 38–2 moles of ATP obtained on oxidative degradation of 2 moles of pyruvate supplied by glycolysis, it will be found that with a relative involvement of 20% of the oxidative metabolism in glucose degradation $0.2 \times 36 = 7.2$ moles of ATP will be formed by oxidation, compared with $1.0 \times 2 = 2$ moles of ATP formed during glycolysis. These figures show that in spite of the relative minor participation of the oxidative glucose degradation in the thrombocytes the oxidative phosphorylation (theoretically) accounts for as much as 78% of the entire ATP yield, and they are an effective reflection of the significance of the oxidative metabolism in thrombocytes.

The high *enzyme activities of the glycolytic metabolism* (Waller et al., 1959; Löhr et al., 1961a,b; Dastague et al., 1966; Gross, 1967; Gross et al., 1967; Goebell et al., 1968; Ohler, 1968) which correspond to the high glycolytic flow rate additionally seemed to emphasize the significance of glycolysis for the energy metabolism in the thrombocytes. It should, however, be considered in this context that these values that had been determined *in vitro* under optimal substrate conditions actually represent *enzyme capacities* (Rapoport, 1968b) which give no indication per se of the *flow rates* actually obtaining *in vivo*, because in a state of metabolic equilibrium all steps of the reaction have the same throughout, i.e., the same number of molecules will be converted. Allowing for the enzyme capacity, hexokinase actually would appear to be the limiting enzyme in the glycolytic flow rate of the thrombocytes (Grignani and Löhr, 1960). However, in many instances the available enzyme capacities are utilized only in part *in vivo*, all those enzymes determining the metabolic rate which are far from the thermodynamic equilibrium conditioned by the law of mass action. As *"controlled" enzymes* they are governed by the substrate supply and product inhibition, and in particular by allosteric reaction mechanisms (for a review, refer to Krause, 1969). Due to the distinct and clear experimental conditions available, particular attention has been given to the study of metabolic regulations in red blood cells (Rapoport, 1968b), but these relations may also be demonstrated in a similar fashion in other cells, because of the concordance in the metabolic systems (for a review, refer to Caputto *et al.*, 1967). It has thus been seen that controlled enzymes, in addition to hexokinase (Grignani and Löhr, 1960), mainly involve phosphofructokinase, pyruvate kinase, and lactate dehydrogenase (Rapoport, 1968b). On the other hand, "uncontrolled" enzymes are only dependent on the substrate supply. This will explain why the activity of an enzyme determined *in vitro* under optimal reaction conditions does not necessarily furnish an indication of the conversion rate taking place *in vivo*. It should be remembered here that in the platelet metabolism pyruvate kinase and lactate dehydrogenase are the enzymes having the highest capacities (Waller *et al.*, 1959).

Lactate dehydrogenase, which is present in the thrombocyte with a high capacity, has great metabolic significance. This is due, on the one hand, to its ability of recovering the NAD reduced during glycolysis by reduction of pyruvate. On the other hand, the LDH isoenzyme pattern of a cell seems to permit some insight into the type of metabolism present (for a review, see Markert, 1968).

The formation of the isoenzymes of the lactate dehydrogenase is due to the fact that two genetically determined polypeptide chains with varying structures combine to form tetramers in the enzymically active molecule. The resultant combination possibilities determine the structure of the five isoenzymes. Combination of the subunits takes place in different organs at a varying proportion of the two components and results in the formation of regular organ patterns. Preponderance of the anionic isoenzymes LDH-1 and LDH-2 in the heart muscle, brain, and kidney and of the cationic isoenzymes LDH-4 and LDH-5 in skeletal muscle and liver seemed to suggest a certain correlation between the type of metabolism in the cell and the distribution pattern of the LDH-isoenzymes. It was assumed that isoenzymes LDH-1 and 2 predominate in cells with a primarily aerobic metabolism, while isoenzymes 4 and 5 are prevailing in cells showing a mainly glycolytic metabolic pathway. Studies on enzyme kinetics seemed to support this theory; they revealed that the anionic isoenzymes show more pronounced substrate inhibition by pyruvate than do the cationic isoenzymes. This would mean, however, that in case of a high pyruvate yield and predominance of anionic isoenzymes due to the substrate inhibition obtaining the reduction to lactate is blocked and that the metabolic functions are thus channeled toward terminal oxidation via an increased decarboxylation of pyruvate. The particularly high proportion of isoenzymes 1 and 2 in cells undergoing oxidative metabolism would be compatible with this view (G. Pfleiderer and Wachsmuth, 1961; Kaplan and Ciotti, 1961; Cahn et al., 1962; Dawson et al., 1964; Lindy and Rajasalmi, 1966). Human erythrocytes and thrombocytes, which in the past had been considered to undergo a primarily glycolytic energy metabolism—notwithstanding the prevalent anionic LDH-isoenzyme pattern—did not seem to fit into this scheme. For this reason it was argued by Vesell (1965b) that the LDH-isoenzyme pattern observed in human platelets furnishes ample proof of a metabolic dependence. He also demonstrated (Vesell and Pool, 1966) that the varying kinetic properties of the isoenzymes are temperature-dependent and that the substrate concentrations which exert an inhibitory action in vitro are not attained in vivo.

Using exchange chromatography and polyacrylamide disk electrophoresis we found a pronounced proportion of bands 2 and 3 in human platelets, whereas LDH-1 was demonstrable only to a minor degree, and LDH-4 and LDH-5 were present in traces, if any (Schneider et al., 1968a; Schumacher et al., 1968). Similar patterns with slight variations, which were probably due to the method used, have been described by Bezkorovainy and Rafelson (1964), Vesell (1965b), Cohen and Larson (1966), and Hule (1966). Differences in enzyme kinetics could also be demonstrated for the LDH-isoenzymes in human platelets at 37°C. It was of particular interest to note that high substrate concentrations inhibited lactate oxidation, this inhibition increasing rapidly from LDH-1 to LDH-3. Similar differences were not found to exist in the behavior of the LDH-isoenzymes from human thrombocytes to high pyruvate concentrations (Schneider et al., 1968a). It is still uncertain at this time whether the varying inhibitory behavior may be responsible, at least in part, for the unusually high lactate–pyruvate ratio, which is demonstrable in thrombocytes following incubation and which may be as high as 20 (Waller et al., 1959). Respective investigations have shown that a correlation between the LDH-isoenzyme pattern and the cellular metabolism can be assumed on reliable grounds; it is considered, however, that such dependence would probably not take the previously proposed simplified form, but rather become effective via the redox potential of the cell and its compartments (Schneider et al., 1968a).

The multiple influences exerted on enzyme activities by low molecular substances and metabolites, respectively, will serve to illustrate that metabolic studies on thrombocytes are being affected appreciably by the *conditions of incubation.* These in turn are influenced by the fact that a constant hydrogen ion concentration is dependent on the use of a buffer since otherwise there might be a very pronounced fall in pH (E. C. Rossi, 1967b). It was seen, however, that utilization of a certain buffer following resuspension of isolated thrombocytes may severely impair the metabolic situation. Using resuspended rat platelets in an imidazole containing buffer system, it was thus found by E. C. Rossi (1967b, 1968) that glucose consumpiton and lactate formation had increased. In view of the simultaneous fall in ATP to 38%, stimulation of the membrane ATPase was considered to be the cause.

It was seen at the same time that the fall in ATP could not be compensated by glycolysis although its flow rate had increased. An entirely identical metabolic behavior was found to occur under the influence of substances that block the oxidative metabolism (Schneider, 1969). We therefore studied in addition the respiration in a tris buffer containing synthetic medium of resuspended human platelets to which had been added increasing imidazole concentrations and could actually demonstrate a fall in respiration which was strictly proportional in concentration to the imidazole concentration (Schneider, 1970). It thus appears probable that respiration is primarily influenced by the action of imidazole, while the alterations which were assumed to take place on the membrane (E. C. Rossi, 1967b, 1968) are influenced secondarily, if at all, by imidazole.

In contrast to erythrocytes, metabolic platelet investigations invariably require the presence of a substance binding divalent cations in order to prevent the formation of spontaneous aggregates as these, on their part, would also initiate significant regulatory mechanisms and metabolic alterations (Gross and Schneider, 1968; Karpatkin and Langer, 1968). It has thus been found that the number of platelets decreases more rapidly in *citrated platelet-rich* plasma than in EDTA-containing plasma (E. C. Rossi, 1967a). These differences are thought to be due to the spontaneous aggregation tendency observed in citrated blood. In addition, citrate involves the disadvantage that it may inhibit certain metabolic segments, primarily the phosphofructokinase reaction; its inhibition by citrate has been evidenced by Garland *et al.* (1964) for the heart muscle, by Passonneau and Lowry (1963) for the brain and liver, and by Parmeggiani and Bowman (1963) for skeletal muscle. It was considered that experiments involving blocking of the citrate cycle by means of fluoroacetate might yield some information of a similar inhibition occurring in human platelets. This gives rise to the formation of fluorocitrate which evidently also inhibits the phosphofructo-kinase in the thrombocytes, as has been evidenced by the distinct rise in fructose-6-phosphate (Gross and Schneider, 1968). On the other hand, citrate can apparently be metabolized as a substrate in the citrate cycle and may therefore reduce the formation of lactate due to stimulation of the oxidative metabolism via increased decarboxylation of pyruvate (Kar-patkin, 1967). While no $^{14}CO_2$ formation was found to occur when using ^{14}C-labeled citrate (E. C. Rossi, 1967a), this finding could be due to the apparently active gluconeogenesis in the thrombocytes which is associ-ated with the carboxylation of pyruvate and the increased radioactivi-ty of labeled substrates in the glycogen (Seitz, 1965; Warshaw et al., 1966).

Use of *EDTA* as a chelating agent for the divalent cations which are present in the plasma and cause disintegration of the platelets, equally involves considerable drawbacks. It has thus been seen that addition of EDTA produces certain morphological alterations as manifested by loss of discoid shape (Zucker and Borelli, 1954), alterations in ultrastructure (Skjørten, 1968; White, 1968a), increase in platelet volume (Bull and Zucker, 1965), as well as impaired function (Zucker and Borelli, 1958; Ozge et al., 1964) and diminished platelet yield on reinfusion (Aster and Jandl, 1964). Similar influences on the metabolic situation have also been demonstrated in other cells (for more recent findings, refer to Settlemire et al., 1968). It is therefore not surprising that the cellular platelet meta-bolism is also adversely affected, such impairment including a rise in glucose consumption and lactate formation (E. C. Rossi, 1967a) which is thought to be due to a blocking of the oxidative metabolism by increasing Ca and Mg withdrawal. Platelets obtained from a donor at one and the same time from blood containing varying EDTA concentrations (0.1–0.5%) and resuspended immediately in the same synthetic medium show a slight fall of the glycolytic flow rate which is proportionate in concentration to the EDTA fraction added to the blood. This is accompanied by a much more distinct fall in respiration (Schneider, 1969).

EDTA, on the other hand, significantly depresses the spontaneous ag-gregation tendency of the platelets. When measuring the oxygen consump-tion in thrombocytes which had been resuspended in EDTA-containing media, the values obtained were particularly high (Bettex-Galland and Lüscher, 1960; Gross and Schneider, 1968; Kitchens and Newcomb, 1968). However, this effect might also be correlated with the action of EDTA on the membrane as shown by a depletion of divalent cations, a resultant increase in membrane permeability, and stimulation of the oxidative phosphorylation (Manery, 1968).

Experience has shown that platelets kept in citrate-containing medium at pH 6.2–6.4 remain capable of function for a longer period and that their rates and times of survival upon reinfusion are prolonged (Aster and Jandl, 1966). In platelets obtained from ACD plasma it is seen, however, that the oxygen consumption is increased (Campbell *et al.*, 1956) and that the oxidative metabolism maintains its proper function for a longer period (Engel, 1966) so that under these conditions considerable deviations in cellular metabolism also have to be reckoned with.

Contrary to citrate and EDTA, *heparin* does not essentially influence the divalent cations of the plasma. This might offer an explanation for the increased adhesiveness of human and rat platelets in heparinized plasma as compared with citrated plasma. This assumption receives further support by evidence that the aggregation tendency is lowered as the citrate content in plasma increases (Nordøy and Odegaard, 1963). The observation of O'Brien *et al.* (1969) that the adhesive behavior of thrombocytes in heparinized blood agrees with that of thrombocytes from native blood is also compatible with this view. By contrast, addition of citrate caused an inhibition of the adhesiveness. By the same token, the first phase of ADP- and adrenaline-induced aggregation was shown to be more pronounced in heparinized plasma than in citrated plasma, the extent of the reaction going parallel with the content of free calcium ions in the suspension medium. When adding collagen or adrenaline, the second phase of the aggregation reaction in heparinized plasma was seen to be less marked than in citrated plasma. It is concluded from these findings that heparin, while it does not inhibit the adhesion processes, still brakes the liberation reaction. In this connection it is of interest to note that heparin simultaneously suppresses the increase in lactate formation obtained by thrombin action on platelet-rich citrated or EDTA plasma. With respect to this mechanism it might be significant that all aggregation processes involve a release of platelet factor 4 which evidently possesses the properties of a cationic polypeptide and is neutralized by heparin (Niewiarowski *et al.*, 1968).

The above indications clearly reflect the difficulty arising in metabolic studies on thrombocytes to provide experimental conditions which are in keeping with the physiological situation, and they will also help to explain why the metabolic events differ according to the method employed. This was also illustrated by the studies of Kim and Baldini (1968) who showed that in platelets prepared from citrated blood the substrate levels of the glycolytic metabolites are different from those obtained from EDTA-containing blood. Additional investigations of the *metabolite content of the glycolytic metabolic sequence* have been conducted in platelets by Campbell *et al.* (1957); more recent studies have been presented by Chernyak (1965) and Detwiler (1969). Using anaerobic conditions, Chernyak and Timofeyeva (1968) determined the dependence of the flow rate on the substrate and nucleotide content and on the NAD–NADH$_2$ ratio during the individual steps of glycolysis.

The *starting substrate of the glycolytic cycle* is glucose. It is assumed that due to a respiratory ratio of 1.0 the thrombocytes are subjected to a pure carbohydrate metabolism (Campbell *et al.*, 1956; Waller *et al.*, 1959; Seitz, 1965; Gross and Schneider, 1968). *Glucose uptake* essentially depends on the conditions of incubation and is higher in EDTA-containing than in citrated plasma (E. C. Rossi, 1967a). However, platelets obtained from EDTA-containing blood also show certain differences, depending on whether or not the spontaneous aggregation tendency of platelets resuspended in synthetic media is suppressed by addition of EDTA (Gross and Schneider, 1968). The values given for the *glucose consumption* therefore vary according to the conditions of incubation and have been reported to be 35–45 μmoles/ 10^{11} for platelets obtained from 0.1% human EDTA-containing blood following resuspension in an EDTA-containing medium (Gross and Schneider, 1968), and 75 μmoles/10^{11} platelets after resuspension in a bicarbonate–Ringer–glucose solution (Waller *et al.*, 1959). The reported values frequently are difficult to compare due to different reference values and use of hydrogen ion concentrations varying from the physiological range (Karpatkin and Siskind, 1967; Karpatkin and Langer, 1968). It is, however, the pH of the incubation medium (refer to p. 130) which, together with the selection of the buffer used for resuspension, is of particular importance (E. C. Rossi, 1968).

When using labeled substrates, it has been possible to demonstrate glucose and also degradation of *mannose* and *fructose* by human platelets. As the sole substrate they are metabolized at equal conversion rates. In the presence of equimolar glucose concentrations (5.5 mM) the conversion rate with mannose falls by one half and it regresses virtually completely with fructose (Warshaw *et al.*, 1966). If the mannose or fructose proportions are lower, the converted relative percentage is higher. With respect to retraction, glucose and mannose are shown to be equivalent, while fructose, D-galactose, D-ribose, saccharose, and lactose were ineffective (Corn *et al.*, 1960). From the densitometric studies of McDonagh *et al.* (1968) it was seen that pentoses enter human platelets by free diffusion, while hexoses are subject to a specific temperature-dependent diffusion mechanism. The *penetration rates* for hexoses show distinct differences; they are smallest for D-glucose, while L-sorbose and D-galactose are classed among the hexoses showing the most rapid permeation. According to Zieve and Solomon (1967, 1968), glycerol and amino acids also may enter human platelets owing to an active transport mechanism.

A common feature in all studies of glycolytic metabolism is the pronounced *formation of lactate* in the thrombocyte which under the experimental conditions employed by Waller *et al.* (1959) amounts to 76 μmoles/10^{11} thrombocytes/hour and accounts for 50% and more of the glucose consumed. Similar results have been obtained by Karpatkin and Langer (1968). Loder *et al.* (1968) have stated that formation of lactate is a sensitive indicator of the glycolytic flow rate in thrombocytes. It is more sensitive and less subject to technical interference than is the glucose consumption. For the same reason Gross and Schneider (1968) and Schneider (1969) when conducting studies on thrombocytes have used lactate formation to serve as a measure of the glycolytic metabolism.

The glycolytic metabolic rate, however, is interdependent with the oxidative energy metabolism. This is confirmed by the presence of a *Pasteur effect* which is reflected by a fall in lactate formation when adding oxygen and which could also be demonstrated in thrombocytes (Wu *et al.*, 1964; Chernyak, 1965; Seitz, 1965). The Pasteur effect comprises a series of regulatory mechanisms that are released by inorganic phosphate. They produce stimulation of hexokinase and phosphofructokinase, relief of the product inhibition exercised by glucose-6-phosphate on hexokinase, relief of the ATP inhibition on phosphofructokinase, and stimulation of glyceraldehyde phosphate oxidation. These effects overlap with the competition between the glycolytic and the oxidative compartment for a substrate that may be phosphorylated in the form of ADP (Uyeda and Racker, 1965; for a review, see Caputto *et al.*, 1967). In human thrombocytes, the fall in glycolysis under aerobic incubation has been given with 33% (Seitz, 1965). This finding is equally suggestive of the occurrence of a significant oxidative energy metabolism in the thrombocytes because coupling between the oxidative phosphorylation and the Pasteur effect appears to represent a general biological law (Seitz, 1961).

Another metabolic correlation that is based on the same regulatory principles is given by the *Crabtree effect*. It entails that if glucose is present in the incubation medium, the oxygen consumption of suspended cells is lower than in a substrate-free medium. The Crabtree effect has also been detected in thrombocytes by various authors. In the course of polarographic oxygen measurements using 1 or 2% glucose in the incubation medium, Kitchens and Newcomb (1968) found a drop in respiration by more than 50%. Similar results which partly involved less significant differences have been reported by Luganova *et al.* (1958), Bettex-Galland and Lüscher (1960), Chernyak *et al.* (1960a, b), Chernyak (1965), and by Seitz (1965). By contrast, Campbell *et al.* (1956), as well as Gross and Schneider (1968), did not observe any fall in respiration following addition of glucose. To our belief, these differences might be caused by the respective incubation conditions: In the synthetic medium employed in our studies, the stimulation of the glycogen breakdown in the glucose-free mixture apparently is not appreciably greater than that observed in the presence of glucose; lactate and pyruvate formation in the substrate-free mixture accordingly are essentially lower than in the glucose-containing control (Gross and Schneider, 1968). Karpatkin and Langer (1968) also observed a considerably lower lactate formation in the glucose-free mixture. This, however, reduces the substrate supply to the oxidative metabolism so that the intimate coupling of systems, which seems to exist in the thrombocytes between glycolysis and oxidative metabolism a as result of the pure carbohydrate metabolism, prevents an increase in respiration. The existence of such a correlation in thrombocytes is also suggested by findings (Gross and Schneider, 1968) implying that specific blocking of glycolysis by 2-deoxy-glucose does not only produce reduced glycolysis, but is also followed by a simultaneous drop in oxygen consumption. Findings obtained from studies on other cells equally are in support of a possible significance of glucose metabolites in the formation of the Crabtree effect: In Ehrlich ascites tumor cells the action of glucose in the direction of a Crabtree effect is observed only after addition of lactate and pyruvate (Ibsen and Fox, 1965), and investigations on Novikoff ascitic hepatoma cells have shown that in such cells consumption of glucose metabolites and ATP during the course of the glycogen synthesis does not produce an inhibition in respiration due to glucose uptake (Nigam, 1966). It is assumed that the continuous sequence of the glycogen synthesis (Scott, 1967) might also play an important role in thrombocytes.

A *stimulation of the glycolytic flow rate*, as measured by the formation of lactate, may be demonstrated under the influence of various substances producing platelet aggregation. We have invariably observed a distinct increase in lactate formation both when initiating aggregation by means of magnesium ions and calcium ions in concentrations releasing only a reversibile aggregation, and when using basic polypeptides (protamine sulfate) and thrombin and calcium ions. Probably as a result of the concomitant increase in the substrate supply to the oxidative metabolism it was found simultaneously that the oxygen consumption in reversible aggregation reactions was increased slightly or distinctly, while under the action of thrombin, and thus in the presence of irreversible platelet aggregation induced by calcium ions, the respiration was always found to be lower than that of the corresponding controls within 1 hour after addition of the aggregating substances (Gross and Schneider, 1968). Since measurements were carried out by the manometric method, detection of a transient increase in the oxygen consumption as described by Hussain and Newcomb (1964) and by Mürer (1968) was not possible due to technical reasons. A fall in oxygen consumption in human platelets due to thrombin action had been reported previously by Bettex-Galland and Lüscher (1960) who carried out manometric measurements over a prolonged period. These authors, as well as Warshaw *et al.* (1966) and Karpatkin (1967), equally reported that an increase in glucose consumption and lactate formation with an attendant fall in ATP is produced in thrombocytes when initiating aggregation by means of thrombin. Karpatkin and Siskind (1967) observed an increase in the glycolytic flow rate, as measured by raised formation of lactate, to occur under the action of thrombin, adrenaline and aggregation-promoting antibodies in the absence of glucose as a substrate. Antibodies, however, only provoked a rise in glycolysis if there was aggregation; this increase was not detectable when the antibodies caused binding to the platelet surface. While in the presence of glucose the increase in the glyco-lytic metabolism was unchanged, by the action of thrombin and adrenaline, this was not true in the case of aggregating platelet antibodies, although glucose consumption continued to show a distinct rise. It is considered by the authors that this finding seems to suggest an activation of a glucose-consuming, nonglycolytic pathway by the aggregating antibodies in the presence of glucose. In analogy to our interpretation of the findings of Warshaw *et al.* (1966) it would appear that here, too, the substrate is being channeled into the direction of neoglucogenesis via an intensified pyruvate carboxylation and formation of oxaloacetate. This process might be par-ticularly conceivable under the action of agglutinative antibodies since in this case the mitochondrial compartment where pyruvate carboxylation has to proceed is not being impaired. Resulting from this, the formation of lactate in this compartment is particularly insignificant. Another situation prevails under thrombin and calcium ions action: Irreversible changes affecting especially the mitochondria will rapidly occur due to the active storage of Ca phosphate which provokes uncoupling of the oxidative phosphorylation. Gluconeogenesis from pyruvate is thus prevented and lactate will accumulate. By contrast, adrenaline action is assumed to stimulate glycogenolysis to such an extent that lactate formation will also be enhanced.

A similar, if fleeting, stimulation of lactate formation under the aggregating action of connective tissue, or collagen preparations, was found to exist by Loder *et al.* (1968) and by Puszkin and Jerushalmy (1968). The same phenomenon was also demonstrated in bovine platelet aggregation induced by simultaneous addition of ADP and fibrinogen (De Vreker and De Vreker, 1965). The authors observed that lactate formation in bovine platelets was not enhanced when adding only ADP, and similar results were obtained by Corn (1966) for human platelets. Loder *et al.* (1968) also could find no evidence of an increased lactate formation neither under ADP action nor when adding calcium ions in concentrations ranging from 0.2 to 2.0 mM. The difference in calcium ions action as compared with our findings (Gross and Schneider, 1968) might be explained by the varying EDTA concentration which was, according to the above authors, double that used in our experiments.

Disregarding ADP-induced platelet aggregation, it thus appears that the metabolic behavior is about identical for almost all aggregation forms involving a stimulation of glucose uptake and lactate formation with a demonstrable drop in the ATP and ADP values. Since at the same time the respiration is normal or even increased, this behavior cannot be caused by a Pasteur effect which might occur, for instance, after difficult oxygen diffusion as a result of aggregation. Viewed over a prolonged period, such a situation presumably would arise only in thrombin-induced platelet aggregation due to the ultimate processes of disintegration. On the other hand, the increased rate of glycolysis in reversible platelet aggregations probably has to be attributed to a sudden rise in the intracellular inorganic phosphate concentration produced by ATP dephosphorylation; with the aid of glycolytic regulatory mechanisms also involved in the Pasteur effect (see p. 134), this increased concentration then produces a stimulation of the metabolic functions. The observation that such increased glycolysis apparently does not occur in ADP-released platelet aggregation; since this would not involve, at least not in the beginning, a sudden intracellular rise in inorganic phosphate might be consistent with this explanation. In this context Holmsen (1965) has pointed out that an immediate fall in the intracellular ATP content is obtained also in ADP-released platelet aggregation, but that this is accompanied by the formation of a corresponding amount of ADP. The fact that the fall in ATP involves a fraction of high specific activity, which had been labeled by preceding incubation with ^{32}P, might suggest that this process takes place in the nucleotide compartment which is characterized by a high rate of phosphorylation while nucleotide liberation is slight or even absent. The compartment involved might be the mitochondrial compartment (Holmsen, 1967; Ireland, 1967).

The studies of Kerby and Taylor (1967) have shown that a *decrease in the glycolytic flow rate*, manifested by diminished formation of lactate, is obtained by incubating platelets with ATP. Simultaneous addition of magnesium ions tends to produce a further "braking" of the glycolytic cycle. These results are compatible with other findings which had revealed that addition of thiamine pyrophosphate (5–10 mmoles) to resuspended human platelets likewise causes decreased formation of lactate and an increase in glucose utilization, the latter reaction being accompanied, possibly in the direction of a Crabtree effect, by a fall in oxygen consumption and a simultaneous rise in ATP (Schneider and Niemeyer, 1968). An effect of pH of thiamine pyrophosphate was excluded since, according to the findings of Campbell *et al.* (1956) and Engel (1966), such an effect would rather have brought about an increase in oxygen consumption. These results might be indicative of a participation of energy-rich phosphates, probably interacting with divalent cations and proteins, in the reactions proceeding at the membrane. In view of their significance, these energy-rich phosphoproteins will be discussed in detail in one of the following chapters.

Inhibition of glycolysis can also be produced by various *inhibitors*. It should be considered in this respect that the excessive attention that has been given for a considerable period of time to the participation of glycolysis in the supply of energy to the thrombocytes is largely due to the vigorous action exercised by such inhibitors on platelet function and metabolism. It has thus been shown that "glycolytic" inhibitors, such as monoiodoacetate, severely depress the ATP content and the retractability of the platelets (Bettex-Galland and Lüscher, 1960; Löhr *et al.*, 1961; Mürer, 1968). With regard to monoiodoacetate it should, however, be remembered that this substance does not only block glycolysis via degradation of glyceraldehyde phosphate, but also reacts with other sulfhydryl groups. It is therefore not surprising that substances that block sulfhydryl groups exert a distinct influence on platelet structure and its metabolic functions (Koppel *et al.*, 1959). It has been shown by recent studies that they do not only inhibit glycolysis, but also affect membrane function (Salzman and Chambers, 1964; Born, 1968), oxidative phosphorylation (Haugaard *et al.*, 1969) and probably in association with these processes also influence intracellular potassium concentration (Buckingham and Maynert, 1964). In view of the complex metabolic effects of such inhibitors blocking sulfhydryl groups, it is not possible to draw any conclusions on their implication in specific metabolic pathways (Mürer, 1968).

Measured by the decrease in glucose consumption and by the formation of lactate and pyruvate more specific inhibitors of glycolysis, e.g., 2-deoxyglucose, cause a concentration-dependent blocking of glycolysis in the platelet metabolism (Gross and Schneider, 1968) which is paralleled by a distinct fall in oxygen consumption (Gross and Schneider, 1968), most probably due to a reduced substrate supply (pyruvate) to the oxidative metabolism. This decreased oxygen consumption is based on the pure carbohydrate metabolism of platelets having a respiratory quotient of 1.0 (Campbell et al., 1956; Waller et al., 1959; Seitz, 1965). The attendant fall in ATP observed during such glycolytic inhibition (Gross and Schneider, 1968) might thus be caused by a reduced substrate phosphorylation, but because of the essentially higher effectivity of the oxidative phosphorylation (see p. 127) it is much more likely to be attributable to the simultaneous fall in respiration (Schneider, 1969).

2. PENTOSE–PHOSPHATE SHUNT

Although the significance of the pentose–phosphate shunt has not been conclusively elucidated, there are various indications pointing to a *correlation with the fatty acid synthesis*. This relationship is ultimately limited by the cellular requirements of high-energy phosphates to be utilized for other functions (for a review, see Caputto et al., 1967). The involvement of the hexose–monophosphate cycle in glucose metabolism may thus be approximated with the glucose–carbon demands required for fatty acid synthesis. The observation that feeding in starved animals produces a sharp rise in glucose utilization with a concomitant increase of the flow rate in the Dickens-Horecker shunt, and that the amount of labeled glucose recovered in the fatty acids is 45%, fits in with the above concept (Katz et al., 1966). On the other hand, adrenaline which also increases glucose utilization, inhibits both the flow rate in the pentose–phosphate shunt and fatty acid synthesis.

Since, however, the $NADPH_2$ generated in the pentose–phosphate shunt is possibly insufficient for fatty acid synthesis (Flatt and Ball, 1964), it is proposed that a mitochondrial, energy (ATP)-dependent transhydrogenase (Lee and Ernster, 1966; Van Dam and Ter Welle, 1966) might facilitate utilization of the reduction equivalents of $NADH_2$. The availability of such a mechanism would simultaneously provide a satisfactory explanation for the energy-dependent control of the fatty acid synthesis.

According to information outlined by Majerus *et al.* (1969) thrombocytes are the only formed constituents in the blood capable of effecting a *de novo* synthesis of fatty acids. In this context the enzymic capacity for fatty acid synthesis in human platelets, calculated on the basis of protein, is of the same order of magnitude as that for human liver. This is in agreement with the observation that the enzyme activities of the pentose–phosphate shunt may also be detected in human platelets (Waller *et al.*, 1959; Gross, 1967; Goebell *et al.*, 1968; Ohler, 1968; Schneider, 1969). It appears that their genetic coupling with the corresponding enzymes in other blood cells, primarily in the erythrocytes which because of the frequency of genetic defects (particularly of G-6-PDH) are of particular interest in this connection, has been established in individual cases (Ramot *et al.*, 1959; Wurzel *et al.*, 1961; Waller *et al.*, 1966; Schulz and Dabels, 1968). By contrast, studies concerning hexokinase activity of platelets in Down's syndrome, where trisomy of the chromosome 21 with a 50% elevation of the erythrocyte enzyme activity had been observed, have found no higher activities (Doery *et al.*, 1968).

Formation of $^{14}CO_2$, which can be demonstrated distinctly when employing $1\text{-}^{14}C$-glucose as a substrate, also supports the view that glucose is converted in the pentose–phosphate shunt. In human platelets formation of $^{14}CO_2$ is proportionate to the substrate concentration employed. Under standardized conditions involving incubation for 140 minutes at 37°C, it was seen that 10^9 platelets formed 42.8 nmoles of $^{14}CO_2$ from $1\text{-}^{14}C$-glucose, the respective value for $6\text{-}^{14}C$-glucose being 14.0 nmoles (Warshaw *et al.*, 1966). These findings prove that the Embden-Meyerhof pathway and the Dickens-Horecker shunt in platelets are both capable of metabolizing glucose, but they also overemphasize the pentose–phosphate shunt. This is considered to be due to the fact that after decarboxylation the C-atom labeled in position 6 is presumably utilized for syntheses involving primarily glycogen, as gluconeogenesis proceeds. The findings of Warshaw *et al.* (1966) seem to be in support of this theory in that, according to these authors, $^{14}Co_2$ formation under the action of thrombin will occur only after a lag period of 30 minutes, while on the other hand it is exactly this phase which shows the most pronounced formation of lactate (Bettex-Galland and Lüscher, 1960; Warshaw *et al.*, 1966; and various other workers), a transient stimulation (Hussain and Newcomb, 1964; Mürer, 1968) with subsequent fall in the oxidative metabolism (Bettex-Galland and Lüscher, 1960; Gross and Schneider, 1968), and in pyruvate oxidation (Warshaw *et al.*, 1966). The findings of Seitz (1965) who when using $u\text{-}^{14}C$-glucose observed only very slight formation of $^{14}CO_2$ amounting to not more than 6–10% of the theoretical CO_2 formation calculated on the basis of the oxygen consumption, lend convincing support to this interpretation which implies a reincorporation of the 6-^{14}C-glucose atom into glycogen, Seitz (1965) concludes from his findings that glucose could not possibly constitute the direct substrate of the oxidative substrate of the oxidative metabolism in the thrombocytes. Instead, he successfully furnished evidence of a rapidly increasing radioactivity in glycogen. From these findings it seems probable that in resting thrombocytes the oxidation of pyruvate accounts for only a small fraction of the metabolic sequence, while the main flux proceeds via pyruvate carboxylation to oxaloacetate and is thus channeled by way of gluconeogenesis into the glycogen synthesis. The stimulation of the "6-^{14}C-glucose oxidation" which according to Warshaw et al. (1966) is observed only after a lag period of approximately 30 minutes under the action of thrombin also seems to lend support to the above concept. This stimulation has to be attributed of necessity to enhanced glycogenolysis initiated by the labeled C-atom after its incorporation into glycogen during the preceding phase of increased glucose utilization and lactate formation. This type of mechanism which involves a thrombin-induced initial increase in the synthesis of glycogen will be explained, on the one hand, by the stimulation of the mitochondrial metabolism in association with a higher supply of lactate and a burst in oxygen consumption (Mürer, 1968) and, on the other hand, by the finding of Zieve and Greenough (1969) who postulated that thrombin inhibits the adenylate cyclase in human platelets. This would produce an initial stimulation of the glycogen synthesis, an intensified glycogenolysis being possible only after regression of the thrombin action and breakdown of the mitochondrial compartment required for gluconeogenesis. This displacement of phases during the regulating segments of the respective metabolic cycles seems to be of fundamental importance for retraction which, it is assumed, may possibly depend on the glycogenolytic production of energy.

From the values given by Warshaw et al. (1966) it may be seen in any case that the pentose–phosphate shunt is a highly significant factor in thrombocytes. On the basis of their experimental values yielding 42.8 nmoles [14]CO_2 from 1-^{14}C-glucose, and 14.0 nmoles from 6-^{14}C-glucose per unit time, and allowing for the findings of Seitz (1965), who had indicated that not more than 6–10% of the value to be expected for labeled CO_2 had been recovered from experiments with u-^{14}C-glucose, the glucose fraction metabolized in resting platelets in the pentose–phosphate shunt accounts for approximately 15–25%. A stimulation induced, for instance, by thrombin, will intensify the increase in the Embden-Meyerhof pathway so that a displacement of the relative fraction will be obtained. Stimulation of the fatty acid synthesis might produce a displacement in the opposite direction.

The fact that erythrocytes not capable of a *de novo* fatty acid synthesis (Majerus *et al.*, 1969) also have a low conversion rate, might by itself support the view that the pentose–phosphate shunt is coupled with lipid synthesis (for a review, see Caputto *et al.*, 1967). Another finding implying that incubation of human platelets in a synthetic medium with the addition of glucose and acetate as substrates (10 and 1.5 mM, respectively) will produce a distinct increase in the oxygen consumption, but also a fall in ATP, might equally endorse such a correlation (Schneider, 1970). It is conceivable that fatty acid synthesis also requires the additional energy-dependent formation of $NADPH_2$ (Flatt and Ball, 1964, 1966).

3. GLYCOGEN METABOLISM

As has been shown by various authors, human platelets are subject to a vigorous glycogen metabolism (Waller *et al.*, 1959; Gross, 1967), and a large number of findings point to a dependence of certain platelet functions, particularly of retraction, on glycogen as an energy store (Löhr *et al.*, 1961a,b; Scott, 1967; Mürer, 1968). It is, therefore, not surprising that thrombocytes, in contrast to erythrocytes which do not have to fulfill such functions, contain relatively large amounts of glycogen. According to Löhr *et al.* (1961a,b), the *glycogen content* is 28.4 μmoles/10^{11} platelets. Seitz (1965) gives a similar figure of 1.5% of the dry weight, and a recently published value referring to 34 $\pm$ 10 μmoles/10^{11} platelets also fits into this range (Schneider, 1969). Compared with other blood cells, it is seen that the glycogen content of leukocytes is equivalent to some 30–50% of the above values, that of the granulocytes to approximently 50–70%, while lymphocytes which are poor in glycogen contain not more than 4–5% of the platelet glycogen content. (Olsson *et al.*, 1963). Brief mention has already been made of the continuous *glycogen synthesis* proceeding in the platelets. Its glycogen content remains relatively stable under the most varied conditions (Seitz, 1965; Scott, 1967), despite the highly metabolic activity that is linked with the platelet function (Seitz, 1965). The glycogen synthesis could be demonstrated by incorporating labeled glucose into platelet glycogen (Seitz, 1965; Scott, 1967). It has also been possible to furnish evidence of the enzymic activity of UDP-glucose glycogen synthetase (Seitz, 1965) and to determine the enzymic kinetic properties of the enzyme from pig thrombocytes (Vainer and Wattiaux, 1968). With the help of this enzyme, the thrombocytes are able to build up themselves the required glycogen stores, instead of having to depend on a glycogen reserve supplied by the mega-karyocyte, as has been assumed originally. Since platelets contain virtually *no creatine phosphate* and *no creatine phosphokinase*, glycogen constitutes the principal energy store (Waller *et al.*, 1959; Gross, 1961; Schmitz *et al.*, 1962).

A *rise in the platelet glycogen content* is observed in certain forms of glycogen storage disease in conjunction with a drop in glucose-6-phosphate activity. Determination of this enzyme and of the platelet glycogen content thus facilitate the diagnosis (Löhr *et al.*, 1961a,b; Linneweh *et al.*, 1963).

The glycogen content of the platelets can be mobilized, as need arises via a complex enzyme system. Even slight membrane alterations as they are obtained, for instance, when resuspending platelets in synthetic media, will produce an activation of the *glycogen phosphorylase* (Scott, 1967). Activation is less pronounced when platelets are resuspended in plasma. In this case two components of glycogen phosphorylase may be distinguished; one of them is AMP-dependent and shows only a transient rise and constant activity after 20–30 minutes. However, this enzyme accounts for not more than about 10% of the entire phosphorylase activity, while the main portion is represented by an enzyme that is susceptible to stimulation by AMP and shows a constant increase in activity when incubated for 60 minutes (Scott, 1967). This pronounced tendency of the platelet phosphorylase to undergo activation by AMP agrees with the property of phosphorylase b from skeletal muscle, while liver phosphorylase is hardly influenced by AMP (Cori *et al.*, 1943; Wosilait and Sutherland, 1956). Interestingly, the behavior of the leukocyte enzyme is identical to that of the liver enzyme (Yunis and Arimura, 1964, 1966a, b). An accurate analysis of the platelet activity has shown, however, that the demonstrable properties do not agree in all details with those of the skeletal muscle enzyme, but show various differences. Intermediary properties have been shown to occur, as manifested by the tendency to undergo activation by AMP following Mg-ATP activation, and by the behavior to anti-rabbit-muscle-phosphorylase-globin; these features have thus pointed to the presence of an inactive enzyme which does not undergo stimulation by AMP in the platelets (Yunis and Arimura, 1968). As a matter of fact it has been possible, when employing polyacrylamide disk electrophoresis, to demonstrate 3 different isoenzymes in the platelet extract. By its rate of migration the mean band corresponded to the skeletal muscle enzyme. Leukocytes equally showed 3 bands, their relative proportion, however, being entirely different. Karpatkin and Langer (1969) have also confirmed the presence of a component of phosphorylase activity that was not stimulated by AMP but showed intensive activation when incubated with Mg-ATP at 37°C. It has in addition been possible to furnish evidence of the presence of inactive monomeric and dimeric forms in the platelet cytolysate; these forms are converted by incubation with Mg-ATP into phosphorylase a and phosphorylase b, and might possibly offer an explanation with regard to the two other isoenzymes that have been detected by electrophoresis (Yunis and Arimura, 1968). *Adenylate cyclase* is another enzyme that might be indirectly concerned with the breakdown of glycogen, causing conversion of ATP into cyclic AMP and contributing to the activation of phosphorylase by adrenaline (Sutherland and Robison, 1966). This enzyme was also detected in human platelets (Zieve and Greenough, 1969) and has been shown to display some interesting properties, e.g., liability to inhibition by thrombin, adrenaline, or serotonin and liability to activation by fluoride or glucagon. On the basis of these properties some relationship to platelet function might be conceivable because it is known that substances activating adenylate cyclase simultaneously block aggregation while conversely inhibitors of the enzyme (thrombin, adrenaline, serotonin) will release aggregation. The exact significance of this enzyme in platelets has not yet been elucidated.

Stimulation of the phosphorylase activity when resuspending platelets in synthetic media causes a continuous decrease in glycogen (Scott, 1967; Gross and Schneider, 1968) which goes parallel with a fall in ATP and hence increasingly affects retraction (Scott, 1967). While it is true that under the action of thrombin the fall in the glycogen content in pig thrombocytes is more rapid than that of the controls (Weber and Unger, 1964), glycogen synthesis in human platelets remains detectable even under the influence of thrombin (Scott, 1967).

B. Metabolic Reaction Sequences Encompassing Two Compartments

1. NUCLEOTIDE METABOLISM

Platelets contain adenine, guanine, uracil, and cytosine nucleotides (Fantl and Ward, 1956; Mizuno *et al.*, 1960; Schmitz *et al.*, 1962). Adenine nucleotides, particularly ATP and ADP, account for the major portion of these nucleotides. In most assays for ATP, the values obtained ranged from 4 to 8 μmoles/10^{11} platelets, with an ATP:ADP ratio varying from 1.5 to 3.0, depending on whether the nucleotides were determined in platelet-rich plasma or in washed thrombocytes. In washed platelets the values obtained were always lower (Born, 1956; Fantl and Ward, 1956; Luganova *et al.*,

1958; Waller *et al.*, 1959; Bettex-Galland and Lüscher, 1960; Detwiler *et al.*, 1962; Schmitz *et al.*, 1962; Holmsen, 1967; Melchinger and Nemerson, 1967; Gross and Schneider, 1968; Karpatkin and Langer, 1968; Moser *et al.*, 1968; Pitney *et al.*, 1968; Mills and Thomas, 1969).

The very high values for human platelets reported by some workers (Waller *et al.*, 1959; Schmitz *et al.*, 1962; Moser *et al.*, 1968) are presumably due to the various methods used. Values for ATP:ADP:AMP were found to attain as much as $56.9:22.0:1.4$ μmoles/10^{11} platelets for calf thrombocytes (Mizuno *et al.*, 1960). The actual occurrence of such high ATP values, at least in human platelets, seems unlikely in that the Mg-ATPase activity determined in the cytolysate has a sharp substrate optimum at 3 mM ATP (Schneider, 1970). When converting the mean of 6 μmoles ATP/10^{11} platelets into a concentration, using a conversion factor according to which 1 gm of the platelet wet weight is equivalent to 4–5×10^{10} platelets (Maupin, 1954; Fantl and Ward, 1956; Luganova *et al.*, 1958; Marcus and Zucker, 1966), a figure of exactly 3 mM will be obtained which is precisely the optimal substrate concentration of Mg-ATPase in human platelets. Upward or downward variations in concentration will immediately produce a distinct fall in ATPase activity. When increasing the ATP concentration three- or fourfold, thus attaining values that would be equal to the higher concentrations detected in thrombocytes (Waller *et al.*, 1959; Schmitz *et al.*, 1962; Moser *et al.*, 1968), the ATPase activity will decrease by more than 50% (Schneider, 1970), while inhibition of Mg-ATPase under different conditions (exposure to cold, basic polypeptides) will invariably enhance the aggregation tendency. It should be noted, however, that the above calculation can be considered to be only a rough estimate, because it does not take into account that the Mg-ATPase activity in human platelets comprises at least 2 isoenzymes (Schneider, 1970) with probably varying kinetic properties. Moreover, the ATP content of platelets is most likely distributed to two cellular compartments (R. J. Haslam, 1964, 1967; Holmsen, 1965; Ireland, 1967) in much the same way as is probably also the Mg-ATPase activity (Schneider, 1970). But there is some indication, though suggesting a mechanism, which by regulating the endogenous ATP content of human platelets makes it possible to control the Mg-ATPase activity. On manometric determination of oxygen using the two-flask method in the Warburg apparatus (for method, refer to Waller *et al.*, 1959) we observed that the platelets resuspended in a large volume tend to aggregate rapidly. Systematic investigations of this phenomenon gave the following results: When resuspending 3×10^9 human platelets in a synthetic medium containing the electrolytes in physiological concentrations (for method, refer to Schneider *et al.*, 1968b) in varying volumes of 2, 4, 6, 8 and 10 ml and incubating for 60 minutes with shaking, pronounced platelet aggregations will be found to occur at first after 10–15 minutes in the large volumes that are followed at regular intervals by similar aggregations decreasing in the descending order in the smaller volumes, with only the smallest samples being exempt from aggregation. Since the volumes differ from each other maximally by the factor 5, the contact surfaces with siliconized glass, however, only by the factor 2, and considering the presence of EDTA in the medium, it seems unlikely that aggregation is released via a contact-activated plasmatic coagulation system traces of which may still be present in the synthetic medium. On the other hand, the "thickness" of the sample layers increases rapidly with rising volumes. In consequence, the gas diffusion in the samples is increasingly interfered with, resulting in a reduced oxygen consumption as the volumes become larger and a simultaneous fall in oxygen saturation. This again will produce a drop in ATP (Gross and Schneider, 1968; Schneider and Niemeyer, 1968) which by way of a decrease in Mg-ATPase from the optimal substrate range may lead to platelet aggregation and to the release of nucleotides, potassium, and serotonin detectable in the supernatant by spectrophotometric and fluorescence determinations, respectively. When simultaneously determining the Mg-ATPase activity in the cytolytic platelet sediments obtained from the samples with varying volumes, using the procedure outlined by Waller *et al.* (1959), a steadily growing enzyme inactivation that increases from the smaller to the largest volumes is shown to occur. This fall in activity which is considered to result from conformational alterations at the molecule, due to decreasing ATP-, Mg-, or Ca-linkage, might release aggregation via an increased flow of potassium from the platelets and a subsequent higher entry of calcium. *In vitro* inactivation of this Mg-dependent ATPase may be demonstrated in much the same fashion by incubating the thrombocytes under study in the cold over several hours, or by adding protamine sulfate (Schneider, 1970). The sensitivity to cold of an Mg-dependent ecto-ATPase in platelets had been evidenced before by Salzman *et al.* (1967).

The above finding gives some indication of the decisive significance of the ATP content in the thrombocytes for their hemostatic functions, probably by way of influencing the membrane permeability. The correlation that exists especially with regard to retraction has been extensively studied (Bettex-Galland and Lüscher, 1960; Gross, 1961; Löhr *et al.*, 1961a, b; Scott, 1967; Mürer, 1968; Schneider and Niemeyer, 1968). Using antiplatelet serum and whole-body irradiation, it has been shown (Detwiler *et al.*, 1962) that rat platelets decrease in size during the *in vivo* aging and lose some of their retraction ability, probably in conjunction with a loss of ATP. On the other hand, the adhesiveness to glass is supposed to depend neither on the ATP content, nor on the oxygen consumption or the size of the platelets (Melchinger and Nemerson, 1967).

Regeneration of purine nucleotides using 2-^{14}C-glycine has not been detectable in human thrombocytes (Holmsen and Rozenberg, 1968b). Studies on the fate of ^{14}C-adenine in platelet-rich plasma and when added to washed platelets, as well as in the platelet cytolysate, have shown that adenine is taken up quantitatively and incorporated into the platelets (Holmsen and Rozenberg, 1968b). Adenine uptake proceeded along saturation–kinetic lines and could be inhibited by adenosine. The platelet cytolysates contained an adenine-phosphoribosyl-transferase that gave rise to the generation of AMP in the platelets and could be inhibited by ATP, AMP, and pyrophosphate. On the other hand, attempts at generating 5-phosphoribosyl-pyrophosphate from ATP and ribose-5-phosphate in human platelets proved unavailing.

When incubating platelets in 10-^{14}C-adenosine, it has been seen that approximately 30% of the radioactivity is accepted and may subsequently be detected in the platelets in the form of labeled ADP and ATP. The remainder is broken down to inosine and hypoxanthine. The presence of an adenine-amino-hydrolase could be proved neither in human platelets nor in plasma. AMP was not accepted across the platelet membrane, but had first to be dephosphorylated to adenosine in the plasma. It has been possible, however, to demonstrate the conversion of 10-^{14}C-adenosine to labeled AMP, ADP, and ATP in the presence of ATP and magnesium ions in the platelet cytolysate. AMP that was converted by adenylate kinase to ATP and ADP within a few seconds was the immediate reaction product. In the platelet cytolysates, no formation of adenine nucleotides from 8-^{14}C-adenine was seen to occur in the presence of ribose-1-phosphate and inorganic phosphate so that it has to be assumed that formation of AMP from adenosine is dependent on the presence of adenosine kinase (Holmsen and Rozenberg, 1968a). Upon further addition of ADP, platelets incubated with ADP lose their reactivity. This *loss of aggregation ability* does not result from the formation of adenosine, but is rather due to a direct influence exerted on the platelets. By contrast, it is proposed that the ATP-induced inhibition may be caused in part by the uptake of adenosine during the breakdown of ATP. It was seen, however, that the sequence of platelet disaggregation following ADP-released aggregation remained uninfluenced even when preventing the formation of adenosine by adding adenosine desaminase to the incubation mixture (Rozenberg and Holmsen, 1968a). Platelet disaggregation also correlated poorly with the slow degradation of ADP in this system. On the other hand, addition of adenylate kinase to the incubation medium consisting of ADP-aggregated thrombocytes produced a rapid disaggregation of human platelets (Rysanek *et al.*, 1969). When adding potato apyrase to ADP-aggregated platelets in plasma, a rapid degradation of ADP was seen to occur which gave rise to an accelerated and comprehensive dissolution of the platelet aggregates (Rozenberg and Holmsen, 1968b). The ADP-induced platelet aggregation in plasma could be inhibited by AMP and adenosine esters only after hydrolysis to adenosine had taken place. The adenosine concentration in plasma did not reveal any correlation to the inhibition achieved, but it has been possible to correlate the inhibition with the phosphorylation rate of adenosine. The inhibition remained demonstrable even after removal of all of the adenosine from the plasma by means of adenosine desaminase.

These recent findings of Holmsen and Rozenberg (1968b) readily supplement and confirm those of Chambers *et al.* (1968) who summarized their results in a separate review. These authors equally could establish that when incubating platelets in citrated plasma with addition of 8-^{14}C-ADP a sharp increase in activity is found in the platelets which is dependent on the logarithm of the concentration (Salzman and Chambers, 1965). The increase in activity is dependent on the time and temperature; it will diminish on preliminary incubation with EDTA and is reduced in an ACD-containing medium, this reduction, however, not being equal in extent to the concurrent decline of the ADP-induced aggregation. Labeled adenosine and AMP equally produce an incorporation of radioactivity within the platelets, but a mutual inhibition is shown to occur on simultaneous addition.

The platelets are aggregated upon addition of ^{32}P-ADP, but there is no uptake of activity, nor does phosphate-labeled AMP produce an incorporation of activity, so that the radioactivity demonstrated in the thrombocytes under the action of 8-^{14}C-ADP constitutes a dephosphorylation product. Extraction with acid and chromatographic analysis of the activity within the thrombocytes yields ATP, ADP, AMP, and adenosine; it is therefore concluded that exogenous adenosine may give rise to a nucleotide phosphorylation in the thrombocytes (Salzman *et al.*, 1966b; Spaet and Lejnieks, 1966). When *resuspending platelets not in plasma, but in synthetic media*, the dephosphorylating plasma enzymes are lacking. Under these conditions adenosine will be incorporated unchanged, while this is not true for all other nucleotides. ^{14}C-labeled ADP will not produce an increase in the intracellular ^{14}C-ATP activity. In contrast to ^{3}H-labeled adenosine, ^{3}H-labeled ADP will be taken up with a certain delay, a finding which gives some indication of the time required for dephosphorylation in plasma

(Ashford *et al.*, 1967). Addition of cyanide will prevent the dephosphorylation of ADP in plasma (Salzman *et al.*, 1966a) without, however, imparing aggregation. This shows that the *release of aggregation* is not dependent on dephosphorylation. The action of ADP most probably effects the inhibition of an ecto-ATPase on the thrombocyte surface (Chambers *et al.*, 1967; White and Krivit, 1965; Robison *et al.*, 1965). This enzyme is sensitive to cold and with respect to kinetic properties shows surprising agreement with the contractile protein of the thrombocytes demonstrated by Bettex-Galland and Lüscher (1961). Inhibitors of this enzyme provoke a swelling of the platelets with an associated high-grade extension of the surface. It is proposed that resulting from this, previously blocked binding sites may become vacant to accept fibrinogen cleavage products or other polypeptides so as to form protein bridges. The availability of a heat-labile, nondialysable plasma cofactor required for ADP-released aggregation might provide support for this concept (Born and Cross, 1964).

Interestingly, the ADP-released aggregation could be blocked by simultaneous *addition of substances inhibiting glycolysis and oxidative metabolism*. This equally produced a distinct inhibition of the formation of labeled nucleotides from labeled adenosine (Rozenberg and Holmsen, 1968a). An inhibitory action on the uptake of labeled adenosine following addition of 8-^{14}C-ADP to platelet-rich plasma, as well as blocking of the formation of labeled nucleotide by cyanide, has also been described by Salzman *et al.* (1966). This clearly reflects once again the dependence of these reactions on the energy metabolism. An interesting possible explanation for this phenomenon is sketched by Rozenberg and Holmsen (1968a): The cellular ATP possibly might not be available for the aggregation reaction during the intracellular transport and phosphorylation of adenosine, respectively. This tentative explanation seems particularly significant inasmuch as studies of various types of mitochondria have revealed that they store large amounts of calcium and phosphate and are simultaneously capable of binding considerable ATP and ADP reserves within the mitochondria (Carafoli *et al.*, 1965; Pullman and Schatz, 1967; C. Rossi *et al.*, 1967; C. S. Rossi *et al.*, 1967; Wenner and Hackney, 1967; Scarpa and Azzi, 1968; Gear and Lehninger, 1968; Scarpa and Azzone, 1968). The ratio of the ATP and ADP binding is conditioned by the calcium content and thus by the uptake of calcium, but the multiple prevalence of the ADP-binding becomes invariably evident (Carafoli *et al.*, 1965). The *nucleotide binding* is most pronounced in the presence of calcium ions and phosphate. The incorporation of adenine nucleotides is blocked by inhibitors of the oxidative metabolism and by agents uncoupling oxidative phosphorylation

(Carafoli *et al.*, 1965). The observation by Rozenberg and Holmsen (1968a) of an inhibition of ADP-released aggregation occurring only upon simultaneous addition of an inhibitor of the glycolytic and oxidative metabolism might be due to the different methods used in that these workers did not employ isolated mitochondria, but used whole platelets. This means that an additional factor aggravating permeation had to be overcome in the platelet membrane. It is also conceivable that in addition substrates of the oxidative metabolism, such as amino acids or acetate, might be taken up and metabolized from the plasma in blocked glycolysis since the experiments had been performed in platelet-rich plasma. The significance of metabolic compartmentation in this context has been evidenced by the findings of Holmsen (1967). He was able to show that incubation of human or rabbit platelets with ^{32}P-phosphate, apart from giving rise to the formation of labeled nucleotides in thrombocytes, also provides convincing evidence of a *distribution of the adenosylphosphatides* (*ATP and ADP*) *to two compartments*. The specific radioactivity of the nucleotides entering the incubation medium during a collagen-induced release reaction is slight. It was concluded from these studies that varying adenine nucleotide compartments occur in the platelets, one of them showing metabolic inactivity and representing the depot of the nucleotides liberated during the collagen reaction, while the other one undergoes an intense nucleotide metabolism, but does not cause a liberation of these nucleotides. In the collagen- or ADP-induced aggregation *dephosphorylation from ATP to ADP* was simultaneously demonstrable. However, the ADP thus formed was retained in the intracellular space (Holmsen, 1965, 1967). In independent studies Ireland (1967), who verified the presence of radioactive ATP or ADP following incubation of human platelets with 8-^{14}C-adenosine or 8-^{14}C-ADP, arrived at similar results. In analogy to the findings described above, it was seen again that incubation of washed platelets containing the labeled nucleotides with thrombin caused the release of significant amounts of ATP and ADP, most of the labeled nucleotides, however, not being released. The unlabeled fraction liberated by the action of thrombin accounted for approximently 45% of the entire ATP + ADP content with an ATP:ADP ratio of 0.7:0.8, while the proportion of the nonliberated nucleotides in the labeled compartment was about 55% (Ireland, 1967). This latter finding is of particular interest when viewed in the light of the observation reported by Gross (1961) that the retraction ability of the platelets is lost as soon as its ATP content drops by more than 50% due to preservation or addition of metabolic inhibitors.

The investigations of R. J. Haslam (1964, 1967, 1968) have equally shown that platelets contain 2 metabolic compartments for nucleotides.

When adding thrombin, ATP and ADP will be liberated, the ADP fraction being larger than that of the ATP dephosphorylated to ADP; this suggests that during the liberation reaction preformed ADP apparently is the main source. The intracellular ATP:ADP ratio is 3:2, and 3:4 in the case of the liberated nucleotide.

The above findings without exception reflect the existence of two nucleotide metabolic compartments within the thrombocytes, one of them showing a high phosphorylation rate with an ATP:ADP ratio above 6.0 (Mills and Thomas, 1969). It might correspond to the *mitochondrial compartment* which undergoes active phosphorylation. On the other hand, the second *compartment*, which might be *cytoplasmic or membrane-oriented*, shows only a very slight phosphorylation rate, if any, and has an ATP:ADP ratio of 0.7:0.8 (Ireland, 1967; R. J. Haslam, 1964, 1967, 1968; Mills and Thomas, 1969). Each compartment contains approximately one half of the nucleotides available as ATP and ADP (Ireland, 1967; Mills and Thomas, 1969). The observation of Salzman *et al.* (1966b) that the uptake of labeled adenosine obtained after incubation of platelets with 8-^{14}C-ADP as well as the subsequent synthesis to labeled nucleotides are susceptible to inhibition, likewise supports an involvement of the oxidative metabolism in the direction of oxidative phosphorylation due to cyanide activity. It might be argued however, that phosphorylation of adenosine to ATP does not appear to be sensitive to 2,4-dinitrophenol (Chambers, *et al.*, 1968). 2.4-Dinitrophenol, however, does not only inhibit oxidative phosphorylation, but also results in considerable membrane effects which in turn give rise to an interference affecting the intracellular electrolyte balance (Bielawski *et al.*, 1966; Carafoli and Rossi, 1967; Kimmich and Rasmussen, 1967). It is clear that such disturbances aggravate an assessment of the inhibitory action of the substance.

2. POTENTIAL SIGNIFICANCE OF PHOSPHOPROTEINS

As mentioned in an earlier chapter (see p. 138), incubation of thrombocytes with ATP (Kerby and Taylor, 1967) or thiamine pyrophosphate (Schneider and Niemeyer, 1968) may reduce the aggregation tendency in thrombocytes and thus also their lactate production. The implication of these findings is that *energy-rich phosphates may interact with membrane proteins* by forming complexes with divalent cations and that they may stabilize the platelet membrane due to a change in configuration (Koketsu, 1965; Abood, 1966; Manery, 1968). This would result in a decreased adhesion and aggregation tendency. With regard to phosphoproteins demonstrated in other mitochondria-containing cells, these findings are of greatest significance. According to the definition of Siliprandi et al. (1966), the phosphoproteins involved, which show no further chemical characterization, contain alkali-labile and acid-stable phosphate groups esterified with the hydroxyl groups of serine and threonine. More recently Ahmed and Judah (1965) could evidence the presence of radioactive serine phosphate in an ATPase preparation so that a possible *interrelation* might be conceivable *between phosphoprotein and the ATPase activity*. A series of additional findings imply that ATPase preparations are susceptible to phosphorylation, the inhibition of this reaction by EDTA being of particular interest in this context (a review has been prepared by Albers, 1967). The phosphorylation is catalyzed by a protein phosphokinase (Burnett and Kennedy, 1954; Rabinowitz and Lipman, 1960) which causes the reversible transfer of a phosphate group from ATP to phosphoprotein and thus implies that the energy potential of this prosphoprotein is of the same order as that of ATP. Ahmed et al. (1961) and Judah (1961) were led to the conclusion that in addition to ATP other energy-rich intermediates of oxidative phosphorylation may equally cause binding of the energy-rich phosphate group, while extra-mitochondrial phosphoproteins, for instance those of the cytoplasmic type (Livanova, 1962), are strictly dependent on the mitochondrial ATP synthesis and on the release of the involved ATP into the extramitochondrial compartment. In this connection the phosphorylation of the extramito-chondrial phosphoproteins is critically dependent on the cellular content of "external," i.e., cytoplasmic, ATP but not on mitochondrial ATP (Siliprandi et al., 1966). These findings are of significance inasmuch as Seitz (1965) also detected phosphoproteins in thrombocytes, although at lower concentrations. The conclusion that these phosphoproteins influence the *permeability of the membrane* by changing its conformation in the phosphorylated and nonphosphorylated state, respectively, might provide an explanation for a considerable number of findings relative to platelet metabolism which are still obscure. It has thus been shown by the studies of Ahmed et al. (1961) and of Judah (1961) that Benadryl (diphenhydramine hydrochloride) blocks the mitochondrial conversion of phosphoproteins. The same substance inhibits aggregation in thrombocytes (O'Brien, 1964), an effect which conceivably might be brought about by a stabilization of the phosphoproteins and hence of the membrane. In addition 2,4-dinitrophenol inhibits the uptake of ^{32}P-phosphate into the phosphoproteins without, however, interfering with the mitochondrial regeneration of ATP (refer to p. 151) (Ahmed et al., 1961; Judah, 1961). This would furnish an adequate explanation for the finding in thrombocytes (Gross and Schneider, 1968) to the effect that 2,4-dinitrophenol, while blocking respiration (which is not unusual in view of the high concentrations of 0.001 M utilized by us), does not adversely affect the ATP content of the platelets, in contrast to the action exercised by other inhibitors. In accordance with these findings, alterations of the membrane properties due to high dinitrophenol concentrations have also been reported to take place in other cells (Kimmich and Rasmussen, 1967; Carafoli and Rossi, 1967).

The resultant postulate that the membrane permeability of the thrombocytes is also dependent on the state of phosphorylation of a phosphoprotein in the form of an ATPase, would allow some highly interesting conclusions to be drawn on the underlying mechanisms of platelet aggregation. It is of significance in this connection that there is considerable evidence pointing to the existence of two metabolic compartments for nucleotide conversion in the thrombocyte. It is presumed from the individual properties that one of them corresponds to the mitochondrial, and the other one to the cytoplasmic compartment (see p. 151). Since the cited investigations have shown that due to the reversibility of the protein-phosphokinase reaction (see p. 152) the state of phosphorylation of the ATPase and thus the properties of the cell membrane are at equilibrium with the ATP content of the cytoplasmic compartment (which in turn is at equilibrium with the ATP content of the mitochondrial compartment), it will be seen that any interference with the oxidative metabolism is liable to produce changes of the membrane properties. As a matter of fact, we have been successful in demonstrating aggregation of platelets released by imparied oxygen diffusion (Schneider, 1970; see pp. 145–146). Conversely, it has been seen that inhibition of the activity of the membrane ATPase due to ADP, adrenaline, cationic polypeptides, etc., may cause a fall in potassium (Kimmich and Rasmussen, 1967) and the potential release of nucleotides, thus influencing the oxidative phosphorylation and also exerting a secondary effect on the membrane properties. In contrast to the above substances (Chambers *et al.*, 1968) thrombin displays no direct influence on the Mg-ATPase activity extractable from thrombocytes (Schneider, 1970). Its efficacy might therefore be due to the proteolytic liberation of cationic polypeptides from plasma proteins (fibrinogen) or platelet proteins (platelet factor 4) (Morse *et al.*, 1967; Niewiarowski *et al.*, 1968) and cause platelet aggregation by this route. The fact that the platelet aggregation initiated by cationic polypeptides apparently is the only reaction of this type requiring neither calcium ions nor a protein as cofactors (Brossmer and Pfleiderer, 1966; Pfleiderer and Brossmer, 1967; Schneider *et al.*, 1968b) might well emphasize the basic significance of polypeptides in initiating aggregation.

The explanation for the *inhibitory action* particularly *of adenosine* on ADP-released platelet aggregation would thus appear to be found in an increased phosphorylation potential of the mitochondria and the resultant elevated phosphorylation rates of the phosphoproteins. This would also explain the necessity for preliminary incubation. It may also be of interest to consider the aspects derivable from the acid stability and alkali lability of the phosphate groups of the phosphoproteins. It is well conceivable that they may be correlated with the reduced aggregation tendency of the platelets on slight acidification of the incubation medium (ACD-containing medium) and the associated increase in respiration, oxidative phosphorylation, and phosphoprotein conversion (Engel, 1966). On the other hand, the alkali lability of the phosphate groups, by producing a rapid decrease in respiration with a corresponding fall in the oxidative phosphorylation and phosphoprotein phosphorylation (Engel, 1966), may lead to an enhanced aggregation tendency. This would be in accord with the observation of Salzman *et al.* (1968) that poisoning of the platelets by means of cyanide favors aggregation. It should also be noted that while respiration is intact, hydrogen ions are continuously released from the mitochondria of a cell in exchange for potassium ions. This will slightly displace the value of pH in the intact cell to less than 7.4. However, when the respiration is blocked, the pH will rise and OH ions will be liberated from the mitochondria into the cytoplasm (for a review, see Pullman and Schatz, 1967). Similar displacements of the values of pH at rest and under the action of cyanide were also shown to take place in platelets (Zieve and Solomon, 1966). Reversible and irreversible aggregations would accordingly differ from each other only by the respiration-dependent uptake of calcium ions. This aspect will be described in detail in connection with platelet respiration.

The question of whether such phosphorylation of proteins is correlated with the action of adenylate cyclase also detectable in the platelets (Zieve and Greenough, 1969) and the adenylate cyclase catalyzed conversion of ATP to cyclic AMP has not been resolved so far. But there still seems to exist an intimate relationship with the processes occurring at the membrane as manifested by adhesion and aggregation (see p. 144).

C. Mitochondrial Metabolic Pathways

Platelets vary from erythrocytes by a number of specific properties which account for their metabolic similarity to leukocytes (Seitz, 1965) and which are considered to be due to the mitochondrial content of the thrombocytes. Apart from rendering the platelets capable of *respiration* and probably also of *oxidative phosphorylation*, these properties additionally account for the ability of the platelets to carry out certain *syntheses* which in turn are intimately related with the function of the hemostatic mechanism. Such syntheses may encompass protein synthesis, possibly fatty acid synthesis and, as is assumed on reliable grounds, neoglycogenesis which partially proceeds within the mitochondria and leads to glycogen synthesis and most likely permits retraction. All of these syntheses show a relatively high energy demand and are consequently controlled by the energy supply, on the one hand, as has been seen before in connection with fatty acid synthesis and its interdependence with the generation of NADPH in the pentosephosphate shunt and with energy-dependent mitochondrial transhydrogenation (refer to pp. 139ff.). On the other hand, these syntheses also influence by themselves the extent of the energy metabolism. This probably explains the high glycolytic flow rate obtaining in the thrombocytes (see p. 127). Such metabolic performances that in turn form the basis of platelet functions are thus made possible by the availability of a respiratory system which has been recognized for some time, the true significance of which has, however, not been grasped until recently. It is presumed that such respiration also is a regulatory factor in platelet metabolism and is thus indirectly concerned with platelet functions. The various syntheses performed have been studied increasingly only during recent years.

1. Platelet Respiration

Respiration in human platelets was demonstrated at a relatively early date (Tullis, 1953; Maupin, 1954) and was confirmed later by a number of authors (Campbell *et al.*, 1956; Luganova *et al.*, 1958; Waller *et al.*, 1959; Bettex-Galland and Lüscher, 1960; Chernyak *et al.*, 1960a; Estes *et al.*, 1962; De Luca, 1964; Hollard and Servoz-Gavin, 1964; Hussain and Newcomb, 1964; Servoz-Gavin and Hollard, 1964; Seitz, 1965; Melchinger and Nemerson, 1967; Gross and Schneider, 1968). Systematic measurements of *oxygen consumption* using the polarographic method were carried out by Kitchens and Newcomb (1968) who compared the resultant values with those available in the previous literature. Although the methods of determination varied, including both manometric and polarographic technics, the results which ranged from 4.5 to 13.5 nmoles O_2/minute for 10^9 platelets were found to be in relatively good agreement. The values found by Kitchens and Newcomb (1968) under optimal experimental conditions following resuspension of platelets from EDTA-containing blood in tris buffer, gave a mean oxygen consumption of 12.9 nmoles O_2/minute for 10^9 platelets

Appreciably higher values were obtained only by Chernyak *et al.* (1960a) and by Estes *et al.* (1962) who reported values of 17 and 29.5 nmoles O_2/minute for 10^9 platelets.

The *significance of respiration* for the energy metabolism has frequently been underrated since on the one hand the enzyme capacities in glycolysis (see p. 127) are very high, while on the other hand not more than approximently 20% of the glucose metabolized by human thrombocytes are degraded oxidatively to CO_2 and water (Waller *et al.*, 1959). Making allowance for the relative proportion and also for the effectivity of the ATP yield in the various metabolic pathways, it will be seen, however, that the situation is directly reversed and that the oxidative generation of ATP with a (theoretical) yield of close to 80% is now predominating (see p. 127). Various authors (Warshaw *et al.*, 1966; Lüscher, 1968; R. J. Haslam, 1968; Schneider *et al.*, 1969) have called attention to the significance of such a correlation.

Alterations in the oxygen consumption of the thrombocytes may occur as a function of the glucose content in the incubation medium. This phenomenon, termed the Crabtree effect, which involves a reduction of cellular respiration in the glucose-containing incubation media, has been discussed exhaustively in an earlier chapter in connection with the glycolytic regulatory mechanisms of glycolysis (see p. 134).

Various authors have reported changes in the oxygen consumption of human platelets to occur under the *action of thrombin*. In their respective investigations involving manometric measurement and incubation for 1 hour at 37°C with addition of thrombin, Bettex-Galland and Lüscher (1960) and Gross and Schneider (1968) have observed a fall in the oxidation rate to approximently 50%. This reduction might be due to disturbed oxygen diffusion in the thrombocytes which had been irreversibly clumped under the action of thrombin. On the other hand, it is conceivable that the essential changes in the membrane permeability of the thrombocytes due to thrombin action (Grette, 1962) might cause an endogenous blocking of the oxidative metabolism by incorporation of metabolic products. Such uncoupling of oxidative phosphorylation with resultant functional platelet defects has first been discussed by Lasch (1961). The observation of Grette (1962) that the release reaction at thrombocytes constitutes a two-phase process might be in support of this theory. According to this author, the first phase would be characterized by alterations in the membrane permeability due to the action of thrombin, while the second calcium-dependent phase would involve their transition to irreversible changes at the thrombocyte. On the other hand, it has been realized that incorporation of large amounts of calcium may produce a loss of respiratory control, uncoupling of oxidative phosphorylation, and pronounced morphological alterations at the mitochondria (Greenawalt et al., 1964; Brierley and Slauterback, 1964).

The observation that low calcium concentrations tend to release a reversible platelet aggregation, while the aggregation would be irreversible in case of higher calcium concentrations (Niemeyer et al., 1967) would appear to lend support to the above concept. By the same token, the findings of Hussain and Newcomb (1964) and of Mürer (1968) might be suggestive of such uncoupling of oxidative phosphorylation. Shortly after having added thrombin, these workers observed a rapid increase in the oxygen consumption as it is known to occur upon uptake of calcium (for a review, refer to Pullman and Schatz, 1967) and when studying oxidative phosphorylation in the mitochondria of other cells (Gurban and Cristea, 1965).

According to the findings of Mürer (1968) the increase in oxygen consumption which can be distinctly reduced by adding a combination of glycolytic and oxidative metabolic inhibitors thus seems to be dependent on the energy metabolism. On the other hand, addition of KCN will not inhibit these sudden bursts in oxygen consumption (Detwiler, 1967; Mürer, 1968) a dependence on terminal oxidation would thus appear to be questionable. On the basis of his experimental findings, Mürer (1968), therefore, concludes that the eruption in oxygen consumption is not correlated with the platelet respiration per se, but is rather associated with processes similar to the ones produced by leukocytes during phagocytosis (Sbarra and Karnovsky, 1959; Iyer et al., 1961; Zatti and Rossi, 1965, 1966). On the other hand, Detwiler (1967) and also Kitchens and Newcomb (1968) consider that the phenomenon of increased oxygen consumption under the action of thrombin should be attributed to the respective experimental conditions.

The above interpretation would, however, not be in contrast with the findings of Bettex-Galland and Lüscher (1960) and Gross and Schneider (1968) who carried out their experiments by manometric methods and thus did not detect transient changes lasting for only fractions of a minute.

It has been pointed out by various authors who had engaged in studying the interrelation between the glycolytic and oxidative energy metabolism that inhibition of certain platelet functions can only be obtained by simultaneous addition to the thrombocyte-containing incubation mixture of substances inhibiting glycolysis and oxidative metabolism (Gorstein et al., 1967; Mürer et al., 1967; Hellem, 1967; Rozenberg and Holmsen, 1968). Clearly the effects obtained are particularly pronounced and may therefore be detected even in relatively insensitive functional tests. The findings of

Gross and Schneider (1968) and of Schneider and Niemeyer (1968) who reported a drop in the platelet ATP content and a reduced functioning ability when merely adding inhibitors of glycolysis are in apparent contrast to the above theory. Identical results have been published somewhat earlier by Bettex-Galland and Lüscher (1960) and by Löhr et al. (1961a, b). The explanation for these divergent results is probably to be found in the fact that the latter investigators worked with a synthetic medium containing glucose as the only substrate and that inhibition of glycolysis, in view of the reduced substrate supply, will in turn cause a simultaneous decrease of the oxidative metabolism. This type of system would actually comply with the situation which, as has been postulated by Mürer et al. (1967), will effect a blocking of the two metabolic pathways. It should be noted that in contrast to the above experiments Mürer et al. (1967) conducted their studies in platelet-rich plasma that contained besides glucose in the form of glutamine, serine, and glycine, other substances possibly serving as substrates for the oxidative metabolism (Rapoport and Jacobasch, 1968). Mere blocking of glycolysis in this system might in consequence be compensated by the degradation of substrates of the oxidative metabolism; considering the high effectivity of oxidative energy production it would thus exert no outward effect. The findings of Gorstein et al. (1967) which revealed that liberation of labeled potassium is obtained only on simultaneous addition of an inhibitor suppressing both glycolysis and oxidative metabolism have proved that such an interpretation is fully justified. Use of anaerobic incubation, instead of a substance inhibiting the oxidative metabolism, proved to be equally effective. When replacing anaerobic incubation by gassing with oxygen while maintaining glycolytic inhibition, intracellular potassium ion accumulation which to our belief mirrors the significance of the oxidative metabolism was shown to occur again. It was seen in addition that on glycolytic inhibition substrates of the oxidative metabolic cycle may reimprove the ATP content of the platelets and their function (Karpatkin, 1967; Gross and Schneider, 1968). At the same time these findings should prompt reconsideration of the concept of a "pure" carbohydrate metabolism (Waller et al., 1959).

2. OXIDATIVE PHOSPHORYLATION

Although a number of unequivocal and varied indications are available indicative of the fundamental significance of respiration for the platelet metabolism, attempts at demonstrating an oxidative phosphorylation *in vitro* with thrombocyte fractions have not been successful (Chernyak and

Guseinov, 1960; Chernyak and Totskaya, 1963; Chernyak, 1965; Rock and Nemerson, 1969). There are numerous indications though which point to the existence of oxidative phosphorylation, such indications comprising the presence of protein synthesis, the action exerted by various inhibitors of the glycolytic and oxidative metabolic cycle (Gross and Schneider, 1968), and primarily the existence of a Pasteur effect in the thrombocytes (Wu et al., 1964; Chernyak, 1965; Gross and Schneider, 1968). The coupling between the Pasteur effect and oxidative phosphorylation seems to represent a universal biological law (Seitz, 1959, 1961) because complete uncoupling of oxidative phosphorylation is associated with a loss of the Pasteur effect, a feature which will be more clearly understood when considering its underlying reaction mechanisms (see p. 134).

The contradiction that seems to exist between indirect indications of oxidative phosphorylation and the failure so far to provide evidence of such a reaction occurring in vitro is considered to be due to various experimental aspects. On the one hand, it should be considered that the extraction of intact mitochondria from platelets has proved to be especially difficult in view of the high content in human platelets of α-granules, which at about equal size and density contain various desmolases. On the other hand, previous investigations (similar to the experiments with mitochondria-free erythrocytes) invariably involved processing of platelets under "careful" cooling, although metabolic and functional alterations in thrombocytes under the action of cold have been reported for some time. Following the initial observations of Aynaud (1909, 1911), it was established by Zucker and Borelli (1954) that platelets prepared at 37°C from citrated or oxalated blood retain their native discoid form, while this feature is lost when working at lower temperatures. The same authors (Zucker and Borelli, 1960) also observed that cooling to +4°C favors formation of aggregates in platelet-rich plasma, while in a similar plasma that had not been allowed to cool the formation of aggregates occurred with a considerable delay shortly before the onset of coagulation. It would appear that this finding is consistent with the phenomenon that has been referred to as "incubation resistance" and investigated systematically by Niemeyer et al. (1967) and Reuter et al. (1967). When cooling platelets obtained from ACD-containing blood, Bull and Zucker (1965) by determining the individual sizes with the Coulter Counter also detected an increase in volume varying between 15 and 30%. Mann and Krankenhagen (1969) referred again to the aggregation tendency which was enhanced at low temperatures and became particularly pronounced in heparinized plasma, but was reduced in citrated plasma and not demonstrable at all in EDTA-containing plasma.

In *ultrastructural investigations* the thrombocytes that had been prepared in the cold show rapid formation of pseudopodia (Skjørten, 1968), loss of discoid form with disappearance of the marginal bundle of the microtubuli, and increasing adhesion tendency. On rewarming these alterations could initially be reversed (White and Krivit, 1967). When incubating for a prolonged period, alterations involving in particular the mitochondria of the thrombocyte became noticeable under the action of cold (Firkin *et al.*, 1965).

In this connection the findings of Zucker-Franklin *et al.* (1967) and Zucker-Franklin (1969) are of particular interest. It may be seen from their studies that the microfibrils, which can be detected on ultrastructural observation, have to be allocated to the contractile platelet protein as a morphological equivalent, and that further microtubuli and microfibrils are equivalent to varying polymerization steps of the same structural protein that is pooled in the cytoplasm (Behnke, 1967a,b). These authors also claim that depolymerization may be obtained, among other things, by low temperatures. An interesting relationship thus emerges in that the contractile protein of the thrombocytes, the *thrombosthenin* (for a review, see Lüscher and Bettex-Galland, 1968; Grette, 1962), involves an Mg-ATPase that has been shown to be sensitive to cold (Chambers *et al.*, 1967).

In view of the very pronounced instability and aggregation tendency of the thrombosthenin, *investigations of its protein chemistry* met with considerable difficulties. But it was possible to demonstrate that the highly asymmetrical molecule has a sedimentation constant of 36 S and may be divided at high ionic strength into subunits of 18 and 7 S (Ganguly, 1969). Here, too, ultrastructural and biochemical findings were found to show good agreement.

The above findings are particularly significant in that it has also been realized from the study of mitochondrial metabolism that coupling factor I which is sensitive to cold involves a protein with Mg-ATPase activity which under the action of cold is broken down into its 10 monomeric subunits and thus loses its enzymic activity (Penefsky and Warner, 1965; Pullman and Schatz, 1967). In view of the overall agreement of the various findings we were led to search for an *uncoupling of oxidative phosphorylation* in the thrombocytes due to the action of cold, and for factors indicative of an increased glycolysis in the direction of a Pasteur effect. We were able to demonstrate that after incubation over several hours at $+4°C$ platelets that had been prepared in the cold show a distinct reduction in oxygen consumption and a parallel fall in ATP. It is believed that as a result of a Pasteur effect, involving an impaired oxidative metabolism, a concurrent increase in lactate formation may occur in the samples that had been in-cubated in the cold and examined at 37°C; on the other hand, the controls that had been kept at 37°C both during the preliminary incubation and the actual testing period, showed neither a fall in the oxygen consumption or the ATP content, nor an increase in lactate formation (Gross and Schneider, 1968). Rock and Nemerson (1969) equally concluded from their experi-mental results that an uncoupling of oxidative phosphorylation would seem to be at work in the platelets prepared under common experimental condi-tions (in the cold). Such uncoupling by means of cooling might become effective via defective function of the ecto-ATPase with associated distur-bance of the intracellular electrolyte balance (Chambers *et al.*, 1967) and might thus produce a sensitivity to cold of the coupling factor I of oxidative phosphorylation which is sensitive to cold (Penefsky and Warner, 1965); or else it might also be associated with findings according to which ATP at a temperature of 5°C is no longer capable of catalyzing active transport processes (J. M. Haslam and Griffiths, 1968). It has also been observed that the translocation of adenine nucleotides between the cytoplasmic and the mitochondrial compartment is blocked at low temperatures (Heldt and Klingenberg, 1968) in much the same way as the uptake of adenosine by the thrombocytes is dependent on the temperature (Chambers *et al.*, 1968). The reversible nature of the dissociation in both cases, provided the cooling phase is not excessively protracted, is also consistent with the biochemical findings pointing to a dissociation of coupling factor I into its subunits at the thrombocyte. Rewarming will initially lead to the recovery of the full metabolic activity and thus produce the phenomenon of "incuba-tion resistance" due to a decreasing aggregability (Niemeyer *et al.*, 1967; Reuter *et al.*, 1967). Upon prolonged cooling, however, the alterations observed are irreversible. This might furnish an explanation for the observa-tion that a particularly active glycolytic energy metabolism in the platelets was described, with oxidative metabolism being delegated to a minor position, whenever the cooling phase was particularly prolonged, as was the case in the experiments of Bettex-Galland and Lüscher (1960), Chernyak (1965), and Warshaw *et al.* (1966). The findings of Murphy and Gardner (1969) are consistent with the conclusion that cooling should be avoided to maintain the structure and function of mitochondria-containing cells. These authors have shown that under standardized conditions the survival time of ^{51}Cr-labeled platelets which had been cooled to $+4$°C before reinfusion is distinctly diminished compared with that of the samples kept at 22°C. The survival time *in vivo* was seen to decrease as the duration of the cooling phase was prolonged (the incubation times employed were 0,

8, and 18 hours). It is concluded by the authors that cooling must be avoided when preparing and storing platelets.

Interestingly, the outlines of present understanding of the metabolic events in the leukocytes have also taken new shape. Here again vigorous aerobic glycolysis was first detected (Beck, 1958; Frei, 1961). However, this was recognized to be due to an impaired oxidative metabolism while the cells were prepared under the action of cold (Warburg et al., 1958), and attempts at demonstrating oxidative phosphorylation (Foster and Terry, 1967) eventually proved successful, thus vindicating the theory of Seitz (1965) that there is essential agreement between leukocytes and thrombocytes. It is seen again that the mitochondrial content of both types of cells is responsible for the observed agreement.

Active depletion of divalent cations obviously may influence the platelet metabolism in the same direction as does cooling. It has been possible to demonstrate that the morphological (Zucker and Borelli, 1954; Skjørten, 1968; White, 1968a) and functional alterations (Zucker and Borelli, 1960; Bull and Zucker, 1965) described above for cooling also occur in much the same way after addition of EDTA. The initial EDTA concentration in the blood before isolation of thrombocytes is sufficient by itself to exert a considerable influence on the metabolic behavior of the isolated platelets when resuspended in identical incubation media (Schneider, 1969): Platelets which had been isolated from 0.1 to 0.5% EDTA-containing blood by adding identical volumes of isotonic EDTA solutions of varying concentration to native donor blood show a slight decrease in the consumption of glucose and the formation of lactate and pyruvate following resuspension in the same synthetic medium. This decrease is brought about by a diminished glycolytic flow rate most probably due to magnesium deprivation. At the same time, however, there will be an essentially more rapid decrease in oxygen consumption which is associated with a fall of the ATP content in the platelets isolated from this blood and resuspended in the same medium. It thus seems probable that the impairment of platelet metabolism and function by EDTA—an observation which has been recognized for some time and which has led to the widespread use of platelets from ACD-containing blood—may be traced to a defect of the oxidative energy metabolism and resultant mitochondrial damage. It is now appreciated that EDTA produces intracellular potassium loss (Riggs et al., 1958) and particularly gives rise to potassium losses from the mitochondria (Settlemire et al., 1968). Potassium loss will in turn lead to respiratory depression (Kimmich and Rasmussen, 1967) with subsequent impairment of platelet function. The findings of Kitchens and Newcomb (1968) that the oxygen consumption of resuspended platelets using the polarographic method in the presence of EDTA will yield extremely high measuring values are only in apparent contrast to these indications. It is believed that their results comply with those of Bettex-Galland and Lüscher (1960) and Gross and Schneider (1968) indicating an increased oxygen consumption of the platelets in EDTA-containing media when employing manometric methods. This finding may be interrelated with the very low tendency in EDTA-containing blood to form spontaneous aggregates (Mann and Krankenhagen, 1969); disturbed oxygen diffusion in the measuring arrangement which might occur due to formation of aggregates thus would not interfere with the reaction. Since, on the other hand, the oxygen consumption is increased despite release of aggregation by calcium ions, magnesium ions, or basic polypeptides (Gross and Schneider, 1968), unless there is irreversible aggregation, further, since the measuring arrangement is not affected by reversible formation of aggregates at least on manometric measurement, this phenomenon is considered to be of minor importance only. We are, therefore, led to the assumption that loss of divalent cations will produce an increased membrane permeability which brings about an increased ATP consumption at the membrane due to elevated flow rates for monovalent cations and that as a result respiration will be enhanced by way of elevated ATP dephosphorylation.

3. ENERGY-DEPENDENT EXCHANGE OF CATIONS

The functional impermeability of the cellular membranes to electrolytes and the resultant formation of *ionic and metabolite gradients at the membranes* involving high intracellular potassium and low sodium values is of fundamental importance for cellular metabolism. Depending on the energy supply such an ionic gradient can be maintained with the help of ATP and is not linked with oxidative metabolism. A pertinent example is furnished by the mature erythrocyte which, despite the lack of mitochondria, is able to maintain its high *potassium content* in dependence of the formation, of ATP by substrate phosphorylation during glycolysis (Cooley and Cohen 1967a). Erythrocytes, however, are characterized by a relatively stable membrane which increases still further in stability during the transition from the reticulocyte to the mature red blood cell (Rapoport, 1968a). The average potassium loss of these cells per unit time is accordingly relatively low while that of the thrombocytes is more than twice the erythrocyte value (Cooley and Cohen, 1967a). In contrast to erythrocytes, platelets react sensitively to thrombin and other proteolytic enzymes by loss of potassium (Buck-

ingham and Maynert, 1964; Zieve *et al.*, 1964). Potassium loss in thrombocytes can also be obtained by employing SH reagents (Buckingham and
Maynert, 1964) and local anaesthetics (Aledort and Niemetz, 1968).

In view of the dependence of many platelet functions, e.g., incorporation
of serotonin (Da Prada *et al.*, 1967; Cooley and Cohen, 1967a; Rysanek
et al., 1967) or retraction (Mey and Sundermann, 1966) on a high potassium
content of the platelets, sensitive regulatory mechanisms are required to
maintain constant conditions. As far as the energy-dependent, and not the
concentration-dependent potassium uptake is concerned, these regulatory
mechanisms were shown to be dependent on the glycolytic energy metabolism (Cooley and Cohen, 1967a). Incubation of platelets in a glucose-free
medium produced a slight fall in potassium which when compared with the
controls was quite distinct. Monoiodoacetate and sodium fluoride caused
a sharp decrease in potassium which became even more pronounced when
adding calcium. Ouabain equally inhibited the influx of potassium and
thus produced a distinct fall in the potassium concentration.

Under the action of cold, a potassium loss resembling that obtained in
other cells is seen both in the erythrocyte and the thrombocyte (Buckingham
and Maynert, 1964; Cooley and Cohen, 1967a) so that the impairment due
to low temperatures is considered to involve an inhibition of the membrane
ATPase (see p. 160) and does not necessarily result from a defect of the
mitochondrial metabolism.

On the basis of these results it is possible to compare *two different inhibitory mechanisms*: On the one hand inhibitors such as ouabain, sulfhydryl reagents, and cold cause an inactivation of the potassium- and
sodium-dependent Mg-ATPase and are thus followed by intracellular loss
of potassium. These substances are confronted by metabolic inhibitors,
e.g., monoiodoacetate, sodium fluoride, or anaerobic incubation, which
give rise to a loss of potassium by producing a fall in the energy potential
of the cell. Although anaerobic incubation was associated with only a
slight potassium loss throughout the cited investigations, it is considered
that such studies do not furnish conclusive evidence of the sole dependence
of the potassium transport mechanisms on the substrate phosphorylation
in thrombocytes because monoiodoacetate also may react with sulfhydryl
groups and thus exert a direct influence on oxidative phosphorylation and
the ion transport dependent on it (Haugaard *et al.*, 1968). Using PCMBS
to inhibit sulfhydryl groups, Cooley and Cohen (1967a) demonstrated a
distinct intracellular loss of potassium. Due to the intimate coupling between the glycolytic and the oxidative metabolism in thrombocytes a
blocking of glycolysis by sodium fluoride produces a concomitant im-

pairment of the oxidative metabolism and thus an indirect inhibition of oxidative phosphorylation and the dependent transport of cations.

A distinction between the active cationic transport that also takes place under anerobic conditions and is dependent on the cellular ATP content, and the cationic transport made possible by oxidative phosphorylation, is of particular interest in order to characterize the various functions proceeding in the thrombocyte. It has become evident by a large number of investigations that mitochondria are capable of a particularly rapid and intensive ion accumulation (Pullman and Schatz, 1967; Albers, 1967). They consequently exert a regulatory action on the ionic milieu not only in the mitochondrial compartment but in the entire cell (Sallis et al., 1963; Lehninger, 1964; Chance, 1965; Rasmussen, 1966; Pullman and Schatz, 1967). The cellular and mitochondrial potassium content are interdependent so that potassium loss is associated with a fall in respiration (Kimmich and Rasmussen, 1967). Specific studies of a possible dependence of the potassium uptake on the oxidative mitochondrial metabolism of the thrombocytes have not yet become available. Some indirect indications may, however, be obtained from the findings of Gorstein et al. (1967) (see p. 158). Using the radioactive nuclide ^{42}K these authors presented highly convincing evidence pointing to the distribution of the intracellular potassium to two cellular compartments. Using a different method, Zieve et al. (1964) had arrived earlier at similar results. Beyond this, Gorstein et al. (1967) established that concurrent inhibition of the glycolytic and oxidative metabolic cycles using iodoacetate and cyanide, and iodoacetate and anaerobic incubation, respectively, results in an increasing release of potassium from the thrombocytes. When anaerobic incubation in this system involving glycolytic inhibition is discontinued and replaced by gassing with oxygen, a recurrent intracellular accumulation of potassium will be observed which indicates, to our belief, that in this case oxidative phosphorylation, and thus the mitochondrial metabolism, are of prime importance. The differences which were obtained for the various preparations in this experimental series and which in part only served to demonstrate the availability of one potassium compartment, might be attributed to exposure to cold of varying duration with beginning uncoupling of oxidative phosphorylation.

In contrast to these findings the implication in the studies of Cooley and Cohen (1967a), who had established the sole dependence of the potassium gradient on the glycolytic metabolism, necessarily is that in all cases an appreciable uncoupling of oxidative phosphorylation due to cold or to the relatively high pH of 7.6 in the incubation mixture must have taken place so that an additional blocking in the oxidative metabolic cycle could not become effective. The fact that Gorstein *et al.* (1967) utilized a pH of 6.2–6.4 in the incubation mixture would appear to lend support for such an explanation of the different findings of the two groups. For it has been established by the investigations of Engel (1966) that platelet respiration in a weakly acid pH down to pH 6.0 is maintained for a considerably longer period, while it decreases rapidly with higher pH values. This observation might also illustrate the significance of using ACD-containing plasma in that this medium ensures more satisfactory maintenance of the oxidative metabolic functions of the platelets and thus of the intracellular regulatory mechanisms than is obtained with physiological pH values, uncoupling of oxidative phosphorylation probably also occurring essentially later in the weakly acid range.

The energy-dependent cellular potassium uptake is invariably coupled with the *release of protons* from the mitochondria (Pullman and Schatz, 1967; Albers, 1967) and might be responsible for the finding that the cellular pH of metabolically intact platelets is always slightly lower than that of the incubation medium. This would also be compatible with the results of Zieve and Solomon (1966) indicating an increase of the cellular pH when blocking of the platelet metabolism has occurred due to para-chloromercuribenzoate, thrombin or cyanide action. It is proposed that in this process parachloromercuribenzoate might effect a direct blocking of the sulfhydryl groups that are involved in oxidative phosphorylation (Haugaard *et al.*, 1969), while cyanide by inhibiting the terminal oxidation, might equally affect oxidative phosphorylation. The action of thrombin which in contrast is quite complex has been studied intensively by Grette (1962). A two-phase action involving a thrombin-catalyzed, proteolytic reaction with resultant increased membrane permeability was seen to occur during the first phase. This was followed by a calcium-dependent reaction which by way of releasing the contraction of the contractile platelet protein led to the liberation of platelet components and thus initiated the liberation reaction per se. Here again an indirect relationship is seen to exist between the action of thrombin and calcium, this correlation also being evidenced in terms of a fall in the potassium level (Zieve *et al.*, 1964). In the investigations of Zieve and Solomon (1966) thrombin interfered with the maintenance of a hydrogen gradient and was seen to cause an intracellular pH which was higher than that of the controls. This finding might suggest that mitochondria are incapable to function under the action of thrombin. In this context increasing significance has attached to findings revealing an association between the release of protones during mitochondrial cation translocation with the *uptake of calcium* (Chance, 1965; Albers, 1967; Pullman and Schatz, 1967; C. Rossi *et al.*, 1967; C. S. Rossi *et al.*, 1967; Wenner and Hackney, 1967; Gear and Lehninger, 1968; Manery, 1968; Scarpa and Azzone, 1968). If the respiration is blocked, the calcium uptake may take place by binding on the mitochondrial surface, resumption of respiration producing a translocation of the calcium molecules to the internal mitochondrial segments. The process of calcium storage consequently is a respiration- and mitochondria-dependent reaction. In this reaction capacity to bind calcium is partially determined by the ATP content of the cell: A high ATP content at a concentration of up to 20 mM thus will effect an increase in the binding capacity for potassium and sodium and a decrease in the calcium and magnesium binding (Manery, 1968). Calcium, monovalent cations, and local anaesthetics eject each other from the binding sites (Scarpa and Azzi, 1968; Scarpa and Azzone, 1968) and are thus responsible for the low calcium binding in intact cells with a high potassium content. However, if mitochondrial respiration is being blocked, loss of potassium from the cell will give rise to the attachment of calcium to the vacant binding sites. While in the resting cell an equilibrium is maintained by slight conversion of calcium (Pullman and Schatz, 1967; Albers, 1967), blocking of the membrane ATPase or of the oxidative metabolism in conjunction with release of potassium will induce a very rapid explosive uptake of calcium involving up to 99% of the calcium available in the incubation medium (Pullman and Schatz, 1967). Under aerobic conditions acceptance of this calcium into the mitochondria is accompanied by a substantial burst in the oxygen consumption and will produce deposition of calcium phosphate with a rapid increase in concentration; calcium phosphate, in turn, will give rise to irreversible mitochondrial damage with a simultaneous uncoupling of oxidative phosphorylation. Calcium binding is supposed to be due to phospholipids (Chappel *et al.*, 1963; Silver, 1965; Manery, 1968; Scarpa and Azzi, 1968). The calcium can be mobilized, however, and liberated in the presence of energy-yielding reactions.

The *reaction sequence* involved *in the uptake of calcium* thus proceeds in two phases: Binding of calcium basically is associated with a fall in the intracellular ATP content and a resultant decrease in potassium without involvement of the oxidative metabolism. This process may therefore also take place in mitochondria-free cells, such as the erythrocytes, and has in fact already been described (Weed, 1967). In mitochondria-containing cells, however, the entry of calcium will further produce a sudden burst in oxygen consumption with rapid translocation of the calcium into the mitochondrial space where it is deposited in the form of calcium phosphate. The resultant irreversible mitochondrial damage with an uncoupling of the oxidative phosphorylation and an immediate reduction of the energy potential of the cell will effect the liberation of the stored calcium in the next step of the reaction.

These findings that have been found to apply to mitochondria containing widely varying types of cells may be readily extended to the study of platelets, as has been evidenced primarily by the experiments of Grette (1962): Normal thrombocytes without evidence of damage due to cold are characterized by a high potassium content *in vivo* and slight permeability of the membrane due to the presence of calcium ions (Manery, 1968). If the mitochondrial metabolism is intact, there is an equilibrium between the low calcium ion uptake and the calcium ions liberated from the cell (Pullman and Schatz, 1967), and aggregation therefore does not take place. On the other hand, substantial depletion of calcium ions from the incubation medium produces a distinct increase in the *in vitro* permeability (Manery, 1968) so that inhibition of the membrane ATPase by ADP, low calcium ion concentrations, or basic polypeptides (Brossmer and Pfleiderer, 1966; T. Pfleiderer and Brossmer, 1967; Schneider, 1968b) effects potassium exit and rapid inflow of calcium ions. The same result can be obtained in all reactions causing a blocking of the oxygen consumption and thus an inhibition of the mitochondria-controlled cation exchange, e.g., by action of thrombin (Bettex-Galland and Lüscher, 1960; Gross and Schneider, 1968). This reaction will proceed only if the mitochondrial metabolism is impaired, e.g., by exposure to cold, while at 37°C the mitochondrial metabolism—despite calcium ion deprivation and increased permeability—apparently satisfactorily compensates (Brossmer and Patscheke, 1968) the loss of cations, especially of potassium (Cooley and Cohen, 1967a; Gorstein *et al.*, 1967) and thus gives rise to the "incubation resistance" (Niemeyer *et al.*, 1967; Reuter *et al.*, 1967). The flow of calcium ions into the thrombocytes would, however, result in a burst of the oxygen consumption, as it has also been described by Hussain and Newcomb (1964) and Mürer (1968). It would produce an accumulation of calcium ions in the mitochondria, blocking of respiration (Bettex-Galland and Lüscher, 1960; Gross and Schneider, 1968), uncoupling of oxidative phosphorylation, fall in the energy potential of the cell (Zieve *et al.*, 1964) and the final release of relatively large amounts of calcium ions from the mitochondria. It is proposed that similar to the events occurring in the muscle (Weber, 1958) the calcium ions liberated after blocking of the energy metabolism might well inactivate the "relaxing factor" described by Grette (1963) and thus initiate the contraction processes which are associated with the *release reaction*. This interpretation of the findings obtained from studies in thrombocytes is not only consistent with the results from similar investigations in other types of cells, but also coincides with the theory postulated by White (1967) concerning the *mechanism of the contraction processes* at the thrombocyte. Such interpretation would also readily explain the intracellular occurrence of calcium ions, which to date could only be assumed from various indications (Born, 1968), and the susceptibility to inhibition by local anaesthetics observed during the second phase of aggregation and when the burst in oxygen consumption occurred. As is generally known, uptake of calcium ions into the mitochondria of widely varying cells is blocked by these substances which occupy the sites of calcium ions binding (Scarpa and Azzi, 1968; Scarpa and Azzone, 1968). The above interpretation also sheds some light on a number of divergent findings outlined by Cooley and Cohen (1967a) and Gorstein *et al.* (1967) regarding the energy-dependent uptake of potassium. As indicated in an earlier chapter (see p. 165) the first group of authors who had worked at pH 7.6 did not report a possible dependence of the potassium uptake in thrombocytes on respiration, while the findings of the latter group, who incubated the thrombocytes at pH 6.2–6.4, presented presumptive evidence of such a correlation. The reduced number of binding sites available for calcium ions which has been seen in an acid medium (C. Rossi *et al.*, 1967) complicates the uncoupling of oxidative phosphorylation by calcium ions, but at the same time provides support for the finding of Engel (1966) that platelet respiration is maintained for a considerably longer period in a weakly acid range.

It is still obscure at this time whether the *primary action of thrombin* on the release of aggregation proceeds via liberation of ADP (R. J. Haslam, 1964), the presence of cationic polypeptides inhibiting the membrane ATP-ase (Schwartz, 1965; Epstein and Whittam, 1966; Yoshida *et al.*, 1965), an inhibition of the oxygen consumption due to protein absorption at specific binding sites of the platelet surface, or whether thrombin effects a release of calcium-containing peptides (Manery, 1968). The fact that the aggregation reaction released by cationic polypeptides does not require any further cofactors (Brossmer and Pfleiderer, 1966; T. Pfleiderer and Brossmer, 1967; Schneider *et al.*, 1968b) might serve to emphasize its fundamental importance. It is interesting to note in this context that when investigating the uncoupling of oxidative phosphorylation increasing attention has most recently focused on the proteins and their conformational changes (Weinbach and Garbus, 1969). The ability to release aggregation by various processes points to all possibilities which may induce increased uptake of calcium ions via loss of potassium. It would thus appear that oxidative phosphorylation is acquiring increasing significance for the study of aggregation (refer to Lasch, 1961).

The *processes involving the uptake of sodium ions and magnesium ions* are intimately related with the potassium and calcium ion cationic transport sketched above (Pullman and Schatz, 1967; Albers, 1967). With respect to thrombocytes it is important to note that all processes involving loss of potassium simultaneously cause an increase in sodium which in turn decisively influences the changes in volume occurring under exposure to cold or under the action of EDTA (Albers, 1967). This transport of sodium presumably is dependent on ATP, but not on the oxidative metabolism and consequently not on the mitochondrial content of a cell. Seen in broad perspective, the uptake of monovalent and divalent cations seems to be subject to competitive inhibition according to the number of binding sites available.

4. Anionic Permeability, Citrate Cycle, and Gluconeogenesis

Study of the anionic permeability of varying biological and synthetic phospholipoid membranes (Eccles, 1964) has evidenced that the membranes are permeable to anions with a hydratational diameter smaller than 2.9 Å. This is, however, not true in the case of mitochondrial membranes (possibly due to the different generation of the membranes, particularly of the inner membrane, in the course of autonomic, mitochondrial protein synthesis). It appears that the presence of malate is required both for the introduction of tricarboxylic acids into the mitochondria and for their metabolic conversion (Chappel and Haarhoff, 1967), while fumarate and oxalacetate virtually may not pass the mitochondrial membrane (Lardy et al., 1965; Haynes, 1965; J. M. Haslam and Krebs, 1968). As far as human thrombocytes are concerned, it has been possible to demontrate an increased incorporation of ^{32}P-orthophosphate into phosphatide fractions in the presence of malate, citrate, and succinate. It was seen that uptake of phosphate was severely inhibited by malonate and that it is thus dependent on the citrate cycle and again on the oxidative metabolism (Grossman and Bartos, 1968).

It is of significance to note that besides citrate, large amounts of malate are also detectable in the thrombocytes (Detwiler, 1969). In the case of citrate Karpatkin (1967) had established that it may be metabolized as a substrate in the Krebs cycle and will lead to the *resynthesis of ATP by the oxidative route*. This finding came as a surprise in that major attention had previously focused on the glycolytic energy metabolism in platelets (Waller et al., 1959; Bettex-Galland and Lüscher, 1960; Chernyak, 1965; Cooley and Cohen, 1967a); Waller et al. (1959) had called attention, however, to the involvement of the citrate cycle; in contrast to various other workers

(Bettex-Galland and Lüscher, 1960) they also stressed the efficacy of oxidative metabolic inhibitors (Löhr et al., 1961a, b) and determined the most important enzyme activities of the citrate cycle (Waller et al., 1959; Löhr et al., 1961a, b). It has been seen that in a number of instances the enzyme activities effective in glycolysis are higher than those of the mitochondrial metabolism, an observation that was equally confirmed by the assays for activity conducted by Goebbell et al. (1968). Before drawing any conclusions from these enzyme capacities assayed in vitro under optimal substrate conditions about the significance of the different metabolic pathways in thrombocytes, it should be considered that frequently only fractions of the available capacities are utilized (see p. 127). A comparison of cytoplasmic and mitochondrial enzyme capacities should also take into account that the glycolytic enzymes, which are freely dissolved in the cytoplasm or accumulate in a few instances as aggregates, require essentially higher activities for attaining identical conversion rates than the mitochondrial enzymes, which are structurally organized in an optimal (lipid) medium to form functional units. For the latter group it has been seen that in most cases an entire metabolic segment is available in a morphologically tightly assembled structural unit. This ensures that very short reaction times may be attained at minimal substrate concentrations. In view of the alignment resulting from such structural functional units, the enzymes of such a metabolic pathway are also referred to as "vectorial" enzymes (Criddle et al., 1962; Green and Fleischer, 1963; Green, 1964; Pette, 1966). It will be understood from these indications that the in vitro enzyme capacity of a mitochondrial vectorial enzyme released from its structural assembly may apparently be lower than would correspond to its conversion rate in vivo. There is thus no justification to conclude from a mere comparison of the in vitro activities to a prevalence of the glycolytic metabolic pathways in blood platelets.

The fact that many enzyme activities encompass the individual activities of varying isoenzymes with different kinetic properties constitutes another aspect appreciably complicating the assessment of simple enzyme capacities. It should be considered in this connection that the different isoenzymes may be located in various cell compartments thus interacting only by way of membrane processes. Malate dehydrogenase is a representative enzyme of this group. Previous studies in other types of cells have revealed that its intracellular overall activity includes two isoenzymes, one of them being assigned to the cytoplasmic and the other one to the mitochondrial cellular compartment (Delbrück et al., 1959a,b; Thorne, 1960; Siegel and Englard, 1961; Englard and Breiger, 1962; Thorne et al., 1963; Neumeister et al.,

1965; Kitto and Kaplan, 1966; Blonde *et al.*, 1967; Kitto and Lewis, 1967; Pette, 1968; and various other authors). When determining the enzyme activities within the thrombocytes, it was noted that the overall activity of the malate dehydrogenase (compared with the activities of the other enzymes of the citrate cycle) is particularly high (Waller *et al.*, 1959; Goebell *et al.*, 1968). A comparison of the malate dehydrogenase activity of a platelet homogenate obtained by mechanical cytolysis in which the cellular organelles are still essentially intact, with the much higher activity of a homogenate prepared by multiple freezing of the cytolysate already suggested a partially particular location of the enzyme. In this determination the particle-bound portion of the total activity is not assayed in the noncytolyzed cellular organelles because of the impermeability of the membrane to oxalacetate as substrate, while in the frozen cytolysate the full activity may be detected. Using DEAE cellulose exchange chromatography the presence of two distinctly isolated isoenzymes of the malate dehydrogenase was successfully demonstrated (Schneider and Schumacher, 1969). Under the experimental conditions employed, one isoenzyme appeared as a cationic protein in the effluent and accounted for about one third of the overall activity, while the activity of the second isoenzyme was eluted only after having increased the ionic strength. By purifying the activity of the cationic isoenzyme in the mitochondria-containing fraction and appropriately increasing the activity of the anionic isoenzyme in the cytoplasmic supernatant we could provide conclusive evidence, which was further supplemented by a comparison with the properties of isoenzymes from other cells, that the cationic isoenzyme represents the mitochondrial, and the anionic isoenzyme the cytoplasmic isoenzyme. The two isoenzymes differ characteristically in their kinetic properties; while the mitochondrial isoenzyme shows a distinctly higher affinity to oxalacetate as substrate, no significant differences were found to exist with regard to malate as substrate. The inhibitory behavior of the two isoenzymes caused by higher substrate concentrations was shown to be particularly typical. After having exceeded an optimal substrate concentration (oxaloacetate being used as substrate), the mitochondrial isoenzyme showed rapidly increasing inhibition, while the cytoplasmic isoenzyme was seen to remain uninfluenced even at very high oxaloacetate concentrations. When using malate as a substrate, the effects observed were reversed: The mitochondrial isoenzyme was slightly influenced even at high concentrations, while the cytoplasmic isoenzyme was markedly inhibited at increasing substrate concentrations. From studies in other cells, it was seen that the malate dehydrogenase isoenzymes located in the cytoplasmic and mitochondrial compartment are of great significance as regards the distribution of reduction equivalents and carbon chains between the cytoplasmic and mitochondrial compartment across the mitochondrial membrane (Greville, 1966; Krebs, 1967; J. M. Haslam and Krebs, 1968; McElroy et al., 1968).

Malate dehydrogenase isoenzymes thus form part of a control system that is a significant factor in determining whether the glycolytic degradation products are metabolized oxidatively in the direction of an optimal energy yield in the form of ATP, or whether, after having returned as malate to the cytoplasmic compartment, they enter into the *glyconeogenesis* by way of oxaloacetate and phosphoenolpyruvate.

On the other hand, the fact that the malate content within the thrombocytes is relatively high (Detwiler, 1969), while the overall activity of the malate dehydrogenase equally is very high (Waller et al., 1959; Löhr et al., 1961a, b; Goebell et al. (1968) would appear to offer support for the hypothesis that this metabolic pathway is of great importance also in the thrombocyte. But its true significance will only be grasped when considering the particularly high ATP content of the thrombocytes (Born, 1956; Born and Esnouf, 1959; Waller et al., 1959; Bettex-Galland and Lüscher, 1960; Löhr et al., 1961a, b; Schmitz et al., 1962; Detwiler et al., 1962; Holmsen, 1967; Pitney et al., 1968; Moser et al., 1968; Gross and Schneider, 1968). As has been pointed out by Hathaway and Atkinson (1965), a high ATP content will, however, effect an inhibition of the citrate synthase, which is a key enzyme in the citrate cycle, catalyzing, in the presence of acetyl-CoA and oxaloacetate, the formation of citrate. There will be a resultant accumulation of acetyl-CoA which, on the one hand, inhibits the oxidative decarboxylation of pyruvate (Garland and Randle, 1964), and on the other hand, stimulates the carboxylation of pyruvate to oxaloacetate (Krebs et al., 1965). In this way there will be an increased formation of oxaloacetate which cannot be metabolized any further, due to blocking of the citrate synthase in the citrate cycle. On the other hand, it cannot be released from the mitochondria, owing to the impermeability of the membrane to oxaloacetate (Lardy et al., 1965; Haynes, 1965; J. M. Haslam and Krebs, 1968). After nicotinamide adenine dinucleotide dependent reduction to malate, it can pervade the mitochondrial membrane in this form and is reconverted to oxaloacetate in the cytoplasm by the action of the cytoplasmic malate dehydrogenase isoenzyme to be subsequently channeled via phosphoenolpyruvate into the glyconeogenesis. It is envisaged that in this way the height of the ATP level in thrombocytes might regulate, via an alternate blocking of the citrate synthase, the transition from the glycolytic to the oxidative metabolic pathway and/or from glycolysis to neoglucogenesis, certain segments of the citrate cycle within the mitochondrion serving as intermediate links. In this process the malate dehydrogenase isoenzymes would be assigned the important function of serving as a *compensatory mechanism for the carbon chains and reduction equivalents* between the mitochondrial and the cytoplasmic compartment if the oxidative metabolism is essentially braked by the high ATP content of the platelets (Schneider and Schumacher, 1969). The metabolic flow would be directed toward gluconeogenesis resulting in a continuous synthesis of glycogen within the resting thrombocytes, as could be experimentally verified (Scott, 1967). The importance of this intramitochondrial segment for the glycogen synthesis might be illustrated by the fact that the mitochondria-free erythrocyte shows virtually no glycogen synthesis (Rapoport, 1968a,b).

The existence of such a regulatory mechanism might explain why increasing significance is finally being attached, though hesitantly, to the oxidative metabolism in the thrombocyte after many years of intensive studies. Due to the high ATP content, the oxidative metabolic routes of the thrombocyte are essentially blocked at rest and the metabolic flow is consequently channeled into the gluconeogenesis cycle after having passed through glycolysis and the oxaloacetate–malate segment of the Krebs cycle. This has been demonstrated by the findings of Seitz (1965) who, after incubation of thrombocytes in u-^{14}C-glucose, observed only 6–10% of the expected CO_2 formation when compared with the oxygen taken up. Instead, the platelet glycogen content showed a rapid increase in labeling substance. It is emphasized by Seitz (1965) that this glycogen synthesis was seen to take place approximately to the same degree both under aerobic and anaerobic conditions. It might be postulated that under aerobic conditions a favorable effect is exerted on the glycogen synthesis which would operate in the described manner via inhibition of the citrate synthase due to a high ATP content in the thrombocyte and resultant accumulation of oxaloacetate; on anaerobic incubation the same effect would be achieved by stimulation of glycolysis due to the Pasteur effect (Wu *et al.*, 1964; Chernyak, 1965) leading via an increased formation of lactate to a sufficiently pronounced negativation of the cellular redox potential to favor the reductive carboxylation of pyruvate.

In the same way the findings of Warshaw *et al.* (1966) confirmed the availability of a vigorous gluconeogenesis. Using 1-^{14}C-glucose and 6-^{14}C-glucose these workers investigated the action of thrombin on glucose oxidation in human platelets via the generation of $^{14}CO_2$. Pertinent details of their findings have been discussed in detail on p. 140. In this context it is considered significant that under the action of thrombin blocking of the oxidative metabolism (Bettex-Galland and Lüscher, 1960; Warshaw *et al.*, 1966; Gross and Schneider, 1968) causes a stimulation of glucose oxidation and lactate formation in the direction of a Pasteur effect. Since the oxidation rate diminishes simultaneously, as is evidenced by the decreasing utilization of pyruvate (Warshaw *et al.*, 1966), a displacement of the cellular redox potential due to increased lactate formation with a favoring of gluco-neogenesis is obtained. Simultaneous blocking of the adenylate cyclase in human platelets due to the action of thrombin which has been shown to occur by recent investigations (Zieve and Greenough, 1969) and which probably causes an additional increase in the net synthesis of glycogen might promote the above process. It is well conceivable that the increase in glucose oxidation described by Warshaw *et al.* (1966) might be obtained over a period of 30 minutes, proceeding by way of a thrombin-induced fall in ATP (Zieve *et al.* (1964) and a concomitant decrease of the thrombin-induced adenylate cyclase inhibition. Due to the preceding vigorous glycogen synthesis with labeled glycogen (Seitz, 1965), the formation of labeled CO_2 increases during the ensuing glycogenolysis. Since in the meantime the fall in ATP has relieved the inhibition of the citrate synthase, the lactate accumulation observed over the initial 30 minutes will decline slowly. The observation by Warshaw *et al.* (1966) that stimulation of glucose oxidation does not recede, although the protein synthesis has been blocked by puromycin, might be due to the fact that the blocking effect of puromycin on the protein synthesis also extends to phosphodiesterase (Butcher and Sutherland, 1962) which normally inhibits in turn the previously stimulated glycogenolysis.

The apparently highly active gluconeogenesis within the thrombocyte that has been demonstrated by the described findings is presumed to be highly significant for retraction and would appear to represent the only energy reserve still available at this point of the hemostatic mechanism, provided our hypothesis postulating an uncoupling of oxidative phosphory-lation by intramitochondrial calcium ion uptake should prove to be correct. By the same token such an interpretation would explain the divergent findings which point to a dependence of retraction on the glycolytic metabolism, on the one hand, (Bettex-Galland and Lüscher, 1960; Löhr *et al.*, 1961; Mürer, 1968), and on the oxidative ATP supply, on the other (Schneider and Niemeyer, 1968), since in the latter case blocking of the oxidative metabolism will produce a simultaneous inhibition of gluconeogenesis and thus a reduction of the glycogen stores, resulting in a secondary impairment of retraction.

5. Mitochondrial Syntheses

Various properties resulting from the mitochondrial content of the platelets decisively influence their energy metabolism. They include the *fatty acid synthesis* which depends on the availability of nicotinamide adenine dinucleotide phosphate and hence is interrelated with the pentose–phosphate shunt (see p. 139).

Another synthesis that has been properly appreciated only during the last few years is *protein synthesis* in the thrombocytes. On account of its high energy demand it seems to be basically dependent on the oxidative metabolism and thus also appears to be essentially linked with the presence of mitochondria within the cell. This dependence is exemplified by the mature erythrocyte which toward the end of the hemoglobin synthesis also loses its mitochondria (Rapoport, 1968a). By contrast, thrombocytes retain their mitochondria and even if they did not appear to be capable of performing the protein synthesis due to the absence of a nucleus, Luganova *et al.* (1958) and Seitz (1965) were successful in demonstrating the incorporation of a small amount of radioactivity into a fraction which could be precipitated by trichloroacetic acid, when incubating platelets in u-^{14}C-glucose. Following up this observation, it was found by Warshaw *et al.* (1966, 1967) that platelets are capable of incorporating labeled leucine into material which could be precipitated by trichloroacetic acid. It can be degraded by proteolytic enzymes, but not by desoxyribonuclease or ribonuclease. In the acidified hydrolysate of this product leucine could be demonstrated by means of chromatography. In contrast to actinomycin D, puromycin inhibits the incorporation of leucine. Booyse and Rafelson (1967a, b) arrived at the same conclusions; they established in addition that as much as 20–37% participate in the synthesis of the contractile platelet protein (Booyse and Rafelson, 1968). Protein synthesis in the platelets may proceed if the following requirements are fulfilled: presence of numerous amino acid (Gerok and Gross, 1959; Gross and Gerok, 1961); amino acid incorporation from the surrounding medium into the platelets (Cooper and Firkin, 1968); ability to accept certain amino acids actively against a concentration gradient from the surrounding medium [a process which apparently is specifically dependent on the oxidative metabolism, as is shown by its susceptibility to inhibition by cyanide and dinitrophenol (Zieve and Solomon, 1968)]; and availability of ribosomes (Porter and Bonneville, 1963; Booyse *et al.*, 1968). The availability of peptidases (Kocholaty, 1962; Balogh, 1963) and protease activity may perhaps be contributing factors (Nachman and Ferris, 1968). The protein synthesis in the thrombocytes is, however, primarily dependent on ATP and an ATP-regenerating system, and in a cell-free medium requires additionally a soluble enzyme system (Booyse and Rafelson, 1968). This enzyme system, however, apparently loses some of its activity on aging of the platelets and might thus limit the life-span of the platelets by producing a fall in the contractile protein synthesis and of structural protein (Steiner and Baldini, 1969). It was seen, however, that the adhesion capacity of ^{51}Cr-labeled platelets is not impaired on glass (Rolovic and Baldini, 1969).

DNA could not be reliably demonstrated in platelets (Maupin and Gineste, 1968), but the presence of DNase has been described (Connolly et al., 1962). A coding of the proteins regenerated in the platelets by a particularly stable RNA having a life of several days is therefore assumed (Booyse and Rafelson, 1967a).

The protein synthesis which has been shown to proceed in the platelets is of particular interest with respect to the presence of mitochondria. The properties thus observed most strikingly resemble the autonomous mitochondrial protein synthesis demonstrated in other cells (for a review, refer to Wagner, 1969). It depends on the presence of autonomous, mitochondrial DNA and RNA which are characterized by a high degree of stability and are confined to the synthesis of only a few peptide sequences belonging to the structural protein (Gibor and Granick, 1964; Granick and Gibor, 1967; Wagner, 1969; Bielka, 1969). It has thus been possible to demonstrate mitochondrial DNA in various cells with a particularly high mitochondrial content (Corneo et al., 1968). The substance appears to be present in all plant and animal mitochondria described to date (Nass et al., 1965). They account, however, for not more than 15% of the RNA located in these cellular organelles (Bielka, 1969); considering the low mitochondrial content of the thrombocytes, mitochondrial DNA would appear to be below the demonstrable limit (Booyse and Rafelson, 1968). As mitochondria are present in the platelet, a mitochondrial DNA, and thus a mitochondrial protein synthesis, have to be assumed for the thrombocyte. The finding of Seitz (1965) who when incubating thrombocytes in a u-^{14}C-glucose-containing medium recovered radioactivity not only in the platelet protein, but also detected an almost identical portion in the RNA formed, provides support for this theory. It does, however, not fit in with the observation of Warshaw et al. (1967) and Booyse and Rafelson (1967a) who observed no blocking of the protein synthesis in the thrombocytes by actinomycin D. But even in the absence of DNA, it might still be envisaged that a protein synthesis dependent on a stable mitochondrial RNA proceeds in the thrombocyte.

However, from the assumption of a mitochondrial protein synthesis a fascinating relationship between a small number of mitochondria, on the one hand, and a very high content of contractile protein in the thrombocytes, on the other hand, might emerge. Since the autonomous protein synthesis of the mitochondria is restricted to a few structural proteins (Zahler *et al.*, 1968; Wagner, 1969), while most of the soluble mitochondrial proteins are coded within the cellular nucleus, formed in the cytoplasm and have to migrate into the newly forming mitochondria (Wagner, 1969), the resynthesis of intact mitochondria occurring in other cells cannot reasonably be envisaged to take place in the thrombocytes in the absence of a nucleus. Instead, it might be assumed that due to the lack of a nucleus the absence of a controlling system and repression of the protein synthesis might account for the unusually high content of contractile structural protein. A similar process is found to occur in yeast cultured under anaerobic conditions, where structures in the form of "promitochondria" are obtained. These are composed of structural protein and mitochondrial DNA and are synthesized to typical mitochondria only on transition to the aerobic phase (Schatz, 1965). The possibility of a *mitochondrial genesis of the contractile platelet protein* receives further support from the demonstration of a contractile, actomyosinlike protein with ATPase activity from other mitochondria (Ohnishi and Ohnishi, 1962; Neifakh and Kazakova, 1963). Beyond this, Kalf and Grece (1964) demonstrated that isolated lambs' heart mitochondria incorporate labeled amino acids into a specific protein which can be isolated from the mitochondria with 0.6 M KCl and which shows the properties of a contractile protein. The contractile protein of the platelets is isolated under quite similar conditions (Bettex-Galland and Lüscher, 1959). It is now conceivable that in view of its slight solubility this structural protein might deposit in the thrombocytes in the form of microtubuli or microfibrils (Behnke, 1965; Behnke and Zelander, 1967; White, 1967, 1968c, e; Zucker-Franklin, 1969). The mitochondrial genesis of the microfibrils and microtubules is again supported by the demonstration of such structures in nucleated erythrocytes which thus also contain mitochondria (Fawcett, 1959, 1962; Fawcett and Witebsky, 1964; Maser and Philpott, 1964).

The unusually high content of structural protein which could be of importance for all functions (White, 1967, 1968b, d) in the platelets (Bettex-Galland and Lüscher, 1961; Grette, 1962) might therefore be attributable to the quite unusual feature of platelets of *possessing mitochondria, but no cell nucleus.* Contractile properties and formation of complexes with nucleotides have also been demonstrated for the mitochondrial structural proteins in other cells (Zahler *et al.*, 1968) and might provide a basis for all adhesion and aggregation processes (B. M. Jones, 1966; P. C. T. Jones, 1966).

III. CONCLUSIONS

The demonstration of high enzyme capacities involved in the glycolytic metabolic pathway (Waller *et al.*, 1959), active formation of lactate (Waller *et al.*, 1959); Bettex-Galland and Lüscher, 1960; Chernyak, 1965; Karpatkin and Langer, 1968; Löhr, 1968; Ohler, 1968), and the pronounced action of substances inhibiting the glycolytic metabolic cycle have led investigators of platelet metabolism until very recently to focus their main interest on the significance of glycolysis within the platelet metabolism. The biochemical knowledge elucidated during recent years, extending mainly to metabolic regulation of enzyme capacities in the metabolic sequences, compartmentation of cellular metabolism, and functional co-ordination of the individual compartments, and quite particularly the newly derived concepts of the structure- and function-dependent control of the mitochondrial metabolism and its significance for other cellular segments, has helped to bring about a gradual change. In view of the above decisive preliminaries and the increasing knowledge of syntheses proceeding in the thrombocytes (such as the protein synthesis, fatty acid synthesis and glycogen synthesis), the new aspects of metabolic compartmentation and of control and coordination as a function of the mitochondrial compartment in the platelets have now increasingly come to the forefront of current re-search. The existing differences relating especially to metabolic events at rest might be explained by the unusual feature found in human platelets of possessing mitochondria, but no nucleus. It seems that respiration—an apparently significant factor in human platelet metabolism—still seems to be capable of regulating the other metabolic sequences and to provide the basis for the various syntheses. Respiration thus acquires increasing sig-nificance also for platelets in that it supplies the required energy in the form of ATP, while glycolysis at least in part seems to exercise the functions of making available oxidizable substrates and of supplying carbon structures for the individual syntheses.

REFERENCES

Abood, L. G. (1966). *Int. Rev. Neurobiol.* **9**, 223.
Ahmed, K., and Judah, J. D. (1965). *Biochim. Biophys. Acta* **104**, 112.
Ahmed, K., Judah, J. D., and Gallagher, C. H. (1961). *Nature* **191**, 1309.
Albers, R. W. (1967). *Annu. Rev. Biochem.* **35**, 727.
Aledort, L. M., and Niemetz, J. (1968). *Proc. Soc. Exp. Biol. Med.* **128**, 658.
Ashford, T. P., Salzman, E. W., Chambers, D. A., and Neri, L. L. (1967). *Blood* **30**, 540.
Aster, R. H., and Jandl, J. H. (1964). *J. Clin. Invest.* **43**, 843.

Aynaud, M. (1909). Thesis, Paris.

Aynaud, M. (1911). *Ann. Inst. Pasteur, Paris* **25**, 56.

Balogh, K. (1963). *Nature* **199**, 1196.

Beatty, C. H., Peterson, R. D., Basinger, C. M., and Boeck, R. M. (1966). *Amer. J. Physiol.* **210**, 404.

Beck, W. S. (1958). *J. Biol. Chem.* **232**, 251.

Behnke, O. (1965). *J. Ultrastruct. Res.* **13**, 469.

Behnke, O. (1967a). *J. Cell Biol.* **34**, 697.

Behnke, O. (1967b). *J. Ultrastruct. Res.* **19**, 147.

Behnke, O., and Zelander, T. (1967). *J. Ultrastruct. Res.* **19**, 147.

Bettex-Galland, M., and Lüscher, E. F. (1959). *Nature* **184**, 276.

Bettex-Galland, M., and Lüscher, E. F. (1960). *Thromb. Diath. Haemorrh.* **4**, 178.

Bettex-Galland, M., and Lüscher, E. F. (1961). *Biochim. Biophys. Acta* **49**, 536.

Bezkorovainy, A., and Rafelson, M. E. (1964). *J. Lab. Clin. Med.* **64**, 212.

Bielawski, J., Thompson, T. E., and Lehninger, A. L. (1966). *Biochem. Biophys. Res. Commun.* **24**, 948.

Bielka, H. (1969). "Molekulare Biologie der Zelle." Fischer, Stuttgart.

Blonde, D. J., Kresack, E. J., and Kosicki, G. W. (1967). *Can. J. Biochem.* **45**, 641.

Booyse, F. M., and Rafelson, M. E. (1967a). *Biochim. Biophys. Acta* **145**, 188.

Booyse, F., and Rafelson, M. E. (1967b). *Nature* **215**, 283.

Booyse, F. M., and Rafelson, M. E. (1968). *Biochim. Biophys. Acta* **166**, 689.

Booyse, F. M., Hoveke, T. P., and Rafelson, M. E. (1968). *Biochim. Biophys. Acta* **157**, 660.

Born, G. V. R. (1956). *Biochem. J.* **62**, 33.

Born, G. V. R. (1968). *Plen. Sess. Pap., 12th Congr. Int. Soc. Hematol.*, 1968, p. 95.

Born, G. V. R., and Cross, M. J. (1964). *J. Physiol. (London)* **170**, 397.

Born, G. V. R., and Esnouf, M. P. (1959). *Proc. 4th Int. Congr. Biochem.*, 1958, p. 97. Pergamon Press, New York.

Brierley, G. P., and Slauterback, D. B. (1964). *Biochim. Biophys. Acta* **82**, 183.

Brossmer, R., and Patscheke, H. (1968). *In* "Stoffwechsel und Membranpermeabilität von Erythrozyten und Thrombozyten" (E. Deutsch, E. Gerlach, and K. Moser, eds.), p. 215. Thieme, Stuttgart.

Brossmer, R., and Pfleiderer, T. (1966). *Naturwissenschaften* **53**, 464.

Buckingham, S., and Maynert, E. W. (1964). *J. Pharmacol. Exp. Ther.* **143**, 332.

Bull, B. S., and Zucker, M. B. (1965). *Proc. Soc. Exp. Biol. Med.* **120**, 296.

Burnett, G., and Kennedy, E. P. (1954). *J. Biol. Chem.* **211**, 969.

Butcher, R. W., and Sutherland, E. W. (1962). *J. Biol. Chem.* **237**, 1244.

Cahn, R. D., Kaplan, N. O., Levine, L., and Zwilling, E. (1962). *Science* **136**, 962.

Campbell, E. W., Small, W. J., and Dameshek, W. (1956). *J. Lab. Clin. Med.* **47**, 835.

Campbell, E. W., Small, W. J., Lo Pilato, E., and Dameshek, W. (1957). *Proc. Soc. Exp. Biol. Med.* **94**, 505.

Caputto, R., Barra, H. S., and Cumar, F. A. (1967). *Annu. Rev. Biochem.* **36**, 211.

Carafoli, E., and Rossi, C. S. (1967). *Biochem Biophys. Res. Commun.* **29**, 153.

Carafoli, E., Rossi, C. S., and Lehninger, A. L. (1965). *J. Biol. Chem.* **240**, 2254.

Chambers, D. A., Salzman, E. W., and Neri, L. L. (1967). *Arch. Biochem. Biophys.* **119**, 173.

Chambers, D. A., Salzman, E. W., and Neri, L. L. (1968). *Exp. Biol. Med.* **3**, 62.

Chance, B. (1965). *J. Biol. Chem.* **240**, 2729.

Chappel, J. B., and Haarhoff, K. N. (1967). *In* "Biochemistry of Mitochondria" (E. C. Slater, Z. Kaniuga, and L. Wojtczak, eds.), p. 75. Academic Press, New York.

Chappel, J. B., Cohn, M., and Greille, G. D. (1963). *In* "Energy-linked Functions of Mitochondria" (B. Chance, ed.), p. 219. Academic Press, New York.

Chernyak, N. B. (1965). *Clin. Chim. Acta* **12**, 244.

Chernyak, N. B., and Guseinov, C. S. (1960). *Dokl. Akad. Nauk SSSR* **133**, 476.

Chernyak, N. B., and Timofeyeva, L. M. (1968). *In* "Stoffwechsel und Membranpermeabilitat von Erythrozyten und Thrombozyten" (E. Deutsch, E. Gerlach, and K. Moser, eds.), p. 239. Thieme, Stuttgart.

Chernyak, N. B., and Totskaya, A. A. (1963). *Fed. Proc., Fed. Amer. Soc. Exp. Biol.* Suppl. 23, T326.

Chernyak, N. B., Svensitskaya, M. B., and Guseinov, C. S. (1960a). *Byull. Eksp. Biol. Med.* **49**, 251.

Chernyak, N. B., Svensitskaya, M. B., and Guseinov, C. S. (1960b). *Probl. Gematol. Pereliv. Krovi* **9**, 39.

Cohen, L., and Larson, L. (1966). *N. Engl. J. Med.* **275**, 465.

Connolly, J. H., Herriott, R. M., and Gupta, S. (1962). *Brit. J. Exp. Pathol.* **43**, 392.

Cooley, M. H., and Cohen, P. (1967a). *J. Lab. Clin. Med.* **70**, 69.

Cooley, M. H., and Cohen, P. (1967b). *Arch. Intern. Med.* **119**, 345.

Cooper, I. A., and Firkin, B. G. (1968). *Abstr. 12th Congr. Int. Soc. Hematol.*, 1968, p. 201, Art. ZZ-3.

Cori, C. F., Cori, G. T., and Green, A. A. (1943). *J. Biol. Chem.* **151**, 39.

Corn, M. (1966). *J. Appl. Physiol.* **21**, 62.

Corn, M., Jackson, D. P., and Conley, C. L. (1960). *Bull. Johns Hopkins Hosp.* **107**, 90.

Corneo, G., Zardi, L., and Polli, E. (1968). *J. Mol. Biol.* **36**, 419.

Criddle, R. S., Bock, R. M., Green, D. E., and Tisdale, H. (1962). *Biochemistry* **1**, 827.

Da Prada, M., Tranzer, J. P., and Pletscher, A. (1967). *J. Pharmacol. Exp. Ther.* **158**, 394.

Dastague, P., Bastide, P., and Plat, M. (1966). *Nouv. Rev. Fr. Hematol.* **6**, 265.

Dawson, D. H., Goodfriend, T. L., and Kaplan, N. O. (1964). *Science* **143**, 929.

Delbrück, A., Zebe, E., and Bucher, T. (1959a). *Biochem. Z.* **331**, 273.

Delbrück, A., Zebe, E., and Bucher, T. (1959b). *Biochem. Z.* **331**, 297.

De Luca, F. (1964). *Riv. Gastro-Enterol.* **16**, 39.

Detwiler, T. C. (1967). *Arch. Biochem. Biophys.* **120**, 721.

Detwiler, T. C. (1969). *Biochim. Biophys. Acta* **177**, 161.

Detwiler, T. C., Odell, T. T., and McDonald, T. P. (1962). *Amer. J. Physiol.* **203**, 107.

Deutsch, E., and Gerlach, E., and Moser, K. (1968). "Stoffwechsel und Membranpermeabilität von Erythrozyten und Thrombozyten" (E. Deutsch, E. Gerlach, and K. Moser, eds.), Thieme, Stuttgart.

De Vreker, G. G., and De Vreker, R. A. (1965). *Rev. Belge. Pathol. Med. Exp.* **31**, 79.

Doery, J. C. G., Hirsh, J., Garson, O. M., and De Gruchy, G. C. (1968). *Lancet* II, 894.

Eccles, J. C. (1964). "The Physiology of Synapses." Springer, Berlin.

Engel, P. F. (1966). *Acta Physiol. Scand.* **66**, 282.

England, S., and Breiger, H. H. (1962). *Biochim. Biophys. Acta* **56**, 571.

Epstein, F. H., and Whittam, R. (1966). *Biochem. J.* **99**, 232.

Estes, J. W., McGovern, J. J., Goldstein, R., and Rota, M. (1962). *J. Lab. Clin. Med.* **59**, 436.

Fantl, P., and Ward, H. A. (1956). *Biochem. J.* **64**, 747.

Fawcett, D. W. (1959). *Anat. Rec.* **133**, 379.

Fawcett, D. W. (1962). *Circulation* **26**, 1105.

Fawcett, D. W., and Witebsky, F. (1964). *Z. Zellforsch. Mikrosk. Anat.* **62**, 785.

Firkin, B. G., O'Neill, J., Dunstan, B., and Oldfied, R. (1965). *Blood* **25**, 345.

Flatt, J. P., and Ball, E. G. (1964). *J. Biol. Chem.* **239**, 675.

Flatt, J. P., and Ball, E. G. (1966). *J. Biol. Chem.* **241**, 2862.

Foster, J. M., and Terry, M. L. (1967). *Blood* **30**, 168.

Frei, J. (1961). *In* "Biological Activity of the Leukocyte" (G. E. W. Wolstenholme, ed.), p. 86. Little, Brown, Boston, Massachusetts.

Ganguly, P. (1969). *Blood* **34**, 511.

Garland, P. B., and Randle, P. J. (1964). *Biochem. J.* **91**, 60.

Garland, P. B., Randle, P. J., and Newsholme, E. A. (1963). *Nature* **200**, 169.

Gear, A. R. L., and Lehninger, A. L. (1968). *J. Biol. Chem.* **243**, 3953.

Gerok, W., and Gross, R. (1959). *Thromb. Diath. Haemorrh.* **3**, 654.

Gibor, A., and Granick, S. (1964). *Science* **145**, 890.

Goebell, H., Bickel, H., Bode, C., Egbring, R., and Martini, G. A. (1968). *Klin. Wochenschr.* **46**, 526.

Gorstein, F., Carroll, H. J., and Puszkin, E. (1967). *J. Lab. Clin. Med.* **70**, 938.

Granick, A., and Gibor, A. (1967). *Progr. Nucl. Acid Res. Mol. Biol.* **6**, 143.

Green, D. E. (1964). *Sci. Amer.* **210**, 63.

Green, D. E., and Fleischer, S. (1963). *Biochim. Biophys. Acta* **70**, 554.

Greenawalt, J. W., Rossi, C. S., and Lehninger, A. L. (1964). *J. Cell Biol.* **23**, 21.

Grette, K. (1962). *Acta Physiol. Scand.* **56**, Suppl., 195.

Grette, K. (1963). *Nature* **198**, 488.

Greville, G. D. (1966). *In* "Regulation of Metabolic Processes in Mitochondria" (I. M. Tager *et al.*, eds.), p. 86. Elsevier, Amsterdam.

Grignani, F., and Löhr, G. W. (1960). *Klin. Wochenschr.* **38**, 796.

Gross, R. (1961). *In* "Blood Platelets" (S. A. Johnson *et al.*, eds.), p. 407. Little, Brown, Boston, Massachusetts.

Gross, R. (1967). *In* "Platelets: Their Role in Hemostasis and Thrombosis," p. 143. (K. M. Brinkhous *et al.*, eds.). Schattauer, Stuttgart.

Gross, R., and Gerok, W. (1961). *Thromb. Diath. Haemorrh.* **6**, 462.

Gross, R., and Schneider, W. (1968). *In* "Stoffwechsel und Membranpermeabilität von Erythrozyten und Thrombozyten" (E. Deutsch, E. Gerlach, and K. Moser, eds.), p. 206. Thieme, Stuttgart.

Gross, R., Löhr, G. W., and Waller, H. (1967). *In* "Biochemistry of Blood Platelets" (F. Kowalski and S. Niewiarowski, eds.), p. 81. Academic Press, New York.

Grossman, C. M., and Bartos, F. (1968). *Arch. Biochem. Biophys.* **128**, 231.

Gurban, C., and Cristea, E. (1965). *Biochim. Biophys. Acta* **96**, 195.

Haslam, J. M., and Griffiths, D. E. (1968). *Biochem. J.* **109**, 921.

Haslam, J. M., and Krebs, H. A. (1968). *Biochem. J.* **107**, 659.

Haslam, R. J. (1964). *Nature* **202**, 765.

Haslam, R. J. (1967). *In* "Physiology of Hemostasis and Thrombosis" (S. A. Johnson and W. H. Seegers, eds.), p. 88. Thomas, Springfield, Illinois.

Haslam, R. J. (1968). *Plen. Sess. Pap., 12th Congr. Int. Soc. Hematol.*, 1968, p. 198.

Hathaway, J. A., and Atkinson, D. E. (1965). *Biochem. Biophys. Res. Commun.* **20**, 661.

Haugaard, N., Lee, N. H., Kostrzewa, R., and Horn, R. S. (1969). *Biochim. Biophys. Acta* **172**, 198.

Haynes, R. C. (1965). *J. Biol. Chem.* **240**, 4103.

Heldt, H. W., and Klingenberg, M. (1968). *Eur. J. Biochem.* **4**, 1.

Hellem, A. J. (1967). *In* "Platelets: Their Role in Hemostasis and Thrombosis," p. 193. (K. M. Brinkhous *et al.*, eds.). Schattauer, Stuttgart.

Hollard, D., and Servoz-Gavin, M. (1964). *Rev. Fr. Etud. Clin. Biol.* **9**, 1078.

Holmsen, H. (1965). *Scand. J. Clin. Lab. Invest.* **17**, 230.

Holmsen, H. (1967). *In* "Biochemistry of Blood Platelets" (F. Kowalski and S. Niewiarowski, eds.), p. 81. Academic Press, New York.

Holmsen, H., and Rozenberg, M. C. (1968a). *Biochim. Biophys. Acta* **155**, 326.

Holmsen, H., and Rozenberg, M. C. (1968b). *Biochim. Biophys. Acta* **157**, 266.

Hule, V. (1966). *Clin. Chim. Acta* **13**, 431.

Hussain, Q. Z., and Newcomb, T. F. (1964). *J. Appl. Physiol.* **19**, 297.

Ibsen, K. H., and Fox, J. P. (1965). *Arch. Biochem. Biophys.* **112**, 580.

Ireland, D. M. (1967). *Biochem. J.* **105**, 857.

Iyer, G. Y. N., Islam, D. M. F., and Quastel, J. H. (1961). *Nature* **192**, 535.

Jones, B. M. (1966). *Nature* **212**, 362.

Jones, P. C. T. (1966). *Nature* **212**, 362.

Judah, J. D. (1961). *Biochim. Biophys. Acta* **53**, 375.

Kalf, G. F., and Grece, M. A. (1964). *Biochem. Biophys. Res. Commun.* **17**, 674.

Kaplan, N. O., and Ciotti, M. M. (1961). *Ann. N.Y. Acad. Sci.* **94**, 701.

Karpatkin, S. (1967). *J. Clin. Invest.* **46**, 409.

Karpatkin, S., and Langer, R. M. (1968). *J. Clin. Invest.* **47**, 2158.

Karpatkin, S., and Langer, R. M. (1969). *J. Biol. Chem.* **244**, 1953.

Karpatkin, S., and Siskind, G. W. (1967). *Blood* **30**, 617.

Katz, J., Landau, B. R., and Bartsch, G. E. (1966). *J. Biol. Chem.* **241**, 727.

Keitt, S. A. (1966). *Amer. J. Med.* **41**, 762.

Kerby, G. P., and Taylor, S. M. (1967). *J. Lab. Clin. Med.* **69**, 194.

Kim, B. K., and Baldini, M. (1968). *Abstr. 12th Congr. Int. Soc. Hematol.*, 1968, p. 202, Art. ZZ-9.

Kimmich, G. A., and Rasmussen, H. (1967). *Biochim. Biophys. Acta* **131**, 413.

Kitchens, C. S., and Newcomb, T. F. (1968). *J. Appl. Physiol.* **35**, 581.

Kitto, B., and Kaplan, N. O. (1966). *Biochemistry* **5**, 3966.

Kitto, G. B., and Lewis, R. G. (1967). *Biochim. Biophys. Acta* **139**, 1.

Kocholaty, W. (1962). *Thromb. Diath. Haemorrh.* **7**, 295.

Koketsu, K. (1965). *Perspect. Biol. Med.* **9**, 54.

Koppel, J. L., Novak, L. V., and Olwin, J. H. (1959). *Proc. Soc. Exp. Biol. Med.* **100**, 227.

Kowalski, E., Kopec, M., Wegrzynowicz, Z., Hurwic, M., and Budzynski, A. Z. (1966). *Thromb. Diath. Haemorrh.* **16**, 134.

Kowalski, E., Kopec, M., Wegrzynowicz, Z., Hurwic, M., and Budzynski, A. Z. (1967). *In* "Biochemistry of Blood Platelets" (F. Kowalski and S. Niewiarowski, eds.), p. 91. Academic Press, New York.

Krause, E. G. (1969). *In* "Molekulare Biologie der Zelle," p. 203. (H. Bielka ed.). Fischer, Stuttgart.

Krebs, H. A. (1967). *In* "Biochemistry of Mitochondria" (E. C. Slater, Z. Kaninga and L. Wojtcrak, eds.), p. 105. Accademic Press, New York.

Krebs, H. A., Speake, R. N., and Hems, R. (1965). *Biochem. J.* **94**, 712.

Lardy, H. A., Paetkau, V., and Walter, P. (1965). *Proc. Nat. Acad. Sci. U.S.* **53**, 1410.

Lasch, H. G. (1961). *In* "Blood Platelets" (S. A. Johnson *et al.*, eds.), p. 430. Little, Brown, Boston, Massachusetts.

Lee, C. P., and Ernster, L. (1966). *In* "Regulation of Metabolic Processes in Mitochondria" (I. M. Tager *et al.*, eds.), p. 218. Elsevier, Amsterdam.

Lehninger, A. L. (1964). "The Mitochondrion." Benjamin, New York.

Lindy, S., and Rajasalmi, M. (1966). *Science* **153**, 1401.

Linneweh, F., Löhr, G. W., Waller, H. D., and Gross, R. (1963). *Enzymol. Biol. Clin.* **2**, 188.

Livanova, N. B. (1962). *Vop. Med. Khim.* **8**, 429.

Loder, P. B., Hirsh, J., and De Gruchy, G. C. (1968). *Brit. J. Haematol.* **14**, 563.

Löhr, G. W., Waller, H. D., and Gross, R. (1961a). *Deut. Med. Wochenschr.* **86**, 897.

Löhr, G. W., Waller, H. D., and Gross, R. (1961b). *Deut. Med. Wochenschr.* **86**, 946.

Luganova, S., Seitz, I. F., and Teodorovich, V. I. (1958). *Biochemistry (USSR)* **23**, 379.

Lüscher, E. F. (1968). *Schweiz. Med. Wochenschr.* **98**, 1629.

Lüscher, E. F., and Bettex-Galland, B. (1968). *In* "Stoffwechsel und Membranpermeabilität von Erythrozyten und Thrombozyten" (E. Deutsch, E. Gerlach, and K. Moser, eds.), p. 246. Thieme, Stuttgart.

McDonagh, R. P., Burns, M. J., Delaimi, K. E., and Faust, R. G. (1968). *J. Cell Physiol* **72**, 77.

McElroy, F. A., Wong, G. S., and Williams, G. R. (1968). *Arch. Biochem. Biophys.* **128**, 563.

Majerus, P. W., Smith, M. B., and Clamon, G. H. (1969). *J. Clin. Invest.* **48**, 156.

Manery, J. F. (1966). *Fed. Proc., Fed. Amer. Soc. Exp. Biol.* **25**, 1804.

Manery, J. F. (1968). *Exp. Biol. Med.* **3**, 24.

Mann, H., and Krankenhagen, B. (1969). *Pfluegers Arch.* **307**, R1.

Marcus, A. J., and Zucker, M. B. (1966). "The Physiology of Blood Platelets." Grune & Stratton, New York.

Markert, C. L. (1968). *Ann. N.Y. Acad. Sci.* **151**, 14.

Maser, M. D., and Philpott, C. W. (1964). *Anat. Rec.* **150**, 365.

Maupin, B. (1954). *C. R. Soc. Biol.* **148**, 439.

Maupin, B., and Gineste, J. (1968). *Exp. Biol. Med.* **3**, 29.

Melchinger, D., and Nemerson, Y. (1967). *J. Appl. Physiol.* **22**, 197.

Mey, U., and Sundermann, A. (1966). *Folia Haematol. (Leipzig)* **85**, 90.

Mills, D. C. B., and Thomas, D. P. (1969). *Nature* **222**, 991.

Mills, D. C. B., Robbs, I. A., and Roberts, G. C. K. (1968). *J. Physiol. (London)* **195**, 715.

Mizuno, N. S., Sautter, J. H., and Schultze, M. O. (1960). *J. Biol. Chem.* **235**, 2109.

Morse, E. E., Jackson, D. P., and Conley, C. L. (1967). *J. Lab. Clin. Med.* **70**, 106.

Moser, K., Lechner, K., and Vimazzer, H. (1968). *Thromb. Diath. Haemorrh.* **19**, 46.

Mürer, E. H. (1968). *Biochim. Biophys. Acta* **162**, 320.

Mürer, E. H., Hellem, A. J., and Rozenberg, M. C. (1967). *Scand. J. Clin. Lab. Invest.* **19**, 280.

Murphy, S., and Gardner, S. H. (1969). *N. Engl. J. Med.* **280**, 1095.

Nachman, R. L., and Ferris, B. (1968). *J. Clin. Invest.* **47**, 2530.

Nass, M. M. K., Nass, S., and Afzelius, B. A. (1965). *Exp. Cell Res.* **37**, 516.

Neifakh, S. A., and Kazokova, T. B. (1963). *Nature* **197**, 1106.

Neumeister, E., Otto, P., Schmidt, E., and Schmidt, F. W. (1965). *Med. Welt* **27**, 1479.

Niemeyer, G., Reuter, H., and Gross, R. (1967). *Klin. Wochenschr.* **45**, 1142.

Niewiarowski, S., Farbiszewski, R., Poplawski, A., and Lipinski, B. (1968). *In* "Stoffwechsel und Membranpermeabilität von Erythrozyten und Thrombozyten" (E. Deutsch, E. Gerlach, and K. Moser, eds.), p. 314. Thieme, Stuttgart.

Nigam, V. N. (1966). *Biochem. J.* **99**, 413.

Nordøy, A., and Ødegaard, A. E. (1963). *Scand. J. Clin. Lab. Invest.* **15**, 399.

O'Brien, J. R. (1964). *J. Clin. Pathol.* **17**, 275.

O'Brien, J. R., Shoobridge, S. M., and Finch, W. J. (1969). *J. Clin. Pathol.* **22**, 28.

Ohler, W. G. A. (1968). *Klin. Wochenschr.* **46**, 737.

Ohnishi, Tsuyoshi, and Ohnishi, Tomoko (1962). *J. Biochem. (Tokyo)* **51**, 380.

Olsson, I., Dahlqvist, A., and Norden, A. (1963). *Acta Med. Scand.* **174**, 123.

Ozge, A., Baldini, M., and Goldstein, R. (1964). *J. Lab. Clin. Med.* **63**, 378.

Parmeggiani, A., and Bowman, R. H. (1963). *Biochem. Biophys. Res. Commun.* **12**, 268.

Passonneau, J. V., and Lowry, O. H. (1963). *Biochem. Biophys. Res. Commun.* **13**, 372.

Penefsky, H. S., and Warner, R. C. (1965). *J. Biol. Chem.* **250**, 4694.

Pette, D. (1965). *Naturwissenschaften* **52**, 597.

Pette, D. (1966). *In* "Regulation of Metabolic Processes in Mitochondria" (I. M. Tager *et al.*, eds.), p. 28. Elsevier, Amsterdam.

Pette, D. (1968). *In* "Praktische Enzymologie," p. 15. (H. Aebi *et al.*, ed.). Huber, Bern.

Pfleiderer, G., and Wachsmuth, E. D. (1961). *Klin. Wochenschr.* **39**, 352.

Pfleiderer, T., and Brossmer, R. (1967). *Thromb. Diath. Haemorrh.* **18**, 674.

Pitney, W. R., Hinterberger, H., and Potter, M. (1968). *Thromb. Diath. Haemorrh.* **19**, 36.

Porter, K. R., and Bonneville, M. A. (1963). "An Introduction to the Fine Structure of Cells and Tissues." Lea & Febiger, Philadelphia, Pennsylvania.

Pullman, M. E., and Schatz, G. (1967). *Annu. Rev. Biochem.* **36**, 539.

Puszkin, E., and Jerushalmy, Z. (1968). *Proc. Soc. Exp. Biol. Med.* **129**, 346.

Rabinowitz, M., and Lipman, F. (1960). *J. Biol. Chem.* **235**, 1043.

Ramot, B., Szeinberg, A., Adam, A., Sheba, C., and Gafni, D. (1959). *J. Clin. Invest.* **38**, 1659.

Rapoport, S. (1968a). *Folia Haematol. (Leipzig)* **89**, 105.

Rapoport, S. (1968b). *Bibl. Haematol.* **29**, 133.

Rapoport, S., and Jacobasch, G. (1968). *In* "Stoffwechsel und Membranpermeabilität von Erythrozyten und Thrombozyten" (E. Deutsch, E. Gerlach, and K. Moser, eds.), p. 1. Thieme, Stuttgart.

Rasmussen, H. (1966). *Fed. Proc., Fed. Amer. Soc. Exp. Biol.* **25**, 903.

Reuter, H., Niemeyer, G., and Gross, R. (1967). *Klin. Wochenschr.* **15**, 1147.

Riggs, T. R., Walter, L. M., and Christensen, H. N. (1958). *J. Biol. Chem.* **233**, 1479.

Robison, C. W., Kress, S. C., Wagner, R. H., and Brinkhous, K. M. (1965). *Exp. Mol. Pathol.* **4**, 457.

Rock, R. C., and Nemerson, Y. (1969). *J. Lab. Clin. Med.* **73**, 42.

Rolovic, Z., and Baldini, M. G. (1969). *Scand. J. Haematol.* **6**, 25.

Rossi, E. C. (1967a). *J. Lab. Clin. Invest.* **69**, 204.

Rossi, E. C. (1967b). *J. Lab. Clin. Med.* **70**, 1010.

Rossi, E. C. (1968). *Thromb. Diath. Haemorrh.* **19**, 53.

Rossi, C., Azzi, A., and Azzone, G. F. (1967). *J. Biol. Chem.* **242**, 951.

Rossi, C. S., Siliprandi, N., Carafoli, E., Bielawski, J., and Lehninger, A. L. (1967). *Eur. J. Biochem.* **2**, 332.

Rozenberg, M. C., and Holmsen, H. (1968a). *Biochim. Biophys. Acta* **155**, 342.

Rozenberg, M. C., and Holmsen, H. (1968b). *Biochim. Biophys. Acta* **157**, 280.

Rysanek, K., Svehla, C., and Doubravova, J. (1967). *Arch. Nerv. Sup. (Praha)* **9**, 414.

Rysanek, K., Svehla, C., Spankova, H., and Mlejnkova, M. (1969). *Experientia* **25**, 31.

Sallis, J. D., De Luca, H. F., and Rasmussen, H. (1963). *Biochem. Biophys. Res. Commun.* **10**, 266.

Salzman, E. W., and Chambers, D. A. (1964). *Nature* **204**, 698.

Salzman, E. W., and Chambers, D. A. (1965). *Nature* **206**, 727.

Salzman, E. W., Chambers, D. A., and Neri, L. L. (1966a). *Nature* **210**, 167.

Salzman, E. W., Chambers, D. A., and Neri, L. L. (1966b). *Thromb. Diath. Haemorrh.* **15**, 52.

Salzman, E. W., Chambers, D. A., and Neri, L. L. (1967). *Fed. Proc., Fed. Amer. Soc. Exp. Biol.* **26**, 759.

Sbarra, A. J., and Karnovsky, M. L. (1959). *J. Biol. Chem.* **234**, 1355.

Scarpa, A., and Azzi, A. (1968). *Biochim. Biophys. Acta* **150**, 473.

Scarpa, A., and Azzone, G. F. (1968). *J. Biol. Chem.* **243**, 5132.

Schatz, G. (1965). *Biochim. Biophys. Acta* **96**, 342.

Schmitz, H., Schleipen, T., and Gross, R. (1962). *Klin. Wochenschr.* **40**, 13.

Schneider, W. (1969). "Untersuchungen zum Energiestoffwechsel menschlicher Blutplättchen." Habilitationsschrift, Köln.

Schneider, W. (1970). Unpublished findings.

Schneider, W. (1970). To be published.

Schneider, W., and Niemeyer, G. (1968). *In* "Stoffwechsel und Membranpermeabilität von Erythrozyten und Thrombozyten" (E. Deutsch, E. Gerlach, and K. Moser, eds.), p. 254. Thieme, Stuttgart.

Schneider, W., and Schumacher, K. (1969). *Verh. Deut. Ges. Inn. Med.* **75**, 470.

Schneider, W., Schumacher, K., Thiede, B., and Gross, R. (1968a). *Thromb. Diath. Haemorrh.* **20**, 301.

Schneider, W., Kübler, W., and Gross, R. (1968b). *Thromb. Diath. Haemorrh.* **20**, 314.

Schneider, W., Schumacher, K., and Gross, R. (1969). *Thromb. Diath. Haemorrh.* **22**, 208.

Schulz, K., and Dabels, J. (1968). *Klin. Wochenschr.* **46**, 447.

Schumacher, K., Schneider, W., and Gross, R. (1968). *Thromb. Diath. Haemorrh.* **19**, 430.

Schwartz, A. (1965). *Biochim. Biophys. Acta* **100**, 202.

Scott, R. B. (1967). *Blood* **30**, 321.

Seitz, I. F. (1959). *Vop. Med. Khim.* **5**, 714.

Seitz, I. F. (1961). "Interaction of Respiration and Glycolysis in the Cell." Medgiz, Leningrad (in Russian).

Seitz, I. F. (1965). *Advan. Cancer Res.* **9**, 303.

Servoz-Gavin, M., and Hollard, D. (1964). *Nouv. Rev. Fr. Hematol.* **4**, 699.

Settlemire, C. Z., Hunter, G. R., and Brierley, G. P. (1968). *Biochim. Biophys. Acta* **162**, 487.

Siegel, L., and Englard, S. (1961). *Biochim. Biophys. Acta* **54**, 67.

Siliprandi, N., Moret, V., Pinna, L. A., and Lorini, M. (1966). *In* "Regulation of Metabolic Process in Mitochondria" (I. M. Tager *et al.*, eds.), p. 247. Elsevier, Amsterdam.

Silver, M. J. (1965). *Amer. J. Physiol.* **209**, 1128.

Skjorten, F. (1968). *Scand. J. Haematol.* **5**, 401.

Spaet, T. H., and Lejnieks, J. (1966). *Thromb. Diath. Haemorrh.* **15**, 36.

Steiner, M., and Baldini, M. (1969). *Blood* **33**, 628.

Sutherland, E. W., and Robison, G. A. (1966). *Pharmacol. Rev.* **18**, 145.

Thorne, C. J. R. (1960). *Biochim. Biophys. Acta* **42**, 175.

Thorne, C. J. R., Grossman, L. I., and Kaplan, N. O. (1963). *Biochim. Biophys. Acta* **73**, 193.

Tullis, J. L. (1953). "Blood Cells and Plasma Proteins: Their State in Nature". Academic Press, New York.

Uyeda, K., and Racker, E. (1965). *J. Biol. Chem.* **240**, 4689.

Vainer, H., and Wattiaux, R. (1968). *Nature* **217**, 951.

Van Dam, K., and Ter Welle, H. F. (1966). In "Regulation of Metabolic Processes in Mitochondria" (I. M. Tager *et al.*, eds.), p. 235. Elsevier, Amsterdam.

Vesell, E. S. (1965a). *Progr. Med. Genet.* **4**, 128.

Vesell, E. S. (1965b). *Science* **148**, 1103.

Vesell, E. S. (1965c). *Science* **150**, 1735.

Vesell, E. S., and Pool, P. E. (1966). *Proc. Nat. Acad. Sci. U.S.* **55**, 756 (1966).

Wagner, R. P. (1969). *Science* **163**, 1026.

Waller, H. D., Löhr, G. W., Grignani, F., and Gross, R. (1959). *Thromb. Diath. Haemorrh.* **3**, 520.

Waller, H. D., Löhr, G. W., and Gayer, J. (1966). *Klin. Wochenschr.* **44**, 122.

Warburg, O., Gawehn, K., and Geissler, A. W. (1958). *Z. Naturforsch.* B**13**, 515.

Warshaw, A. L., Laster, L., and Shulman, N. R. (1966). *J. Clin. Invest.* **45**, 1923.

Warshaw, A. L., Laster, L., and Shulman, N. R. (1967). *Biol. Chem.* **242**, 2094.

Weber, H. H. (1958). "The Motility of Muscle and Cells." Harvard Univ. Press, Cambridge, Massachusetts.

Weber, H. H., and Unger, W. (1964). *Biochem. Pharmacol.* **13**, 23.

Weed, R. J. (1967). *J. Clin. Invest.* **46**, 1130.

Weinbach, E. C., and Garbus, J. (1969). *Nature* **221**, 1016.

Wenner, C. E., and Hackney, J. H. (1967). *J. Biol. Chem.* **242**, 5053.

White, J. G. (1967). *Blood* **30**, 539.

White, J. G. (1968a). *Scand. J. Haematol.* **5**, 241.

White, J. G. (1968b). *Blood* **31**, 604.

White, J. G., (1968c). *Blood* **32**, 148.

White, J. G. (1968d). *Blood* **32**, 324.

White, J. G. (1968e). *Blood* **32**, 638.

White, J. G., and Krivit, W. (1965). *Blood* **26**, 554.

White, J. G., and Krivit, W. (1967). *Blood* **30**, 625.

Wosilait, W. D., and Sutherland, E. W. (1956). *J. Biol. Chem.* **218**, 469.

Wu, R., Sessa, G., and Hamerman, D. (1964). *Biochim. Biophys. Acta* **93**, 614.

Wurzel, H., McCreary, T., Baker, L., and Gumerman, L. (1961). *Blood* **17**, 314.

Yoshida, H., Fujisawa, H., and Ohi, Y. (1965). *Can. J. Biochem.* **43**, 841.

Yunis, A. A., and Arimura, G. K. (1964). *Cancer Res.* **24**, 489.

Yunis, A. A., and Arimura, G. K. (1966a). *Biochim. Biophys. Acta* **118**, 325.

Yunis, A. A., and Arimura, G. K. (1966b). *Biochim. Biophys. Acta* **118**, 335.

Yunis, A. A., and Arimura, G. K. (1967). *Blood* **30**, 859.

Yunis, A. A., and Arimura, G. K. (1968). *Biochem. Biophys. Res. Commun.* **33**, 119.

Zahler, W. L., Saito, A., and Fleischer, S. (1968). *Biochem. Biophys. Res. Commun.* **32**, 512.

Zatti, M., and Rossi, F. (1965). *Biochim. Biophys. Acta* **99**, 557.

Zatti, M., and Rossi, F. (1966). *Experientia* **22**, 758.

Zieve, P. D., and Greenough, W. B. (1969). *Biochem. Biophys. Res. Commun.* **35**, 462.

Zieve, P. D., and Solomon, H. M. (1966). *J. Clin. Invest.* **45**, 1251.

Zieve, P. D., and Solomon, H. M. (1967). *Amer. J. Physiol.* **213**, 1275.
Zieve, P. D., and Solomon, H. M. (1968). *Amer. J. Physiol.* **215**, 650.
Zieve, P. D., Gamble, J. L., and Jackson, D. P. (1964). *J. Clin. Invest.* **43**, 2063.
Zucker, M. B., and Borelli, J. (1954). *Blood* **9**, 602.
Zucker, M. B., and Borelli, J. (1958). *J. Appl. Physiol.* **12**, 453.
Zucker, M. B., and Borelli, J. (1960). *Thromb. Diath. Haemorrh.* **4**, 424.
Zucker-Franklin, D. (1969). *J. Clin. Invest.* **48**, 165.
Zucker-Franklin, D., Nachman, R. L., and Marcus, A. J. (1967). *Science* **157**, 945.

5

MEMBRANE GLYCOPROTEINS

OF BLOOD PLATELETS*

G. A. JAMIESON and D. S. PEPPER

Blood platelets are relatively rich in carbohydrate (Table I) and have a surface density of sialic acid about tenfold greater than that on the red cell (Madoff *et al.*, 1964). When this sialic acid is removed by brief treatment with neuraminidase, their internal structures appear unchanged in

* Contribution No. 190 from The American National Red Cross Blood Research Laboratory.

Much of the unpublished work reported in this review has been supported, in part, by USPHS Grants GM-13057 and AI-09017.

TABLE I

CARBOHYDRATE CONTENT (W/W DRY WEIGHT) OF HUMAN PLATELETS

Hexose	Hexosamine	Uronic acid	NANA	Pentose	Reference
4.41	2.67	present	0.72	0.67	Woodside and Kocholaty, 1960
n.d.[a]	n.d.	n.d.	0.5	n.d.	Nunnari and Cristaaldi, 1966
n.d.	0.6	0.10	0.38	n.d.	Manley and Mullinger, 1967
n.d.	n.d.	n.d.	0.72	n.d.	Madoff *et al.*, 1964
4.8	1.4	0.15	0.54	n.d.	Barber *et al.*, 1969

[a] n.d., not determined.

the electron microscope (Hovig, 1965), although they will readily aggregate in homologous plasma. Rather unexpectedly, neuraminidase *in vivo* renders mice thrombocytopenic within 20 hours (Gasic *et al.*, 1968). This removal of platelets from the circulation implies that there is some recognition process based on very specific configurations of surface sugars, particularly sialic acid.

The glycoproteins of the platelet membrane play other important roles in its biochemical and physiological processes; certain aspects of platelet adhesion and aggregation are mediated by sialic acid (Wilson *et al.*, 1967; Hellem, 1968), as is serotonin uptake (Michal, 1969). In addition glyco-proteins may be determinants of platelet isoantigens (Shulman *et al.*, 1964) and may be involved in congenital platelet defects such as paroxysmal nocturnal hemoglobinuria (Pepper and Jamieson, 1970) and in macro-thrombocytic thrombocytopenia (Gröttum and Solum, 1969), and in allo-graft rejection (Lowenhaupt and Nathan, 1968).

Despite this, relatively little is known about the function and biosynthesis of these structures and a number of basic questions remain largely unans-wered. This chapter attempts to summarize present knowledge of these membrane glycoproteins and of the other complex carbohydrates of the human platelet such as glycosaminoglycans (mucopolysaccharides), poly-saccharides, and glycolipids. A number of outstanding general reviews have recently discussed certain aspects of the carbohydrate chemistry of platelets and their structure and function (Johnson *et al.*, 1961; Marcus and Zucker, 1965; Brinkhous *et al.*, 1967; Johnson and Seegers, 1967; Kowalski and Niewiarowski, 1967; Born, 1968; Haslam, 1968; Jensen and Killman, 1968; Schulz, 1968).

I. ELECTROKINETIC CHARGE

The surfaces of all cells so far studied, including the platelet, appear to possess a net negative charge. That is, they move toward a positive electrode in neutral buffered solution. The technical problems of measuring platelet mobility are open to a number of theoretical criticisms but the difficulty of interpreting results is more serious. The basic (normally positive) groups which might occur at the platelet surface include the amino and imino groups of amino acids, nucleic acids, and phospholipids. The acidic (normally negative) groups which might occur include the carboxyl, phosphoric or sulfate groupings of sialic acids, uronic acids, amino acids, nucleic acids, phospholipids, sulfated polysaccharides, and glycoproteins. Although no direct experimental evidence is available a small number of free amino groups may be contributed by amino sugars which are normally *N*-acetylated.

It is only when the above charged groups are present in the outermost layer of the platelet (perhaps only 10 Å in depth) that they contribute effectively to the electrokinetic charge, or zeta potential. Obviously, any change in the arrangement of the platelet surface macromolecules is going to bring a new mosaic of charged groups into the outermost layer. Such changes are to be expected during platelet aggregation or after contact with thrombin, collagen, or glass (Hampton, 1966; Hampton and Mitchell, 1966; Seaman, 1966). Since the outer layer attached to the platelet membrane may be anything from 100–500 Å thick (Behnke, 1968a; Hovig, 1968) only a small proportion of all charged groups will contribute to the zeta potential at any one time.

A useful approach to determining which groups are responsible for surface charge is to treat the platelet with specific enzymes such as the neuraminidases, the phospholipases, or ribonuclease. Any resulting change in calculated charge may then be ascribed to the loss of that particular substrate (e.g., sialic acid, phospholipid phosphate ester, or RNA). However, a number of practical considerations alter this simple picture, in particular, the possibility that the enzyme may penetrate the cell as has been shown for neuraminidase with various types of cultured cells (Nordling and Mayhew, 1966).

With platelets, most of the published work concerns the effect of neuraminidase on electrophoretic mobility (Jerushalmy *et al.*, 1961; Madoff *et al.*, 1964; Bray and Alexander, 1969). It is a common finding that more sialic acid (NANA) is found in the supernatant by chemical assay of such digests than is expected from the change in electrophoretic mobility. This may be explained in a number of ways. If neuraminidase penetrates between the macromolecules of the surface coat, although not to the inside of the cell, then any sialic acid released will not have contributed to the zeta potential. Sialic acids (pK 1.9–2.6), which are the dominant group on the platelet surface, exert a considerable repulsive force on each other. When they are removed by neuraminidase conformational changes are to be expected with a resultant unpredictable change in the apparent surface charge. No specific evidence has been produced for groups other than carboxyl at the platelet surface. However, in view of the observed isoelectric (zero mobility) point of platelets at ca. pH 3.9 (Madoff *et al.*, 1964), it is reasonable to assume that amino groups are also present. The electrophoretic mobility of thrombosthenic platelets is identical with normal platelets (Zucker and Levine, 1963) even after incubation with ADP (Hampton and Hardisty, 1967) and probably reflects a defect in ADP binding in these cells. However, the reduced electrophoretic mobility observed in congenital macrothrombocytic thrombopenia has been related to low sialic acid, possibly reflecting a defect in the platelet membrane (Gröttum and Solum, 1969).

In all experiments at extremes of pH, cell lysis can only be overcome by tanning with formaldehyde or other agents which block amino groups, and this requires appropriate corrections in calculations of the isoelectric point. An alternative approach (Barber *et al.*, 1970) is to isolate and purify stable membrane vesicles of platelets and subject these to isoelectric focusing (Svensson, 1967). Under these conditions, the membranes form a discrete, narrow band with an isoelectric point of 3.9–4.2, in good agreement with the values obtained by classic mobility methods.

II. VIRAL RECEPTOR SITES

The mechanism whereby a virus penetrates and multiplies inside a living cell proceeds in several stages, the first of which is adsorption on to the cell coat. In the case of the myxoviruses (influenza, Newcastle disease virus, etc.) this is known to be mediated by sialic acid (Formula I) when present in glycoproteins or glycolipids.

$$CH_3COHN \quad \begin{array}{c} H \\ | \\ H-C-OH \\ H-C-OH \\ | \\ CH_2OH \end{array} \quad \begin{array}{c} O \\ OH \\ COOH \end{array}$$

In species other than the human, the terminal sialic acids have acetyl or *N*-glycolyl groups on the 5-amino nitrogen and may have *O*-acetyl groups in positions 4, 7, 8, or 9.

The influenza viruses possess a hemagglutinin (for adsorption) and a neuraminidase (for release) both directed toward a single specific type of sialic acid on the cell surface. When platelets are incubated *in vitro* with live or heat-killed virus at 4°C, complete adsorption of virus onto platelets takes place. On warming to 37°C, most of the live virus will elute (65–95%), but some is phagocytosed within the platelets, losing its outer coat to the platelet and causing degranulation (Danon *et al.*, 1959; Jerushalmy *et al.*, 1961; Broun and Broun, 1962; Schulz and Landgraber, 1966; Terada *et al.*, 1966). This may be the basic mechanism behind the common observation of thrombocytopenia during viral infections (Broun and Broun, 1962). Schulz (1968) has observed high concentrations of mouse leukemia virus (Maloney) in association with the demarcation membranes of mouse megakaryocytes which may indicate that Maloney virus also binds to carbohydrate on cell membranes in view of the known carbohydrate concentration in this region (Behnke, 1968b). It is not known whether platelets will support the multiplication of any virus, although from theoretical considerations it is possible for RNA viruses to replicate within platelets (Green, 1969).

Jerushalmy and co-workers (1962) studied the effect of influenza virus and Newcastle disease virus (NDV) on the thromboplastin generation time and clot retraction of platelets. NDV shortened clotting times but influenza virus had no effect. The clot retraction of NDV-treated platelets was only 16% of control and that of influenza-treated only 60%.

The isolation of an active receptor molecule from crude platelet membranes was achieved by solubilization in aqueous (33% v/v) pyridine (Pepper and Jamieson, 1968), although Uhlenbruck (1961) had noted the presence of hemagglutination inhibition (HI) activity in platelets. The chemical analysis of partially purified glycoprotein inhibitor (apparent mol. wt. $\geq$ 200,000) was protein, 68%; phospholipid, 18%; hexose, 2.5%; NANA, 1.4%; N-acetylglucosamine, 0.9%. Highly purified platelet membranes also show HI activity, the highest titres being obtained with A_2 (Singapore) and ROB strains of influenza virus (Barber et al., 1970).

III. CARBOHYDRATE ULTRASTRUCTURE

Because of the difficulty of obtaining pure, fresh platelet preparations in large quantities, it is natural that earlier studies on the carbohydrate structure of platelets should have used a histochemical or electron microscopic approach rather than direct analysis. Of the electron dense stains which have been used for the identification of sugar polymers, periodic acid/silver ammine, phosphotungstic acid, and ruthenium red/osmium tetroxide appear to be the most specific.

In the rat 50 different cell types, including the megakaryocyte, show a diffuse surface coating of carbohydrate-rich material using periodic acid and silver metheneammine (Rambourg and Leblond, 1967, 1969). Furthermore, the demarcation membrane of the mature megakaryocyte (which is later destined to become the outer coat of the platelet (Schulz, 1968) is rich in carbohydrate on the basis of its reaction with phosphotungstic acid (Behnke, 1968b). Negative staining of whole platelets in phosphotungstic acid showed a considerable number of dense, hexagonal particles spilling from the outer membrane that were thought to be carbohydrate in view of their affinity for the reagent (Bull, 1966). Ruthenium red/osmium tetroxide visualized a layer 150–200 Å thick on the outer surface of the platelet possibly composed of sulfated polysaccharides and sialylglycoproteins or glycolipids (Behnke, 1968a; Nakao and Angrist, 1968). After incubation with trypsin or pronase, the staining reaction of the surface coat was largely abolished although any staining present in the surface canal system remained. Hovig (1968) concluded that the outer membrane mediates contact between platelets during adhesion and viscous metamorphosis and possesses a carbohydrate layer up to 500 Å thick. This outer layer has also been observed to bind colloidal iron and thorium oxides, but these are more indicative of acidic groups ($pK < 2$) than carbohydrate per se. Carbohydrate staining reactions have also been observed within the surface connected canal system of traumatized platelets (Behnke, 1968a). No evidence has been obtained for carbohydrate components within the platelet cytoplasm other than glycogen, soluble glycoproteins, and glycosaminoglycans.

The question of what compounds these stains are detecting is very pertinent to any histochemical work. Periodic acid followed by silver salts should detect mainly cis-diol groups characteristic of carbohydrates, but considerable nonspecific staining with silver alone is observed in practice (Rambourg and Leblond, 1967). Phosphotungstic acid is capable of forming many hydrogen bonds simultaneously to an array of hydroxyl groups, and is found to be quite specific for carbohydrates. This may be due to the rigid conformation of hydroxyls in each sugar and the fixed shape of the phosphotungstic acid moiety (Gautier *et al.*, 1963; Pease, 1966; Behnke, 1968b). Ruthenium red (a polyammine trinuclear complex of ruthenium oxychloride) probably reacts with acidic polysaccharides via a combination of electrostatic and hydrogen bonds. The resultant complex is insoluble and is an effective way of fixing acidic polysaccharides *in situ* (Luft, 1966, 1969). Precipitates are observed *in vitro* with purified preparations of heparin, polymethacrylic acid, and pectin.

In our own experience, native platelets do not take up ruthenium red (or its oxidized form ruthenium brown) alone or in the presence of osmium tetroxide. However, if the platelets are traumatized in plasma (e.g., by hypotonic shock, sonication, or treatment with ammonium oxalate or glutaraldehyde) rapid staining does occur. We believe that the staining is due primarily to the precipitation of chondroitin sulfate, hyaluronic acid, and possibly heparin on the surface of the platelet immediately following trauma. Control experiments using erythrocytes and a spectrophotometric assay for ruthenium red showed that there is no interaction between sialylglycoproteins or glycolipids and ruthenium red. The appearance of electron density, as opposed to a visible chromogen, is dependent on both ruthenium red and osmium tetroxide; Luft (1966, 1969) has suggested that each ruthenium red molecule acts as a catalyst for the reduction of osmium tetroxide. Additionally, the ruthenium red may act as a fixative for the highly soluble acidic polysaccharides which themselves can react with osmium.

IV. POLYSACCHARIDES

The only neutral polysaccharide so far detected in platelets from any species is glycogen. In fresh preparations of platelets this appears as dense, tetrahedral aggregates in localized fields in the electron microscope. Both the total hexose and glycogen content of platelets vary depending on the time since phlebotomy (Woodside and Kocholaty, 1960; Olsson *et al.*, 1963). Although the exact mechanism underlying this loss is not known, it is clearly related to platelet metabolism and is connected with the viability of platelets when transfused. The glycogen content of depleted platelets is regained *in vivo* following transfusion (Murphy and Gardner, 1969), probably due to platelet glycogen synthetase (Vainer and Wattiaux, 1968). The metabolic state of platelets in the "resting state" appears to be a mixture of aerobic and anaerobic but when stimulated, e.g., in viscous metamorphosis, there is a large burst of anaerobic metabolism. Although there have been no reports of the isolation of morphologically intact glycogen tetrahedra from platelets, Bezkorovainy and Rafelson (1964) obtained a soluble complex of 70% carbohydrate and 22% protein which was not retained on a column of DEAE-cellulose; they inferred that this was a complex of glycogen in a matrix of protein.

V. GLYCOSAMINOGLYCANS (MUCOPOLYSACCHARIDES)

Platelets are known to contain chondroitin-4-sulphate, hyaluronic acid, and possibly heparin or keratan sulphate (Olsson and Gardell, 1967). These investigators used lyophilized human platelets which were subjected to solvent extraction, papain digestion and, finally, to discontinuous elution from a column of ECTEOLA-cellulose. Odell and Anderson (1957; Anderson and Odell, 1958) have studied the acidic polysaccharides of rat platelets including the incorporation of radioactive sulfate. Manley and Mullinger (1967) isolated a proteolytic digestion product of atherosclerotic plaques which they suggested was a platelet-specific acidic polysaccharide and later showed (Mullinger and Manley, 1968) that chromatography of proteolytic digest of pig platelets produced two fractions, one being chondroitin sulphate but the other of glycoprotein origin.

In view of the importance of acidic polysaccharides in both the structural and secretory elements of cells, it is surprising that they have only recently been observed histochemically in intact platelets (Dunn and Spicer, 1969). They are stored in the granules of the platelets from which they are released during viscous metamorphosis (Ridell and Bier, 1965) via the surface-connected canal system (Behnke, 1968a). This has been confirmed by the isolation of glycosaminoglycans from the outer surface of platelets which have undergone the release reaction as the result of exposure to proteolytic enzymes (Jamieson and Pepper, 1970).

VI. GLYCOPROTEINS

Glycoproteins are the largest component of the complex carbohydrates of the blood platelet (Olsson and Gardell, 1967) although their presence was deduced on the basis of earlier analytical data (Woodside and Kochalaty, 1960; Bezkorovainy and Doherty, 1962). Fibrinogen and γG are the main cytoplasmic glycoprotein components of human platelets together with unidentified α- and β-globulins of platelet-specific origin detected by immunodiffusion and immunoelectrophoresis (Bezkorovainy and Rafelson, 1964). A glycopeptide fraction containing galactose (16.5%), fucose (1.2%), hexosamine (15%), and sialic acid (9.6%) has been isolated from pig platelets (Mullinger and Manley, 1968), although it is not known what proportion of this is derived from soluble glycoproteins and what from structural units.

A major problem in these studies is to separate platelets into pure, morphologically intact fractions in good yield; this ideal has not been realized. Probably the best techniques available are various modifications of the method of Marcus *et al.* (1966) in which platelets are homogenized and the subunits separated by density gradient centrifugation to isopycnic equilibrium. A number of modifications have been proposed in both techniques of disruption and in centrifugation (Nachman *et al.*, 1967b; Pepper and Jamieson, 1968, 1969a; Day *et al.*, 1969). Varying results have been obtained following disruption of platelets by homogenization, explosive decompression, freeze-thawing, or sonication. A particularly useful technique involves the loading of the platelet with glycerol and its subsequent hypotonic lysis. Over 80% of the cells are destroyed, and a simplified density step method provides an excellent yield of membranes containing a fourfold increase (2%) in NANA over the intact platelet (Barber *et al.*, 1970). This membrane fraction may be subfractionated on a continuous density sucrose gradient (15–40%) into two bands (d, 1.09 and 1.12) which differ in their phospholipid content but both of which possess identical activity in the thromboplastin generation test and in hemagglutination inhibition. Both bands contain a range of enzyme activities, including the UDP-*N*-acetylglucosamine transferase involved in glycoprotein biosynthesis, but the heavier band is selectively enriched in esterase and β-*N*-acetylglucosaminidase, two enzymes of lysosomal or granular origin. The nature of these two membrane fractions is under active investigation, but two platelet membrane fractions have been obtained in other cases by different techniques (Boosye and Rafelson, 1969; Saba *et al.*, 1969).

In order to identify the outer surface and the location of the two membranes, platelets have been labeled in plasma while still fresh with colored or fluorescent dyes such as fluorescein mercuric acetate (FMA), trinitro-benzene sulfonic acid (TNBS), and stilbene isothiocyanate sulfonic acid (SITS). These colored probes bind only to the macromolecules of the outer surface via -SH or NH_2 groups and do not penetrate within the cell. Using the fractionation procedure described previously it is relatively simple to obtain glycoprotein fractions which have been specifically labeled as coming from the plasma membrane (Barber et al., 1969). However, it is necessary to exclude the possibility of dye exchange in studies of this type.

A. Soluble Glycoproteins

A soluble fraction has been obtained from bovine platelets which gave eight platelet-specific precipitin lines in immunoelectrophoresis and 20 bands on disk-acrylamide gel electrophoresis (Lopaciuk and Solum, 1969). Although not so identified, some of these bands must correspond to the glycoprotein fractions observed by earlier workers. A thrombin-labile β_2-globulin has been observed in disk gels of human platelet cell sap (Ganguly and Moore, 1967; Ganguly, 1969a) which has a potent antithrombin effect (Ganguly, 1970), but it is not known whether this is a glycoprotein. Several studies have been made on the soluble macromolecules of platelets although relatively few are specifically concerned with glycoproteins. The best characterized protein is platelet fibrinogen, although the fundamental question of its identity with plasma fibrinogen is still unresolved.

B. Platelet Fibrinogen

The term *platelet fibrinogen* has been used to designate the thrombin-clottable protein identified in extracts of washed platelets (Roskam, 1923; Ware et al., 1948). However, these extracts appear to contain several thrombin-labile proteins (Salmon and Bounameaux, 1958; Davey and Lüscher, 1966; Ganguly and Moore, 1967; Ganguly, 1969a). One of these has been reported to become thrombin resistant in thrombosthenia (Nachman, 1966), although this has not been confirmed (Caen et al., 1967; Weiss and Kochwa, 1968).

Fibrinogen has been reported to comprise 14% of the platelet dry weight (Bezkorovainy and Rafelson, 1964) and occurs in both the intracellular and membrane-adsorbed extracellular compartments of the platelet. The extracellular fibrinogen may be partly removed with chelating agents for calcium (Castaldi and Caen, 1965; Kopec et al., 1966) and platelet fibrinogen appears to be mainly of intracellular origin (Sokal, 1962; Gocken and Yunis, 1963). The soluble cell sap contains three-quarters of the intracellular fibrinogen, the remaining quarter being in the granules (Nachman *et al.*, 1967b). In view of the trauma involved, it is not certain that this represents the distribution in the intact platelet, since it is evulsed in a selective release reaction effected by thrombin or trypsin (Grette, 1962; Davey and Lüscher, 1967; Holmsen and Day, 1968).

Platelet fibrinogen has been isolated by precipitation with cold ethanol (Grette, 1962) by ammonium sulfate followed by gel filtration (Davey and Lüscher, 1967) or with ethanol/glycine and dimethylformamide (Solum and Lopaciuk, 1969a); this last procedure yielded protein which was 91–98% clottable.

Platelet and plasma fibrinogens have been reported to be identical on immunoelectrophoresis and cellulose acetate electrophoresis as well as by monodimensional high voltage paper electrophoresis of their tryptic digests (Bezkorovainy and Rafelson, 1964) and on ultracentrifugation, gel electrophoresis, and *N*-terminal amino acid analysis (Davey and Lüscher, 1967; Solum and Lopaciuk, 1969b). However, differences have been reported in intrinsic viscosity, carbohydrate content, and rate of thrombin polymerization for bovine platelet and plasma fibrinogens (Solum and Lopaciuk, 1969b). Some of the reported values for the two proteins are summarized in Table II.

The decreased clottability of platelet fibrinogen and its increased carbohydrate content parallel a similar relation in a soluble form of plasma fibrinogen which probably arises by partial proteolysis of the parent protein

TABLE II

Reported Values for Bovine Plasma and Platelet Fibrinogens[a]

	Plasma fibrinogen	Platelet fibrinogen
Intrinsic viscosity (dl/qm)	0.26	0.48
$S_{20,w}$	————8.2————	
N-Terminal amino acids	———Tyr,Glu,Asp———	
Sialic acid (*N*-glycolyl neuraminic acid)	0.53	0.56
Hexose (Gal:Man = 1:2)	1.01	1.56
Hexosamine (as GlcN)	1.09	1.37

[a] Solum and Lopaciuk, 1969b.

(Mosesson et al., 1967), although no proteinase activity at neutral pH has been found in bovine (Solum and Lopaciuk, 1969b) or human (Beese et al., 1966) platelet extracts.

Ganguly, in this laboratory, has recently undertaken an extensive examination of the soluble proteins of human platelets (Ganguly and Moore, 1967; Ganguly, 1969–1970). His work has demonstrated the modification of the structure of platelet albumin and platelet fibrinogen by lysosomal proteases with maximum activity around pH 5. In particular, his results emphasize that an *essential* control in all comparisons of platelet and plasma proteins is the reisolation of the plasma protein after its addition to platelet extracts. In the particular case of platelet fibrinogen (Ganguly, 1969c), low molecular weight products are split from the parent molecule during storage, and the starch gel immunoelectrophoretic pattern of plasmin digests of isolated platelet fibrinogen differs from that obtained with digests of plasma fibrinogen (Jamieson and Gaffney, 1968). Although attempts to remove the proteolytic activity were unsuccessful, recent results, using suitable inhibitors, indicate that platelet and plasma fibrinogens are, in fact, identical (Ganguly, 1969f).

C. Structural Glycoproteins

Following separation of cell components by the procedures described above, the various structures must then be solubilized before any meaningful data can be obtained on their constituent molecules. There are two basic approaches to the problem of the solubilization of structural components: (1) dissolution in organic solvents; and (2) digestion with hydrolytic enzymes.

Organic solvents, such as aqueous pyridine (33%) (Pepper and Jamieson, 1968), aqueous phenol (90%), and acidified 2-chloroethanol (90%), and nonionic detergents, such as Triton X-100 (Pepper and Jamieson, 1969c), have all been used with varying degress of success. Recent results (Nachman and Ferris, 1970) have shown that delipidated platelet membranes can be solubilized in 1% sodium dodecylsulfate and resolved by gel filtration or gel electrophoresis into a series of components of molecular weight 20,000–90,000 one of which retained antigenic characteristics similar to those found in intact platelets (Nachman and Marcus, 1968).

The second approach, solubilization with proteolytic enzymes, has so far provided much more information on the glycoproteins of the platelet surface. Prolonged proteolysis (3 days) of crude platelet membranes with a combination of trypsin and pronase, followed by gel filtration and chromatography on DEAE-Sephadex led to the isolation of a series of glycopeptides devoid of alkali-labile carbohydrate linkages, containing glucosamine as the sole hexosamine and with small but significant differences in their content of galactose and mannose (Pepper and Jamieson, 1969a).

Further studies have shown that glycopeptides are released in a remarkably short time from the outer surface of the intact platelet compared with the digestion of soluble glycoprotein (Masek *et al.*, 1969; Pepper and Jamieson, 1969b, 1970) and that 30–50% of total cell sialic acid is released within 30 minutes. Since approximately 60% of platelet sialic acid, comprising both glycoproteins and glycolipids, is on the outer surface (Madoff *et al.*, 1964), a very high release of membrane glycoproteins is indicated.

The glycopeptides so released fall into three distinct classes designated GP-I, GP-II, and GP-III (Pepper and Jamieson, 1969b, 1970). The molecular weight of GP-I was calculated to be 120,000 on the basis of gel filtration and ultracentrifugal data (Pepper and Jamieson, 1970). Since this value is about tenfold higher than that of the glycopeptides of the erythrocyte membrane (Winzler, 1969) and greater than that of several intact glycoproteins, the term *macroglycopeptide* has been coined for this membrane component.

Relatively more of the macroglycopeptide GP-I was released by trypsin while the lowest molecular weight glycopeptide, GP-III (mol. wt., 5000), was preferentially released by either pronase or papain. The intermediate glycopeptide, GP-II (mol. wt., 22,500), was obtained in small amounts by either proteolytic procedure. GP-I was resistant to further proteolysis and GP-I and GP-II gave single peaks on chromatography on DEAE-Sephadex, while GP-III could be subfractionated into several components identical with those obtained by prolonged proteolysis of isolated platelet membranes (Pepper and Jamieson, 1969a).

The macroglycopeptide contained ca. 22% sialic acid, 16% galactose, and equal amounts of glucosamine and galactosamine (15% each). Proline (6%) was the principal amino acid with similar amounts of threonine (5.5%) and serine (3.5%). About half of the hexosamine was in alkali-labile linkage. GP-III contained ca. 18% sialic acid, 15% galactose, 10% mannose, and 33% glucosamine; it was devoid of galactosamine and of alkali-labile carbohydrate. GP-II was intermediate in properties between these two glycopeptides but was not related to GP-I in a degradative sequence; the small amounts available precluded extensive structural characterization.

Thus, the macroglycopeptide has many of the properties of a mucin and may extend as a semiflexible rod from the surface of the platelet. It may be related to the fuzzy coat seen in electron photomicrographs of platelet thin sections (Hovig, 1968) and may be involved in platelet adhesion during hemostasis and in platelet immune lysis (Aster and Enright, 1969).

Of particular interest is the orientation of these glycopeptide structures on the outer surface of the platelet membrane. One possibility is that GP-I, II, and III are released simultaneously from a single precursor. This would require a total glycopeptide chain of molecular weight approximately 300,000 and a very definite segregation of glycopeptide structures and protease susceptibility. Another possibility is that we have a single glycoprotein in the platelet membrane which produces the macroglycopeptide, GP-I, on proteolytic digestion and this is then sequentially converted to GP-II and GP-III on further proteolysis. However, this seems to be unlikely since GP-I is resistant to further proteolytic attack and since GP-I, GP-II, and GP-III have different analytical and structural characteristics. At present, the weight of evidence favors the third possibility, namely, that the glycoprotein precursors of GP-I and GP-III and, possibly, GP-II (although this point cannot yet be settled because of the limited amount of material available) are individual units on the platelet surface.

A number of changes in platelet function are observed following proteolysis. Trypsinized platelets show an increased ability to aggregate (Wilson et al., 1967) but a decreased ability to adhere to collagen (Hellem, 1968). Of particular interest is the observation (Aster and Enright, 1969) that brief treatment of platelets with papain results in a greatly increased sensitivity to immune lysis by quinidine-dependent antibodies mimicing that observed in platelets from patients suffering from paroxysmal nocturnal hemoglobinuria (PNH). This could be interpreted as indicating a membrane glycoprotein defect in PNH platelets. Although no direct evidence is available, it is possible that the HL-A antigens of platelets contain carbohydrate (Shulman et al., 1964). However, these antigens could not be detected in the glycoprotein-enriched fraction isolated by pyridine solubilization (Pepper and Jamieson, 1968).

VII. GLYCOLIPIDS

Platelet membrane sialic acid can also occur in glycolipids (cerebrosides, hematosides) which probably constitute about 1% of total platelet lipid (Marcus, 1970). Evidence is accumulating both in the platelet (Michal, 1969) and other cells (Woolley and Gommi, 1964; Carrol and Sereda, 1968; Wesemann and Zilliken, 1968; Wesemann, 1969) that receptors for serotonin contain bound sialic acid as an essential prosthetic group. Conflicting evidence at the moment is more strongly in favor of the receptors as being glycolipids rather than glycoproteins. There is obviously a fruitful field of research in elucidating the contribution of the sialylglycolipids and glycoproteins to platelet function and immunology.

REFERENCES

Anderson, B., and Odell, T. T., Jr. (1958). *Proc. Soc. Exp. Biol. Med.* **99**, 765.

Aster, T. H., and Enright, S. E. (1969). *J. Clin. Invest.* **48**, 1199.

Barber, A. J., Pepper, D. S., and Jamieson, G. A. (1969). *Fed. Proc., Fed. Amer. Soc. Exp. Biol.* **28**, 575.

Barber, A. J., Pepper, D. S., and Jamieson, G. A. (1970). Unpublished experiments.

Beese, J., Farr, N., Grunner, E., and Haschen, R. J. (1966). *Klin. Wochenschr.* **44**, 1049.

Behnke, O. (1968a). *J. Ultrastruct. Res.* **24**, 51.

Behnke, O. (1968b). *J. Ultrastruct. Res.* **24**, 412.

Bezkorovainy, A., and Doherty, D. G. (1962). *Arch. Biochem. Biophys.* **86**, 412.

Bezkorovainy, A., and Rafelson, M. E. (1964). *J. Lab. Clin. Med.* **64**, 212.

Booyse, R. M., and Rafelson, M. E. (1969). *In* "Dynamics of Thrombus Formation and Dissolution" (S. A. Johnson and M. Guest, eds.), pp. 149–71. Lippincott, Philadelphia, Pennsylvania.

Born, G. V. R. (1968). *Proc. 12th Congr. Int. Soc. Hematol.*, 1968, p. 95.

Bray, B. A., and Alexander, B. (1969). *Blood* **34**, 523.

Brinkhous, K. M., Wright, I. S., Soulier, J. P., Roberts, H. R., and Hinnom, S. (eds.) (1967). "Platelets: Their Role in Hemostasis and Thrombosis." Schattauer, Stuttgart.

Broun, G. D., and Broun, G. O. (1962). *Proc. 8th Int. Congr. Hematol.*, 1960, p. 1756.

Bull, B. S. (1966). *Blood* **28**, 901.

Caen, J., Vainer, H., and Gautier, A. (1967). *Thromb. Diath. Haemorrh.* **26**, 223.

Carrol, P. M., and Sereda, D. D. (1968). *Nature (London)* **217**, 667.

Castaldi, P. A., and Caen, J. (1965). *J. Clin. Pathol.* **18**, 579.

Danon, D., Jerushalmy, Z., and de Vries, A. (1959). *Virology* **9**, 719.

Davey, M. G., and Lüscher, E. F. (1966). *Thromb. Diath. Haemorrh.* **16**, Suppl. 283.

Davey, M. G., and Lüscher, E. F. (1967). *In* "Biochemistry of Blood Platelets" (E. Kowalski and S. Niewiarowski, eds.), p. 9. Academic Press, New York.

Day, H. J., Holmsen, H., and Hovig, T. (1969). *Scand. J. Haematol.* Suppl. 7.

Dunn, W. B., and Spicer, S. S. (1969). *J. Histochem. Cytochem.* **17**, 668.

Ganguly, P. (1969a). *Blood* **33**, 590.

Ganguly, P. (1969b). *Biochim. Biophys. Acta* **188**, 78.

Ganguly, P. (1969c). *Clin. Chim. Acta* **23**, 514.

Ganguly, P. (1969d). *Blood* **35**, 511.

Ganguly, P. (1969e). *Clin. Chim. Acta* **25**, 33.

Ganguly, P. (1969f). Unpublished experiments.

Ganguly, P. (1970). *Fed. Proc., Fed. Amer. Soc. Exp. Biol.* (in press).

Ganguly, P., and Moore, R. (1967). *Clin. Chim. Acta* **17**, 153.

Gasic, G. J., Gasic, T. B., and Stewart, C. S. (1968). *Proc. Nat. Acad. Sci. U.S.* **61**, 46.

Gautier, A., Jean, G., Probst, M., and Falcao, L. (1963). *Arch. Ital. Anat. Istol. Patol.* **37**, 503.

Gocken, M., and Yunis, E. (1963). *Nature* (*London*) **200**, 590.

Green, R. (1969). *In* "Dynamics of Thrombus Formation and Dissolution" (S. A. Johnson and M. Guest, eds.), p. 72. Lippincott, Philadelphia, Pennsylvania.

Grette, K. (1962). *Acta Physiol. Scand.* Suppl. 195, 56.

Grottum, K. A., and Solum, N. O. (1969). *Brit. J. Haematol.* **16**, 277.

Hampton, J. R. (1966). *Brit. Med. J.* **0**, 1074.

Hampton, J. R., and Hardisty, R. M. (1967). *Nature* (*London*) **213**, 490.

Hampton, J. R., and Mitchell, J. R. A. (1966). *Nature* (*London*) **209**, 470.

Haslam, R. J. (1968). *Proc. 12th Congr. Int. Soc. Hematol.*, 1968, p. 198.

Hellem, A. J. (1968). *In* "Blood Platelets" (K. J. Jensen and S. A. Killmann, eds.), pp. 99–145. Williams & Wilkins, Baltimore, Maryland.

Holmsen, H., and Day, H. J. (1968). *Nature* (*London*) **219**, 760.

Hovig, T. (1965). *Thromb. Diath. Haemorrh.* **13**, 84.

Hovig, T. (1968). *In* "Blood Platelets" (K. J. Jensen and S. A. Killman, eds.), pp. 3–64. Williams & Wilkins, Baltimore, Maryland.

Jamieson, G. A., and Gaffney, P. J. (1968). *Biochim. Biophys. Acta* **154**, 96.

Jamieson, G. A., and Pepper, D. S. (1970). Unpublished experiments.

Jensen, K. J., and Killman, S. A. (1968). *Ser. Haematol.* **1**, No. 2.

Jerushalmy, Z., Kohn, A., and de Vries, A. (1961). *Proc. Soc. Exp. Biol. Med.* **106**, 462.

Jerushalmy, Z., Adler, A., Rechnic, J., Kohn, A., and de Vries, A. (1962). *Pathol. Biol.* **10**, 41.

Johnson, S. A., and Seegers, W. H., eds. (1967). "Physiology of Hemostasis and Thrombosis." Thomas, Springfield, Illinois.

Johnson, S. A., Monto, R. W., Rebuck, J. W., and Horn, R. C., eds. (1961). "Blood Platelets." Little, Brown, Boston, Massachusetts.

Kopec, M., Budzynski, A., Stachurska, J., Wegrzynowicz, Z., and Kowalski, E. (1966). *Thromb. Diath. Haemorrh.* **15**, 476.

Kowalski, E., and Niewiarowski, S., eds. (1967). "Biochemistry of Blood Platelets." Academic Press, New York.

Lopaciuk, S., and Solum, N. O. (1969). *Thromb. Diath. Haemorrh.* **21**, 132.

Lowenhaupt, R., and Nathan, P. (1968). *Nature* (*London*) **220**, 822.

Luft, J. H. (1966). *Fed. Proc. Fed. Amer. Soc. Exp. Biol.* **25**, 1773.

Luft, J. H. (1969). Personal communication.

Madoff, M. A., Ebbe, S., and Baldini, M. (1964). *J. Clin. Invest.* **43**, 870.

Manley, G., and Mullinger, R. N. (1967). *Brit. J. Exp. Pathol.* **48**, 529.

Marcus, A. J. (1969). *N. Engl. J. Med.* **280**, 1213, 1278, and 1330.

Marcus, A. J. (1970). *Blood* **34**, 521.

Marcus, A. J., and Zucker, M. B. (1965). "The Physiology of Blood Platelets." Grune & Stratton, New York.

Marcus, A. J., Zucker-Franklin, D., Safier, L. B., and Ullman, H. L. (1966). *J. Clin. Invest.* **45**, 41.

Masek, K., Libanska, J., Nosal, R., and Raskova, H. (1969). *Naunyn-Schmiedebergs Arch. Pharmakol. Exp. Pathol.* **262**, 419.

Michal, F. (1969). *Nature* (*London*) **221**, 1253.

Mosesson, M. W., Alkjaersig, N., Sweet, B., and Sherry, S. (1967). *Biochemistry* **6**, 3279.

Mullinger, R. N., and Manley, G. (1968). *Biochim. Biophys. Acta* **170**, 282.

Murphy, S., and Gardner, F. H. (1969). *Blood* **34**, 544.

Nachman, R. L. (1966). *J. Lab. Clin. Med.* **67**, 411.

Nachman, R. L., and Ferris, B. (1970). *Biochemistry* **9**, 200.
Nachman, R. L., and Marcus, A. J. (1968). *Brit. J. Haematol.* **15**, 181.
Nachman, R. L., Marcus, A. J., and Zucker-Franklin, D. (1967). *J. Lab. Clin. Med.* **69**, 51.
Nakao, K., and Angrist, A. (1968). *Nature (London)* **217**, 960.
Nordling, S., and Mayhew, E. (1966). *Exp. Cell Res.* **44**, 552.
Nunnari, A., and Cristaaldi, R. (1966). *Boll. Soc. Ital. Biol. Sper.* **42**, 685.
Odell, T. T., Jr., and Anderson, B. (1957). *Proc. Soc. Exp. Biol. Med.* **94**, 151.
Olsson, I., and Gardell, S. (1967). *Biochim. Biophys. Acta* **141**, 348.
Olsson, I., Dahlqvist, A., and Norden, A. (1963). *Acta Med. Scand.* **174**, 123.
Pease, D. C. (1966). *J. Ultrastruct. Res.* **15**, 555.
Pepper, D. S., and Jamieson, G. A. (1968). *Nature (London)* **219**, 1252.
Pepper, D. S., and Jamieson, G. A. (1969a). *Biochemistry* **8**, 3362.
Pepper, D. S., and Jamieson, G. A. (1969b). *Blood* **34**, 522.
Pepper, D. S., and Jamieson, G. A. (1969c). Unpublished experiments.
Pepper, D. S., and Jamieson, G. A. (1970). *Biochemistry* **9**, 3706.
Rambourg, A., and Leblond, C. P. (1967). *J. Cell Biol.* **32**, 27.
Rambourg, A., and Leblond, C. P. (1969). *J. Microsc. (Paris)* **8**, 342.
Riddell, P. A., and Bier, A. M. (1965). *Nature (London)* **205**, 711.
Roskam, J. (1923). *Arch. Int. Physiol.* **10**, 241.
Saba, S. R., Rodman, N. F., and Mason, R. G. (1969). *Amer. J. Pathol.* **55**, 225.
Salmon, J., and Bounameaux, Y. (1958). *Thromb. Diath. Haemorrh.* **2**, 96.
Seaman, G. V. F. (1966). *Arch. Biochem. Biophys.* **117**, 10.
Schulz, H. (1968). "Electron Microscopy of Blood Platelets and Thrombosis." Springer, Berlin.
Schulz, H., and Landgraber, E. (1966). *Klin. Wochenschr.* **44**, 998.
Shulman, N. R., Marder, V. J., Hiller, M. C., and Collier, E. M. (1964). *Progr. Hematol.* **4**, 222.
Sokal, G. (1962). *Acta Haematol.* **28**, 313.
Solum, N. O., and Lopaciuk, S. (1969a). *Thromb. Diath. Haemorrh.* **21**, 419.
Solum, N. O., and Lopaciuk, S. (1969b). *Thromb. Diath. Haemorrh.* **21**, 478.
Svensson, H. (1967). *Protides Biol. Fluids Proc. Colloq.* **15**, 515.
Terada, H., Baldini, M., Ebbe, S., and Madoff, M. A. (1966). *Blood* **28**, 213.
Uhlenbruck, G. (1961). *Z. Immunitaetsforsch. Exp. Ther.* **121**, 420.
Vainer, H., and Wattiaux, R. (1968). *Nature (London)* **217**, 951.
Ware, A. G., Fahey, J. L., and Seegers, W. H. (1948). *Amer. J. Physiol.* **154**, 140.
Weiss, H. J., and Kochwa, S. (1968). *J. Lab. Clin. Med.* **71**, 153.
Wesemann, W. (1969). *FEBS Letters* **3**, 80.
Wesemann, W., and Zilliken, F. (1968). *Z. Physiol. Chem.* **349**, 823.
Wilson, P. A., McNicol, G. P., and Douglas, A. S. (1967). *Thromb. Diath. Haemorrh.* **18**, 66.
Winzler, R. J. (1969). *In* "Red Cell Membrane—Structure and Function" (G. A. Jamieson and T. J. Greenwalt, eds.), pp. 157–171. Lippincott, Philadelphia, Pennsylvania.
Woodside, E. E., and Kocholaty, W. (1960). *Blood* **16**, 1173.
Woolley, D. W., and Gommi, B. W. (1964). *Nature (London)*, 1074.
Zucker, M. B., and Levine, R. U. (1963). *Thromb. Diath. Haemorrh.* **10**, 1.

6

PLATELET PROTEINS*

RALPH L. NACHMAN

* Supported by grants from the American Heart Association, USPHS, the Krakower Fund, and the Kreizel Foundation.

I. HISTORICAL BACKGROUND

Approximately 50 years ago Roskam (1922) first called attention to the protein constituents associated with platelets. He proposed the presence of a "plasmatic atmosphere" consisting of adsorbed plasma proteins. Since this time considerable evidence has accumulated supporting the concept that this microplasmatic environment plays an important role in partly mediating the role of the platelet in hemostasis, blood coagulation, and thrombosis (Bounameaux, 1957; Adelson et al., 1961; Bull, 1966; Horowitz and Fujimoto, 1965; Ware et al., 1948). This external protein coat of the platelet is easily visualized as a dense phosphotungstic acid positive halo on electron microscopy (Bull, 1966). Initially, it was felt that the adsorbed membrane layer resulted from a sponge-like effect; however, in recent years the evidence strongly suggests that the phenomenon more probably represents a selective adsorptive process (Nachman, 1968). Thus the clotting factors V and XI and fibrinogen are found in high concentrations on the

TABLE I

HUMAN PLATELET PROTEIN

Plasma proteins
  Fibrinogen
  Albumin
  γG-Globulin
  γM-Globulin
  Plasminogen
  Prealbumin
  Fibrin stabilizing factor
  Complement C3, C4
  β-Lipoprotein

Procoagulants
  (II, V, VII, VIII, IX, X, XI, XII)

Platelet specific
  Thrombosthenin
  Glycoprotein
  α-Globulin
  β-Globulin
  Cationic permeability factor(s)
  Platelet factor 2: fibrinogen activator
  Platelet factor 4: antiheparin
  Antiplasmin
  Protease (cathepsin A)

---

platelet surface despite extensive washing procedures (Horowitz and Fuji-moto, 1965). On the other hand, the procoagulants—factors II, VII, VIII, and XII which have been identified on the platelet surface—are washed off with relative ease. It therefore appears likely that the platelet membrane exhibits differential binding affinitives for various plasma proteins.

In addition to the plasma proteins of the periplatelet atmosphere, it has become clear in recent years that certain platelet specific proteins mediate important steps in the normal platelet physiologic processes. Table I lists the major protein constituents of the human platelet. Certain of these such as the contractile protein, thrombosthenin, are dealt with extensively in this volume, Chapter 7 by Lüscher and Bettex-Galland.

II. METHODOLOGY AND GENERAL CONSIDERATIONS

Protein comprises approximately 60% of the dry weight of platelets (Maupin, 1961). 1500 μq of protein can be obtained from 10^9 normal platelets (Nachman, 1968). Most of the recent work relating to the specific characterization of various platelet proteins has involved immunochemical analysis of platelet sonicates and extracts. These studies have employed extensively washed platelets so as to ensure maximal removal of the loosely adsorbed plasma proteins. We have utilized platelet protein solubilized by ultrasonic vibration and subsequently concentrated by ultrafiltration pro-cedures. Various antisera absorbed and nonabsorbed with lyophilized platelet-free human plasma have been utilized to characterize the solubilized platelet protein. It should be noted that in studies such as these, care should be taken to avoid prolonged ultrasonic treatment of the washed cell suspen-sions. Thus prolonged ultrasonic exposure of plasma fibrinogen leads to significant denaturation of the molecule (Searcy et al., 1965). Generally the sonic extraction on platelets performed in our immunochemical studies was carried out over 10 seconds which is appreciably less than the times used to denature fibrinogen (Searcy et al., 1965). Frozen and thawed as well as mechanically homogenized cell preparations have also been used with success. An example of an immunoelectrophoretic analysis of platelet sonicate is shown in Fig. 1. The polyvalent antihuman platelet serum revealed multiple precipitins. The univalent antifibrinogen serum clearly identified the fibrinogen component in the platelet protein mixture. Thus by utilizing various antisera, different components in the sonicate were specifically identified. Utilizing quantitative immunologic methods based on the measurement of precipitin ring diameters, it was possible to estimate the amount of various proteins in the normal platelet sonicate (Table II). Fibrinogen was found to represent approximately 10–12% of the total platelet protein. Albumin and γG-globulin (biclonal) were present in amounts equal to 2–4% of the total protein.

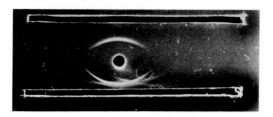

FIG. 1. Immunoelectrophoresis of platelet sonicate protein. Antiplatelet serum at bottom. Antifibrinogen at top. The anode is toward the right.

In addition to the above immunochemical techniques, DEAE chromatography and polyacrylamide gel electrophoresis have been used to clarify the platelet protein population in greater detail. An example of such an approach is shown in Fig. 2, where 180 mg of soluble platelet protein was subjected to DEAE chromatography. The heterogeneity of the various protein peaks was demonstrated by polyacrylamide gel electrophoresis of the major peaks. This particular study was designed to characterize the intracellular platelet proteases particularly cathepsin A which was localized to the peak 4 material (Nachman and Ferris, 1968). The highly sensitive acrylamide gel system has allowed a much more precise analysis of the various platelet proteins. By these techniques up to 20 separate platelet proteins have been demonstrated (Nachman, 1968; Lopaciuk and Solum, 1969).

TABLE II

PLATELET PROTEIN QUANTITATION IN 10^9 PLATELETS[a]

Protein	μg
Fibrinogen	150–180 (10–12%)
Albumin	30–45 (2–3%)
γG-Globulin	38–55 (2–4%)

[a] Modified from Nachman and Marcus (1968).

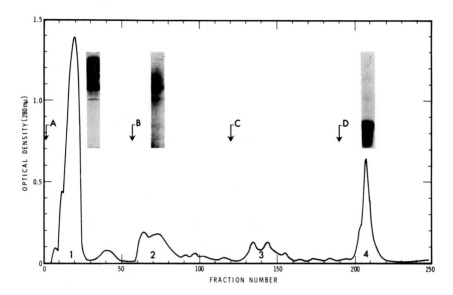

Fig. 2. DEAE chromatography of soluble platelet protein. Batch elution of major protein peaks using increasing salt concentration at B, C, and D. The acrylamide gel patterns of the separate peaks is shown. (From Nachman and Ferris, 1968.)

Clotting factor assays of various platelet preparations using substrate with specific factor deficiencies have been quite useful in identifying specific platelet associated procoagulants (Horowitz and Fujimoto, 1965).

III. PLASMA PROTEINS ASSOCIATED WITH PLATELETS

A. Fibrinogen

One of the most clearly defined and extensively studied platelet antigens is a thrombin clottable protein which is immunologically identical to fibrinogen (see Fig. 1). Roskam (1922) and Ware *et al.* (1948) described the clottable platelet protein. Salmon and Bounameaux (1958) first using immunochemical techniques identified fibrinogen in bovine platelets after extensive washing. They concluded that the protein was part of the intracellular structure. On the other hand, Schmidt *et al.* (1962) who were unable to detect the clottable protein after the exposure of the platelets to trypsin concluded that the fibrinogen was essentially a surface component. Grette (1962) chemically extracted the thrombin clottable protein from trypsinized platelets and concluded that fibrinogen was therefore an intracellular constituent. This work was confirmed by Gocken and Yunis (1963) using fluorescent antibody techniques who reported the presence of fibrinogen in trypsin and plasmin treated platelets and in megakaryocytes as well. We similarly demonstrated that a thrombin clottable protein, immunologically identical to fibrinogen was present in the solubilized protein derived from trypsinized platelets (Nachman, 1965). These enzyme treated platelets did not form aggregates in the presence of thrombin suggesting that the surface fibrinogen was essentially digested. Subsequently direct immunochemical analyses of isolated intracellular granules have clearly demonstrated the presence of an intracellular compartment of the platelet fibrinogen (Nachman et al., 1967b). Approximately 25% of the total platelet fibrinogen was intimately associated with the intracellular granule, mitochondrial fraction isolated following sucrose density gradient ultracentrifugation of the cell homogenate (Table III).

TABLE III

SUBCELLULAR PLATELET FIBRINOGEN[a]

	mg
Total platelet protein on gradient	25.5
Fibrinogen in soluble fraction	2.1
Fibrinogen in granule fraction	0.7
Fibrinogen in membrane fraction	0.0

[a] Modified from Nachman et al. (1967b).

It is of interest that the granule fibrinogen formed a poor flocculent clot upon the addition of a thrombin calcium mixture. Castaldi and Caen (1965) also reported that intracellular platelet fibrinogen showed impaired clottability. In considering these studies, it is important to note that platelet granules contain proteases (Nachman and Ferris, 1968) which have the capacity to alter the clottability as well as the immunochemical integrity of the intracellular protein. Castaldi and Caen (1965) using radioisotopically labeled fibrinogen demonstrated that plasma fibrinogen exchanged with adsorbed surface fibrinogen on the platelet; there was no exchange with the intracellular compartment. Thus, it appears likely that there are two platelet fibrinogen compartments: one extracellular, adsorbed to the external membrane; and the other intracellular, primarily associated with granules. It remains to be determined whether these two separate compartmental molecular systems have functionally different activities.

It is thus of great interest and importance to determine whether the intracellular and extracellular fibrinogens are truly identical. Solum and Lopaciuk (1969a,b) working with bovine platelets have provided the most extensive data in this regard. They purified bovine platelet fibrinogen by application of the plasma fibrinogen methods of Blombach and Blombach. The platelets used for these studies were carefully washed four times. The extractable bovine fibrinogen represented approximately 14% of the total platelet protein obtained following freeze thawing. These authors stated that the platelet fibrinogen in their studies was mainly "of intracellular origin," however, the possibility must be considered that a significant percentage represented adsorbed bovine plasma fibrinogen. The most highly purified platelet fibrinogen fraction contained 91–98% thrombin clottable protein. No significant differences were found between platelet and plasma fibrinogen as to sedimentation behavior, electrophoretic mobility, or light absorption spectra. The amino acid composition and the N-terminal acids were the same. However, distinct significant differences were found in intrinsic viscosity, carbohydrate content, and clotting behavior. It was concluded that denaturation during purification was not a likely cause of the observed biochemical differences. The findings of Castaldi and Caen (1965) relating to absence of exchange of plasma and platelet fibrinogen together with Solum's demonstration of a biochemical uniqueness of platelet fibrinogen compared to plasma fibrinogen raises the interesting possibility of a separate functional role for the intracellular platelet fibrinogen. Further studies in this area will be awaited with great interest particularly in view of the growing body of evidence suggesting the innate biochemical heterogeneity of normal plasma fibrinogen (Finlayson and Mosesson, 1963).

B. Albumin and γG-Globulin

These plasma proteins were present in solubilized platelet protein preparations in approximately equal concentrations (Table II). The γG-globulin which was biclonal was not detected in preparations derived from trypsinized platelets suggesting that this is entirely a component of the external periplatelet atmosphere (Nachman, 1968).

γM-globulin was first identified as an associated platelet protein by Salmon (1958). Anti-γM has been shown to agglutinate platelets at 4°C as well as inhibit clot retraction and prolong clot lysis of diluted whole blood (Taylor and Müller-Eberhard, 1967). In these studies whole blood was diluted 1:10 with buffer at 4°C and then the platelets were separated by centrifugation.

Platelet albumin was still detected immunochemically in sonicates obtained from trypsinized cells suggesting that this component occupies at least in part an intracellular compartment (Nachman, 1968). Electrophoretic as well as immunologic studies suggest that platelet albumin is essentially identical to serum albumin (Ganguly, 1969a).

C. Complement

C3 and C4 components of human complement have been identified on the platelet surface under the same circumstances as described above for γM. Antisera to C3 and C4 caused impaired clot retraction and retarded lysis of diluted whole blood. These antisera also agglutinated washed platelets and inhibited platelet fusion in clot sections 2 hours after the addition of thrombin (Taylor and Müller-Eberhard, 1967). These authors concluded from these studies that platelets in diluted whole blood at 4°C adsorb a γM globulin which subsequently initiates a complement reaction on the platelet surface involving the components C1 through C4. The physiological significance of these findings remains to be determined.

D. Fibrin Stabilizing Factor

This plasma protein which renders fibrin clots insoluble in certain solvents, such as urea and monochloracetic acid, has been identified in high concentration in human platelets (Kiesselbach and Wagner, 1966). The platelet associated protein has antigenic and enzymic activity similar to the circulating protein. Fibrin stabilizing factor is thrombin labile and loses its antigenic characteristics after exposure to thrombin. Thus it no longer forms a precipitin arc when allowed to diffuse against its specific antibody following thrombin treatment. The mechanism of the loss of the immunoprecipitate is not known, but presumably is related to the proteolytic activity of thrombin on the fibrin stabilizing factor substrate with resultant structural alterations. Platelet fibrin stabilizing factor has been shown to possess antiplasmin activity presumably due to the cross-linking of the fibrin clot (McDonagh et al., 1969a).

Recent data suggest that platelet fibrin stabilizing factor has a smaller molecular weight than the plasma factor (McDonagh et al., 1969a). Mc-

Donagh *et al.* (1969b) studied a patient with congenital fibrin stabilizing factor deficiency. Transfusion of fresh frozen plasma led to the expected appearance of the clotting factor in the plasma in 24 hours; however, no fibrin stabilizing factor was detected in platelets obtained at the same time. The experiment implies that the plasma factor was not transported across the platelet membrane in measurable quantities. The authors raised the possibility that platelet fibrin stabilizing factor is a true platelet component originating in the megakaryocyte. Thus platelet fibrinogen and platelet fibrin stabilizing factor appear to have some rather interesting biochemical analogies when compared to the plasma counterpart: (1) The platelet proteins may not represent transferred plasma products; and (2) both platelet proteins appear to have slight structural differences when compared to the plasma factors. The proof of the rather unique properties of platelet fibrin stabilizing factor as well as platelet fibrinogen must rest on a complete structural analysis of the purified proteins.

E. β-Lipoprotein

Davey and Lüscher (1968) reported that β-lipoprotein was released from platelets after thrombin exposure. This protein reacted with a specific plasma β-lipoprotein antiserum. This released platelet β-lipoprotein showed procoagulant activity in a Russell's viper venom clotting system. The authors speculated that this activity may represent Horowitz's "nonsedimentable platelet factor 3" (1965).

IV. PLATELET SPECIFIC PROTEINS

In recent years great attention has focused on platelet-specific proteins. It is clear that some of these proteins play important roles in various steps of the hemostatic process. One of the most interesting proteins in this category, thrombosthenin, the contractile protein, is the subject of Chapter 7 by Lüscher and Bettex-Galland. As many as 8 different platelet protein antigens have been identified by immunochemical techniques using anti-platelet protein antiserum absorbed with plasma (Lopaciuk and Solum, 1969). The specific functional roles of these proteins is still not known. Many of these proteins have been superficially characterized as a function of immunoelectrophoretic properties.

The platelet glycoprotein described by Bezkorovainy and Rafelson (1964) moved with the same mobility as γ-globulin but failed to react with γ-

globulin antisera. This protein contained 64% hexose and smaller amounts of hexosamine, fucose, and hexuronic acid. Davey and Lüscher (1968) identified platelet specific γ- and β-globulins in the supernatant following the thrombin release reaction.

A. Platelet Factor 2: Fibrinogen Activator

Platelet factor 2 is a heat stable low molecular weight protein which is precipitated in the presence of Zn^{2+} ions (Niewiarowski et al., 1967). The protein has been purified by DEAE chromatography and acrylamide gel electrophoresis. Platelet factor 2 accelerates fibrinogen clotting by thrombin, aggregates platelets and neutralizes antithrombin III. The protein is not released in the generalized platelet release reaction and is presumably a cytoplasmic constituent (Stormorken, 1969).

B. Platelet Factor 4: Antitheparin

Platelet factor 4 is also a heat stable low molecular weight protein precipitable by Zn^{2+} ions (Niewiarowski et al., 1967). This protein has been purified by DEAE chromatography and acrylamide gel electrophoresis. This protein has interesting properties and causes neutralization of heparin and fibrinogen breakdown products. Aggregation induced by thrombin, ADP, collagen, and adrenaline cause a release of a large portion of platelet factor 4 (Niewiarowski et al., 1968; Stormorken, 1969). The protein is presumably a granule constituent. This protein also causes paracoagulation of soluble fibrin monomer complexes. It has been postulated that platelet factor 4 may function in the adherence of platelets to fibrin threads and in the consolidation of the platelet plug (Niewiarowski et al., 1968). It seems clear that this platelet-specific protein may be an important component of early hemostatic reactions.

C. Cationic Permeability Factor(s)

A cationic protein extract obtained from isolated platelet granules, increased vascular permeability in mouse and rabbit skin (Nachman et al., 1970). The permeability effect appeared to be related to a mastocytolytic activity similar to that which has been described for a leukocyte cationic permeability factor. The cationic protein was nondializable, relatively heat stable, and trypsin sensitive. It is still not clear how many separate cationic proteins are involved in the mediation of the permeability effect. The possibility should be considered that other inflammatory effects such as chemotaxis and antibacterial activity may be mediated by the cationic fraction.

D. Cathepsin A

Intracellular platelet granules similar to the lysosomes of other cells contain numerous enzymes including potent proteases (Nachman and Ferris, 1968). Cathepsin A activity has been identified in a DEAE fraction of soluble platelet protein. The enzyme activity which was heat labile and not blocked by standard inhibitors of plasmin, hydrolyzed the synthetic substrate N-carbobenzoxy-α-L-glutamyl-L-tryosine. An identical proteolytic activity was found when the proteins derived from isolated platelet granules were examined. This platelet protease fraction was localized to the albumin–prealbumin region of the platelet soluble protein mixture (peak 4 in Fig. 2). It is of interest that the cathepsin A protease fraction caused marked proteolysis of purified plasma fibrinogen. Thus this platelet proteolytic activity may function in the early stages of platelet plug dissolution.

V. SUBCELLULAR PROTEIN DISTRIBUTION

Marcus and associates (1966) first described the successful analysis of the subcellular fractions of human platelets using a sucrose density gradient ultracentrifugation technique. This approach has greatly facilitated the systematic analysis of the intracellular architecture of the platelet. Immunochemical analyses of the separated washed sucrose gradient fractions has permitted a reasonably accurate assignment of several proteins to specific subcellular compartments. A summary of the platelet proteins identified in isolated subcellular fractions is listed in Fig. 3. Fibrinogen, fibrin stabilizing factor, γG-globulin, albumin, and plasminogen as well as specific α- and β-globulins have been identified in soluble "cell sap" fraction. Platelet factor 2 is also presumably a soluble component. Fibrinogen and two unidentified platelet antigens C and D were demonstrated immunologically in the granule fraction (Nachman and Marcus, 1968). In addition, the cationic permeability factor was extracted from platelet granules. It should be noted also that the granule compartment is rich in several enzyme systems including cathepsin A. Two unidentified platelet

antigens A and B were detected immunologically in the membrane fraction
(Nachman and Marcus, 1968). Thrombosthenin, the platelet contractile
protein, was extracted from both the subcellular granule and membrane
fractions (Nachman *et al.*, 1967a). Platelet aggregation studies using antithrombosthenin sera strongly suggest that contractile protein bears a close
relationship to the plasma membrane and is sterically available to surface

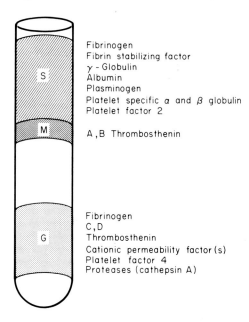

Fibrinogen
Fibrin stabilizing factor
γ - Globulin
Albumin
Plasminogen
Platelet specific α and β globulin
Platelet factor 2

A , B Thrombosthenin

Fibrinogen
C , D
Thrombosthenin
Cationic permeability factor (s)
Platelet factor 4
Proteases (cathepsin A)

FIG. 3. Subcellular distribution of the major platelet proteins. S, soluble or cell sap
layer; M, membrane layer; G, granule layer, as obtained on sucrose density gradient
ultracentrifugation. (Modified from Nachman and Marcus, 1968.)

reacting antisera. The possibility must be considered that the thrombosthenin
which is extracted from the granular layer represents contaminating material
resulting from the separation technique (Lüscher and Bettex-Galland,
1968).

Specific Membrane Proteins

We have recently analyzed in more detail the biochemical properties of
the proteins derived from the isolated membranes of washed human platelets
(Nachman and Ferris, 1970). The protein was solubilized in sodium dodecyl
sulfate and analyzed by acrylamide gel disk electrophoresis. The prepara-

tions obtained from intact as well as lipid extracted membranes contained a heterogeneous population of 10–15 molecules with a predominant molecular weight range of 20,000–90,000 (Fig. 4). It was of interest that one of the membrane proteins appeared to retain antigenic specificity in both delipidated and nonlipid extracted membrane preparations. It was not possible to identify fibrinogen or other known platelet surface components in these denatured membrane preparations.

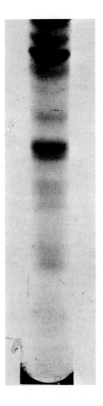

Fɪɢ. 4. Acrylamide gel disk electrophoresis of purified platelet membrane protein solubilized in 1% sodium dodecyl sulfate.

Pepper and Jamieson (1969) have analyzed the glycoprotein content of a partially purified platelet membrane fraction. They characterized a series of glycopeptides obtained by proteolytic digestion of the membrane fraction. The glycoproteins appeared to form an integral part of the membrane and were composed of a variety of complex heterosaccharide units which differed significantly from those isolated from erythrocytes.

VI. THROMBIN LABILE PROTEINS

In recent years attention has been drawn to the fact that thrombin has pronounced effects on several platelet proteins in addition to fibrinogen. The importance of these reactions have been emphasized in view of the key role that thrombin plays in initiating platelet hemostatic reactions. In addition, further data suggest that the thrombin platelet reaction is probably mediated in fact by a nonfibrinogen substrate. Davey and Lüscher (1965) compared the action of various snake venoms on washed platelets and fibrinogen solutions to the effects produced by thrombin and concluded that fibrinogen was not the essential substrate leading to "platelet metamorphosis." Salmon and Bounameaux (1958) and Nachman (1965) have previously shown that mobility of a platelet β-globulin is altered in starch gel electrophoresis following thrombin addition to the platelet protein. The nonfibrinogen effect can also be demonstrated by acrylamide gel electrophoresis and by immunochemical analyses (Nachman, 1968; Ganguly, 1969b). In fact multiple changes in the platelet protein pattern following thrombin exposure have been noted. In Fig. 5 at least two separate platelet antigens have been markedly altered following thrombin treatment. The antiserum used to detect these changes was absorbed with lyophilized platelet free human plasma, thus these immunologic changes are presumably effecting proteins other than fibrin stabilizing factor or fibrinogen. Davey and Lüscher (1967) noted additional nonfibrinogen thrombin effects including attenuation of an α-globulin and cathodal shift of a platelet specific β-globulin. Of great interest are the recent findings of Cohen *et al.* (1969) reporting a marked structural alteration in thrombosthenin M following thrombin exposure. Incubation of purified thrombosthenin M with thrombin resulted in the appearance of one mole of carboxyl terminal arginine per

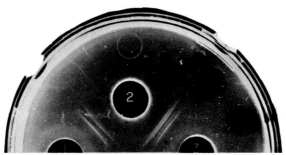

FIG. 5. Immunochemical analysis of thrombin effect on platelet protein. Well 1, platelet protein plus thrombin; well 3, platelet protein; well 2, antiplatelet serum absorbed with plasma. Thrombin has altered the antigenic reactivity of at least 2 platelet proteins.

10^5 g of thrombosthenin M. Incubation of platelets with thrombin resulted in the disappearance of the electrophoretic band corresponding to thrombosthenin M. It is thus clear that the mechanism of the thrombin–platelet reaction remains to be defined. It is tempting to speculate that hydrolytic cleavage of a non fibrinogen substrate on the platelet surface serves to initiate the early reactions of the hemostatic process.

VII. PROTEIN SYNTHESIS

One of the most exciting new chapters in platelet protein physiology is the recent demonstration of protein synthesis in platelets. This observation was first reported by Warshaw *et al.* (1966, 1967) and subsequently confirmed by others (Booyse and Rafelson, 1967a). Human platelets contain small amounts of RNA, but have no nucleus and no DNA (Maupin *et al.*, 1962). Thus the platelet may resemble the reticulocyte possessing a preformed protein synthetic apparatus. Booyse and Rafelson (1967a) described the incorporation of labeled amino acids into the contractile protein thrombostenin using a washed human platelet incubation system. These same workers described the presence of a stable mRNA directing the *de novo* synthesis of contractile proteins in platelets (Booyse and Rafelson, 1967b). It should be noted that the rate of protein synthesis in Booyse's washed platelet system was quite small on the order of 50- to 100-fold less protein synthesized compared to actively synthesizing normal cells. Additional studies have also reported the synthesis of platelet fibrinogen in the circulating platelet (Cooper and Firkin, 1967). At the present time, the significance of protein synthesis in circulating peripheral blood platelets remains obscure.

VIII. FUNCTIONAL CONSIDERATIONS

A. Hemostasis

It is tempting at present to relate most if not all of the characteristic platelet responses to ADP, collagen, and thrombin to specific membrane associated phenomena. These reactions, however, probably involve several different protein systems some of which in part represent adsorbed plasma components such as fibrinogen. This phenomenon is exemplified by the marked differences between two major congenital bleeding disorders— thrombasthenia and afibrinogenemia. These diseases are both characterized by grossly deficient platelet fibrinogen; thrombasthenia in addition represents a more profound aberration of intrinsic platelet constituents (Nachman and Marcus, 1968). Administration of intravenous fibrinogen completely corrects the hemostatic defect in afibrinogenemia, while the plasma fibrinogen in thrombasthenia is qualitatively and quantitatively normal. Thus fibrinogen must be present in the external platelet atmosphere, if the normal hemostatic platelet plug is to form; however, other platelet protein constituents probably specific membrane receptors are required for the successful completion of a hemostatic plug. It is logical to expect that the unique physiologic platelet responses to the classic "hemostatic triggers" ADP, thrombin and collagen will be eventually correlated with specialized structural features of individual membrane proteins. The possibility that thrombosthenin, which is closely associated with the cell membrane, regulates membrane steric conformation through an enzymic pathway raises many interesting functional considerations (Salzman et al., 1966). These have been dealt with in a separate chapter.

B. Clot Retraction

Clot retraction, an in vitro phenomenon, illustrates another complex protein interaction which plays a role in platelet physiology. Disrupted cells do not support clot retraction, thus the contractile protein, thrombosthenin, must retain a specific steric configurational relationship in the cell in order to participate in the retraction process. Platelet fibrinogen is also necessary for clot retraction. It has been reported that enzymic splitting of fibrinopeptide B by thrombin is a necessary prerequisite for clot retraction (Morse et al., 1967). Clot retraction represents the culmination of several complex biochemical steps including (1) energy production in an intact platelet, (2) proteolytic digestion of membrane associated platelet fibrinogen, and (3) sterochemically intact thrombosthenin. The fact that antithrombosthenin which inhibits clot retraction also blocks the ATPase activity of the contractile protein suggests that the enzymic site may be important in the retraction process.

C. Participation in the Inflammatory Process

Platelets accumulate in blood vessels adjacent to areas of tissue damage and inflammation (Cotran, 1965). Mustard and associates (1965) first demonstrated that platelets contribute directly to the inflammatory response accompanying tissue injury by releasing intracellular constituents which increase vascular permeability. Our demonstration of a cationic extract in human platelet granules which increases vascular permeability draws an analogy between the circulating platelet and exudative polymorphonuclear leukocytes. The platelet granule fraction similar to the rabbit leukocyte mastocytolytic lysosomal cationic protein is extracted in weak mineral acid and is retained in the cationic fraction precipitated by 20% ethanol.

Various stimuli, including circulating antigen–antibody complexes, endotoxin, and bacteria as well as endothelial cell damage may lead to platelet aggregation and degranulation with lysosomal discharge of the mastocytolytic cationic protein. It is of interest that platelet granules also contain potent proteases including cathepsin A. These proteolytic activities may also contribute to additional phases of the early cell mediated inflammatory response. One difference should be stressed when comparing the circulating human platelets to exudative leukocytes. No lysosomal cationic permeability activity has been detected in circulating leukocytes. The vascular permeability enhancing activity previously described in leukocytes has been isolated from fractions obtained from exudative cells. It thus appears that the platelet may be a unique circulating cell with a precommitted exudative function which permits it to mediate early blood vessel responses adjacent to focal inflammatory stimuli. In this sense, the platelet represents a rapidly mobilizable efferent pharmacologic arm of the inflammatory response.

REFERENCES

Adelson, E., Rheingold, J. J., and Crosby, W. H. (1961). *Blood* **17**, 767.

Bezkorovainy, A., and Rafelson, M. E., Jr. (1964). *J. Lab. Clin. Med.* **64**, 212.

Booyse, F., and Rafelson, M. (1967a). *Nature* **215**, 283.

Booyse, F., and Rafelson, M. (1967b). *Biochim. Biophys. Acta* **145**, 188.

Bounameaux, Y. (1957). *Rev. Fr. Etud. Clin. Biol.* **2**, 52.

Bull, B. S. (1966). *Blood* **28**, 901.

Castaldi, P. A., and Caen, J. (1965). *J. Clin. Pathol.* **18**, 579.

Cohen, I., Bohak, Z., De Vries, A., and Katchalski, E. (1969). *Eur. J. Biochem.* **10**, 388.

Cooper, I. A., and Firkin, B. G. (1967). *Proc. Aust. Soc. Med. Res.* **2**, 106.

Cotran, R. A. (1965). *Amer. J. Pathol.* **46**, 589.

Davey, M. G., and Lüscher, E. F. (1965). *Nature* **207**, 730.

Davey, M. G., and Lüscher, E. F. (1967). *In* "Biochemistry of Blood Platelets" (E. Kowalski and S. Niewiarowski, eds.), pp. 9–20. Academic Press, New York.

Davey, M. G., and Lüscher, E. F. (1968). *Biochim. Biophy. Acta* **165**, 490.

Finlayson, J. S., and Mosesson, M. W. (1963). *Biochemistry* **2**, 42.

Ganguly, P. (1969a). *Biochim. Biophys. Acta* **188**, 78.

Ganguly, P. (1969b). *Blood* **33**, 590.

Gocken, M., and Yunis, E. (1963). *Nature* (*London*) **200**, 590.

Grette, K. (1962). *Acta Physiol. Scand.* **56,** Suppl., 195.

Horowitz, H. I. (1965). *Thromb. Diath. Haemorrh.* Suppl. **17,** 243.

Horowitz, H. I., and Fujimoto, M. M. (1965). *Proc. Soc. Exp. Biol. Med.* **19,** 487.

Kiesselbach, T. H., and Wagner, R. H. (1966). *Amer. J. Physiol.* **211,** 1472.

Lopaciuk, S., and Solum, N. O. (1969). *Thromb. Diath. Haemorrh.* **31,** 409.

Lüscher, E. F., and Bettex-Galland, M. (1968). *In* "Metabolism and Membrane Permeability of Erythrocyte and Thrombocytes" (E. Deutsch, E. Gerlach, and K. Moser, eds.), pp. 247–253. Verlag, Stuttgart.

McDonagh, J., Kiesselbach, T. H., and Wagner, R. H. (1969a). *Amer. J. Physiol.* **216,** 508.

McDonagh, J., McDonagh, R. P., Delage, J. M., and Wagner, R. H. (1969b). *J. Clin. Invest.* **48,** 940.

Marcus, A. J., Zucker-Franklin, D., Safier, L. B., and Ullman, H. L. (1966). *J. Clin. Invest.* **45,** 14.

Maupin, B. (1961). *Hemostase* **1,** 29.

Maupin, B., Saint-Blancard, J., and Storck, J. (1962). *Rev. Fr. Etud. Clin. Biol.* **7,** 169.

Morse, E. E., Jackson, D. P., and Conley, C. P. (1967). *J. Lab. Clin. Med.* **70,** 106.

Mustard, J. F., Movat, H. Z., MacMouve, D. R. C., and Senyi, A. (1965). *Proc. Soc. Exp. Biol. Med.* **119,** 988.

Nachman, R. L. (1965). *Blood* **25,** 703.

Nachman, R. L. (1968). *Semin. Hematol.* **5,** 18.

Nachman, R. L., and Ferris, B. (1968). *J. Clin. Invest.* **47,** 2530.

Nachman, R. L., and Ferris, B. (1970). *Biochemistry* **9,** 200.

Nachman, R. L., and Marcus, A. J. (1968). *Brit. J. Haematol.* **15,** 181.

Nachman, R. L., Marcus, A. J., and Safier, L. B. (1967a). *J. Clin. Invest.* **46,** 1380.

Nachman, R. L., Marcus, A. J., and Zucker-Franklin, D. (1967b). *J. Lab. Clin. Med.* **69,** 651.

Nachman, R. L., Weksler, B., and Ferris, B. (1970). *J. Clin. Invest.* **49,** 274.

Niewiarowski, S., Farbiszewski, R., and Poplawski, A. (1967). *In* "Biochemistry of Blood Platelets" (E. Kowalski and S. Niewiarowski, eds.), pp. 35–45. Academic Press, New York.

Niewiarowski, S., Poplawski, A., Lipinski, B., and Farbiszewski, R. (1968). *Exp. Biol. Med.* **3,** 121.

Pepper, D. S., and Jamieson, G. A. (1969). *Biochemistry* **8,** 3362.

Roskam, J. (1922). *Arch. Int. Physiol.* **20,** 241.

Salmon, J. (1958). *Schweiz. Med. Wochenschr.* **88,** 1047.

Salmon, J., and Bounameaux, Y. (1958). *Thromb. Diath. Haemorrh.* **2,** 93.

Salzman, E. W., Chambers, D. A., and Neri, L. L. (1966). *Nature (London)* **210,** 167.

Schmid, H. J., Jackson, D. P., and Conley, C. L. (1962). *J. Clin. Invest.* **41,** 543.

Searcy, R. L., Berquist, L. M., Simms, N. M., Johnston, D., and Foreman, J. A. (1965). *Nature (London)* **206,** 795.

Solum, N. O., and Lopaciuk, S. (1969a). *Thromb. Diath. Haemorrh.* **31,** 419.

Solum, N. O., and Lopaciuk, S. (1969b). *Thromb. Diath. Haemorrh.* **31,** 428.

Storrmorken, H. (1969) *Scand. J. Clin. Lab. Invest.* **107,** Suppl. 1, 115.

Taylor, F. B., and Müller-Eberhard, H. (1967). *Nature (London)* **216,** 1023.

Ware, A. G., Fahey, J. L., and Seegers, W. H. (1948). *Amer. J. Physiol.* **154,** 140.

Warshaw, A. L., Laster, L., and Shulman, N. R. (1966). *J. Clin. Invest.* **45,** 1923.

Warshaw, A. L., Laster, L., and Shulman, N. R. (1967). *J. Biol. Chem.* **242,** 2094.

7

THROMBOSTHENIN

ERNST F. LÜSCHER and M. BETTEX-GALLAND

I. INTRODUCTION

The spontaneous, active contraction of newly formed clots from whole blood or platelet-rich plasma is a phenomenon which for a long time has been, and still is, a challenge to research workers (for review, see Budtz-Olsen, 1951). The essential participation of platelets was already recognized in the last century, but whether they exert their effect by acting on a contractile fibrin or whether they are themselves carriers of the contractile principle remained controversial for a long time. This seems the more remarkable as the work of Bizzozero (1882), Eberth and Schimmelbusch (1886), and particularly of Wright and Minot (1917) clearly demonstrates that, independent of fibrin formation, platelets in the course of so-called viscous metamorphosis show active contraction of the primarily loose aggregates formed under the influence of thrombin. More recently this contraction of platelet aggregates in relation to fibrin formation has been studied in detail by Sokal (1960), and again it became quite clear that fine protrusions or pseudopodia which link individual platelets together must possess contractile properties.

Clot retraction is an energy-dependent process, and the consumption of ATP in the course of viscous metamorphosis is its prerequisite (Bettex-Galland and Lüscher, 1960). It therefore seemed logical enough to search for a contractile platelet constituent, and the result of these efforts was the isolation from human blood platelets of an actomyosin-like protein by Bettex-Galland and Lüscher (1959). This finding was confirmed by Grette in 1962 by the extraction of a comparable material from pig platelets. Subsequently Bettex-Galland and Lüscher proposed the name thrombosthenin for the contractile protein from platelets, a term which today has found wide acceptance.

II. PROPERTIES OF THROMBOSTHENIN

A. Biochemical Properties

1. SOLUBILITY

The extraction of thrombosthenin from disrupted platelets is based on its solubility at ionic strengths above 0.25 μ. At lower salt concentrations the protein is insoluble and this property has been used for its purification by repeated precipitation and redissolution (Bettex-Galland and Lüscher, 1959, 1961, 1965). It should be noted, however, that such preparations, as well as those obtained by Grette's method by precipitation with Mg^{2+} ions, still contain impurities, in particular, lipoprotein and fibrinogen of platelet origin. Further purification is best achieved by gel-filtration and density-barrier ultracentrifugation (Probst, 1970; Ganguly, 1969).

As evidenced by other members of the actomyosin family of contractile proteins, the solubility of thrombosthenin is enhanced by the presence of

ATP. At high ionic strength this is connected with a drop in viscosity which must be interpreted as the dissociation of the thrombosthenin complex into its constituents. On the other hand, the addition of ATP to thrombosthenin at low ionic strength, and in the presence of Mg^{2+} ions leads to the active contraction of the formed precipitate, a process termed "superprecipitation." The resulting coarse precipitate is no longer soluble at high ionic strength (cf. Bettex-Galland and Lüscher, 1961).

2. ATPase Activity

Thrombosthenin is an ATP-splitting enzyme; it is activated to a small extent by magnesium, and much more by calcium-ions (Bettex-Galland and Lüscher, 1961; Grette, 1962). It is inhibited by sulfhydryl-reagents, in particular by the mercurial Salyrgan. The Michaelis constant for purified thrombosthenin has been determined as $2.4 \times 10^{-5}M$ (Chambers et al., 1967) or, more recently as $3.6–5.0 \times 10^{-4}M$ (Rossi, 1969).

Solutions of ATP-dissociated thrombosthenin at high ionic strength regain spontaneously their original high viscosity due to the breakdown of the nucleotide by the preparation.

3. Thrombosthenin A and M

Thrombosthenin A corresponds to the actin moiety of muscle actomyosin; it can be prepared either from thrombosthenin or directly from acetone-dried platelets by the methods described for actin of muscular origin (Bettex-Galland et al., 1962, 1963). Thrombosthenin A may be prepared in the two interconvertible forms which correspond to actin G and F, i.e., the monomeric, globular, or the polymerized, fibrillar form. Electron microscopy shows that the tertiary structure of the F form of thrombosthenin A consists of long, beaded subfilaments, two of them being helically intertwined. The monomeric subunit, however, seems to be smaller than muscle actin G (Bettex-Galland et al., 1969; cf. Fig. 1).

Thrombosthenin M is either prepared by the methods used for muscle actin (cf. Bettex-Galland et al., 1962, 1963), or directly from lysed platelets by extraction at low ionic strength at alkaline pH in the presence of pyrophosphate, as described recently by Cohen et al. (1969). These authors have obtained a preparation which appeared homogeneous according to several criteria. In the ultracentrifuge most of the material showed a sedimentation constant of 7.2 S; about 10% were higher polymers. Thrombin altered this protein with respect to both its mobility in disk electrophoresis and to its N-terminal amino acid.

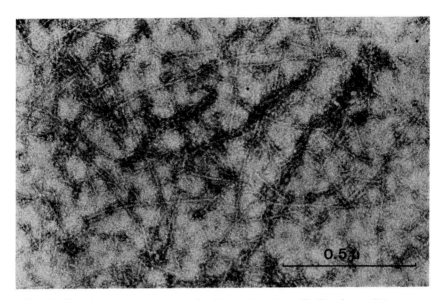

Fig. 1. Negative contrast micrograph of the polymeric or fibrillar form of thrombosthenin A. (Bettex-Galland *et al.*, 1969.)

Thrombosthenin M is the carrier of the ATPase property of thrombosthenin, the activity of the enzyme being considerably enhanced by combination with thrombosthenin A (Bettex-Galland *et al.*, 1963). The thrombosthenin M enzyme is exclusively activated by calcium-ions; its activity is not altered after treatment with thrombin (Cohen *et al.*, 1969).

It is of interest that enzymically active preparations which show the typical viscosity effect upon addition of ATP in solution are also obtained in hybrids from muscle actin and thrombosthenin M, or thrombosthenin A and muscle myosin. This experiment leads to positive results even if the muscle proteins are prepared from striated rabbit muscle and recombined with their counterparts obtained from human platelets (Bettex-Galland *et al.*, 1962, 1963). This would imply a rather far-reaching similarity of these subunits, which at present is difficult to reconcile with the smaller dimensions of thrombosthenin A as compared to muscle actin.

4. COMPARISON OF THROMBOSTHENIN WITH OTHER ACTOMYOSINS

The question arises, to what extent thrombosthenin is an entity of its own, and not just muscle actomyosin localized in platelets. Similarities and dissimilarities of the actomyosins from striated and smooth muscle with thrombosthenin and contractile proteins of other than muscle cells have been discussed in detail (see Bettex-Galland and Lüscher, 1965). As compared to actomyosin from striated muscle, thrombosthenin is soluble at somewhat lower ionic strength; it furthermore is a much weaker ATPase than actomyosins from striated, and even from smooth muscle. There can be no doubt, however, that contractile proteins comparable to thrombosthenin are present in a wide variety of other cells. This is suggested by the observations by Hoffmann-Berling (1956) on certain tumor cells, by the similarities of the ultrastructure of contractile protein in fibroblasts (Keyserlingk, 1969; Schäfer-Danneel and Weissenfels, 1969) and finally by the close resemblance of an actomyosin-like protein from leucocytes to thrombosthenin (Senda et al., 1969). Thus it seems justified to consider thrombosthenin as the prototype of a contractile protein of nonmuscular origin.

B. Ultrastructure of Thrombosthenin and Its Subunits

1. MICROFIBRILS

Electronmicrographs of normal platelets show no evidence for the presence of a preformed contractile system comparable to the one found in striated muscle. Under special conditions, however, the cytoplasm of platelets shows large amounts of microfibrils with a diameter of 80–100 Å, and variable lengths up to 0.5 μ (Zucker-Franklin and Nachman, 1967; Zucker-Franklin et al., 1967; for review, see also Lüscher, 1970). Recently, direct proof for the identity of this material with thrombosthenin has been offered by electronmicroscopy of glycerol-treated platelets in the relaxed and contracted state (Bettex-Galland et al., 1969): In the first case many fibrils of the F form of thrombosthenin A (cf. Fig. 1) and the small, nondiscernible subunits of thrombosthenin M form a flexible, loose network (Fig. 2a); upon addition of ATP thrombosthenin M polymerizes to stiff, often spindle-shaped needles which intermingle with the thrombosthenin A filaments (Fig. 2b). Figure 3 leaves no doubt that thrombosthenin is present in the platelet cytoplasm; there is no evidence for the involvement of either the platelet membrane, or of organelles in the contraction of this material. This does not yet entirely exclude the possibility of a structure-bound portion of the contractile material as postulated by Nachman et al. (1967). In fact, it appears improbable that the contraction of cytoplasmic thrombosthenin would not somehow exert a direct effect on the cell membrane and therefore that some link must exist between membrane structures and contractile protein.

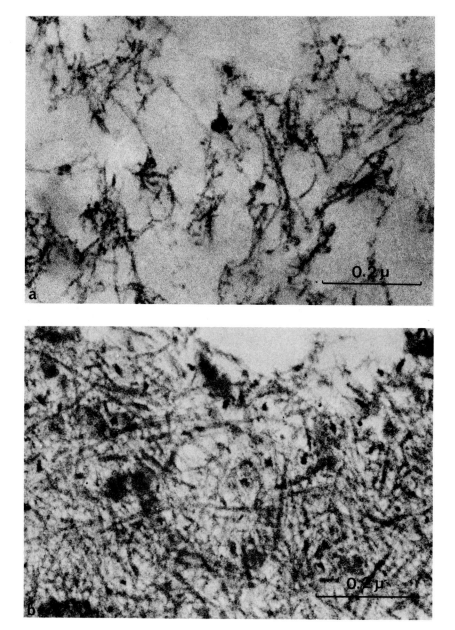

FIG. 2. Ultrathin section of fixed and contrasted thrombosthenin precipitate. (a) Non-contracted precipitate, showing mainly the loose, filmlike aspect of thrombosthenin A polymer. (b) ATP-superprecipitated form of same extract with characteristic thrombos-thenin M needles. (Bettex-Galland *et al.*, 1969.)

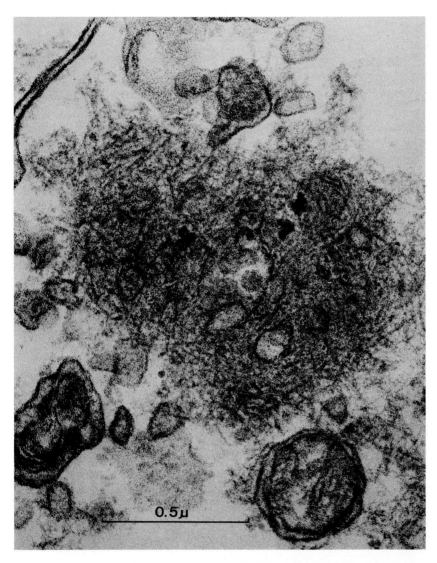

FIG. 3. Ultrathin section of glycerin-extracted platelet after incubation with ATP at low ionic strength, showing characteristic aspect of thrombosthenin superprecipitate. Upper left two adjacent platelet membranes; lower right, mitochondrion. (Bettex-Galland *et al.*, 1969.)

2. Microtubules

Microtubules in platelets have first been described by Behnke (1965) and by Bessis and Breton-Gorius (1965). Since then the presence of these intriguing structures has been confirmed many times. Microtubules show a filamentous substructure (Behnke and Zelander, 1967a,b; White, 1968), and these microfilaments in turn are most likely composed of globular subunits of 35–40 Å periodicity. Although microfilaments show no indication of a helical arrangement, it nevertheless seems probable that their subunits might bear a relationship to thrombosthenin A. Zucker-Franklin (1969) has observed that microfibrils appear whenever microtubules disappear, as after osmotic shock or after the addition of $10^{-4}M$ ADP to platelets (cf. also the discussion by Bettex-Galland et al., 1969). Similar conclusions were reached by Shepro et al. (1969) and by Puszkin et al. (1969). Finally, Mohri (1968) has described that the microtubules of sperm flagella can be dissociated to an actinlike material which will combine with muscle myosin to give a contractile complex. Although this experiment has not yet been repeated with platelet material, it suggests, together with all the other evidence presented, that microtubules could indeed, besides their role as a cytoskeleton, act as a reservoir for thrombosthenin A.

C. Biosynthesis of Thrombosthenin

There can be no doubt that thrombosthenin is synthesized by the megakaryocyte; in fact, in view of the pronounced motility of these cells it is not astonishing to find large amounts of it in their fragmented cytoplasm. For a long time platelets were considered to be unable to synthesize protein: They contain no DNA, and only negligible amounts of RNA. In 1967 Booyse and Rafelson (1967a) were able to demonstrate that platelets nevertheless incorporate labeled amino acids into the contractile protein. The same authors (1967b,c) explained this finding by the presence of a stable messenger RNA, persisting in young platelets and endowing them with synthetic activity; later (1967c), they succeeded in bringing about the synthesis of thrombosthenin by a cell-free in vitro system. This observation was extended by Steiner (1969) whose preliminary report suggests the simultaneous synthesis of the A and M moieties of thrombosthenin.

According to Booyse and Rafelson (1967c) the site of this synthetic activity is the cell membrane; that this is the exclusive site appears improbable in view of the finding by Tsao (personal communication) that ribosomes are found in young platelets in the cytoplasmic compartment.

As interesting as this unexpected activity of the platelet may be, there can be little doubt that it is a remainder of an activity of the parent cell, and most likely without functional significance.

III. FUNCTION OF THROMBOSTHENIN

A. Relaxing Factor

Thrombosthenin could play a role in platelet function in at least three different ways: as a contractile element; as an ATP-degrading enzyme; and, related to the first activity, by contributing to alterations in surface properties as a consequence of allosteric effects linked to the contraction process.

In every case it must be assumed that an inert, perhaps relaxed form is either transformed into the contractile material, and or that contraction is somehow triggered. Since optimal ATPase activity is found in the intact thrombosthenin A–M complex, contractile activity follows the same pattern.

It seems premature to discuss here a possible incorporation of microtubular material into thrombosthenin. Microtubules are extremly labile, and their temperature sensitivity (cf. Behnke, 1967) suggests a hitherto unknown relationship to the energy metabolism. Even after the formation of the thrombosthenin complex the problem of its activation to contraction remains.

In striated muscle it is generally assumed that the contraction–relaxation cycle is governed by the availability of calcium ions. This implies the presence, first of calcium-sensitive troponine, which up to now has not been found in platelets, and, second, of a regulation of the intracellular calcium level. It should be mentioned that such a mechanism becomes meaningless for thrombosthenin localized on the outside of the platelet membrane.

Grette (1963) has indeed described a relaxing factor in extracts from blood platelets, and Statland *et al.* (1969) have recently confirmed and extended this observation. For these authors the relaxing factor consists of membrane vesicles with the properties of a calcium pump, comparable to the sarcoplasmatic reticulum of muscle. These membranes contain an ATPase, and the inhibition of this enzyme would then lead to the availability of calcium ions and to the initiation of contraction.

It is noteworthy that contractile activity in the platelet is a one-way process; a relaxation phase is not observed. This may be due to the fact that the process which triggers contraction involves serious damage to the cell with subsequent loss or impairment of metabolic activity, on the one hand, and unhampered influx of ions from the outside on the other hand. The role of a "relaxing system" therefore must mainly be limited to the maintenance of a steady state in the resting cell.

B. Thrombosthenin as a Contractile Element

After the initiation of platelet viscous metamorphosis by one of several means, i.e., thrombin, collagen, and ADP in the presence of fibrinogen, platelets rapidly undergo morphological changes: They loose their disk shape, and pseudopod formation begins. Although in this phase large scale contraction is not obvious, local phenomena may nevertheless be essential for the observed transformations. This phase is also characterized by a burst of metabolism, and short-lived increase in ATP. It is followed by progressive reduction of metabolically active ATP and by a period of pronounced contractile activity, which in the case of aggregated platelets, is macroscopically discernible.

C. Thrombosthenin as an Enzyme

The fact that ADP in small amounts is a powerful initiator of platelet aggregation has led to the speculation that it might do so by inhibiting an ATP-splitting enzyme. Thrombosthenin–ATPase is indeed inhibited, although not impressively by ADP; it seemed logical enough to designate it as the target for the dinucleotide on the platelet surface. This localization is essential, since ADP will not penetrate into platelets. Several theories for platelet aggregation by ADP are based on this assumption. Thus, Salzman et al. (1966) postulate the inhibition by ADP of an "ecto-ATPase" (cf. Chambers et al., 1967) with the properties of thrombosthenin. This inhibition would lead to a disturbance of the surface structure with an altered charge distribution, which in turn would be responsible for aggregation. B. M. Jones (1966) and P. T. C. Jones (1966) suggest that a membrane-located, contractile protein is quite generally responsible for cell adhesion, and again its inhibition by ADP leads to alterations of the surface charge as a consequence of the allosteric transformation of the protein. Booyse and Rafelson (1969) finally, assume that an increased ATP level, resulting from the inhibition of a membrane-located ATPase by ADP, combined with an increased production during the "metabolic burst" will lead to a dissociation of thrombosthenin into its components. This offers the possibility of the formation of new thrombosthenin A–M complexes, extending from one platelet to another, again resulting in aggregation. This last hypothesis unfortunately does not explain why ATP itself is unable to aggregate platelets.

In view of the fact that in all these theories the presence of thrombosthenin on the membrane appears crucial, it seems appropriate to review briefly the available evidence for such an assumption. Platelets indeed show ATPase activity (cf. Chambers *et al.*, 1967; Rossi, 1969); there can be no doubt, however, that enzymes other than thrombosthenin must also be taken into consideration. It is noteworthy that platelet membrane fragments obtained by density gradient centrifugation display high magnesium-activated ATPase activity, which is also inhibited by ADP (Käser-Glanzmann, 1970).

Antibodies against thrombosthenin or thrombosthenin M, if applied to intact platelets, will interfere with typical manifestations of platelet activity such as clot retraction (Nachman *et al.*, 1967; Cohen *et al.*, 1969). Unfortunately, retraction is also rather unexpectedly inhibited by an antiserum against γM (Taylor and Müller-Eberhard, 1967); this suggests that the question as to the specificity of such reactions is as yet justified.

Taken all together, the hypotheses on the possible role of the thrombosthenin ATPase as the direct target for ADP in platelet aggregation appear attractive in many respects. There are, however, still several points, such as the nature of the "ecto-ATPase(-s)", which need further clarification before anyone is fully accepted.

IV. THE PHYSIOLOGICAL SIGNIFICANCE OF THROMBOSTHENIN

A. Clot Retraction

There can be little doubt that clot retraction is due to the direct contraction of thrombosthenin, especially as its kinetics, if extrapolated to a fibrin concentration of zero coincides with the speed of superprecipitation of isolated thrombosthenin (cf. Lüscher, 1961). It remains remarkable, though, that inhibitors such as parachloromercuribenzene sulfonate act more strongly on the isolated protein than on a retracting coagulum. This might mean that thrombosthenin does not get through the membrane, and that retraction is effected by the contraction of pseudopodia, although it then seems difficult to explain its considerable magnitude. Last, it should be mentioned that the effect of antithrombosthenin antibody (as questionable as it appeared as a criterion for the localization of the protein) nevertheless supports its importance for retractile activity.

B. Morphological Changes in the Course of the "Viscous Metamorphosis" (VM) of the Blood Platelets

Again it is most probable that thrombosthenin plays an essential role, be it direct or indirect, in the development of morphological platelet alterations. Pseudopod formation, as already mentioned might result from local contractions at the onset of viscous metamorphosis. The breakdown of the microtubules, intimately linked to the sphering of the originally disk-shaped platelet, might also be indirectly related to thrombosthenin. It must be stressed, however, that the participation of the contractile protein in morphological changes most likely is limited to the early phases; later, osmotic effects reflecting the death of the cell, will become predominant.

C. Contraction of Platelet Aggregates in Relation to Hemostasis and Thrombosis

The spontaneous arrest of hemorrhage is characterized by the sudden solidification of the primarily loose hemostatic platelet plug. This is undoubtedly a most important process, particularly since it may be compared to the establishment of an irreversible, obstructing platelet aggregate in thrombosis.

Obviously many factors may contribute to this effect: formation of larger amounts of intrinsic thrombin, accumulation of released substances (ADP, adrenaline, serotonin), and impairment of blood flow which in turn favors the other factors. There is good reason to believe that, in addition, the active contraction of the aggregate due to the activity of thrombosthenin is of prime importance. Again, the time requirement for this process fits very nicely into the frame of the normally observed bleeding times. It might well be that this is one of the most important properties of thrombosthenin.

D. Contractility and Release Reaction

The release of nucleotides and biogenic amines from platelets is a fast reaction. It coincides with degranulation, i.e., the disappearance of the typical storage organelles (for review, see Holmsen et al., 1969). It has been pointed out that the release reaction is an energy-dependent process (Mürer *et al.*, 1967), and it might be that it consists in the activation of a contractile tubular system, i.e., an active transport of substances from a storage pool to the outside of the cell.

Release reactions occur in many parts of the organism, and a closer study shows similarities among all of them (Stormorken, 1969). It is probable that they share a basically identical mechanism, and it seems permissible to speculate about the role of contractile protein in this context. This might also partly explain why so many drugs with affinities to very different target organs are all capable of interfering with platelet activities (see review by Lüscher, 1970).

E. Thrombosthenin and Platelet Aggregation

The possible role of thrombosthenin in platelet aggregation has already been discussed under C. Although a direct participation as the receptor for ADP still awaits confirmation, there are other aspects which may point to an indirect but nevertheless important function. Platelets will aggregate with ADP irreversibly only, if brought into close contact. It may be assumed that under these conditions high enough amounts of released aggregating agents become available to induce irreversibly, the so-called "second phase aggregation." Contracting thrombosthenin undoubtedly favors this situation greatly and helps in this way to propagate its own activation.

Cohen *et al.* (1969) showed that thrombin is capable of splitting thrombosthenin M. This reaction remains without effect on the ATPase activity, furthermore thrombosthenin shows normal superprecipitation in the presence of thrombin. Nevertheless, the possibility that this altered molecule, if located in the membrane, might again give rise to an altered charge distribution and to subsequent aggregation, should at least be taken into consideration.

V. DISCUSSION AND SUMMARY

Thrombosthenin, the contractile protein of blood platelets is closely related to but not entirely identical with the actomyosins of muscular origin. Its properties as a complex protein, composed of the two subunits thrombosthenin A (actinlike) and M (myosinlike), and as an ATP-splitting enzyme have been discussed.

Thrombosthenin undoubtedly plays a major role as the contractile effector in clot retraction and in the development of morphological platelet alterations in the course of so-called viscous metamorphosis. Much more speculative is its possible participation in platelet aggregation by ADP. Recent work has shown that thrombosthenin is mainly located within the cytoplasmatic compartment of the cell. This does not exclude its presence on the platelet surface which must be required for its proposed role as the direct target for ADP in the initiation of aggregation.

Other possible functions of thrombosthenin consist of the essential solidification phase of the hemostatic plug (or of a white thrombus), and perhaps of the active phase of the release reaction.

It has been pointed out that many other cells besides platelets contain comparable contractile proteins, and that therefore the study of the properties and function of thrombosthenin may well lead to results of general importance.

REFERENCES

Behnke, O. (1965). *J. Ultrastruct. Res.* **13**, 469.

Behnke, O. (1967). *Vox Sang.* **13**, 502.

Behnke, O., and Zelander, T. (1967a). *J. Ultrastruct. Res.* **19**, 147.

Behnke, O., and Zelander, T. (1967b). *Exp. Cell Res.* **43**, 236.

Bessis, M., and Breton-Gorius, J. (1965). *Nouv. Rev. Fr. Hematol.* **5**, 657.

Bettex-Galland, M., and Lüscher, E. F. (1959). *Nature (London)* **184**, 276.

Bettex-Galland, M., and Lüscher, E. F. (1960). *Thromb. Diath. Haemorrh.* **4**, 178.

Bettex-Galland, M., and Lüscher, E. F. (1961). *Biochim. Biophys. Acta* **49**, 536.

Bettex-Galland, M., and Lüscher, E. F. (1965). *Advan. Protein Chem.* **20**, 1.

Bettex-Galland, M., Portzehl, H., and Lüscher, E. F. (1962). *Nature (London)* **193**, 777.

Bettex-Galland, M., Portzehl, H., and Lüscher, E. F. (1963). *Helv. Chim. Acta* **46**, 1595.

Bettex-Galland, M., Lüscher, E. F., and Weibel, E. R. (1969). *Thromb. Diath. Haemorrh.* **22**, 431.

Bizzozero, J. (1882). *Virchows Arch. Pathol. Anat. Physiol.* **90**, 261.

Booyse, F. M., and Rafelson, M. E., Jr. (1967a). *Nature (London)* **215**, 283.

Booyse, F. M., and Rafelson, M. E., Jr. (1967b). *Biochim. Biophys. Acta* **30**, 1.

Booyse, F. M., and Rafelson, M. E., Jr. (1967c). *Blood* **30**, 553.

Booyse, F. M., and Rafelson, M. E., Jr. (1969). *Blood* **33**, 100.

Budtz–Olsen, O. E. (1951). "Clot Retraction." Blackwell, Oxford.

Chambers, D. A., Salzman, E. W., and Neri, L. L. (1967). *Arch. Biochem. Biophys.* **119**, 173.

Cohen, I., Bohak, Z., de Vries, A., and Katchalski, E. (1969). *Eur. J. Biochem.* **10**, 388.

Eberth, J. C., and Schimmelbusch, C. (1886). *Virchows Arch. Pathol. Anat. Physiol.* **103**, 39.

Ganguly, P. (1969). *Blood* **34**, 511.

Grette, K. (1962). *Acta Physiol. Scand.* **56**, Suppl. 195.

Grette, K. (1963). *Nature (London)* **198**, 488.

Hoffmann–Berling, H. (1956). *Biochim. Biophys. Acta* **19**, 453.

Holmsen, H., Day, H. J., and Stormorken, H. (1969). *Scand. J. Haematol.* Suppl. **8**,

Jones, B. M. (1966). *Nature (London)* **212**, 362.

Jones, P. C. T. (1966). *Nature (London)* **212**, 365.

Käser–Glanzmann, R. (1970). Unpublished data.

Keyserling, D., Graf (1969). *Protoplasma* **67**, 391.

Lüscher, E. F. (1961). "Blood Platelets," p. 445. Little, Brown, Boston.

Lüscher, E. F. (1970). *Thromb. Diath. Haemorrh.* Suppl. No. 29; p. 439.

Mohri, H. (1968). *Nature (London)* **217**, 1053.

Mürer, E. M., Hellem, A. J., and Rozenberg, M. C. (1967). *Scand. J. Clin. Lab. Invest.*
19, 280.

Nachman, R. L., Marcus, A. J., and Safier, L. B. (1967). *J. Clin. Invest.* **46**, 1380.

Probst, E. (1970). Unpublished.

Puszkin, E., Aledort, L., and Puszkin, S. (1969). *Blood* **34**, 526 (abstr.).

Rossi, E. S. (1969). *Blood* **34**, 543 (abstr.).

Salzman, E. W., Chambers, D. A., and Neri, L. L. (1966). *Nature (London)* **210**, 167.

Schäfer–Danneel, S., and Weissenfels, N. (1969). *Cytobiology* **1**, 85.

Senda, N., Shibata, N., Tatsumi, N., Konda, K., and Hamada, K. (1969). *Biochim.
Biophys. Acta* **181**, 191.

Shepro, D., Belamarich, F. A., and Chao, F. C. (1969). *Nature (London)* **221**, 563.

Sokal, G. (1960). "Plaquettes sanguines et structure du caillot." Arscia, Brussels.

Statland, B. E., Heagan, B. M., and White, J. G. (1969). *Nature (London)* **223**, 521.

Steiner, M. (1969). *Blood* **34**, 526.

Stormorken, H. (1969). *Scand. J. Haematol.* Suppl. 9.

Taylor, F. B., and Müller–Eberhard, H. J. (1967). *Nature (London)* **216**, 1023.

White, J. G. (1968). *Blood* **32**, 638.

Wright, J. H., and Minot, G. R. (1917). *J. Exp. Med.* **26**, 395.

Zucker–Franklin, D. (1969). *J. Clin. Invest.* **48**, 165.

Zucker–Franklin, D., and Nachman, R. L. (1967). *J. Cell Biol.* **35**, 149A.

Zucker–Franklin, D., Nachman, R. L., and Marcus, A. J. (1967). *Science* **157**, 945.

8

FUNCTIONS OF PLATELET MEMBRANES*

AARON J. MARCUS, LENORE B. SAFIER,.and HARRIS L. ULLMAN

I. INTRODUCTION

A. Problems Involved in the Study of Cell Membranes

Several important biological functions have been attributed to cell membranes. They form a barrier between the cytoplasm and external environment (the plasma membrane), and they also surround intracellular

* Research mentioned in this chapter was supported by grants from the National Institutes of Health (HE 09070-06), the Veterans Administration, and the New York Heart Association.

organelles such as mitochondria and lysosomes (intracellular membranes). Plasma membranes are capable of protecting cells from alterations in the composition of the external environment by discriminating between the molecular species that may and may not penetrate the cell wall. Furthermore, plasma membranes possess different types of enzymic mechanisms that are capable of working against concentration gradients to allow materials to pass in or out of the cell. Despite many morphological and biochemical advances in the field of biological membrane research, very little is known about the structure of these vital cell components. This paucity of knowledge has in turn made it difficult to comprehend the nature of membrane function. In the case of blood platelets the situation becomes even more perplexing since the platelet membrane serves the functions previously mentioned and, in addition, appears to play a role in hemostasis, coagulation, and probably arterial thrombosis. As it has already been pointed out that the initial steps of the hemostatic process occur with great rapidity (Marcus, 1969), it is logical to visualize hemostasis as a plasma membrane rather than as an intracellular function. Thrombosis may be an exaggerated or aberrant form of hemostasis and thus also a membrane activity. Finally, we have found that platelet membranes possess potent procoagulant activity.

The problem is even further complicated by our inability to precisely define membrane functions. If whole cells are studied, the conclusion that we have in fact examined a membrane function is largely speculative. If, on the other hand, we attempt to study isolated plasma membranes, other difficulties arise. Isolation of these membranes is laborious and imperfect at best. It invariably involves mechanical trauma to the cell, which can remove crucial substances loosely bound to the membrane. Thus, in studying the chemistry of plasma membranes we are evaluating those materials which were not removed by the cell disruption procedure. The behavior of an isolated plasma membrane in a given test system may very well provide inaccurate and misleading information about the function of the cell itself.

On the basis of their properties in *in vitro* coagulation systems, we have attributed the clot-promoting function of platelets to their plasma membranes (so-called platelet factor 3 in the older literature). Although such conclusions are based on experiments with membranes which have been subjected to homogenization and ultracentrifugation in a hypertonic sucrose gradient, these isolated membrane vesicles nevertheless possess the most efficient clot-promoting properties thus far examined in this laboratory. Of course, this does not necessarily mean that the platelet membrane behaves similarly *in vivo*.

B. Recent Morphological Studies on Platelet Membrane Systems

Behnke (1968b) has introduced a new concept to explain the formation of platelets from megakaryocytes in the bone marrow. It was deduced from earlier studies (see Marcus and Zucker, 1965) that a cytoplasmic membrane system coalesced to form what was called "the demarcation membrane system" (DMS). The DMS was presumed to form the plasma membranes of the platelets which would eventually bud off the megakaryocytes. In fact, such a phenomenon has been proposed to explain the unique behavior of platelet membranes—that is, that they actually ,form in the cytoplasm of another cell. In general, plasma membranes of new cells are thought to originate from the plasma membranes of their precursors. In one group of experiments, rat bone marrow was perfused with ruthenium red or lanthanum nitrate. These stains ordinarily do not penetrate intact plasma membranes. However, the megakaryocyte surface and the DMS were outlined by ruthenium red. Similarly, megakaryocytes fixed in glutar-aldehyde and postosmicated in the presence of lanthanum ions showed an increased density of the surface coat of the megakaryocyte as well as of the DMS membranes. It was also observed that the DMS developed from tubular invaginations at regularly spaced sites of the plasma membrane of the megakaryocyte.

In another experiment, rats were injected intravenously with either horse radish peroxidase or Thorotrast. These substances were taken up by the rat megakaryocytes *in vivo* and were eventually found in the cavities formed by the DMS. The findings complemented those previously mentioned with ruthenium and lanthanum.

Thus, it is concluded that the DMS is actually derived from the plasma membrane of the megakaryocyte. The cavities of this system are continuous with the extracellular space at all stages in its development. Finally, the ruthenium red and lanthanum studies have suggested that the acid muco-polysaccharide surface coat on the platelet membrane (Behnke, 1968a) is not acquired in the circulation but originates in the cytoplasm of the megakaryocyte.

Studies on glutaraldehyde-fixed rat platelets have revealed the presence of two membrane systems in the cytoplasm (Behnke, 1967). One has been called the surface-connected system (SCS), which consists of vacuoles and saccules and is limited by a classic "unit membrane" similar to the plasma membrane. The inner portion of these membranes is coated with the same type of amorphous material as the plasma membrane. Current evidence indicates that this coat consists of acid mucopolysaccharide. The dense tubular system (DTS) is composed of membrane-limited tubules and small vesicles which contain an electron-dense substance. In the dense tubular system there is also a submarginal tubule which courses near the marginal bundle of microtubules but is not a part of that system. There is no evidence that the dense tubular system is connected to the plasma membrane or the surface-connected system. When platelets are exposed to various foreign substances *in vitro* and *in vivo*, there appear to be two stages involved in their uptake. First there is binding to the amorphous coat of the platelets and this is followed by incorporation into the surface-connected system but not the dense tubular system. Furthermore, it has been shown that uptake into the surface-connected system from the plasma membrane is not a phagocytic process.

The aforementioned studies on the origin of platelets from megakaryocytes and observations on the membrane systems in platelets have led to a better understanding of the nature of the surface coating on the plasma membrane (Behnke, 1968a). The well known phenomenon of viral adsorption to platelets (for review, see Marcus and Zucker, 1965; Behnke, 1968a; Pepper and Jamieson, 1969) has provided presumptive evidence that there is a mucoprotein and/or a mucopolysaccharide on the external portion of the plasma membrane. It has already been shown in other cell types that viruses interact with mucoprotein or mucopolysaccharide on the cell surface. Indeed, the platelet surface coat can be seen as a layer continuous with the outer portion of the bimolecular leaflet of the plasma membrane. Behnke (1968a) has pointed out that what is probably observed is an intrinsic plasma membrane coating plus plasma proteins which have become adsorbed to the surface during circulation. Many (but not all) plasma proteins found on the platelet can be removed by repeated washing. However, there is always an "intrinsic" coat which remains attached to the surface. The demarcation membrane system found in the cytoplasm of megakaryocytes —which eventually becomes the plasma membranes of platelets—is also coated with material that appears identical to the external coat of the circulating platelet.

The cationic dye, Alcian blue, is known to stain the surface mucopolysaccharides coating cell surfaces. The dye reacts with negatively charged materials to form a mucopolysaccharide–stain complex. This complex becomes relatively insoluble and more dense, permitting clearer visualization of the surface coat in the electron microscope. The Alcian blue is usually added to the glutaraldehyde fixative. Ruthenium red is another useful stain for the surface coat of platelets. Since the dye does not appear to penetrate intact cell membranes, it produces an area of increased density on the plasma membrane itself. As already mentioned, if a portion of the surface-connected system is connected with the area stained by ruthenium red, the stain can be followed into the interior of the platelet along the channels of the surface-connected system. On the basis of reactivity of the surface coat with Alcian blue, ruthenium red, Thorotrast, and colloidal iron it could be inferred that acidic groups (such as carboxyl and sulfate) are present in the surface coat. Many early observations on the morphology of platelet aggregation showed the presence of a "space" or "gap" between platelet membranes. It now appears that this area is occupied by the platelet surface coat which was at that time incompletely stained (or appeared as a "fuzz") by the techniques used. The surface coat of platelets may play an essential role in the reactions of adhesion and cohesion. It is undoubtedly a "zone of interest" (Behnke, 1968a) important for our understanding of platelet–platelet and platelet–blood vessel interactions.

II. COLLECTION AND PROCESSING OF PLATELETS

The final yield of isolated platelet membranes from a unit of whole blood is relatively small. Between 1 and 2 ml of packed platelets can be recovered from a single unit. The average yield of *membrane* protein after processing is 6–7 mg (Marcus *et al.*, 1966, 1967). Initially it is probably best to accumulate membranes from several consecutive fractionation procedures. They can be safely stored for at least a year at −85°C. If experiments are contemplated using fresh membranes, it is advisable to use two donors simultaneously. Once the exact amount of starting material is known, the collection and processing procedure can be scaled accordingly.

The choice of anticoagulant is governed by the type of experiments to be undertaken. If the platelets are going to be washed and then homogenized, acid-citrate-dextrose (ACD) is satisfactory. If the platelets are to be incubated with isotopes or various biochemical compounds, the pH of the ACD should be reduced to 6.5 (Aster and Jandl, 1964; Deykin and Desser, 1968). Alternatively the blood can be collected with EDTA as the anticoagulant. These precautions are necessary in order to avoid platelet clumping during incubation procedures. Metabolic studies are inaccurate if clumping has taken place. It is always preferable to use donors who have fasted overnight since lipemia can interfere with platelet processing. The platelet count should be above 200,000/mm³ in order to insure an adequate yield. The venipuncture must be perfect and the bag should fill briskly with no interruption in flow. The bag should be gently and continuously inverted throughout the collection period until it is filled to complete capacity. This prevents it from folding over during centrifugation, which is undesirable. If these precautions are not taken, platelet clumping and red cell contamination will occur.

If the platelets are to be homogenized, the bag is centrifuged at 800 g for 20 minutes at 5°C. At this temperature the erythrocytes are sedimented more efficiently. On the other hand, if incubation studies are planned prior to fractionation it is preferable to centrifuge at temperatures ranging between 15° and 20°C. The platelet-rich plasma (PRP) is expressed into 50 ml conical polypropylene tubes, and then centrifuged at 1700 g to prepare a platelet button. We have used two types of media for washing platelets: a tris-buffered saline solution with EDTA (Haslam, 1964), which has also been used by Day et al. (1969); and a phosphate buffer devised by Gaintner et al. (1962). Two washes in the 50 ml tubes are usually satisfactory, but if one wishes to remove traces of plasma protein further washing is necessary.

III. PREPARATION OF PLATELET HOMOGENATES

Preparation of platelet homogenates has proven to be a difficult problem. Washed platelets are extremely resistant to physical disruption, and if one resorts to such drastic procedures as sonication the homogenate does not contain recognizable particles when examined by electron microscopy after thin sectioning techniques. It is difficult if not impossible to monitor a cell disruption procedure by shadow casting electron microscopy because subcellular particles have a tendency to form rounded vesicles which may be misinterpreted as morphological entities.

In addition to evaluating sonication, we have also attempted to prepare platelet homogenates by the following techniques: freeze-thawing, various types of glass homogenizers, macro- and microblenders, osmotic lysis, and a high pressure nitrogen bomb. The results were of two types (as evaluated in the electron microscope by Dr. Dorothea Zucker-Franklin): Platelet disruption was incomplete and the specimen consisted of fragments; or, as already mentioned, there was total destruction of all platelet components. The most satisfactory system thus far devised consists of a "no clearance" Teflon plunger and a clear walled glass tube (No. K88600, size D, Kontes Glass Company, Vineland, New Jersey). The shaft of the plunger is inserted into a heavy duty motor which revolves at a speed of about 1700 rpm.

Details of the procedure as currently employed in our laboratory follow.

All operations should be carried out at 4°C. Washed platelets are packed in a volume of about 1 ml in a conical plastic centrifuge tube. One-half to 1 ml of the desired homogenizing medium is added to the packed cells and the platelets are gently aspirated into the medium by back-and-forth motion with a polyethylene dropping pipette attached to a neoprene bulb. With this technique residual red cells which may have contaminated the platelet button can be left behind. The material is then transferred to the clear walled glass receptacle and is ready to be homogenized. The Teflon plunger is placed at 4°C for at least 10 minutes prior to homogenization. It will then fit the receptacle (if the plunger fits the receptacle at room temperature it does not satisfy the requirement of "no clearance" and should not be used). Experience has shown that a 5-minute homogenization period is most satisfactory. After 3 minutes the receptacle becomes slightly warm and is at that point surrounded by a paper cup filled with ice. Theoretically, homogenization is accomplished through the shearing forces between the sides of the Teflon and the glass tube. The rotating pestle expands into the "no clearance" position and accomplishes cell disruption.

At the end of the 5-minute interval, whatever contents of the tube can be poured are transferred to another container. One ml of homogenizing fluid is added to the original tube, which is then subjected to several additional strokes with the motorized plunger. The contents are added to the original homogenate. This procedure may be repeated once or twice and serves to recover a considerable amount of homogenate that has adhered to the sides of the tube and cannot at first be poured out. In addition, if the glass tube is allowed to stand in the upright position, remaining homogenate will eventually drain to the bottom and can be recovered with a Pasteur pipette. This homogenate can be used "as is" for biochemical studies, but if it is to be fractionated, platelets which have escaped disruption must be removed by a preliminary spin. For this reason, platelets to be fractionated should be homogenized in 0.44 M sucrose (0.001 M EDTA). Centrifugation of the homogenate in about 10 ml of this sucrose solution for 30 minutes at 2000 g will result in a pellet consisting of the "intact" platelets (and some granules) and a supernatant composed of granules, membranes, and the soluble components. If isotonic (0.25 M) sucrose is used for homogenization, almost all of the homogenate will be lost in the preliminary spin.

Further details of this method can be found in previous publications (Marcus et al., 1966, 1967). It is far from perfect, but in our hands it is superior to other methods. Day et al. (1969) have carried out a detailed investigation of several homogenization techniques and have also found this one to be useful.

IV. FRACTIONATION AND COLLECTION OF SUBCELLULAR PLATELET PARTICLES

The procedure of choice for fractionating platelet homogenates is iso-pycnic ultracentrifugation in a continuous sucrose gradient. Unfortunately, hypertonic and viscous sucrose solutions are required. These have a dele-terious effect on the morphological and biochemical integrity of subcellular platelet particles. More research is needed to improve this aspect of platelet fractionation procedures. After ultracentrifugation the fractions are best collected by careful aspiration from above with a Pasteur pipette. This effectively prevents overlapping of particulate fractions, which occasionally occurs during dropwise collections from below. In general, the sucrose must be removed from the particles by either washing or dialysis (Bradlow and Marcus, 1966).

V. SUBCELLULAR PLATELET "COMPARTMENTS"

At this writing over 220 fractionations have been carried out in our laboratory. We have arbitrarily defined three main subcellular "compart-ments." It is known that these compartments are heterogeneous and in the future newer techniques, such as zonal ultracentrifugation, may render this compartmentalization obsolete. At the top of the gradient a soluble fraction is obtained. Many platelet proteins (Nachman, 1968) and enzymes can be found in this layer (Day et al., 1969). It was of interest that cytochrome c oxidase and thrombosthenin were absent and that ATPase activity which could not be inhibited by ouabain or mersalyl was present in this fraction. The soluble fraction also demonstrated clot promoting properties (Horowitz and Papayoanou, 1967). Evaluation of the soluble compartment is fraught with difficulty because some of its components may have originally been particle-bound but set free during homogenization and ultracentrifugation. On the other hand, its content of lactic dehydrogenase can be used as a measure of the effectiveness of cell disruption, since it is a soluble enzyme.

The next compartment, with a density range of 1.12–1.13, consists of platelet membranes in the form of vesicles of varying sizes, as seen in Fig. 1. If the gradient tube is examined with a magnifying glass, at least two discrete bands can be discerned. It is hoped that eventually this membrane population will be further subdivided by more refined techniques. Currently it is thought to consist mainly of plasma membranes and membranes derived from granules and smooth endoplasmic reticulum. It is nevertheless a relatively

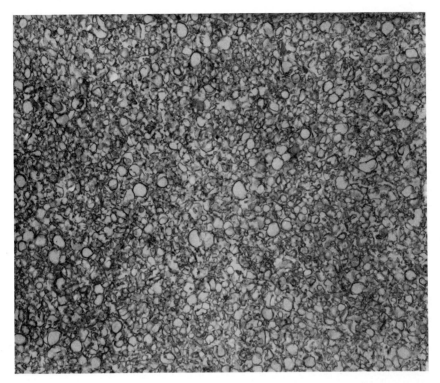

FIG. 1. Electron micrograph of isolated platelet membrane fraction. Membranes are present in the form of vesicles. The background material consists of soluble platelet protein which was precipitated by the fixative. 30,000×. (Micrograph taken by Dr. Dorothea Zucker–Franklin. Photograph reproduced through the courtesy of the *Journal of Clinical Investigation*.)

pure membrane fraction and compares rather favorably in purity with membranes isolated from other tissues.

The third compartment, with a density of 1.17–1.21, consists of platelet granules and mitochondria. Further subfractionation of this compartment is also urgently needed. Lysosomal enzyme activity has been found in the platelet granule fractions and has been studied in great detail (Marcus *et al.*, 1966; Day *et al.*, 1969). Behavior of these enzymes with particular reference to the platelet "release reaction" has been extensively investigated (Holmsen *et al.*, 1969).

It has been suggested by some workers that platelet granules are responsible for the platelet contribution to the coagulation process. The proposed mechanism is a discharge of granules with clot promoting properties into the surrounding medium. Although it is true that granules possess procoagulant activity, evidence from electron microscopic research on the clotting process is that granules are not seen in the surrounding medium *prior to* fibrin formation. *In vitro* clotting tests utilizing isolated platelet granules are positive because of their relatively high lipoprotein content and because they are membrane-bound. We think platelet granules serve mainly metabolic, storage, and lysosomal functions. Furthermore, since granules appear to converge at the center of platelets in the early phases of aggregation (White, 1968), it is difficult to interpret this as a prelude to discharge.

The distribution of enzymes in subcellular platelet compartments has recently been summarized in two excellent publications (Day *et al.*, 1969; Holmsen *et al.*, 1969). It should be pointed out that before the distribution of an enzyme can be localized in a specific compartment it must be shown that its specific activity per unit protein is very high and that only insignificant amounts of it can be found in the other fractions. If these criteria are used, very few platelet enzymes can be regarded as specifically localized. For example, cytochrome c oxidase is a mitochondrial enzyme (Marcus *et al.*, 1966); lactic dehydrogenase is a "soluble" enzyme; 5'-nucleotidase (Holmsen *et al.*, 1969) is probably a membrane enzyme. Most of the other enzymes have been found in more than one compartment, and, of course, this may be a reflection of currently available techniques. At present it is difficult if not impossible to produce a relatively undamaged platelet homogenate and to fractionate it completely.

VI. LIPIDS OF PLATELET MEMBRANES AND GRANULES

Cell membranes consist mainly of lipoprotein. Since the platelet membranes have several unique physiological responses (aggregation by ADP, participation in coagulation, etc.), we reasoned that the platelet membranes might have a unique lipid or fatty acid composition which would at least partially account for these responses. We have therefore carried out a detailed study of the lipid composition of platelet membranes (Marcus *et al.*, 1969). Furthermore, a study of the platelet glycolipids is now in progress.

In terms of dry weight the chemical composition of platelet membranes is as follows: protein, 57%; lipid, 33%; and carbohydrate, 8%. The lipid classes present in platelet membranes are shown in Table I. The principal lipid class in the membranes (as well as in the granules and whole platelets) is the phospholipids. In the isolated state these lipids are active in *in vitro* coagulation systems. As noted in cell membranes of other tissues, lecithin

TABLE I

Lipids in Platelet Membranes

Component	% of total lipids
Cholesteryl esters	0.1
Triglycerides	0.5
Free fatty acids	0.5
Free cholesterol	19.8
Diglycerides	trace
Ethanolamine phosphoglycerides	20.7
Serine phosphoglycerides	6.4
Inositol phosphoglycerides	3.3
Choline phosphoglycerides (lecithin)	32.5
Sphingomyelin	13.4
Lysolecithin	0.2
Cardiolipin	0.2
Gangliosides	0.5

is the predominant phosphatide. The other phospholipids have been found in varying amounts, but in mammalian tissues none has exceeded lecithin. By virtue of their chemical structure phospholipids are particularly suitable as membrane components. In general, the molecules have both polar (hydrophilic) and nonpolar (hydrophobic) portions. Their precise spatial arrangement and relationship to membrane protein is still a subject of controversy, but most workers agree that phospholipoprotein forms the "backbone" of cell membranes.

The major "neutral" lipid in platelet membranes is free cholesterol; in fact, it comprises about 90% of this fraction. The cholesterol component follows a pattern already found in other mammalian cell membranes. It is of interest that bacterial cell membranes do not contain cholesterol. The other neutral lipids of platelets—cholesteryl esters, triglycerides, free fatty acids, and diglycerides—are present in very low amounts. However, they may be important from a metabolic or functional rather than a structural standpoint.

Gas liquid chromatography (GLC) has made it possible to study the fatty acid composition of the lipids of whole platelets as well as the subcellular platelet particles. Since these are present in such small amounts, other analytical procedures would not have been feasible. There was little difference between the fatty acid composition of the phospholipids of platelet membranes, granules, and whole platelets. Each lipid class and subclass did, however, contain a characteristic fatty acid pattern. For example, platelet lecithin contained mainly palmitate and oleate; sphingomyelin was characterized principally by palmitate and behenate. Furthermore, sphingomyelin also had several long chain fatty acids such as lignocerate and nervonate. Newer and more sophisticated gas–liquid chromatography equipment now available to our laboratory may enable us to determine whether even more long chain fatty acids are present in this group of lipids. The ethanolamine phosphoglycerides (PE) had large amounts of arachidonic acid. This species is also notable for its plasmalogen content (Zilversmit et al., 1961). The serine phosphoglycerides (PS)—the most active clot-promoting platelet lipids—have large amounts of stearate, oleate, and

TABLE II

PHOSPHOLIPID FATTY ACIDS AND ALDEHYDES OF PLATELET MEMBRANES[a,b,c]

Component	PE	PS	PI	Lecithin	Sphingomyelin
16:0 DMA[d]	8.7	—	2.0	0.36	—
16:0	3.5	0.36	1.4	31.0	21.9
16:1	0.51	0.51	0.55	1.4	0.15
18:0 DMA	18.2	0.15	—	—	—
18:0	14.1	46.5	44.4	15.7	5.6
18:1 DMA	3.1	—	—	—	—
18:1	5.5	25.0	9.2	27.4	0.72
18:2	2.2	trace	0.33	7.5	0.12
18:3	1.5	—	—	—	—
20:0	0.52	1.7	0.47	0.51	9.8
20:4	31.6	24.7	41.2	12.5	—
22:0	—	—	—	—	31.5
22:1	—	—	—	—	5.8
22:4 (n − 6)	3.8	—	—	—	—
22:5	1.1	trace	—	0.81	—
22:6	1.2	trace	—	trace	—
23:0	—	—	—	—	2.1
24:0	—	—	—	—	7.7
24:1	—	—	—	—	12.0

[a] Fatty acids are designated by chain length: number of double bonds. Besides those shown, the following acids were detected in small (<1.5) percentages: 12:0, 14:0, 15:0, 17:0 DMA, 17:0, 20:1, 20:2, 20:3, and one with a probable carbon number of 22 on Apiezon.

[b] Marcus et al., 1969.

[c] All units in weight %.

[d] Dimethyl acetal(s).

arachidonate. Finally, the inositol phosphatides (PI) were characterized by a high level of stearate and contained the largest quantity of arachidonate (Table II).

There have recently been several very interesting studies on the metabolism of lipids and fatty acids in whole platelets. These have added a new dimension to our knowledge of platelet lipids, which in the past has been more descriptive than dynamic (Deykin and Desser, 1968; Majerus et al., 1969; Lewis and Majerus, 1969; Cohen et al., 1970; Cohen and Wittels, 1970). Data presented by these authors indicates that lipid metabolism in platelets is a relatively autonomous process. This is in contrast to lipid metabolism in leukocytes and erythrocytes.

Studies on the fatty acids of neutral lipid fractions of platelet membranes did show quantitative differences between these and granules and whole platelets. At first glance these might have been attributed to plasma lipids

TABLE III

NEUTRAL LIPID FATTY ACIDS OF PLATELET MEMBRANES[a,b]

Component	Cholesteryl esters (weight %)	Triglycerides (weight %)	Free fatty acids (weight %)
12:0	0.21	0.60	0.71
14:0	1.6	4.0	3.7
14:0[c]	4.7	1.6	0.51
15:0	2.9	1.6	1.4
15:0[c]	1.2	0.57	0.29
16:0	17.4	22.7	26.4
16:1	37.3	7.5	4.4
17:0	4.4	0.81	1.2
17:0 anteiso	trace	1.5	1.2
?	trace	0.96	1.4
18:0	4.4	13.6	22.6
18:1	26.0	30.1	27.8
18:2	—	7.8	3.5
18:3	—	0.45	0.30
20:0	—	2.2	1.6
20:1	—	1.4	1.1
20:3	—	0.58	1.7
20:4	—	2.2	0.20

[a] Fatty acids designated by chain length: number of double bonds.
[b] Marcus et al., 1969.
[c] br, branched chain.

which were adsorbed to the membrane surface. However, the patterns did not resemble those of the fatty acids in plasma triglycerides, free fatty acids, or cholesteryl esters (Marcus *et al.*, 1969) (Table III).

We have recently initiated a study of platelet gangliosides, since we believe that glycolipids may eventually be shown to be of functional importance in platelet physiology (Marcus *et al.*, 1970). Gangliosides contain sphingosine, fatty acid, hexoses, and sialic acid. They are thought to be cell membrane components (Lehninger, 1968), and in the central nervous system have been postulated to be the serotonin receptors (Woolley and Gommi, 1964). Lehninger has proposed that the negatively charged gangliosides may extend beyond the surface coat of the plasma membrane into the surrounding medium. Furthermore, he has also suggested that the sialic acid portion of membrane gangliosides may serve as calcium binding sites. Gangliosides were first identified in brain tissue, and more recently they have been found in many organs outside of the central nervous system. In general, the extraneural gangliosides are less polar than those found in nerve tissue—a property which is useful for thin layer chromatographic analysis. We have detected at least three ganglioside species in platelet lipid extracts. The major platelet ganglioside appears to be "hematoside," which is the species most frequently found in extraneural tissues. Studies on further purification and structure of platelet gangliosides are in progress.

VII. PROTEIN AND LIPID RELATIONSHIPS IN PLATELET MEMBRANES

It has been postulated that quantitative relationships between proteins and lipids of a cell membrane may be related to the metabolic capacity of the membrane in question (Ashworth and Green, 1966). Highly specialized cell membranes which are metabolically active have a high content of protein in proportion to lipid. In intestinal microvilli the phospholipid to protein ratio is 0.11. Brain myelin, which is relatively inert metabolically, has a ratio of 0.92. Platelets, with a ratio of 0.39, are in an intermediate position on this scale (Marcus *et al.*, 1969).

Quantitative relationships between cholesterol and phospholipid are also of interest. Many early studies on cell membranes were carried out on erythrocytes and myelin. The molar ratio of cholesterol to phospholipid in these tissues was very close to 1. This was initially thought to mean that all cell membranes had a similar lipid composition. However, as more and more highly purified membrane preparations became available and were analyzed, this ratio did not appear to hold. The platelet membrane is a typical example, wherein the molar ratio of cholesterol to phospholipid is 0.53 (Marcus *et al.*, 1969).

Unfortunately, the information thus far obtained on the biochemistry of cell membranes has furnished little insight into how these membranes are constructed or precisely how they function. We can only reiterate the problems outlined in the introduction to this chapter.

VIII. *IN VITRO* COAGULATION STUDIES ON PLATELET MEMBRANES AND GRANULES

Although the role of platelets in primary hemostasis is probably their most important function, they also contribute to intrinsic [and possibly extrinsic (Biggs *et al.*, 1968)] prothrombin activation (Marcus, 1969). As platelets aggregate and their plasma membranes come into contact with each other as well as with the blood vessel wall, a previously inactive membrane lipoprotein surface interacts with plasma coagulation factors. The precise mechanism of this "availability" phenomenon is not known. In addition, a basically incorrect and misleading terminology persists in the literature. This clot promoting activity has been inaccurately called a platelet factor, when in reality there is no such identifiable biochemical substance. The misnomer arose after it was discovered that phospholipids were capable of shortening the coagulation time of platelet-poor plasma in *in vitro* coagulation systems (Marcus, 1966). The error was compounded when platelets were treated by various mechanical and chemical techniques and the resulting product was shown to have clot promoting properties. This product was called "platelet factor 3," and it is doubtful whether this name will ever rightfully be removed from the literature. We showed several years ago that platelet lipoprotein in the form of a membrane vesicle was the most effective *in vitro* substitute for platelets (Marcus *et al.*, 1966). We refer specifically to an activity which appears in the interval *before* thrombin forms. After thrombin has formed, nonspecific lipoprotein substances can be identified in the external milieu which are capable of shortening the clotting time. These substances, however, probably did not contribute to the prothrombin activation process. We view prothrombin activation as a lipoprotein–protein interaction. The use of crude phospholipid preparations (for example, soy bean phosphatides) in *in vitro* clotting systems may not provide accurate insight into the blood coagulation process, although they may furnish valuable information about protein–lipid interactions. The potency of platelet membrane lipoprotein is illustrated clinically by the observation that the whole blood coagulation time is rarely if ever prolonged in thrombocytopenia. We have a patient with idiopathic thrombocytopenic purpura whose platelet count is sometimes in the range of 1000/mm³, yet his coagulation time remains essentially normal.

The literature is replete with descriptions of patients with a hemorrhagic disorder attributed to abnormal so-called platelet factor 3 activity. The important question to be considered is whether a patient can bleed because the clot promoting properties of his platelets are defective. We propose that this rarely if ever occurs. We suggest that these patients bleed because there is some interference with platelet aggregation and/or adhesion to damaged blood vessels or thrombocytopenia. The clot promoting activity of platelets will not manifest itself in the absence of normal aggregation. The platelet disorder thrombasthenia is an excellent example of this phenomenon. Platelet aggregation in this case is defective because of un-responsiveness to ADP. Clot promoting properties of these poorly aggregated platelets are usually abnormal.

It has been proposed that platelet granules play a role in coagulation through a mechanism of discharge, either directly or through the canalicular system, into the external medium. While it is true that isolated platelet granules possess clot promoting properties, we feel this is a nonspecific *in vitro* finding. If platelet granules are found in the surrounding medium it is usually *after* thrombin has formed. We visualize the platelet granule as a membrane-bound, individually functioning biological unit. Granules have the biochemical apparatus with which to store and transport many enzymes and metabolic substances. We have not seen convincing electron microscopic or biochemical evidence for a role of platelet granules in coagulation, nor do we see the need to postulate such a role for them. We are, however, always willing to change our views should more persuasive data to the contrary be presented.

IX. SUMMARY

Cell membrane biochemistry and physiology are an important area in biological research. That plasma membranes are significant functional units is now well established. The platelet membrane appears to have an additional role—involvement in adhesion, aggregation and coagulation. A hemostatic platelet plug is capable of withstanding the hydrostatic pressure exerted upon it by virtue of the adhesive properties of the plasma membrane. How these properties are acquired or "unmasked" is completely unknown. Clearly the process must be governed by a dynamic series of biochemical and functional events.

In this chapter we have described procedures for collecting and processing platelets for studies on subcellular platelet organelles. Many aspects of these techniques are imperfect and require further intensive research. This is especially true for the preparation of platelet homogenates. Three subcellular platelet "compartments" have been defined. These are: (1) platelet membranes, which contain both plasma membranes and membranes derived from granules; (2) platelet granules and mitochondria; and (3) the soluble fraction or "cell sap." All of these fractions will eventually be further subdivided as more refined isolation techniques become available.

The lipid classes of platelet membranes have been studied in great detail. The principal lipid class is the phospholipids (about 78%). The remainder is essentially neutral lipid and ganglioside. Ninety percent of the neutral lipid fraction is free cholesterol. The structure of platelet gangliosides is now under study.

Several quantitative relationships between membrane protein and lipid as well as cholesterol and phospholipid have been established for platelet membranes. This information has demonstrated interesting differences between platelet membranes and membranes of other cell types.

Platelet membranes contribute to the blood coagulation process as they aggregate and form a lipoprotein "surface" which interacts with plasma coagulation factors. This clot promoting activity is not a platelet factor. The so-called platelet factor 3 does not exist as a biochemical entity. Patients rarely if ever bleed because of a deficiency in this clot promoting activity. Hemorrhagic disorders attributable to platelet defects usually result from insufficient numbers, or from an inability of the platelets to form an efficient hemostatic platelet plug.

REFERENCES

Ashworth, L. A. E., and Green, C. (1966). *Science* **151**, 210.
Aster, R. H., and Jandl, J. H. (1964). *J. Clin. Invest.* **43**, 843.
Behnke, O. (1967). *Anat. Rec.* **158**, 121.
Behnke, O. (1968a). *J. Ultrastruct. Res.* **24**, 51.
Behnke, O. (1968b). *J. Ultrastruct. Res.* **24**, 412.
Biggs, R., Denson, K. W. E., Riesenberg, D., and McIntyre, C. (1968). *Brit. J. Haematol.* **15**, 283.
Bradlow, B. A., and Marcus, A. J. (1966). *Proc. Soc. Exp. Biol. Med.* **123**, 889.
Cohen, P., and Wittels, B. (1970). *J. Clin. Invest.* **49**, 119.

Cohen, P., Derksen, A., and van den Bosch, H. (1970). *J. Clin. Invest.* **49**, 128.

Day, H. J., Holmsen, H., and Hovig, T. (1969). *Scand. J. Haematol.* Suppl. 7, 1.

Deykin, D., and Desser, R. K. (1968). *J. Clin. Invest.* **47**, 1590.

Gaintner, J. R., Jackson, D. P., and Maynert, E. W. (1962). *Bull. Johns Hopkins Hosp.* **111**, 185.

Haslam, R. J. (1964). *Nature (London)* **202**, 765.

Holmsen, H., Day, H. J., and Stormorken, H. (1969). *Scand. J. Haematol.* Suppl. 8, 1.

Horowitz, H. I., and Papayoanou, M. F. (1967). *J. Lab. Clin. Med.* **69**, 1003.

Lehninger, A. L. (1968). *Proc. Nat. Acad. Sci. U.S.* **60**, 1069.

Lewis, N., and Majerus, P. W. (1969). *J. Clin. Invest.* **48**, 2114.

Majerus, P. W., Smith, M. B., and Clamon, G. H. (1969). *J. Clin. Invest.* **48**, 156.

Marcus, A. J. (1966). *Advan. Lipid Res.* **4**, 1.

Marcus, A. J., (1969). *N. Engl. J. Med.* **280**, 1213, 1278, and 1330.

Marcus, A. J., and Zucker, M. B. (1965). "The Physiology of Blood Platelets: Recent Biochemical, Morphologic and Clinical Research." Grune & Stratton, New York.

Marcus, A. J., Zucker–Franklin, D., Safier, L. B., and Ullman, H. L. (1966). *J. Clin. Invest.* **45**, 14.

Marcus, A. J., Zucker–Franklin, D., Ullman, H. L., and Safier, L. B. (1967). *In* "Physiology of Hemostasis and Thrombosis" (S. A. Johnson and W. H. Seegers, eds.), p. 113. Thomas, Springfield, Illinois.

Marcus, A. J., Ullman, H. L., and Safier, L. B. (1969). *J. Lipid Res.* **10**, 108.

Marcus, A. J., Ullman, H. L., Safier, L. B., and Ballard, H. S. (1970). *Fed. Proc., Fed. Amer. Soc. Exp. Biol.* (abstr.) **29**, 315.

Nachman, R. L. (1968). *Semin. Hematol.* **5**, 18.

Pepper, D. S., and Jamieson, G. A. (1969). *Biochemistry* **8**, 3362.

White, J. G. (1968). *Blood* **31**, 604.

Woolley, D. W., and Gommi, B. W. (1964). *Nature (London)* **202**, 1074.

Zilversmit, R. D., Marcus, A. J., and Ullman, H. L. (1961). *J. Biol. Chem.* **236**, 47.

9

PLATELET AGGREGATION*

LOUIS M. ALEDORT

I. INTRODUCTION

Three factors are responsible for the maintenance of normal hemostasis: the integrity of the vascular endothelium; blood clotting proteins; and platelets. At the site of endothelial damage, platelets leave the mainstream of the blood, adhere to the damaged endothelium, and then aggregate to each other, forming a primary hemostatic plug thereby stopping hemorrhage. This series of events was designated viscous metamorphosis in 1886 by Eberth and Schimmelbusch. Prior to that time platelets, uniquely derived

* This research was supported in part by USPHS Grant No. HE 10905 and USPHS Contract No. PH-43-67-1359 from the National Heart Institute, the Hemophilia Foundation, and by the Albert A. List, Frederick Machlin, and Anna Ruth Lowenberg Funds.

from cytoplasmic fragments of megakaryocytes, were considered to be inert cells.

Platelets have also been implicated as a factor in producing intravascular thrombi. In 1880 Zahn first described the "white thrombus" which was thought to be composed of leukocytes. In 1882 Bizzozero discovered this thrombus to be composed of platelets.

In 1959 Bettex-Galland and Lüscher identified an actomyosin-like protein with ATPase activity, called thrombosthenin, which makes up 15% of the total platelet protein. This protein is most likely responsible for platelet contraction, an energy-dependent process. These biochemical observations, in contrast to earlier morphologic studies, brought recognition that platelets were metabolically active cells with a complexity of functions.

Since that time a large body of literature has accumulated regarding platelet aggregation. Many substances which are capable of either aggregating or deaggregating platelets have been investigated in an attempt to understand the underlying mechanism or mechanisms responsible for platelet aggregation. Many investigators have postulated that a single mechanism exists for all platelet aggregation. There is, however, much data suggesting that there is no final common pathway for all of platelet aggregation. This chapter will present and evaluate, when possible, the various hypotheses which have evolved to explain these mechanisms.

II. AGENTS PRODUCING PLATELET AGGREGATION

The observation of Hellem et al. (1961) that a substance "R" derived from red blood cells, later discovered to be adenosine diphosphate (ADP) (Gaarder et al., 1961) was capable of aggregating platelets strongly implicated ADP in the process of in vivo hemostasis. Since that time a wide range of substances have been investigated because of their ability to produce platelet aggregation. The changes in platelet morphology, physiology, and biochemistry brought about by these substances comprise the bulk of research in this area. At the moment we know a great deal about the events that take place when platelets are aggregated. The causal relationship of these events remains unknown.

A. Adenosine Diphosphate (ADP)

Of the many aggregating agents, the one receiving the most attention is ADP. ADP was the earliest aggregating substance to be described. It is considered to have physiological significance. Many investigators feel that the ADP present in platelets, when released by aggregating agents, is responsible for platelet aggregation. The author shall therefore devote a large portion of this chapter to what is presently known about ADP-induced aggregation.

1. AGGREGATION

a. EFFECT ON PLATELET SHAPE AND VOLUME. Platelets are known to circulate in the blood stream in the form of disks with an average volume of $6.1 \pm 0.5 \, \mu^3$ (Zucker and Zaccardi, 1964; Bull and Zucker, 1965; Aledort et al., 1968). ADP leads to a platelet shape change from a resting state disk to a sphere with protrusions. Electron micrographs (White, 1968) reveal that platelets become irregularly swollen when losing their discoid shape, and develop pseudopods. The normally randomly placed granules move inward and the marginal tubular structure moves toward the interior of the platelet forming a collar around the organelles.

Platelet volume is controlled by many factors. Platelets maintain high intracellular K^+ and low Na^+ concentration which are energy dependent, requiring intact Embden-Myerhoff and monophosphate shunt pathways (O'Brien, 1966; Gorstein et al., 1967). This energy is used to maintain a ouabain sensitive Na^+, K^+, dependent ATPase (Aledort et al., 1968), as well as an ethacrynic acid sensitive pump (Zieve and Solomon, 1968). Platelet volume is temperature dependent (Bull and Zucker, 1965; Mannucci and Sharp, 1967), and a large number of substances will cause platelets to swell: local anesthetics (O'Brien, 1964; Mannucci and Sharp, 1967; Aledort and Niemitz, 1968); EDTA (Bull and Zucker, 1965; Mannucci and Sharp, 1967); and a number of sulfhydryl inhibitors and ouabain (Aledort et al., 1968).

b. EFFECT ON SURFACE CHARGE. The electrophoretic mobility of normal platelets when resting, under various aggregating conditions, and in the presence of metabolic and sulfhydryl inhibitors (Hampton and Mitchell, 1966a,b), have undergone extensive investigation. The platelet membrane surface has a negative charge, and low concentrations of ADP will increase this platelet surface charge. These studies, however, have provided little information as to the relationship between the surface charge of the platelet and aggregation.

c. CHARACTERISTICS OF AGGREGATION. In 1966 Macmillan observed two phases to platelet aggregation produced by ADP. The first, a reversible phase, was seen in all studied normals. It was rapid and direct. A second phase, dependent on maximal stirring of platelet-rich plasma, occurred in many subjects, and differed from the first phase in that it was irreversible. The physiological significance of a secondary wave of aggregation is not clear.

O'Brien in 1964 noted that platelets could become refractory to ADP. This concept of refractoriness has recently undergone reevaluation. Based on measurements of the disappearance of plasma ADP in the presence of adenosine, a potent inhibitor of ADP induced aggregation, it was conceived that platelets exist in three forms: responsive, capable of responding; cohesive, responding (aggregating); and refractory. It was further postulated that primary aggregation was comprised of three phases: an initial phase where most platelets were aggregated with only a few deaggregated cells; a midphase where a balance existed between aggregated and deaggregated platelets; and a final stage wherein refractoriness exceeded responsiveness (Rozenberg and Holmsen, 1968b).

The second phase of ADP-induced platelet aggregation which is irreversible is potentiated by adrenaline and serotonin (5-hydroxytryptamine) (Thomas, 1967). It has been suggested that the catecholamine content of platelets (0.2–0.7 mg/10^8 platelets) may in part be responsible for producing the secondary phase of ADP-induced platelet aggregation. Serotonin antagonists have no effect on secondary aggregation, whereas platelets preincubated with tyramine, a compound capable of replacing platelet catecholamines and 5-hydroxytryptamine, abolishes secondary aggregation. In addition α adrenergic blockers also inhibit secondary aggregation. The potentiation of ADP-induced platelet aggregation by catecholamines raises the possibility that platelet adenyl cyclase activity is stimulated with subsequent activation of phosphorylase kinase making ADP available at the platelet surface (Ardlie et al., 1966). These observations deserve further investigation.

d. RELEASE. The release of platelet aggregating substances, ADP (Macmillan, 1966) and 5-hydroxytryptamine (Zucker and Peterson, 1967), as well as platelet factor 3 (Zucker and Peterson, 1967; Horowitz and Papayoanou, 1968), during aggregation has received a great deal of attention. The relationship of these released compounds to the secondary phase of platelet aggregation is as yet undefined. The release of ADP, however, has been considered to be most important in explaining the secondary phase. To lend support are the following observations: Mills and Roberts (1967) demonstrated that agents such as chlorpromazine, imipramine, and dismethylmipramine, stabilizers of biologic membranes, inhibit the secondary phase of ADP-induced platelet aggregation, and those of Zucker and Peterson (1968) demonstrated that acetylsalicylic acid (ASA) inhibited ADP-induced secondary aggregation by interfering with the release of ADP. These observations do not answer the critical question as to the mechanism of ADP-induced secondary aggregation. Further studies of the role of catecholamine and serotonin in this aggregation are needed.

e. THEORY OF BRIDGES. The mechanism of primary aggregation produced by ADP has undergone careful scrutiny. Many conflicting theories pervade the literature and will be reviewed here. An early, attractive hypothesis was that proposed by Gaarder and Laland (1964) and Hellem and Owren (1964). They postulated that platelets were aggregated by the linkage of platelet membranes to ADP with a plasma factor felt to be absent in von Willebrand's disease (Fig. 1). Gaarder and Laland (1964), recognizing

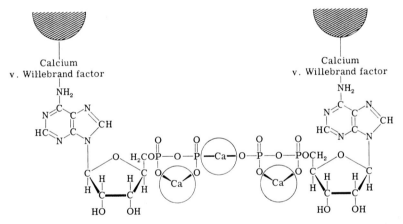

FIG. 1. A proposed model for ADP-induced platelet aggregation. Reproduced with permission of the publisher: Hellem and Owren (1964), The mechanism of the Hemostatic Function of Blood Platelets, *Proc. 9th Congr. Europ. Hemat.*, Lisbon 1963; *Acta Haemat.* **31**, 230–238, 1964 (Karger, Basel New York).

that the amino group of adenine was essential for aggregation, demonstrated the aggregating activity of the following substances: 3-deoxyadenosine diphosphate, 1-N-oxide of adenosine diphosphate, deoxyadenosine diphosphate, and adenosine tetraphosphate. They felt that the α amino group and the N_1 group of the adenine attached to the platelet surface by hydrogen bonding (Fig. 2). If there is an uneven number of negative charges, a greater chance of aggregation exists as calcium is attracted to negative charges. The adenosine diphosphates and tetraphosphate at physiologic pH have three and five negative charges, respectively. Inhibitors of ADP-induced aggregation have either no charge or an even number of charges at physiologic pH, and are thereby less attracted to calcium. They postulated that inhibitors hydrogen-bond to the platelet surface and function as competitive inhibitors. Other investigators have pursued these observations. Skalhegg *et al.* (1964), using metabolic poisons, and Skoza *et al.* (1966), using chelators, adenosine and guanadino compounds, support the concept that the aggregation of platelets by ADP occurs by attaching to the platelet membrane and complexing with calcium ions.

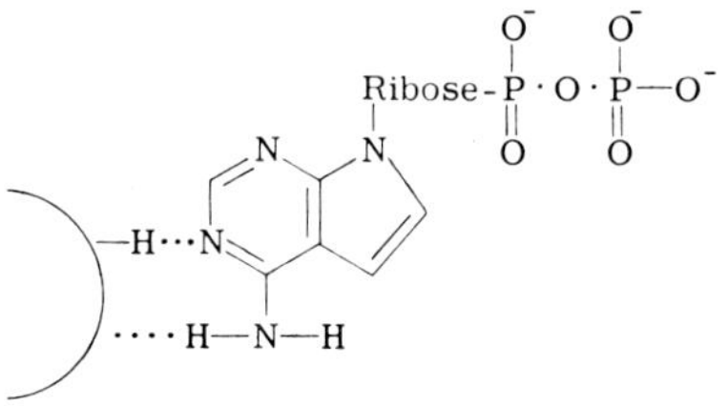

FIG. 2. A model for ADP-induced platelet aggregation based on hydrogen bonding. Reproduced with permission of the publisher (Gaarder and Laland, 1964).

Pursuing these observations, studies were later carried out to determine the number of ADP receptor sites per platelet. Born (1965) using adenosine as an inhibitor of ADP-induced platelet aggregation calculated 2×10^5 ADP receptor sites per cell. Hampton and Mitchell (1966c) calculated the number of ADP molecules capable of changing the electrophoretic mobility of a single platelet, from the postcontact phase to the maximally charged state, to be 0.85×10^5, a figure quite comparable to that of Born. The studies of Salzman *et al.* (1966a), however, seriously challenge the theory of ADP aggregation being caused by platelet–ADP linkage. Using ^{14}C-labeled ADP they showed increasing platelet uptake with increasing ADP concentration and time of incubation. Cyanide (0.01 M) strongly inhibits the platelet incorporation of ^{14}C-ADP while facilitating ADP-induced platelet aggregation. Furthermore, when β-^{32}P-ADP or α, β-^{32}P-ADP aggregate platelets, no incorporation or radioactivity can be measured.

f. CONTROVERSY OF CONTRACTION VS. RELAXATION. Platelets are known to contain proteins with several ATPase activities (Bettex-Galland and Lüscher, 1965; Aledort *et al.*, 1968). Salzman *et al.* (1966b) and Chambers *et al.* (1967) noted that in the presence of whole platelets, ADP inhibited the conversion of ^{32}P-labeled ATP to ADP $+$ P. They interpreted these data to mean that ADP aggregates platelets by inhibiting a membrane ATPase called "ecto-ATPase." This "ecto-ATPase" contained no ouabain-sensitive ATPase. They hypothesized that the energy for the hydrolysis of the terminal phosphate bond was used to maintain the "unsticky state" of the platelet. The inhibition of the platelet membrane ATPase, allowed the platelet to become adhesive by allowing it to relax and to change from a high-energy sticky state. In contrast to these data are the observations that washed canine platelets (Robinson et al., 1965) will agglutinate with methylmercuric nitrate, a sulfhydryl inhibitor, accompanied by a fourfold enhancement of the membrane ATPase activity.

It was also observed that an antithrombosthenin antibody inhibited this "ecto-ATPase" and also produced platelet aggregation (Salzman et al., 1966b; Chambers et al., 1967). Recently Booyse and Raphelson (1967) have shown the presence of contractile ATPase in the platelet membrane. The evidence that this "ecto-ATPase" is identical to the contractile protein thrombosthenin (Bettex-Galland and Lüscher, 1965) remains speculative. Aledort et al. (1968) have found that the platelet protein responsible for clot retraction lies beneath an outer permeability barrier. This has been confirmed by Haslam (1969). Based on morphologic studies, White (1967) suggests that platelets are in a relaxed discoid form when circulating and that ADP causes aggregation by releasing intracellular calcium which then produces platelet contraction which makes platelets sticky. When ADP is removed, the platelet relaxes and deaggregates.

Despite discrepancies in the theory of an "ecto-ATPase" being intimately associated with ADP-induced platelet aggregation, many investigators are further exploring this possibility and have made some interesting observations. B. M. Jones (1966) and P. C. T. Jones (1966), using chick embryo fibroblasts, muscle and liver cells grown in tissue culture, have noted membrane ATPases in these cells and found that ADP inhibits this ATPase activity. Jones postulated that cell adhesion has an inverse correlation with its surface negativity and when the cell surface is in its contracted, or folded, state, the negative charge per unit surface area increases and the cell becomes nonadhesive. The relaxed or unfolded membrane is adhesive. The membrane folding or contraction is dependent on a high concentration of ATP, contractile ATPase and Ca^{2+} ions and is inhibited by ADP, and Ca^{2+} depletion. The relaxing function depends on an intact relaxing factor and the presence of Mg^{2+} and is inhibited by Ca^{2+} ions and high concentrations of Mg^{2+}. A relaxing factor has been isolated from platelets (Grette, 1963).

Davey and Lüscher (1968b) have put forth a theory of platelet aggregation which reincorporates the concept of bridging. They postulate the following: Platelets circulate in a contracted form, relax before aggregation, and may actually form "bridges" with external calcium ions.

g. ADPASE. It is known that plasma contains an inactivator of ADP (Odegaard et al., 1964; Ireland and Mills, 1966). Spaet and Lejnieks (1966) feel that the hydrolysis of ADP to AMP by a platelet membrane ADPase provides the energy for aggregation. On the other hand, Haslam (1966) has shown that ADP per se must be available at the platelet membrane, for in the presence of pyruvate kinase and phosphoenol-pyruvate, aggregation is inhibited. These substances enhance the synthesis of ATP and ADP and lead to the disappearance of ADP as well.

h. SUMMARY. One can readily see that the theories put forth to explain ADP-induced aggregation are at best complex and confusing. The conclusions drawn by one group are frequently diametrically opposed to those of another. It is apparent, therefore, that different approaches to the study of aggregation are needed to resolve these differences. Little work has been done to evaluate the energy dependence of ADP induced aggregation. In 1964 it was noted that in platelet-rich plasma incubated at 37°C for more than 3 or 4 hours the platelets lost their ability to aggregate with ADP (Hellem and Owren, 1964; O'Brien, 1964; Skalhegg et al., 1964). Two laboratories independently showed that it was necessary to block both glycolysis and oxidative phosphorylation in order to inhibit ADP induced aggregation (O'Brien, 1966; Murer et al., 1967). The metabolic requirements for aggregation need further exploration.

Although divalent cations have been considered by most to be an essential in aggregation, there is little information regarding intraplatelet calcium and magnesium. These cations can now be easily measured using atomic energy spectrophotometry (Aledort et al., 1969d). The role of these divalent cations in bringing about aggregation is now ready for investigation.

2. ROLE OF PLATELET FIBRINOGEN IN ADP-INDUCED AGGREGATION

There seems to be general agreement that ADP-induced platelet aggregation requires the presence of divalent cation. However, the requirement for and the nature of a plasma factor remains speculative. It is known that pig platelets in heated plasma have little or no ability to aggregate with ADP. These platelets in serum or plasma defibrinated with thrombin are equally inactive (Cross, 1964). In rabbits, washed, citrated platelets required a heat labile factor for ADP induced aggregation. A plasma fraction precipitated at 0.2% saturated NH_4SO_4, or purified fibrinogen, human or bovine, were equally able to restore the aggregability of these platelets with ADP and calcium ions (McLean et al., 1964). The "von Willebrand factor" has been ruled out as the essential plasma factor, with pig platelets (Cross, 1964) or in humans (Deykin et al., 1965). Solum and Stormorken (1965) using a Chandler loop, and a washed human platelet model, noted that ADP would not aggregate these platelets in heat inactivated plasma. As little as 0.05–0.1 mg of fibrinogen stimulated aggregation. Either removal of fibrinogen by bentonite or tannic acid, as well as treatment of fibrinogen with neuraminidase interfered with the ability of fibrinogen to aggregate these platelets. In contrast, however, is the observation that platelets of patients with congenital afibrinogenemia (Caen, 1965; Rodman et al., 1966) respond normally to ADP. One cannot, however, exclude trace amounts of fibrinogen in the plasma.

The studies of Brinkhous and co-workers have shown a marked synergism of purified human fibrinogen and ADP in the aggregation of human platelets (Brinkhous et al., 1967). This seems to be true in other species as well (Mason and Read, 1967). Barium sulfate absorbed plasma has a factor which is more potent than fibrinogen. It is of interest that this factor is absent in absorbed plasma of afibrinogenemic patients. These investigators postulate another cofactor necessary for ADP-induced aggregation.

Despite a plethora of laboratory observations, the nature of ADP aggregation and the role that fibrinogen plays in aggregation are obscure. A large body of data has been compiled regarding the use of a whole host of agents capable of inhibiting ADP-induced platelet aggregation, in an attempt to help clarify this apparently simple event which in reality is quite complex. These deaggregating agents will now be dealt with.

3. INHIBITORS OF ADP-INDUCED AGGREGATION

Although many theories have been put forth to explain ADP-induced platelet aggregation, the mechanism remains undefined. There has been great interest in deaggregating agents as potential antithrombogenic substances. Recently a deaggregating substance has been described in the plasma of uremic patients which may explain their hemorrhagic diathesis (Horowitz et al., 1970). Various inhibitors of platelet aggregation have been studied in an attempt to shed light on the mechanisms for aggregation and will be dealt with below.

a. SULFHYDRYL INHIBITORS. Sulfhydryl inhibitors (Rozenberg and Holmsen, 1968b; Aledort et al., 1968) such as parachloromercuribenzoate (PCMB), parachloromercuribenzenesulfonate (PCMBS), and N-ethylmaleimide (NEM) have demonstrated that sulfhydryl groups are essential for ADP aggregation. These agents produce a platelet shape change from a disk to a sphere. A "nonpenetrating" (Aledort et al., 1968) sulfhydryl inhibitor parachloromercuribenzenesulfonate is capable of inhibiting aggregation without altering platelet contraction.

b. α AMINO ACIDS. Certain substituted α amino acids such as tosyl arginine methyl ester (Salzman et al., 1964; O'Brien, 1966) can inhibit ADP induced aggregation, as well as disperse preformed aggregates. It is of note that, as with sulfhydryl inhibitors, disk to sphere shape change remains unaltered.

c. LOCAL ANESTHETICS. A large number of local anesthetics have been studied because of their ability to inhibit platelet aggregation (O'Brien, 1964; Aledort and Niemitz, 1968). Several anesthetics will not inhibit ADP-induced aggregation unless they are preincubated with the platelet for longer than 15 minutes. This appears to be related to the lipid permeability of the compound. Local anesthetics affect muscle contraction by increasing the influx of calcium and the available free cation in the cell (Bianchi, 1968). Although many local anesthetics can inhibit platelet aggregation upon long-term incubation, dibucaine (Aledort and Niemitz, 1968) can aggregate platelets at a time when contraction is abolished. This observation, coupled with its corollary parachloromercuribenzenesulfonate (*supra vida*) challenge the interdependence of aggregation and contraction.

d. PROSTAGLANDINS. The prostaglandins are a group of compounds which have the following properties in common: They cause the contraction of smooth muscle and are potent vasodilators (Emmons et al., 1967; Carlson et al., 1968; and Kloeze, 1969). One prostaglandin in particular, PGE_1, has been extensively studied for its effect on platelet aggregation. *In vitro*, it is more effective than adenosine as an inhibitor of ADP-induced platelet aggregation (Carlson et al., 1968; O'Brien, 1968). It inhibits the electrophoretic mobility changes caused by 0.5 mg ADP, but not those by 0.05 mg (Emmons et al., 1967; von Euler and Eliasson, 1967). The inhibitory effects of PGE_1 are counteracted by the addition of Ca^{2+}. The mechanism of action of prostaglandins on smooth muscle is postulated to be that they facilitate the influx and the release of bound calcium (Emmons et al., 1967). Of great interest is that local anesthetics are reported to produce the same changes in smooth muscle, leading to muscle contraction (Bianchi, 1968). Both types of agents inhibit ADP-induced platelet aggregation giving further credence to the importance of the contractile–relaxing mechanism in platelets for aggregation, as well as pointing up the importance of changes in cellular divalent cations.

e. ADENOSINE. Adenosine, a very potent inhibitor of ADP-induced platelet aggregation, has been investigated by many. The inhibition has been thought to be highly specific and competitive (Born, 1967). They also noted that the relative potency of aggregation inhibition corresponds to its potency as vasodilators (Born et al., 1965), similar to the effects of the prostaglandins. Dr. Born and co-workers (1964) have further found that adenosine and some of its analogues are effective in vivo as inhibitors of embolization following blood vessel injury in the rabbit.

Recently, a group of investigators in Norway have carried out a series of elegant experiments studying the metabolic fate of labeled adenosine and AMP during the inhibition of ADP-induced platelet aggregation (Rozenberg and Holmsen, 1968a). Adenosine monophosphate, adenosine monoacetate, and adenoise monoproprionate work only as inhibitors after hydrolysis to adenosine. Using $^{14}C_{10}$-adenosine and $^{14}C_{10}$-AMP, the plasma adenosine concentration and the amount phosphorylated in the platelet during inhibition were measured. The rate of phosphorylation, not the adenosine concentration, correlated with inhibition. Inhibition remained even after the clearance of adenosine by adenosine deaminase. Inhibition and the rate of phosphorylation were saturated at identical adenosine concentrations. A glycolytic inhibitor (D-2-deoxyglucose) together with a mitochondrial inhibitor (actimycin) known to inhibit ADP-induced aggregation, lowered by 50% the rate of adenosine phosphorylation and by 80% the conversion of the labeled adenine to nucleotides.

The experiments carried out suggested that adenosine inhibition may occur after it is transported across the membrane and phosphorylated. The inhibition may be due to competition for the energy necessary for platelet aggregation and the adenosine transport–phosphorylation process.

These data attempt to further characterize the interrelationship between aggregation and platelet energy metabolism. Karpatkin had showed previously that ADP resulted in agglutination, contraction and increased platelet glycogenolysis (phosphorylase activity) (Karpatkin, 1967). He also suggested that "younger" more metabolically active platelets aggregate better with ADP (Karpatkin, 1969). This approach is useful and requires further investigation, promising greater understanding of platelet aggregation.

f. ANTIINFLAMMATORY AGENTS. Of these drugs, only phenylbutazone and ketozone inhibited the platelet aggregation produced by ADP (Svehla *et al.*, 1968).

g. SUMMARY. The observations presented here underscore the varied approaches taken to clarify the mechanism of ADP-induced platelet aggregation. Our knowledge has vastly increased, but the chain of events that causes aggregation remains a mystery.

B. Antigen–Antibody Complexes

It has been recognized for some time that antigen–antibody (an–ab) complexes could produce platelet aggregation (Mustard, 1964; Movat *et al.*, 1965; Packham *et al.*, 1968). This aggregation is accompanied by platelet degranulation and the release of ADP and serotonin. It has also been observed that platelets are capable of phagocytosing these complexes (Mustard and Packham, 1968), that this process itself is calcium dependent, requires intact glycolysis and oxidative phosphorylation, and leads to increased O_2 consumption and CO_2 and lactate production.

During phagocytosis, ^{32}P-labeled orthophosphate shows an increased incorporation into phosphatidic acid, phosphatidyl ethanolamine and phosphatidyl serine, changes also noted during ADP-induced aggregation. These same investigators have shown that during degranulation, there is release of a substance capable of increasing blood vessel permeability (Mustard *et al.*, 1965). It has recently been shown that an–ab complexes can produce primary and secondary aggregation and that the primary reaction is not ADP dependent (Marney and Des Prez, 1969).

Once again we note a strong relationship between platelet aggregation and cell metabolism.

C. Fatty Acids

In the 1960's in several laboratories it was noted that long chain saturated fatty acids were thrombogenic (Conner *et al.*, 1963; Day and Soloff, 1963; Haslam, 1964; Mahadevon *et al.*, 1966) whereas short chain saturated and unsaturated fatty acids were not. Platelet aggregates were a prominent component of these thrombi. Simultaneously in rabbits, high molecular weight saturated fatty acids were observed to produce the release of platelet serotonin (Shore and Alpers, 1963), and probably ADP (Haslam, 1964).

Free fatty acid (FFA) induced platelet aggregation requires calcium ions (Shore and Alpers, 1963; Mahadevon et al., 1966; Hoak et al., 1967), is not inhibited by heparin (Hoak et al., 1967), and is inhibited by high albumin concentrations, most likely due to the binding of free fatty acids to albumin. Recently it was reported (Spector et al., 1969) that platelet membranes rapidly take up unesterified free fatty acid, a process which tapers off over a period of 1 hour. In contrast there is an increasing amount of fatty acids oxidized to CO_2 and incorporated into glycerides and phospholipids. With increasing concentrations of free fatty acid, platelet-free fatty acid content increases, but the incorporation into CO_2 and lipid esters does not increase to the same extent. The free fatty acid uptake does not appear to be temperature dependent and is reversible. These investigators postulate that the induced platelet aggregation may be secondary to changes in the platelet membrane caused by large amounts of free fatty acid.

D. Fibrinogen Split Products

Thrombocytopenia may be seen as a manifestation of defibrination. With defibrination there is an element of compensatory fibrinolysis. Over the past 10 years there has been a considerable amount of interest in the effect of fibrinogen split products (FSP) on platelets. Several investigators (Wilson et al., 1966; Barnhart et al., 1967), have found these fibrinogen split products to produce calcium-dependent platelet aggregation in vitro, in particular the fraction B_2 fibrinogen derivative D (Barnhart et al., 1967). In vivo these fibrinogen split products have produced platelet depletion. In contrast to these observations, the majority of investigators have found these fibrinogen split products to inhibit the ability of platelets to be aggregated by a whole host of agents, as well as interfering with the platelets' release reactions (Kowalski et al., 1964; Wilson et al., 1966; Larrieu et al., 1966; Jerushalmy and Zucker, 1966; Kopec et al., 1966; Barnhart et al., 1967; Kowalski, 1967; Cronberg, 1968; Kowalski, 1968). One group feels that early and late fibrinogen split products are equally effective (Larrieu et al., 1966) whereas another feels that early fibrinogen split products are more effective inhibitors of aggregation (Kowalski, 1968). Arvin, a purified coagulant fraction of Malayan-pit viper venom, was recently studied in seven humans in the treatment of thrombosis. Arvin acts on plasma fibrinogen in producing unstable fibrinogen and fibrinogen split products. In these patients there was no change in platelet count, but in the first 24 hours of treatment, at the peak concentration of fibrinogen split products, the platelets from these patients were significantly less reactive to ADP (Prentice et al., 1969). In a recent review

Kowalski (1968) has attempted to explain the discrepancy in results of the various investigators. There is evidence that fibrinogen split products have a high avidity to form complexes with fibrinogen or fibrin monomer; these complexes are unclottable by thrombin and are soluble. Depending on the relative concentration of the components of the complexes, either aggregation or inhibition of aggregation is seen. Only the complexes found in the presence of low concentrations of fibrinogen split products aggregate platelets. If fibrinogen split products are in excess, aggregates will not form, and when added to aggregating complexes, aggregating ability is abolished.

E. Connective Tissue

In 1959 Bounameaux described the aggregation of platelets by endothelium. These observations were extended by Hughes and Lapiere (1964). *In vivo* experiments with pigs (Geissinger *et al.*, 1962), rabbits (Stehbens, 1965), and rats (Ashford and Freeman, 1967) have shown that endothelial damage leads to platelet aggregation, degranulation, and the formation of fibrin. In contrast, a recent electron microscopic study (Stehbens and Boscoe, 1967) of platelet changes in cat carotid bodies revealed only a few small platelet aggregates, with a rare shape change and only an occasional cell showing pseudopods. Some intraplatelet granules appeared dense but there was no degranulation. There were some closely packed aggregates with little or no change in platelet morphology at the surface of the aggregates and minor changes in the granules.

Collagen or connective tissue is used to study platelet aggregation. As early as 1962, Zucker and Borrelli showed that viscous metamorphosis did not occur with connective tissue. They further showed that connective tissue aggregation was pH and temperature dependent, and that the active part of connective tissue is collagen, as collagenase inactivates its effects. This latter observation was corroborated by Wilner *et al.* (1968).

The ability of collagen to activate Hageman factor (Barth *et al.*, 1966) has been implicated in the mechanism of connective tissue induced platelet aggregation. Recently the ability of collagen to aggregate platelets could be completely dissociated from the activation of Hageman factor (Wilner *et al.*, 1968). These investigators showed that the negatively charged carboxyl groups of glutamic and aspartic acid are critical for Hageman factor activation but not for platelet aggregation. In contrast, however, the positively charged ε amino groups of lysine are critical for platelet aggregation but not for Hageman factor activation.

As early as 1963, Hovig noted that when platelets were aggregated by a tendon extract the supernatant had the ability to aggregate and this aggregation could be inhibited by AMP. He further showed that the morphologic changes in platelets produced by the supernatant were identical to those produced by ADP, and that this aggregating material in the supernatant was, in fact, ADP. Although AMP could interfere with the ability of tendon extract to aggregate platelets, the supernatant in this reaction could still aggregate an untreated platelet preparation.

These observations have led to the assumption that platelets treated with connective tissue release their ADP which aggregates them. This theory has received much support. Drugs, such as aspirin, capable of inhibiting connective tissue-induced platelet aggregation (Weiss *et al.*, 1968) also inhibit the secondary aggregation produced by ADP and epinephrine (Zucker and Peterson, 1968) but not their primary response, by interfering with the release of platelet ADP. Hughes (1968) recently challenged this hypothesis by demonstrating that Prostaglandin E_1 known to inhibit ADP-induced platelet aggregation, did not inhibit connective tissue-induced aggregation. No measurements were performed on the effect of Prostaglandin E_1 on connective tissue-induced release of platelet ADP. Connective tissue, however, will release platelet factor 3 (Spaet and Cintron, 1965) as well as 5-hydroxytryptamine (Zucker and Peterson, 1968; Hovig *et al.*, 1968). Aledort and Niemetz (1969) have pursued the observations of Hughes by studying the effects of local anesthetics on connective tissue, aggregation, and the release of 5-hydroxytryptamine. They have demonstrated that procaine and lidocaine, agents which do not inhibit ADP-induced platelet aggregation, (Aledort and Niemitz, 1968) as well as metycaine which inhibits ADP-induced platelet aggregation, inhibit connective tissue and 5-hydroxytryptamine-induced platelet aggregation. The platelets treated with the local anesthetics and connective tissue are still capable of releasing ADP and 5-hydroxytryptamine. It is of note that the inhibition of connective tissue-induced platelet aggregation by aspirin is accompanied by an inhibition of the release of platelet ADP and 5-hydroxytryptamine (Zucker and Peterson, 1968). These observations suggest that the released ADP may not be the sole mechanism for connective tissue-induced platelet aggregation and raises the possibility that intraplatelet 5-hydroxytryptamine may play a more important role in bringing about platelet aggregation.

Connective tissue does more than aggregate platelets and produce the release of intraplatelet material. Connective tissue aggregation leads to a burst of lactate production. Collagen and connective tissue both lead to lactate production and collagenase inhibits this. Collagen-induced lactate production is sustained for 60 minutes whereas with connective tissue it only lasts for 15 minutes. This difference in lactate production is presumed to be due to the binding of divalent cations by acid mucopolysaccharides present in connective tissue (Puszkin and Jerushalmy, 1968). These experiments raise a question as to the interpretation of results from one laboratory to another. Are there contaminants in connective tissue specimens which may interfere with the function or the biochemical changes produced by the active collagen moiety? The work of Puszkin and Jerushalmy (1968) further illustrates the close relationship between aggregation and energy metabolism. In this vein, Aledort et al. (1969c) have observed that when platelets are depleted of ATP by long-term storage at 37°C they will no longer aggregate with collagen.

F. Thrombin

Thrombin has long been recognized as a potent platelet aggregating agent. Aggregation which is calcium dependent (Skermer et al., 1961; Schmid et al., 1962; Zieve et al., 1964; Morse et al., 1965; Corn, 1967) is accompanied by the release of ADP, 5-hydroxytryptamine and fibrinogen (Haslam, 1964; Morse et al., 1965, Niewiarowski and Thomas, 1966; Davey and Lüscher, 1968a), platelet factor 3 (Corn, 1967), K^+ (Zieve et al., 1964), free amino acids, lipoproteins, acid phosphatase, β glucuronidase, and procoagulant activity (Davey and Lüscher, 1968a).

The role of fibrinogen as an essential factor for thrombin induced platelet aggregation is as yet unresolved Brinkhous et al. (1969) demonstrated that porcine platelets will not aggregate without fibrinogen as a cofactor. Several other investigators (Skermer et al., 1961; Schmid et al., 1962) using trypsinized platelets, demonstrated the need for fibrinogen in platelet aggregation. More recently Morse and co-workers (1965) demonstrated that washed human platelets treated with EDTA, thrombin, trypsin, and papain, all of which lead to the release of 5-hydroxytryptamine and/or ATP, inactivated clottable protein and rendered the platelet unable to be subsequently aggregated by thrombin in the presence of calcium. They concluded that platelet fibrinogen was vital for the reaction of platelets to fibrinogen. In sharp contrast to these data are observations of Davey and Lüscher (1965) and Lüscher (1966). They have been able to dissociate the effects of thrombin on fibrinogen from its effects on platelets by using a snake venom, A-rhondostoma, which has the properties of thrombin. They concluded that it is untenable that thrombin acts on the fibrinogen of platelets just as it acts on plasma fibrinogen to produce platelet aggregation.

It is known that

$$2 \text{ phosphoenolpyruvate (PEP)} + \text{ADP} + \text{H}^+ \underset{\text{K}^+, \text{ Mg}^{++}}{\overset{\text{pyruvate kinase (PK)}}{\rightleftharpoons}} \text{pyruvate and ATP}$$

Haslam (1964) observed that in the presence of K^+, Mg^{2+} phosphoenol-pyruvate plus pyruvate kinase, which removed the formed ADP and led to the accumulation of pyruvate, inhibited thrombin-induced platelet aggregation. He postulated from these data that thrombin induced release of platelet ADP was an essential for platelet aggregation. Niewiarowski and Thomas (1966) demonstrated that although ADP was additive to thrombin in producing human platelet aggregation, adenosine, an inhibitor of ADP induced aggregation, would only partially inhibit thrombin induced platelet aggregation. These data raise serious question as to how essential released ADP is in bringing about thrombin-induced aggregation.

Recently Booyse and Rafelson (1969), proposed an interesting model for platelet aggregation by thrombin wherein they postulate an intimate rela-tionship between energy metabolism and a surface, or near surface ac-tomyosin (Salzman *et al.*, 1966b; Booyse and Rafelson, 1967; Chambers *et al.*, 1967). The authors suggest that thrombin stimulates glycolysis, leading to an increase of platelet ATP which dissociates the actomyosin-like protein into F actin and platelet myosin. Although in the dissociated form the ATPase activity decreases, the ATPase activity of myosin leads to a fall in ATP content. The lowered ATP favors reassociation of the dissociated moieties with a subsequent increase in ATPase activity. They suggest that during reassociation the F actin from one platelet interacts with the myosin of an adjacent platelet forming bridges which contract and lead to aggregates. This remains highly speculative. It is of interest that calcium depletion also leads to the dissociation of actomyosin com-plexes and sulfhydryl groups are essential for aggregation and actomyosin interaction.

G. Serotonin

Zucker (1947) was one of the first to implicate platelet serotonin in hemostasis. The relationship between the low platelet serotonin in myelo-proliferative disorders to the high incidence of hemorrhage remains obscure (Bigelow, 1954; Hardisty and Stacey, 1957). Most investigators have con-cerned themselves with the effect of aggregating agents on the release of serotonin and not with the importance of serotonin as an aggregating agent. Mitchell and Sharp showed in 1964 that low concentrations of 5-hydroxytryptamine could aggregate platelets. Serotonin aggregation, although reversible, produces platelet changes manifested by the release of platelet factor 3 (Horowitz and Papayoanou, 1968). Aspirin inhibits connective tissue aggregation and simultaneously inhibits the release of ADP (Weiss et al., 1968) and 5-hydroxytryptamine (Zucker and Peterson, 1968). Periactin, a potent antiserotonin, is a potent inhibitor of ADP, connective tissue, epinephrine and serotonin induced platelet aggregation (Aledort et al., 1969a). It is conceivable that the release of 5-hydroxytryptamine and its ability to aggregate platelets play more of a role in platelet aggregation than previously recognized. If this is true it then becomes imperative that accurate measurements of 5-hydroxytryptamine release be performed. At present very few measurements of the release of endogenous platelet 5-hydroxytryptamine have been carried out using aggregating agents (Gaintner et al., 1962; Buckingham and Maynert, 1964; Holmsen, 1965).

Recently Aledort et al. (1969b) have raised the possibility that the release of endogenous 5-hydroxytryptamine may not be identical to that of exogenous added radioactive 5-hydroxytryptamine. Stacey (1968) has given further credence to this by showing that ADP will only release endogenous 5-hydroxytryptamine if the platelet is preloaded with 5-hydroxytryptamine.

H. Epinephrine

Epinephrine is a well-known platelet aggregating agent. It may produce a primary and secondary response (Macmillan, 1966) with no change in platelet volume (Bull and Zucker, 1965). These platelets produce pseudopods (Mannucci and Sharp, 1967). Norepinephrine has also been shown to produce platelet aggregation but it is approximately one-tenth as potent.

The platelet response is accompanied by the release of platelet factor 3 (Horowitz and Papayoanou, 1968) and ADP (O'Brien, 1964). The primary response is inhibited by phentolamine (Macmillan, 1966) and the imipramines are capable of inhibiting both the primary and secondary response (Mills and Roberts, 1967). Sulfhydryl inhibitors such as N-ethylmaleimide and parachloromercuribenzoate (Harrison et al., 1966) also inhibit the epinephrine response. Adenosine only partially inhibits the secondary response (Macmillan, 1966) but β adrenergic blockers will inhibit the secondary response (Thomas, 1967). These data raise doubt as to the role of released ADP in bringing about secondary aggregation.

As with ADP, it has been noted that nonstirred platelets incubated with epinephrine will become refractory to this compound when it is added subsequently, and the mixture then agitated (O'Brien, 1964). These platelets are responsive to ADP. Similarly platelets refractory to ADP will respond to epinephrine. The significance of this refractory state is unknown.

The concept of young metabolically more active platelets has been recently investigated (Karpatkin, 1969). The observations that the larger younger platelets are more responsive to epinephrine confirm the earlier observation that epinephrine aggregates the larger platelet (Mannucci and Sharp, 1967). Karpatkin (1967) demonstrated that epinephrine is a potent activator of phosphorylase and Ardlie *et al.* (1966) suggested that adenyl cyclase activation may play a role in aggregation. These observations suggest that the mechanism for epinephrine aggregation is mediated via platelet energy metabolism, and that aggregation occurs at a "high energy" state rather than a "low energy" state ((Salzman *et al.*, 1966b).

III. SUMMARY AND CONCLUSIONS

The bulk of the studies presented have been carried out *in vitro* and only a relatively small proportion *in vivo*. Many attractive hypotheses have evolved from these data. Whether or not the observations discussed here truly represent mechanisms active in bringing about *in vivo* hemostasis remains a moot point. At present, however, we must utilize these experimental models as tools to better understand platelet–platelet interaction.

At this time there appears to be no agreement as to the mechanism of platelet aggregation induced by any agent, or whether there is a final common pathway for all agents. The data of Davey and Lüscher (1968a) and Holmsen *et al.* (1969) clearly demonstrate that different aggregating agents produce different patterns of platelet release reactions, suggesting that agents bring about aggregation by varying mechanisms. Despite the great interest in the released ADP as a final pathway producing aggregation, this remains speculative. However, the possible role of released 5-hydroxytryptamine in producing platelet aggregation has been neglected.

There are some themes running through the literature which require further evaluation. The contractile protein, thrombosthenin, has been regarded by many as either being active or inhibited when platelets aggregate. A large host of inhibitors of platelet aggregation are vasodilators, stimulate muscle contraction and/or effect calcium transport in other cell systems. Little information is known about intraplatelet calcium, its metabolic dependence, its state as the platelet aggregates and how it affects platelet contraction. There seems to be an intimate relationship between aggregation and platelet energy metabolism.

The above mentioned areas appear to the author to be the most fruitful areas of further investigation in the definition of the mechanism of platelet aggregation.

REFERENCES

Aledort, L. M., and Niemetz, J. (1968). *Proc. Soc. Exp. Biol. Med.* **128**, 658.
Aledort, L. M., and Niemetz, J. (1969). Unpublished observation.
Aledort, L. M. Troup, S. B., and Weed, R. I. (1968). *Blood* **31**, 471.
Aledort, L. M., Gellernt, I., and Burrows, L. (1969a). Unpublished observations.
Aledort, L. M., Gilbert, H., and Puszkin, E. (1969b). *Blood* **34**, 535.
Aledort, L. M., Gutfreund, D., Udkow, M., and Puszkin, E. (1969c). Unpublished observations.
Aledort, L. M., Hirsch, K., Udkow, M., and Puszkin, E. (1969d). *Transfusion (Philadelphia)* **9**, 212.
Ardlie, N. G., Glew, G., and Schwartz, C. J. (1966). *Nature (London)* **212**, 416.
Ashford, T. P., and Freiman, D. G. (1967). *Amer. J. Pathol.* **50**, 257.
Barnhart, M. I., Cress, D. C., Henry, R. L., and Riddle, J. M. (1967). *Thromb. Diath. Haemorrh.* **17**, 79.
Barth, P., Kommerell, B., and Pfleiderer, T. (1966). *Thromb. Diath. Haemorrh.* **16**, 378.
Bettex–Galland, M., and Lüscher, E. F. (1959). *Nature (London)* **184**, 276.
Bettex–Galland, M., and Lüscher, E. F. (1965). *Advan. Protein Chem.* **20**, 1.
Bianchi, C. P. (1968). *Fed. Proc., Fed. Amer. Soc. Exp. Biol.* **27**, 126.
Bigelow, F. S. (1954). *J. Lab. Clin. Med.* **43**, 759.
Bizzozero, G. (1882). *Gazz. Osp. Milano* **3**, 162.
Booyse, F. M., and Rafelson, M. E., Jr. (1967). *Nature (London)* **215**, 283.
Booyse, F. M., and Rafelson, M. E. ,Jr. (1969). *Blood* **33**, 100.
Born, G. V. (1965). *Nature (London)* **206**, 1121.
Born, G. V. (1967). *Fed. Proc., Fed. Amer. Soc. Exp. Biol.* **26**, 115.
Born, G. V., Honour, A. J., and Mitchell, J. R. A. (1964). *Nature (London)* **202**, 761.
Born, G. V., Haslam, R. J., and Goldman, M. (1965). *Nature (London)* **205**, 678.
Bounameaux, Y. (1959). *C. R. Soc. Biol.* **153**, 865.
Brinkhous, K. M., Mason, R. G., and Rodman, N. F. (1967). *Thromb. Diath. Haemorrh.* **26**, Suppl. 79.
Brinkhous, K. M., Read, M. S., Rodman, N. F., and Mason, R. G. (1969). *J. Lab. Clin. Med.* **73**, 1000.
Buckingham, S., and Maynert, E. W. (1964). *J. Pharmacol. Exp. Ther.* **143**, 332.
Bull, B. S., and Zucker, M. B. (1965). *Proc. Soc. Exp. Biol. Med.* **120**, 296.
Caen, J. P. (1965). *Nature (London)* **205**, 1120.
Carlson, L. A., Iron, E., and Org, L. (1968). *Life Sci.* **7**, 85.
Chambers, D. A., Salzman, E. W., and Neri, L. L. (1967). *Arch. Biochem. Biophys.* **119**, 173.
Connor, W. E., Hoak, J. C., and Warner, E. D. (1963). *J. Clin. Invest.* **42**, 860.
Corn, M. (1967). *Blood* **30**, 552.
Cronberg, S. (1968). *Thromb. Diath. Haemorrh.* **19**, 474.
Cross, M. J. (1964). *Thromb. Diath. Haemorrh.* **12**, 524.
Davey, M. G., and Lüscher, E. F. (1965). *Nature (London)* **207**, 731.

Davey, M. G., and Lüscher, E. F. (1968a). *Biochim. Biophys. Acta* **165**, 490.
Davey, M. G., and Lüscher, E. F. (1968b). *Semin. Hematol.* **5**, 5.
Day, H. J., and Soloff, L. A. (1963). *Clin. Res.* **11**, 192.
Deykin, D., Pritzker, C. R., and Scolnick, E. M. (1965). *Nature (London)* **208**, 296.
Eberth, J. C., and Schimmelbusch, C. (1886). *Virchow's Arch. Pathol. Anat. Physiol.* **103**, 39.
Emmons, P. R., Hampton, J. R., Harrison, M. J. G., Honour, A. J., and Mitchell, J. R. A. (1967). *Brit. Med. J.* **2**, 468.
Gaarder, A., and Laland, S. (1964). *Nature (London)* **202**, 909.
Gaarder, A., Jonsen, J., Laland, S., Hellem, A., and Owren, P. A. (1961). *Nature (London)* **192**, 531.
Gaintner, J. R., Jackson, D. P., and Maynert, E. W. (1962). *Bull. Johns Hopkins Hosp.* **111**, 185.
Geissinger, H. D., Mustard, J. F., and Rowsell, H. C. (1962). *Can. Med. Ass. J.* **87**, 405.
Gorstein, F., Carroll, H. J., and Puszkin, E. (1967). *J. Lab. Clin. Med.* **70**, 938.
Grette, K. (1963). *Nature (London)* **198**, 488.
Hampton, J. R., and Mitchell, J. R. A. (1966a). *Brit. Med. J.* **1**, 1074.
Hampton, J. R., and Mitchell, J. R. A. (1966b). *Nature (London)* **210**, 1000.
Hampton, J. R., and Mitchell, J. R. A. (1966c). *Nature (London)* **211**, 245.
Hardisty, R. M., and Stacey, R. S. (1957). *Brit. J. Haematol.* **3**, 292.
Harrison, M. J. G., Emmons, P. R., and Mitchell, J. R. A. (1966). *Thromb. Diath. Haemorrh.* **16**, 122.
Haslam, R. J. (1964). *Nature (London)* **202**, 765.
Haslam, R. J. (1966). *Thromb. Diath. Haemorrh.* **15**, 626.
Haslam, R. J. (1969). Personal communication.
Hellem, A., and Owren, P. A. (1964). *Acta Hematol.* **31**, 230.
Hellem, A. J., Borchgrevink, C. F., and Ames, S. B. (1961). *Brit. J. Haematol.* **7**, 42.
Hoak, J. C., Warner, E. D., and Conner, W. F. (1967). *Circ. Res.* **20**, 11.
Holmsen, H. (1965). *Scand. J. Clin. Lab. Invest.* **17**, 239.
Holmsen, H., Day, H. J., and Stormorken, H. (1969). Personal communication.
Horowitz, H. I., and Papayoanou, M. F. (1968). *Thromb. Diath. Haemorrh.* **19**, 18.
Horowitz, H. I., Stein, I. M., Cohen, B. D., and White, J. G. (1970). *Amer. J. Med.* **49**, 336.
Hovig, T. (1963). *Thromb. Diath. Haemorrh.* **9**, 264.
Hovig, T., Jorgensen, L., Packham, M. A., and Mustard, J. F. (1968). *J. Lab. Clin. Med.* **71**, 29.
Hughes, J. (1968). Unpublished observation.
Hughes, J., and Lapiere, C. M. (1964). *Thromb. Diath. Haemorrh.* **11**, 327.
Ireland, D. M., and Mills, D. C. B. (1966). *Biochem. J.* **99**, 283.
Jerushalmy, Z., and Zucker, M. B. (1966). *Thromb. Diath. Haemorrh.* **15**, 413.
Jones, B. M. (1966). *Nature (London)* **212**, 362.
Jones, P. C. T. (1966). *Nature (London)* **212**, 365.
Karpatkin, S. (1967). *J. Clin. Invest.* **46**, 409.
Karpatkin, S. (1969). *J. Clin. Invest.* **48**, 1083.
Kloeze, J. (1969). *Acta Physiol. Pharmacol. Neer.* **15**, 50.
Kopec, M., Budzynski, A., Stachurska, J., Wegrzynowicz, Z., and Kowalski, E. (1966). *Thromb. Diath. Haemorrh.* **15**, 477.
Kowalski, E. (1967). *Thromb. Diath. Haemorrh.* **26**, Suppl. 113.

Kowalski, E. (1968). *Semin. Hematol.* **5**, 45.

Kowalski, E., Kopec, M., and Wegrzynowicz, Z. (1964). *Thromb. Diath. Haemorrh.* **10**, 407.

Larrieu, M. J., Marder, V. J., and Inceman, S. (1966). *Thromb. Diath. Haemorrh.* **19**, Suppl. 26.

Lüscher, E. F. (1966). *Thromb. Diath. Haemorrh.* **15**, 625.

McLean, J. R., Maxwell, R. E., and Hertler, D. (1964). *Nature (London)* **202**, 605.

Macmillan, D. C. (1966). *Nature (London)* **211**, 140.

Mahadevan, V., Singh, H., and Lundberg, W. O. (1966). *Proc. Soc. Exp. Biol. Med.* **121**, 22.

Mannucci, P. M., and Sharp, A. A. (1967). *Brit. J. Haematol.* **13**, 604.

Marney, S. R., and Des Prez, R. M. (1969). *Blood* **34**, 538.

Mason, R. G., and Read, M. S. (1967). *Exp. Mol. Pathol.* **6**, 370.

Mills, D. C. B., and Roberts, G. C. K. (1967). *Nature (London)* **213**, 35.

Mitchell, J. R. A., and Sharp, A. A. (1964). *Brit. J. Haematol.* **10**, 78.

Morse, E. P., Jackson, D. J., and Conley, C. L. (1965). *J. Clin. Invest.* **44**, 809.

Movat, H. Z., Mustard, J. F., Taichman, N. S., and Uriuhara, T. (1965). *Proc. Soc. Exp. Biol. Med.* **120**, 232.

Murer, E. H., Hellem, A. J., and Rozenberg, M. C. (1967). *Scand. J. Clin. Lab. Invest.* **19**, 280.

Mustard, J. F., (1964). *Fed. Proc., Fed. Amer. Soc. Exp. Biol.* **23**, 548.

Mustard, J. F., and Packham, M. A. (1968). *Ser. Haematol.* **1**, 168.

Mustard, J. F., Movat, H. Z., Macmorine, D. R. L., and Senye, A. (1965). *Proc. Soc. Exp. Biol. Med.* **119**, 988.

Niewiarowski, S., and Thomas, D. P. (1966). *Nature (London)* **212**, 1544.

O'Brien, J. R. (1964). *J. Clin. Pathol.* **17**, 275.

O'Brien, J. R. (1966). *Nature (London)* **212**, 1057.

O'Brien, J. R. (1968). *Lancet* **1**, 149.

Odegaard, A. E., Skalhegg, B. A. ,and Hellem, A. J. (1964). *Thromb. Diath. Haemorrh.* **11**, 317.

Packham, M. A., Nishizawa, E. E., and Mustard, J. F. (1968). "Biochemical Pharmacology," 171. Pergamon Press, New York.

Prentice, C. R. M., Hassanein, A. A., Turpie, A. G. G., McNecal, G. P., and Douglas, A. S. (1969). *Lancet* **1**, 644.

Puszkin, E., and Jerushalmy, Z. (1968). *Proc. Soc. Exp. Biol. Med.* **129**, 346.

Robinson, C. W., Jr., Kress, S. C., Wagner, R. H., and Brinkhous, K. M. (1965). *Exp. Mol. Pathol.* **4**, 457.

Rodman, N. F., Mason, R. G., Painter, J. C., and Brinkhous, K. M. (1966). *Lab. Invest.* **15**, 641.

Rozenberg, M. C., and Holmsen, H. (1968a). *Biochim. Biophys. Acta* **155**, 343.

Rozenberg, M. C., and Holmsen, H. (1968b). *Biochim. Biophys. Acta* **157**, 280.

Salzman, E. W., and Chambers, D. A. (1964). *Nature (London)* **204**, 698.

Salzman, E. W., Chambers, D. A., and Neri, L. L. (1966a). *Thromb. Diath. Haemorrh.* **15**, 52.

Salzman, E. W., Chambers, D. A., and Neri, L. L. (1966b). *Nature (London)* **210**, 167.

Schmid, H. J., Jackson, D. P., and Conley, C. L. (1962). *J. Clin. Invest.* **41**, 543.

Shore, P. A., and Alpers, H. S. (1963). *Nature (London)* **200**, 1331.

Skalhegg, B. A., Hellem, A. J., and Odegaard, A. E. (1964). *Thromb. Diath. Haemorrh.* **11**, 305.

Skermer, R. W., Mason, R. G., Wagner, R. H., and Brinkhous, K. M. (1961). *J. Exp. Med.* **114**, 905.

Skoza, L., Zucker, M. B., Jerushalmy, Z., and Grant, R. (1966). *Thromb. Diath. Haemorrh.* **18**, 713.

Solum, N. O., and Stormorken, H. (1965). *Scand. J. Clin. Lab. Invest.* Suppl. **84**, 170.

Spaet, T. H., and Cintron, J. (1965). *Brit. J. Haematol.* **11**, 269.

Spaet, T. H., and Lejnieks, I. (1966). *Thromb. Diath. Haemorrh.* **15**, 36.

Spector, A. A., Hoak, J. C., Warner, E. D., and Fry, G. L. (1969). *Blood* **34**, 524.

Stacey, R. S. (1968). *Experientia* **24**, 908.

Stehbens, W. E. (1965). *Lab. Invest.* **14**, 449.

Stehbens, W. E., and Boscoe, T. J. (1967). *Amer. J. Pathol.* **50**, 219.

Švehla, C., Ryšánek, K., König, J., Štěpánková, H., and Mlejnková, M. (1968). *Cas. Lek. Cesk.* **107**, 757.

Thomas, D. (1967). *Nature* (*London*) **215**, 298.

von Euler, V. S., and Eliasson, R., eds. (1967). "Prostaglandins." Academic Press, New York.

Weiss, H. J., Aledort, L. M., and Kochwa, S. (1968). *J. Clin. Invest.* **47**, 2169.

White, J. G. (1967). *Abstr. 3rd Conf. Blood Platelets*, 1967, p. 7.

White, J. G. (1968). *Blood* **31**, 604.

Wilner, G. D., Nossel, H. L., and LeRoy, E. C. (1968). *J. Clin. Invest.* **47**, 2616.

Wilson, P. A., McNicol, G. P., and Douglas, A. S. (1966). *Thromb. Diath. Haemorrh.* **18**, 66.

Zieve, P. D., and Solomon, H. M. (1968). *Fed. Proc., Fed. Amer. Soc. Exp. Biol.* **27**, 569.

Zieve, P. D., Gamble, J. L., Jr., and Jackson, D. P. (1964). *J. Clin. Invest.* **43**, 2063.

Zucker, M. B. (1947). *Amer. J. Physiol.* **148**, 275.

Zucker, M. B., and Borrelli, J. (1962). *Proc. Soc. Exp. Biol. Med.* **109**, 779.

Zucker, M. B., and Peterson, J. (1967). *Blood* **30**, 556.

Zucker, M. B., and Peterson, J. (1968). *Proc. Soc. Exp. Biol. Med.* **127**, 547.

Zucker, M. B., and Zaccardi, J. B. (1964). *Fed. Proc., Fed. Amer. Soc. Exp. Biol.* **23**, 299.

10

ENDOTHELIAL SUPPORTING FUNCTION OF PLATELETS*

SHIRLEY A. JOHNSON

The petechial and purpuric hemorrhages which appear in the skin and mucous membranes when the number of circulating platelets falls below 50,000/mm³ have been called the thrombocytopenic lesion. Gaydos and associates (1962) showed that spontaneous bleeding may occur in such patients when the platelet count is under 20,000/mm³. Some of these purpuric hemorrhages in thrombocytopenic individuals result from the escape of red blood cells into the interstitial spaces from anatomically intact capillaries.

* Supported by USPHS Project Grant HE 12121-02 and the Veterans Administration.

I. MEASUREMENT OF VASCULAR INTEGRITY

Measurements of capillary integrity are performed by application to the skin of positive or negative pressure. When the platelet count is low, either type of pressure results in formation of petechiae which indicates a weakened capillary wall. According to Kramar (1961) a normal person develops very few petechiae under test conditions.

Red blood cells escape from the blood vessels in abnormal numbers in thrombocytopenic individuals by way of two mechanisms: Either the weakened endothelial cells rupture readily when slightly traumatized allowing blood to flow out into the interstitial spaces or red blood cells escape singly through the intact wall. The gaps in the vessel wall can only be filled by formation of hemostatic plugs from aggregates of transfused platelets.

The hemostatic plugs also contain fibrin and red blood cells, the proportions varying with the size of the vessel (see Chapter 12). Woods and coworkers (1953) quantitated the escape of erythrocytes from blood vessels by serial counting of the red blood cells in the lymph obtained by cannulation of the thoracic duct. Following irradiation, these animals became thrombocytopenic and had grossly bloody lymph. Platelet transfusions decreased the red blood cells in the lymph of rats from 900,000 to 30,000/mm^3 within 6 hours. No depression of erythrocyte counts in lymph was found in control rats receiving plasma only. These experiments clearly showed that thrombocytopenic bleeding, even that produced by total body irradiation, was controlled by transfusions of platelets.

These same techniques were used by Jackson *et al.* (1959) to compare the hemostatic effectiveness of fresh and lyophilized platelets in reducing the output of red blood cells in the lymph of thrombocytopenic dogs. The infusions of lyophilized platelets did not increase the circulating platelet counts nor did they increase the output of red blood cells in the lymph, while the infusions of freshly prepared dog platelets accomplished both. This ability of fresh platelets to prevent escape of erythrocytes from intact capillaries was described by Rebuck (1963) as the endothelial supporting function of platelets.

The first experimental evidence that platelets interact with endothelial cells was reported by Cronkite and associates (1961) using autoradiography. They transfused $^{35}SO_4$-labeled, donor rat platelets into normal and irradiated thrombocytopenic rats. No regular evidence of the deposition of radioactive material was found in the capillary beds of normal animals, whereas in the thrombocytopenic animals a picture of apparent labeling of the capillary beds of numerous organs was found. They concluded that platelets probably interacted with the endothelial cells of the capillaries of thrombocytopenic animals and contributed radiosulfate-labeled material to the endothelial cells.

Although it is usually assumed that circulating platelets are functioning platelets, we have observed an increase in the number of platelets with no improvement of bleeding time and no correction of the poor prothrombin consumption time. Since the donor platelets came from several donors, we considered it a characteristic of the recipient that the donor platelets were viable but nonfunctioning in this respect (Arnaud *et al.*, 1963).

II. MECHANISM OF RED BLOOD CELL ESCAPE FROM INTACT CAPILLARIES IN THROMBOCYTOPENIA

Although erythrocytes are only occasionally seen lying free in the interstitial spaces of the lamina propria of the mucous membranes in normal animals, many are seen in thrombocytopenic animals.

We have described the mechanism by which erythrocytes escape from intact capillaries (Fig. 1) in thrombocytopenic animals following slight trauma (Van Horn and Johnson, 1966; Johnson *et al.*, 1966). In the initial stage the red blood cell in response to being pushed against the weakened endothelial cell puts forth a process which produces an indentation in the endothelium (Fig. 2). In the second stage the process of the red blood cell creates a channel through the endothelial cytoplasm and contacts the basement membrane. In the third stage the red blood cell escapes from the lumen through the endothelial cell. In some instances the red blood cell comes to rest in the basement membrane in stage four; in stage five the endothelial cytoplasm closes the channel and the red blood cell passes into the interstitial spaces.

Our observation of large numbers of erythrocytes lying free in the interstitial spaces correlates with the measurement of the increased numbers of erythrocytes in the lymph of thrombocytopenic dogs and rats. After escaping from capillaries the erythrocytes find their way to the lymph vessels and are either destroyed in the lymph nodes or returned to the circulation by the lymphatic system. In thrombocytopenic animals biopsied 20 minutes after infusion of fresh platelet concentrates, no blood cells have been observed in the act of escaping. A few red blood cells were seen in the interstitial spaces at a distance from the capillaries indicating that they had escaped before the infusion was given.

According to Odland (1961) a space measuring about 200 Å separates

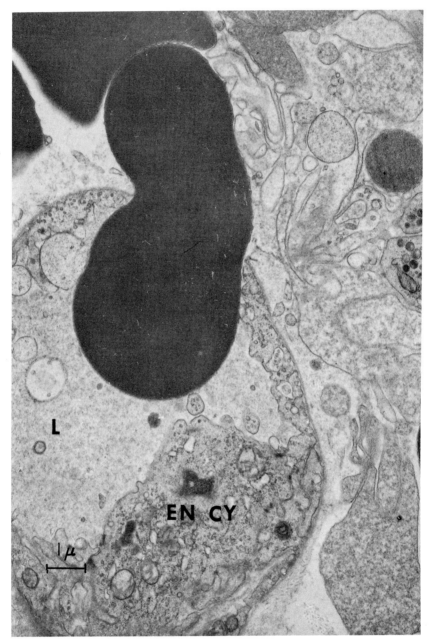

FIG. 1. A red blood cell can be seen escaping from the lumen (L) through the endothelial cytoplasm (EN CY) of a capillary taken from the buccal mucosae of a thrombocytopenic (produced by injection of antiplatelet sera) guinea pig. The tissue was fixed in osmium, sections were stained with uranyl acetate and lead citrate. 10,000×.

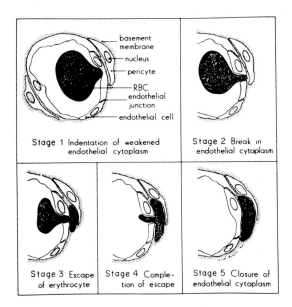

FIG. 2. A diagram showing the mechanism of escape of red blood cells through intact capillary walls in thrombocytopenic guinea pigs. (Taken from Van Horn and Johnson, 1966.)

the plasma membranes of red blood cells in normal animals from the endothelial cells even in vessels distended by erythrocytes. In thrombocytopenic animals when red blood cells were frequently pushed into the endothelial cytoplasm near but not into the intact endothelial junctions, the space of 200 Å disappeared (Johnson *et al.*, 1966). We have seen endothelial nuclei broken by the passage of red blood cells.

Serial sections of the same capillary have been most useful in establishing the sequence of events in the escape of erythrocytes. The indentation in the endothelial cytoplasm made by the process from a red blood cell is not located at the junction between endothelial cells. Since the act of penetration has been observed only a few times in the study of several hundred capillaries, we believe that the escape occurs very quickly (Fig. 1). Using capillary microscopy, Humble (1949) described exudation of blood in thrombocytopenic animals as a shower of red blood cells being "hurled from the capillaries, some traveling three times their diameter before coming to rest." Some electron micrographs suggest that the basement membrane may be a thin gel that flows into the break in the endothelial cell or into the area distorted by the presence of an erythrocyte.

The relatively dense area around the escaping red blood cell could represent the area of contact of plasma and basement membrane. It is possible that this dense material may be hemoglobin that has been squeezed from the erythrocyte during passage through the endothelial wall. The forces which enable the erythrocytes to move around the pericytes and collagen and through the interstitial spaces to the lymph vessels are unknown. The details of the repair of the endothelial cytoplasm consisting of disappearance of the membranes lining the channel are also unknown but the gap is small and closes immediately after the red blood cell squeezes through.

III. PERMEABILITY OF ENDOTHELIUM TO TRACER PARTICLES IN THROMBOCYTOPENIA

Colloidal particles have been used as tracers to delineate either changes in the blood vessel walls or abnormal capillary permeability. Benacerraf and co-workers (1959) demonstrated that a nontoxic stable suspension of colloidal carbon in a gelatin solution was removed by the reticuloendothelial system. It did not localize in the capillary wall unless the reticuloendothelial system had been blocked by previous injections of carbon or of thorotrast.

A. Use of Particles

We chose to study the supposed impaired capillary permeability in thrombocytopenic animals by infusion of ferritin, thorotrast, and colloidal carbon.

B. Behavior of Particles in Normal and Thrombocytopenic Animals

We observed that ferritin escaped through the endothelial cells in both normal and thrombocytopenic guinea pigs. Thorotrast, a particle of different size and physicochemical characteristics, was retained within the vascular system of both types of animals. Only colloidal carbon was handled differentially by the thrombocytopenic endothelium.

C. Mechanism of Escape of Colloidal Particles

Colloidal carbon particles injected into the circulation of normal guinea pigs were retained by the capillaries in the lamina propria of the mucous membrane (Fig. 3a). One hour after the infusion was begun no carbon

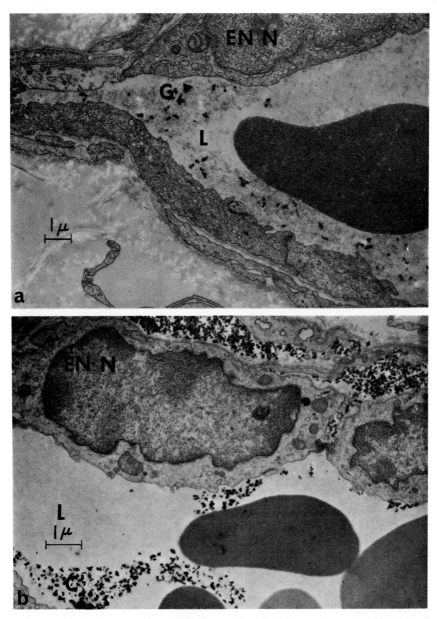

FIG. 3. (a) An electron micrograph of a capillary in the buccal mucosae of a normal guinea pig which was infused with colloidal carbon 20 minutes earlier. No carbon escaped from the vessel. 6500×. (b) An electron micrograph of a capillary in the buccal mucosa of a thrombocytopenic guinea pig who was infused with colloidal carbon 20 minutes earlier. Much carbon has escaped from the vessel. The tissue was fixed in osmium, stained with uranyl acetate and lead citrate. 9800×.

particles were seen in the endothelial cytoplasm, junction, vesicles, basement membrane, or in the interstitial spaces in any of the five normal animals.

In guinea pigs with platelet counts below 20,000/mm³ caused by whole body X-irradiation, injected carbon particles were observed to escape from the capillaries 20 minutes following the initiation of the infusion (Fig. 3b). Carbon particles could be seen lying in the basement membrane surrounding many capillaries. At 1 hour following a carbon infusion, large aggregates of carbon particles were seen surrounding about one-third of the capillaries. Three hours following carbon infusion the plasma was almost cleared of particles. None was seen in the interstitial spaces and only a few particles were present in the phagocytic vacuoles of the pericytes. The manner in which endothelial cells handled colloidal particles was the same whether the thrombocytopenia in the animals had been produced by total body X-irradiation or injection of antiplatelet serum (Van Horn and Johnson, 1968).

D. Effect of Platelet Transfusion

The platelet counts in irradiated animals fell from the normal level of about 400,000 platelets/mm³ to less than 20,000 by the eighth day following irradiation. Platelet transfusions at this time raised the number of circulating platelets above 200,000 but within 1 hour after the transfusion the number of platelets circulating decreased by 15–30% to 133,000/mm³ in one animal and 172,000/mm³ in another. Colloidal carbon particles injected 1 hour after the transfusion of platelets reduced the number of circulating platelets but not to the hemorrhagic level. The presence of carbon particles was evident in the lumen but not in the basement membrane or interstitial spaces 1 hour after the carbon infusion. Platelets were observed in the circulation and in the process of entering the endothelial cytoplasm (Van Horn and Johnson, 1968).

IV. MECHANISM WHEREBY PLATELETS SUPPORT THE ENDOTHELIUM

Since the total number of platelets utilized regularly by the normal endothelium is small [Harker and Finch (1969) showed it to be 35,000/mm³ day] and the area of the vascular endothelium enormous, the chance of observing platelet interaction with the normal lining endothelium is ex-

tremely unlikely. For this reason, we have studied the interaction of transfused platelets in thrombocytopenic recipients. This condition exposes
platelet-deprived vascular endothelium to a large number of viable platelets.
Our experimental design involved producing acute thrombocytopenia in
guinea pigs, usually by total body irradiation but occasionally we have
used antiplatelet serum. Although the antiserum removes the platelets
from the circulation, it leaves the bone marrow relatively unchanged. There
is no way to estimate how deprived the endothelium is because adequate
quantities of platelets may be released into the circulation to support the
endothelium but not enough to cause an increase in the platelet count.
For this reason some patients with few circulating platelets bleed profusely
and others, whose bone marrow continues to produce only enough platelets
to support the endothelium, do not have hemorrhagic problems. The
platelet count is not an accurate means of quantitating thrombopoiesis.
Plateletpheresis is also an effective way to remove platelets from the circulation of an animal but the bone marrow continues to produce platelets
(Johnson *et al.*, 1964).

A. Role of Platelets in Transfusion

A platelet count represents the surplus number of platelets after the
needs of the endothelium and of hemostasis are met. When the platelet
counts dropped below 10,000/mm³ we transfused the animals with donor
platelets and performed biopsies of the buccal mucosae. Platelets were seen
interacting with the endothelial membrane.

Because vascular fragility tests usually improve when a limited number of
platelets are transfused into a thrombocytopenic patient, even though the
bleeding time may not be reduced to normal, we have always stated that
the first use of platelets on entry into the vascular system was support of
the endothelium. Once this need has been met, surplus platelets are available
to form hemostatic plugs to arrest microhemorrhages in a fashion similar
to termination of the bleeding time determination. The remaining platelets
circulate and constitute the platelet count in peripheral blood.

When the plasma membranes of platelet and juxtaposed endothelium
disintegrate, the identification of the platelet becomes difficult (Johnson
et al., 1964). Although adjacent or serial sections (Fig. 4) give additional
information about the interrelationship of platelets with the endothelium,
it was clear that electron autoradiography would have to be used to describe
how the contents of the platelet were incorporated into endothelial cells.

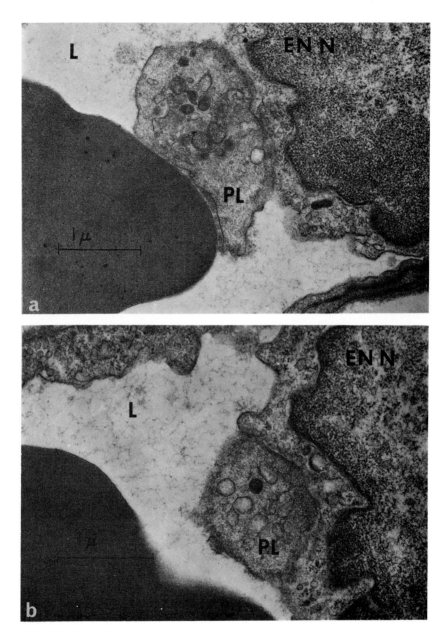

FIG. 4. (a) and (b) These two micrographs are serial sections of a platelet (PL) entering the endothelium [endothelial nucleus (EN N)] in a capillary in the buccal mucosae
in a thrombocytopenic (produced by total body irradiation) guinea pig. The tissue was
biopsied 3 minutes after the platelet transfusion, fixed in osmium, sections were stained
with uranyl acetate and lead citrate. L, lumen 22,700× and 27,000×, respectively.

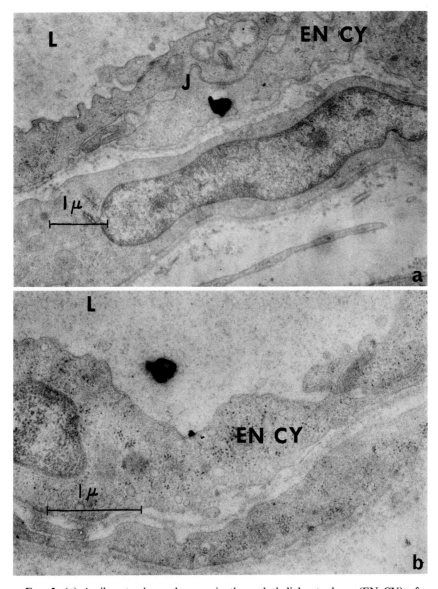

Fɪɢ. 5. (a) A silver track can be seen in the endothelial cytoplasm (EN CY) of a vessel taken from the buccal mucosae of a thrombocytopenic guinea pig (thrombocytopenia produced by total body irradiation) 3 minutes after transfusion of ^{3}H-DFP tagged platelets. Tissue was fixed in glutaraldehyde and osmium, sections were stained with uranyl acetate and lead citrate. (L, lumen) 21,000×. (b) A silver track can be seen in the lumen (L) of a vessel taken from the buccal mucosae of a control thrombocytopenic guinea pig after a transfusion of ^{3}H-DFP tagged plasma. Tissue prepared as above. 26,000×.

B. Autoradiography

Donor guinea pig platelets that had been tagged with tritium-labeled diisopropylfluorophosphonate (^{3}H-DFP) were transfused into thrombocytopenic guinea pigs and the sections prepared for electron autoradiography.

Sections of the platelet button prior to transfusion were also prepared for autoradiography. Using *in vivo* labeling with ^{3}H-DFP other investigators have calculated that less than 50% of the donor platelets became labeled. Our autoradiographs showed that 22% of donor platelets were labeled with ^{3}H-DFP. Some of the platelets seen entering the endothelium in these experiments were labeled and some not.

Much label was found in the endothelial cytoplasm 3 minutes after the end of the transfusion (Fig. 5a) and many platelets could be seen entering the endothelium. Thirty minutes after the end of the transfusion a great deal of label was found in the vascular endothelium with very few platelets in the act of entering. When labeled plasma, containing ten times the amount of radioactivity the labeled platelets had contained, was transfused into thrombocytopenic animals very little label was found in the endothelial cytoplasm. Most was found in the plasma (Fig. 5b) in the lumen of the vessels (Table I). When the endothelium had been deprived of platelets for several days, the transfused platelets entered the endothelial cells immediately on transfusion into the blood vessels (Fig. 6). Clearly the platelets are required to carry the label into the endothelium.

TABLE I

DISTRIBUTION OF ISOTOPE LABEL IN CAPILLARIES IN BUCCAL MUCOSAE FOLLOWING TRANS-FUSION OF EITHER PLATELETS TAGGED WITH ^{3}H-DFP OR PLASMA TAGGED WITH ^{3}H-DFP INTO THROMBOCYTOPENIC GUINEA PIGS

Location	Platelets ^{3}H-DFP		Plasma ^{3}H-DFP	
	Number	%	Number	%
Endothelium	215	86	3	3
Lumen	17	7	104	87
Elsewhere	18	7	13	10
Total	250	100	120	100

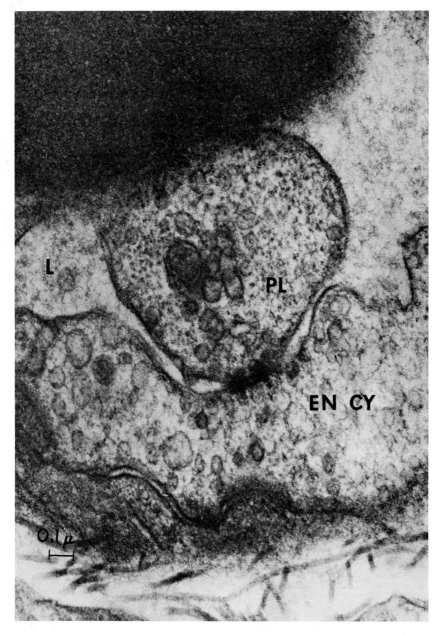

Fɪɢ. 6. A platelet (PL) is seen entering the endothelial cytoplasm (EN CY) of a capillary in the buccal mucosae of a thrombocytopenic (produced by total body irradiation) guinea pig 3 minutes after a transfusion of platelets. Tissue was fixed in osmium, section stained with uranyl acetate and lead citrate. L, lumen. 68,000×

C. Description of Mechanism of Supportive Function

We have described this mechanism of interaction in five stages (Wojcik *et al.*, 1969). *Stage one* consists of formation of dense areas between platelet and endothelial membrane. *Stage two* shows these membranes beginning to disintegrate. *Stage three* shows vesicles forming from the dense areas. The contents still resemble the organelles of the platelet. *Stage four* is characterized by the reappearance of polyribosomes last seen in the mega-karyocyte before the platelet was separated. At *stage five* the platelet has completely disappeared with part of the limiting membrane of the platelet now constituting a portion of the luminal endothelial membrane. Since the interaction of platelets is so rapid following transfusion, we feel that many more platelets support the endothelium than was formerly suspected (Fig. 7).

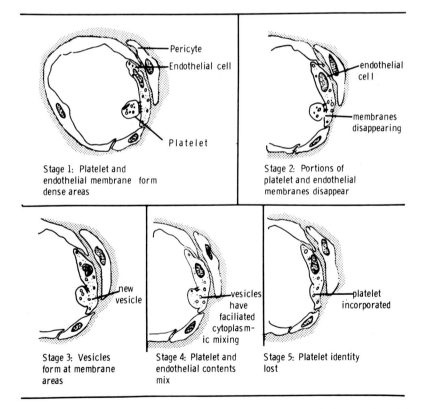

FIG. 7. Diagram of mechanism of a platelet entering the endothelial cytoplasm of a capillary.

We have been surprised to observe the sudden appearance of polyribosomes in the cytoplasm of the platelets after the platelet–endothelial membranes disintegrate. Behnke (1969) has reported disappearance of polyribosomes in platelets as they leave the polyribosome-containing megakaryocytes. Possibly the ribonucleases in the platelet cytoplasm split polyribosomes to ribosomes which are too small to be identified at the magnification most investigators have used. It is possible that some as yet undescribed mechanism exists that causes the polyribosomes to disassemble when the platelets leave the megakaryocytes and to reassemble very rapidly when the platelets join the endothelial cells. Perhaps some material such as an inhibitor of ribonuclease in the endothelial cell stimulates the reassembling of polyribosomes, or possibly the vesicular transport mechanism rapidly carries polyribosomes from the endothelial cytoplasm into the platelet. Vesicles are usually seen arising from the dense areas where the platelets contact the endothelial cell.

We have no evidence that the label leaves the platelet in the time of our experiment (24 hours), although Cooney et al. (1968) have shown about 10% of this label to be reutilized by new platelets 8 days after the transfusion. Even if the label did leave the platelets to enter the plasma, our control experiments show that label in the plasma is not picked up by the endothelium.

Transfusions of platelet fragments, such as lyophilized platelets or the isolated phospholipid, platelet factor 3, into thrombocytopenic recipients do improve vascular fragility. Although we have not yet transfused labeled fragments into thrombocytopenic recipients to study the details of this interaction, previous observations indicate that fragmented platelets enter the endothelium.

Gaps are seldom seen between the endothelial cells either in normal or thrombocytopenic capillaries of the peripheral vascular system. Application of reserpine, histamine, serotonin, or any stressful condition to the capillary wall, may produce these gaps. Majno (1965) hypothesizes that histamine acted directly on the endothelium by loosening the intercellular junctions. According to Tranzer and Baumgartner (1967) circulating platelets may fill the gaps formed following stretching: When the vessels constrict, the platelets move out. This phenomenon is a reversible one as the platelets involved do not degranulate. We consider it neither to be a mechanism whereby platelets normally support the endothelium nor one by which platelets are related to thrombocytopenic bleeding. These authors stated that in capillaries of untreated animals, the endothelial cells completely covered the underlying basement membrane lamina. Certainly if gaps opened between endothelial cells one would expect platelets to be attracted to them.

D. Characteristic of the Endothelial Membrane That Attracts Platelets

We have wondered for some years what characterizes the endothelial membrane of the thrombocytopenic animals to attract a circulating platelet to it. Recently we have observed marked deterioration of the endothelial membrane in juxtaposition to an approaching platelet (Stewart *et al.*, 1970). The endothelial membrane on either side of the area opposite the approaching platelet is intact and healthy in ultrastructure. We suggest that when the endothelial cytoplasm is deprived of platelet material the membrane cannot be reformed and repaired following injury inflicted by turbulent currents of blood. The healthy endothelial membrane has a negative charge that normally repels the negatively charged circulating platelets. When injured, the positively charged endothelial membrane may attract instead of repelling platelets.

V. SUMMARY

We have shown how red blood cells escape from intact vessels in thrombocytopenic individuals by squeezing through the weakened endothelial cells. Colloidal carbon particles escape through intact capillary and venule walls in thrombocytopenic animals but not in normal ones. Transfusions of fresh, whole platelets prevent this escape by being incorporated into the endothelial cells. Donor platelets labeled with tritium tagged diisopropyl-fluorophosphonate were followed by electron autoradiography in the recipient thrombocytopenic animals. The appearance of much label in the endothelial cells when labeled platelets were transfused and by virtually none when labeled plasma was transfused proves that platelet material enters the endothelial cells.

REFERENCES

Arnaud, S. B., Greenwalt, T. J., Pawlowski, J. M., and Johnson, S. A. (1963). *Transfusion (Philadelphia)* **3**, 8.
Behnke, O. (1969). *J. Ultrastruct. Res.* **26**, 111.
Benacerraf, B., McCluskey, R. T., and Patras, D. (1959). *Amer. J. Pathol.* **35**, 75.
Cooney, D. P., Smith, B. A., and Fawley, D. E. (1968). *Blood* **31**, 791.

Cronkite, E. P., Bond, V. P., Fliedner, T. M., Paglia, D. A., and Adamik, E. R. (1961). *In* "Blood Platelets" (S. A. Johnson *et al.*, eds.), p. 595. Little, Brown, Boston, Massachusetts.

Gaydos, L. A., Freireich, E. J., and Mantel, N. (1962). *N. Engl. J. Med.* **266**, 905.

Harker, L. A., and Finch, C. A. (1969). *J. Clin. Invest.* **48**, 963.

Humble, J. G. (1949). *Blood* **4**, 69.

Jackson, D. P., Sorenson, D. K., Cronkite, E. P., Bond, V. P., and Fliedner, T. M. (1959). *J. Clin. Invest.* **38**, 1689.

Johnson, S. A., Balboa, R. S., Dessel, B. H., Monto, R. W., Siegesmund, K. A., and Greenwalt, T. J. (1964). *Exp. Mol. Pathol.* **3**, 115.

Johnson, S. A., Van Horn, D. L., Pederson, H. J., and Marr, J. (1966). *Transfusion (Philadelphia)* **6**, 3.

Kramar, J. (1961). *In* "Blood Platelets" (S. A. Johnson *et al.*, eds.), p. 41. Little, Brown, Boston, Massachusetts.

Majno, G. (1965). *In* "Handbook of Physiology" (Am. Physiol. Soc., V. Field, ed.), Sect. 2, Vol. III, p. 2293. Williams & Wilkins, Baltimore, Maryland.

Odland, G. F. (1961). *Advan. Biol. Skin* **2**, 57–70.

Rebuck, J. W. (1963). *Transfusion (Philadelphia)* **3**, 1.

Stewart, B. C., Wojcik, J. D., Van Horn, D. L., and Johnson, S. A. (1970). *Thromb. Diath. Haemorrh.* **22**, Suppl. (in press).

Tranzer, J. P., and Baumgartner, H. R. (1967). *Nature (London)* **216**, 1126.

Van Horn, D. L., and Johnson, S. A. (1966). *Amer. J. Clin. Pathol.* **46**, 204.

Van Horn, D. L., and Johnson, S. A. (1968). *J. Lab. Clin. Med.* **71**, 301.

Wojcik, J. D., Van Horn, D. L., Webber, A. J., and Johnson, S. A. (1969). *Transfusion (Philadelphia)* **9**, 324.

Woods, M. C., Gamble, F. N., Furth, J., and Bigelow, R. R. (1953). *Blood* **8**, 545.

11

ROLE OF PLATELETS IN BLOOD CLOTTING

WALTER H. SEEGERS

I. INTRODUCTION

One of the encouraging aspects of our contemporary literature is the important contributions made on the subject of blood platelets and their function in blood clotting (Tocantins, 1938, 1948; Budtz-Olsen, 1951; Quick, 1951, 1957, 1966a,b; DeRobertis et al., 1953; Tullis, 1953; Deutsch et al., 1955; Bessis, 1956; S. A. Johnson et al., 1959, 1961; Ferguson, 1960; Seegers, 1962, 1967a,b; Davey and Lüscher, 1963; E. R. Hecht, 1965; Johnson and Greenwalt, 1965; Marcus and Zucker, 1965; S. A. Johnson and Seegers, 1966; Barnhart and Riddle, 1967; Hampton, 1967; Kowalski and Niewiarowski, 1967; Mustard, 1967; Hagen et al., 1968; Johnson and Guest, 1969; Marcus, 1969; Michal and Firkin, 1969). There are divergent points of view which I would like to bring out for review and discussion, but this cannot be done in a single chapter. I like to believe that I have surveyed most of the pertinent literature and whether mentioned or not it is taken into account in this study which is an attempt to present a unified perspective. Platelets have a role at the very beginning of blood coagulation. Their lipoproteins and other components participate in the formation of autoprothrombin C, in the formation of thrombin, and in the formation of fibrin. Before taking up specific functions, a theory of blood clotting is presented.

Definition of Some Terms

(1) *Autoprothrombin III*—Subunit of prothrombin complex, and precursor of autoprothrombin C. Residual quantities found in serum of most species. Activity induced by cathepsin C, trypsin, Russell's viper venom, calcium ions plus thromboplastin, calcium ions plus platelet cofactor I plus platelet lipids, fraction from urine, and by autocatalysis. N-terminal amino acids are glycine and serine (bovine). A modified form has been produced and I propose that it be called autoprothrombin III_m. Its activation characteristics differ from those of autoprothrombin III. Synonyms: factor X, thrombokinase, Stuart factor.

(2) *Autoprothrombin C*—Proteolytic enzyme derived from plasma precursor (autoprothrombin III). Catalyzes thrombin formation. Inactivated by plasma antithrombin and soy bean trypsin inhibitor, diisopropylfluorophosphate, phenylmethanesulfonyl fluoride, and reducing agents. Synonyms: factor X_a, active thrombokinase, active Stuart factor.

(3) *Prothrombin complex*—A complex containing the zymogen (prothrombin) of thrombin and the zymogen (autoprothrombin III) of auto-

prothrombin C. Generates thrombin in two-stage analytical procedure. Generates thrombin and autoprothrombin C in 25% sodium citrate solution. Supplies F-II, VII, IX, and X activity. Synthesis by hepatocytes requires vitamin K. In bovine prothrombin complex the N-terminal amino acid is alanine. Synonym: Prothrombin.

(4) *Prothrombin*—Component of the prothrombin complex. Probably contains two moles of thrombin. Generates thrombin in two-stage analytical procedure. Synthesis by hepatocytes requires vitamin K. N-terminal amino acid is alanine (bovine). Synonyms: factor II, thrombin zymogen.

(5) *Prethrombin*—Derivative of prothrombin complex. A zymogen of thrombin. Does *not* generate thrombin with two-stage analytical reagents. In bovine prethrombin N-terminal amino acids are lysine and isoleucine.

(6) *Thrombin*—Proteolytic enzyme which catalyzes fibrin formation. Has special affinity for arginyl-glycyl bonds of fibrinogen. Inactivated by plasma inhibitors, antithrombin, α_2-antitrypsin, and α_2-macroglobulin or by strong reducing agents, diisopropylfluorophosphate, and phenylmethanesulfonyl fluoride. N-terminal amino acids are threonine and isoleucine (bovine).

(7) *Fibrinogen*—Plasma protein produced by hepatocytes. Composed of three polypeptide chains termed α, β, and γ occurring as dimers. Molecular weight of 330,000. The composition of fibrinogen is indicated as follows: for half the molecule (bovine) $\alpha(A)\beta(B)\gamma$; for the whole molecule $[\alpha(A)\beta(B)\gamma]_2$. A and B refer to peptides removed by thrombin.

(8) *Fibrin monomer*—Protein produced from fibrinogen with thrombin (or certain snake venoms). Enzyme removes A and B peptides from respective α and β polypeptide chains. Fibrinogen $[\alpha(A)\beta(B)\gamma]_2$ becomes fibrin monomer $(\alpha\beta\gamma)_2$.

(9) *Fibrin*—Polymer of fibrin monomer produced from fibrinogen by thrombin or snake venoms. Can be symbolized as $(\alpha\beta\gamma)_n$. Greek letters designate three polypeptide chains of fibrin monomer. Cross-linking by plasma transglutaminase converts to the insoluble form $(\alpha\beta\gamma)_n^x$ commonly seen.

(10) *Ac-globulin*—A labile plasma protein, abbreviated to Ac-G. Accelerates thrombin formation by the enzyme autoprothrombin C. In most species the activity is not found in serum. Plasma deficiency associated with bleeding tendency called parahemophilia. Synonyms: factor V, accelerin, labile factor, proaccelerin.

(11) *Plasma transglutaminase*—Plasma protein closely associated with fibrinogen. Forms branched peptides in fibrin. Produces cross-links between γ-glutamyl residues and ε-amino group of lysine residues with release of

ammonia. The zymogen is activated by thrombin. Synonyms: factor XIII, L-L factor, fibrin stabilizing factor, fibrinoligase.

(12) *Platelet cofactor*—Plasma protein. Functions with platelets, and platelet factor 3 in particular, in the formation of autoprothrombin C. In serum combined with an inhibitor. Synonyms: factor VIII, antihemophilic factor (AHF), antihemophilic globulin (AHG).

(13) *Platelet cofactor II*—Procoagulant derived from prothrombin complex during clotting. Functions with platelets, and platelet factor 3 in particular, in the formation of autoprothrombin C. Active form in serum. Synonyms: factor IX?, plasma thromboplastin component (PTC), autoprothrombin II, hemophilia B factor.

II. BLOOD CLOTTING MECHANISMS

A. Phenomena Requiring Chemical Description

Blood that is carefully drawn with a syringe and transferred to a test tube normally clots in about 10 minutes. If extracts of muscle, lung, heart, brain, or other tissues are mixed with this blood it may clot solid in only 15 seconds. Bleeding from an open wound is another situation. A superficial lancet stab wound on the ear lobe oozes blood that can make red blots on contact with filter paper, but there is a time limit. In about 3 minutes no more red spots form because the bleeding stops. The clotting of blood is concerned with bleeding in a very particular way and is only a part of the physiology of hemostasis which also requires the participation of the blood vessels and platelets (Jaques, 1967; Henry and Steiman, 1968). Fig. 1 represents a view of a vessel wall, a platelet, and a red blood cell. We must account for the fluidity of blood in the circulation, its slow clotting following withdrawal, and its rapid clotting when tissue extracts are added. Three basic chemical reactions are involved; namely,

(1) Formation of autoprothrombin C
(2) Formation of thrombin
(3) Formation of fibrin

Prior to outlining a theory of blood clotting, I will briefly consider conditions which retard coagulation. Removal of calcium ions is the most common and effective way to prevent clotting. This can be done by using a chelating agent such as sodium citrate or ethylenediaminetetraacetate. Oxalates form microcrystalline precipitates with calcium, while heparin leaves the calcium

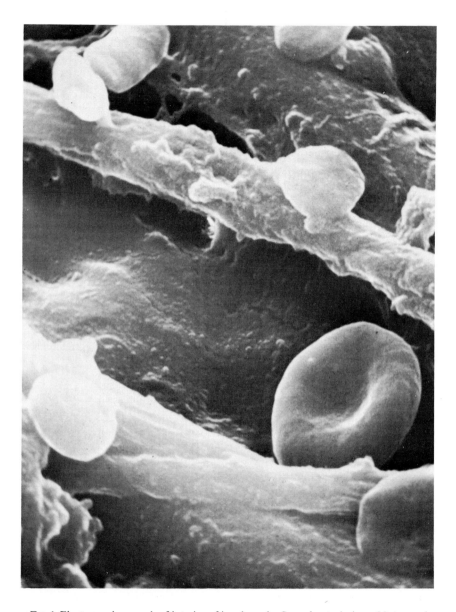

FIG. 1. Electron micrograph of interior of jugular vein. Scanning technique. Note roughness of blood vessel wall, red blood cell, and platelets. Made available through the generosity of Professor Marion I. Barnhart.

alone and blocks protein interactions. In like manner hirudin, obtained from the saliva of the leech, is an anticoagulant. Cooling blood, or centrifuging to remove the formed elements and especially the platelets, leaves the mechanisms of the plasma in a balanced state. Lack of vitamin K in the diet, or its faulty absorption due to bile salt deficiency, is followed by a lowering of plasma prothrombin concentration and reduced clotting power. Reduced liver function due to tissue pathology or inhibition of the metabolic machinery, as with Dicumarol and related compounds, may be associated with restricted supplies of the prothrombin complex in the blood plasma, and slow clotting of the blood. Lytic agents that are capable of destroying fibrinogen can eliminate the very possibility of fibrin formation or remove the fibrin which forms. The surface characteristics of the vessel in which the blood circulates or into which it is received may either promote or retard clotting, depending upon the electric charge, hydrophobic and hydrophilic properties, and wettability. Paraffin-lined or silicone-treated glassware is perhaps the most commonly used surface for maintaining the fluidity of the blood when anticoagulants are not used.

B. Three Basic Reactions in Blood Coagulation

The idea of three basic reactions in blood coagulation is an old one. Following literature surveys it was summarized (Milstone, 1947; Lenggenhager, 1949; Astrup, 1950) as follows:

Prothrombokinase   --------→ Thrombokinase

Prothrombin   --------→ Thrombin

Fibrinogen   --------→ Fibrin

When this perspective was being reviewed Ac-globulin was made a reality in several laboratories and a previously unrecognized bleeding irregularity was repeatedly found and ascribed to blood coagulation. This gave rise to lively enterprise in research for more than a decade, sometimes resulting in confusion, sometimes in misinterpretation and going beyond experimental facts, sometimes in new and inaccurate theories (Davie and Ratnoff, 1964; Macfarlane, 1964; Quick, 1966a,b) and sometimes in advances toward a solution to the riddle of blood clotting. According to T. H. Huxley the greatest tragedy of science was when a beautiful theory was destroyed by an ugly fact. The predictions made at the beginning of this century were upheld by work with purified materials. There are three basic reactions in blood clotting. However, these go so slowly that accessory substances are needed to accelerate them sufficiently for harmonious and useful physiological functioning. First I shall discuss the three basic reactions, and later how they are accelerated.

1. FORMATION OF AUTOPROTHROMBIN C

Autoprothrombin C can arise from its zymogen spontaneously; that is, by autocatalysis. Evidence for this was repeatedly produced in this laboratory in a series of experiments performed over a period of two decades. These experiments were possible because methods were worked out for preparing prothrombin complex. In the basic experiment (Seegers, 1949) purified prothrombin complex was dissolved in 25% sodium citrate solution, and thrombin generated spontaneously (Fig. 2). It was at once evident that all the absolute requirements for thrombin formation were fulfilled. For the first time it was shown that calcium ions and many clotting factors are not necessary. Studies were continued along that line and are in progress even today. An accelerator of thrombin generation was then found in the prothrombin complex itself (McClaughry and Seegers, 1952; Seegers *et al.*, 1955a; Alkjaersig *et al.*, 1955b). Soy bean trypsin inhibitor blocked the development of thrombin activity (Alkjaersig *et al.*, 1955a). The thrombin

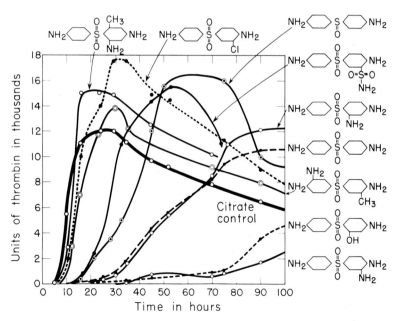

FIG. 2. Activation of purified prothrombin complex in 25% sodium citrate solution (heavy line). Two of the diphenyl sulfones tested inhibited the reaction, because they were competitive inhibitors for autoprothrombin C (Seegers, 1949).

zymogen was shown to be associated with the autoprothrombin C zymogen in the prothrombin complex (Marciniak and Seegers, 1962). We now know that the following occurred in the original experiment:

$$\text{Autoprothrombin III} \xrightarrow{\text{Auto-C}} \text{Autoprothrombin C}$$

$$\text{Prothrombin} \xrightarrow{\text{Auto-C}} \text{Thrombin}$$

The above conclusion was further supported experimentally by the isolation of autoprothrombin III. The purified zymogen transformed to autoprothrombin C in 25% sodium citrate solution (Marciniak and Seegers, 1962; Seegers et al., 1962, 1963a, 1964, 1967). Formation of the enzyme was accelerated by the addition of purified autoprothrombin C (Seegers and Kagami, 1964; Kipfer and Seegers, 1968). Furthermore, 3,4,4'-triamino-diphenyl sulfone, as in the original experiment with prothrombin complex, inhibited the generation of autoprothrombin C on a competitive basis. The autoprothrombin III used in these experiments had the same physical chemical properties as the protein isolated in an independent endeavor (Jackson and Hanahan, 1968). Concentrated ammonium sulfate solutions were even more suitable as a medium for autocatalysis than sodium citrate (Lechner and Deutsch, 1965; Seegers et al., 1966). Among numerous other developments the summary of Milstone's work represents the most extensive effort (Milstone, 1964).

There was another interesting development; namely, a modified form of autoprothrombin III was produced and purified (Seegers et al., 1964; Seegers and Marciniak, 1965). This product, called autoprothrombin III_m, did not convert to autoprothrombin C in suitable concentrated salt solutions, but could be activated by Russell's viper venom. In contrast to the unmodified form of autoprothrombin III, it also failed to correct the prothrombin consumption of hemophilia B plasma (Marciniak and Seegers, 1965; Seegers et al., 1965). This form of the zymogen may thus be of further interest in the study of hemophilia B (Seegers and Marciniak, 1970). In another laboratory, failure to achieve activation in 25% sodium citrate solution was also reported (Papahadjopoulos et al., 1964), but no remarks were made about the possibility of having introduced a modification in the proenzyme.

2. FORMATION OF THROMBIN

Autoprothrombin C alone is sufficient for the formation of thrombin. In connection with this topic it is commonly pointed out that Morawitz postulated a plasma thrombokinase (Morawitz, 1904), capable of generating thrombin. The idea was given much attention (Weidenbauer and Reichel, 1942; Apitz, 1943; Laki, 1943; Astrup, 1944; Milstone, 1947, 1949; Quick, 1957). Milstone considered his experiments as adequate to demonstrate the fact that there is a substance which alone is capable of generating thrombin (Milstone, 1952a,b). His interpretation of the literature and his own data was most fortunate, because he did not use "pure" components in his experiments. Furthermore, the first change in prothrombin produced by autoprothrombin C leaves prothrombin refractory to the two-stage analytical reagents, and practically no thrombin forms (Seegers et al., 1963a; Seegers and Kagami, 1964). Large amounts of purified autoprothrombin C, however, produce changes extending beyond the first reaction and thrombin forms. In 25% sodium citrate solutions the generation of thrombin by autoprothrombin C proceeds far more rapidly than in the absence of the salt (Seegers et al., 1965, 1967).

3. Formation of Fibrin

Thrombin alone is sufficient for the formation of fibrin. In this last of the three basic reactions (Fig. 3) of blood coagulation, thrombin produces fibrin. Since this is perhaps the best known of all the reactions and has been written about repeatedly (Lorand, 1965; Laki, 1968), I summarize without further literature references.

The fibrinogen molecule has an α-polypeptide chain to which there is attached the short A fibrinopeptide chain which is removed by thrombin. The peptide bond broken is between arginine and glycine. For this calcium ions are not essential, but accelerate the rate of fibrin formation. There is also a β-chain with a B peptide attached, and a third γ-chain from which thrombin does not remove a peptide. These three main polypeptide chains

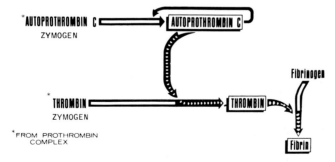

FIG. 3. The three basic reactions in blood coagulation occur in sequence and involve two enzymes. The enzyme precursors are found in the prothrombin complex.

are *almost* duplicated as a dimer. The formula for half a fibrinogen molecule (bovine) can be written: $\alpha(A)\beta(B)\gamma$. For the whole molecule this would be $[\alpha(A)\beta(B)\gamma]_2$. After thrombin removes peptides A and B the fibrin monomer $(\alpha\beta\gamma)_2$ remains, and forms fibrin polymer $[(\alpha\beta\gamma)_2]_n$ by a process of self assembly. In the presence of the fibrin stabilizing factor, which is a plasma transglutaminase, cross-linked fibrin polymers are created. This is indicated as $[(\alpha\beta\gamma)_2]_n^x$. It is interesting that thrombin removes peptide A very rapidly while peptide B is removed slowly, and for the polymer to form it is not even necessary to remove the B peptide. Certain snake venoms produce fibrin without removing peptide B, and this fibrin has been designated as $[(\alpha\beta(B)\gamma)_2]_n$. The removal of peptides by thrombin gives access to the critical sites for plasma transglutaminase action. The fibrin cross-links are formed by a peptide link as a consequence of the liberation of ammonia from the ε-amino group of lysine (donor) and a glutaminyl side chain (acceptor). From the latest reports (Chen and Doolittle, 1969; Lorand *et al.*, 1969) we know that the β-chain of fibrinogen does not participate. The α-chain has both donor and acceptor groups while the γ-chain has only acceptor sites for forming ε-(γ-glutamyl) lysine isopeptide links. γ-Chains link to each other and to α-chains.

C. Autocatalysis and Blood Clotting

Autocatalysis in blood coagulation has been a recurrent theme for decades (Astrup, 1939, 1941, 1944, 1957). It was not possible, however, to conclude whether autocatalysis meant the involvement of autoprothrombin C or thrombin or both. One of the important considerations was reviewed with pertinent conclusions (Astrup, 1950). "...The substance formed autocatalytically in fresh plasma is not thrombin...it is not an *active* substance (thrombin) which is the cause of the autocatalytic reaction, but that an activating substance that can convert prothrombin into thrombin, is present in plasma as a precursor, and may be transformed autocatalytically into the activating substance." It was also said that kinase forms by autocatalysis (Milstone, 1947, 1948a,b, 1949, 1951, 1952a). In the latter paper and others a chain reaction was envisioned.

The activation of purified prothrombin complex in 25% sodium citrate solution (Seegers, 1949; Seegers *et al.*, 1950) was obviously autocatalytic. It was accelerated with purified thrombin, and purified thrombin proved to have procoagulant qualities under various experimental conditions (Fukutake *et al.*, 1958). Autoprothrombin C also accelerated its own formation (Seegers and Kagami, 1964), and the spontaneous generation of auto-

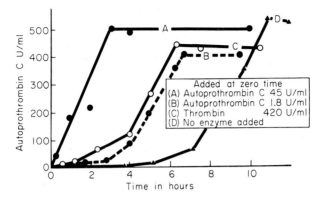

FIG. 4. Generation of autoprothrombin C activity from purified prothrombin complex in 25% sodium citrate solution. Rate was increased by either purified autoprothrombin C or purified thrombin (free of autoprothrombin C) added at zero time.

prothrombin C from highly purified autoprothrombin III in 25% sodium citrate solution was clearly demonstrated (Kipfer and Seegers, 1968). The addition of purified autoprothrombin C at zero time accelerated the reaction. Careful attention was given to the question whether the procoagulant power ascribed to thrombin might not be due to some remaining autoprothrombin C not removed during the purification. This possibility was reduced to the point of negligibility. Thrombin *does* function as a catalyst in the production of thrombin and also in the formation of autoprothrombin C when the purified prothrombin complex is activated (Seegers *et al.*, 1968). Autoprothrombin C also functions in that manner (Figs. 4 and 5).

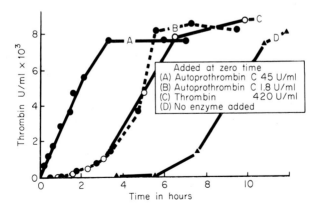

FIG. 5. Spontaneous generation of thrombin activity from purified prothrombin complex in 25% sodium citrate solution. The rate of thrombin formation was accelerated by adding either thrombin or purified autoprothrombin C at zero time.

The term autocatalysis applies to either thrombin or autoprothrombin C, and this is fundamental to blood coagulation theory. Another relevant fact remains to be added.

Autoprothrombin III_m, in purified form, did *not* convert to autoprothrombin C in 25% sodium citrate solution (Seegers *et al.*, 1965, 1969a). However, a mixture of purified prethrombin and autoprothrombin III_m formed thrombin and autoprothrombin C (Seegers *et al.*, 1969a). Thus, neither zymogen alone became active in 25% sodium citrate solution, but the two together generated both enzymes. It was proposed to call this *reciprocal proenzyme activation*.

D. Acceleration of the First Two Basic Reactions

1. ACCELERATION OF THROMBIN FORMATION

When the first two basic reactions were clearly recognized and beautifully demonstrated, *it was realized that the slow rates were inconsistent with physiological requirements*. Accelerators for both reactions had to be found and put in their proper place (Fig. 6). The new question was quite evident. How are the rates governed to meet the requirements of normal health and well being? The reply supplies the answer to the riddle of blood coagulation. In the case of thrombin production, with the enzyme autoprothrombin C, the rate was found to be governed by two types of molecules. One is a protein found in plasma and called accelerator globulin or Ac-globulin, because it is a globulin and functions to accelerate thrombin formation. The other is a phospholipid or phospholipid protein complex, and comes from the blood platelets, and under special conditions also from red blood cells. In the presence of calcium ions, Ac-globulin and lipids, the rate of thrombin production by autoprothrombin C met the requirements of physiological conditions. A detailed report related to kinetics was presented (Baker and Seegers, 1967). Autoprothrombin C serves as the enzyme, Ac-globulin as the "coenzyme", phospholipid (phospholipoproteins) as surface micelle, and calcium ion as complexing agent. Figure 3 can be expanded as in Fig. 6.

2. ACCELERATION OF AUTOPROTHROMBIN C FORMATION

The molecular arrangement for acceleration of autoprothrombin C formation follows the same design as the one for acceleration of thrombin formation, except that two procoagulant systems are involved. It might

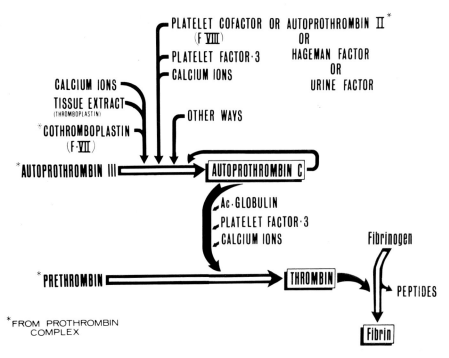

FIG. 6. Accessories accelerate the first two basic reactions of blood coagulation. For effective acceleration two molecules from two anatomic compartments function together. Mixing of "fluids" (plasma + tissues or plasma + platelets or plasma + platelets + tissues) occurs upon injury. Platelets are important for the *formation* and *function* of autoprothrombin C.

be better to say that two prototype reactions illustrate the minimum possibilities. These are the plasma + platelet system and the plasma + tissue system.

a. PLASMA + TISSUE SYSTEM. In response to cuts or bruises, cell membranes are broken and the cell contents and membranes enter into the chemical reactions. The cells contain cathepsin which converts the zymogen to autoprothrombin C, but primarily the thromboplastin (lipoprotein) already known in the past century, produces autoprothrombin C rapidly. That is why blood mixed with tissue extracts can clot in 15 seconds. Practically all of the zymogen is converted to the active form.

A cothromboplastin or factor VII of plasma is very important for this function of thromboplastin. A rapid reaction between F-VII and thromboplastin takes place. This becomes especially evident in experiments where thromboplastin from one species is used to accelerate the clotting of blood from another. This was reviewed recently (Williams, 1969). The main point is that the line of defense at the tissue injury level is very powerful, because the potential autoprothrombin C activity is developed rapidly and completely by tissue extracts (Fig. 6). Later we shall consider that platelets potentiate this.

b. PLASMA + PLATELET SYSTEM. If blood is drawn by a clean venipuncture there is practically no mixing of blood with tissue material and the development of autoprothrombin C activity depends entirely upon the resources in the circulating blood itself. This chemical activity is relatively weak, and only a small amount of the potential autoprothrombin C forms. The rest remains as zymogen in the serum (Macfarlane and Ash, 1964; Reno and Seegers, 1967).

Autoprothrombin C forms slowly in the presence of only platelet factor 3, and more rapidly with platelet factor 3 and platelet cofactor. The lipids and/or lipoproteins come from the platelets and the platelet cofactor is in the plasma. The lipids and the platelet cofactor function together. Here again there are two molecules from two anatomic locations, and injury serves to combine the two. The platelets are target elements for initiating the coagulation of the blood. This has been said many times before, but since I have a notion that it was scarcely heard, it perhaps needs emphasis. As discussed by other authors of this volume, they respond to a variety of stimuli such as surface contact, adenosine diphosphate, collagen, endotoxin, thrombin, and antigen–antibody reactions. Their lipids, primarily in the form of platelet factor 3, then have their function augmented with platelet cofactor and perhaps other proteins (with platelet cofactor activity) in the acceleration of autoprothrombin C formation. Platelets also function with Hageman factor, because the latter protein has platelet cofactor activity (Mammen and Grammens, 1967).

c. DISCUSSION. To recapitulate, the first of our three basic chemical reactions yields autoprothrombin C and proceeds under two sets of conditions. One involves the platelets, while the other relates to cellular materials. One is weak while the other is strong. In responding to cuts, abrasions, or the injury of countless capillaries, the whole procoagulant power of tissue, platelets, and plasma is mobilized. On the other hand, in the injury free condition, the blood flowing through the circulation is not disturbed, unless the platelets and platelet cofactor are involved in a substantial way. Substitution and supplementation for platelet cofactor occurs. The acceleration of autoprothrombin C formation is illustrated by a diagram taken from laboratory notes of Genesio Murano:

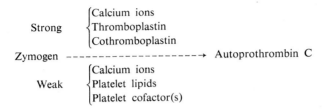

Surface activity has much to do with blood coagulation and this includes the beginning or acceleration of the process (Lister, 1863; Nossel, 1964; Vroman, 1967). A "cascade" or "waterfall" sequence is postulated as comprising stages preceding those described above (Davie and Ratnoff, 1964; Macfarlane, 1964), but there remains the difficulty of discovering and describing the properties of F-XI and F-IX, and until now good experimental evidence still needs to be supplied. The availability of purified Hageman factor serves as a forward step in clarifying this confusing area of research. We already know that platelet factor 3 + Hageman factor can directly accelerate the generation of autoprothrombin C. The cascade hypothesis continues to be examined (Esnouf, 1969; Macfarlane, 1969) and the later stages of it have been rearranged to coincide with the three basic reactions outlined above. The usefulness of what remains of that hypothesis seems to be in the challenge of trying to support it with further investigations of the beginning phases. However, once the platelets are taken into account, the early phases of blood clotting are less mysterious than formerly.

E. Inhibitors and Fibrinolysis

The regulation of blood coagulation is kept under control by the use of inhibitors such as antithrombin, clearing of procoagulants by the reticulo-endothelial system, negative feedbacks, the dissolution of clots by fibrino-lysis, and other mechanisms. Unnoticed, continuous coagulation occurs at all times, and is counterbalanced to maintain homeostasis. However, an extensive discussion of this aspect cannot be undertaken. Instead an attempt was made to create a chart intended as a helpful outline of major considerations together with specific designations for some irregularities that have been encountered (Fig. 7).

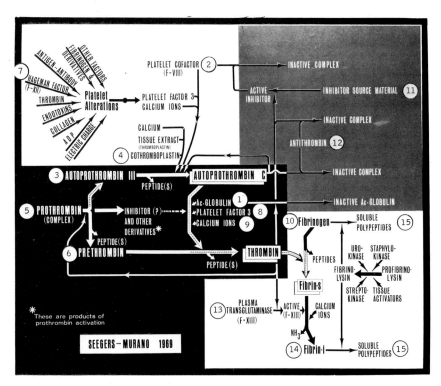

Fig. 7. *Blood clotting mechanisms.* The clotting of blood consists of three main reactions: (1) The formation of autoprothrombin C (F-X_a, thrombokinase, Stuart factor);
(2) the formation of thrombin; and (3) the formation of fibrin. For the formation of
fibrin from fibrinogen only thrombin is necessary. For the formation of thrombin from
prothrombin only autoprothrombin C is necessary, but the formation of autoprothrombin C from autoprothrombin III can occur spontaneously. The *rate* of thrombin formation by autoprothrombin C is *regulated* by plasma Ac-globulin and lipids of platelets
(lipids of thromboplastin are also satisfactory). The *rate* of autoprothrombin C formation
is *regulated* in two ways. Rapid formation occurs with tissue thromboplastin which has
been "activated" by cothromboplastin (F-VII). Slow formation of autoprothrombin C
occurs when the lipids and lipoproteins of platelets function synergistically with platelet
cofactor (F-VIII, AHF). Even by themselves platelets induce the formation of some
autoprothrombin C. Hageman factor also has platelet cofactor activity. Autoprothrombin
II (platelet cofactor II) has the same function as platelet cofactor. The regulatory mechanisms for zymogen activation require calcium ions. Each one of the two molecules
needed to govern the rate of thrombin or autoprothrombin C formation comes from a
separate anatomic compartment (platelets + plasma or tissues + plasma). Consequently,
injury brings them together and accelerates the clotting process. Platelets are especially
labile and respond to a variety of stimuli. Even without injury the clotting mechanisms
are in operation at an imperceptible level. Prothrombin complex and prethrombin are
found in the plasma.

After the removal of peptides from fibrinogen by thrombin, the fibrin polymerizes.

There follows cross-linking reaction(s), due to thrombin activated plasma transglutaminase. This involves a lysine ε-amino group and a γ-glutaminyl group to form a peptide link with liberation of ammonia.

The powerful procoagulants generated during the forward phase of clotting are neutralized by inhibitors, and the product of clotting (fibrin) can be lysed by the fibrinolytic mechanisms and by cellular phagocytosis. Heparin accelerates the neutralization of thrombin by antithrombin, and the neutralization of autoprothrombin C by antithrombin. Thrombin first activates and subsequently inactivates plasma Ac-globulin. Thrombin indirectly inactivates platelet cofactor. Very little thromboplastin and very little transglutaminase are found in serum. The amount of residual autoprothrombin C zymogen in serum is related to rate of clotting.

Irregular blood clotting. The summary refers to the numbers for interpretation; (1) Deficiency (functional or absent) of Ac-globulin (F-V) is called parahemophilia. Poor clotting because any autoprothrombin C (F-X_a, active Stuart factor, thrombokinase) which forms is ineffective without Ac-globulin. (2) Ineffective in classic hemophilia (hemophilia A) due to an inhibitor. Some authors say it is due to absence of the cofactor (F-VIII). Plasma concentration diminished in some patients with von Willebrand's disease. (3) Abnormality in autoprothrombin III activation in hemophilia B. Some postulate a special factor IX. Its function would be to serve as a platelet cofactor. Most likely a prothrombin complex derivative does not readily form in hemophilia B. This is autoprothrombin II (F-IX?) and it functions as a platelet cofactor. Deficiency (functional or absent) of autoprothrombin III in Stuart plasma. Autoprothrombin C activity generates with Russell's viper venom. (4) Perhaps same as factor VII. Decreased or abnormal in factor VII deficiency. Required to interact with thromboplastin before the latter functions in autoprothrombin III activation. Species specific. (5) Contains thrombin and autoprothrombin C zymogens, corrects hemophilia B plasma clotting defect, and factor VII and X deficient plasma. (6) Low concentration in normal plasma. Temporary increase in plasma when coumadin and indanedione drugs are given. (7) Plasma protein, activation surface dependent. Diminished in Hageman trait. Not found in avian plasma. Contributes to platelet aggregation. Serves as a platelet cofactor and as a weak activator of autoprothrombin III. (8) Low concentration in thrombocytopenia. Not released or absent in certain forms of thrombocytopathy. It alone can slowly activate autoprothrombin III. Makes prothrombin two-stage refractory. (9) Plasma levels not diminished to level where clotting is impaired. Removed by chelating agents (citrate, EDTA) or precipitating agents (oxalates). Serves to form complexes with lipids. (10) Afibrinogenemia and hypofibrinogenemia or dysfibrinogenemia (abnormal molecule). (11) Possibly diminished in F-XI or PTA deficiency. (12) Heparin increases rate of autoprothrombin C and thrombin inactivation by antithrombin (heparin cofactor). Heparin retards or blocks autoprothrombin C formation and thrombin formation. Low concentration of antithrombin associated with clotting tendency—thrombophilia. (13) Low activity in plasma associated with bleeding tendency and possibly poor wound healing. (14) Urea insoluble fibrin. Cross-linked fibrin polymer due to formation of peptide bond at lysine ε-amino group and γ-glutaminyl group with liberation of ammonia. (15) Competitive inhibitors of thrombin activity. Interfere with normal fibrin polymerization. (1, 2, 3, 5, 7, 10, 12, and 13) Diminished appreciably, and in some instances reduced to zero activity, in serum and in some patients with disseminated intravascular clotting (consumption coagulopathy). Disseminated intravascular clotting creates a serum mimetic condition. It may be initiated via platelets and/or tissue extract thromboplastin. (3, 4, 5, and 6) Synthesized by liver parenchymal cells. Synthesis dependent upon vitamin K. Vitamin K function inhibited by coumadin and indanedione drugs.

III. PLATELET-POOR PLASMA

Many investigators found it interesting to collect avian blood in paraffin-lined containers to preserve its fluidity. With mammalian blood there was no success, but renewed efforts were made when silicone surfaces were introduced (Jaques *et al.*, 1946). Human blood was collected and when the plasma was recalcified there was no clotting whenever the centrifugation for removal of the formed elements was hard enough. The replacement of platelets was followed by clotting of the recalcified plasma (Brinkhous, 1947; Langdell *et al.*, 1950). The work was done in conjunction with hemophilic plasma and it was postulated that there is a plasma factor required for platelet utilization. This plasma component would correspond to platelet cofactor (AHF, F-VIII, AHG) of contemporary literature. Crude preparations were being made (van Creveld and Mastenbroek, 1946), and it was said that both platelets and a globulin are necessary for a procoagulant effect (Milstone, 1948b; J. F. Johnson *et al.*, 1952). I reviewed this at that time (Seegers, 1951).

Another special effort to obtain incoaguable plasma in siliconed containers was made in this laboratory (Patton *et al.*, 1948). Dog blood was investigated and no anticoagulant was introduced. It was found that plasma would stay fluid for varying periods—in some runs longer than 72 hours at room temperature. Usually, however, some fibrin formed. Much depended upon the length of time the centrifugation was carried out. There were no measurable significant changes in prothrombin concentration (Table I). Evidence for thrombin formation was, however, obtained indirectly from Ac-globulin studies. This was of interest because this protein is changed from plasma type Ac-globulin to serum type Ac-globulin by minute amounts of thrombin, and all the activity disappears with large amounts of thrombin. For example, a quantity of thrombin insufficient to produce a clot in 1 hour can markedly effect plasma Ac-globulin activity. In the platelet-poor plasma which clotted slowly serum Ac-globulin was found, but there was no reduction in Ac-globulin concentration. Thus, although a trace of thrombin activity developed or was there at the outset, the clotting mechanisms practically remained intact in platelet-poor plasma. The experimentalist strains himself with the wish to maintain complete fluidity of the plasma and occasionally succeeds in obtaining it.

On the other hand, nothing spectacular occurred when the principle procoagulant of platelets, platelet factor 3, was added to recalcified bovine plasma. Nor was the result very impressive with the addition of a concentrate of platelet cofactor. The recalcified clotting time of the bovine plasma (Fig.

TABLE I

PROTHROMBIN AND FIBRINOGEN CONCENTRATION IN DOG PLASMA KEPT IN SILICONE TUBES AT ROOM TEMPERATURE[a]

Hours after centrifugation	Percent prothrombin								F[c]
	5[b]	10[b]	15[b]	30[b]	60[b]	120[b]	240[b]	300[b]	150[b]
0	90	78	100	99	96	100	102	105	85
1	77	57	95	104	—	—	103	115	81
1½	—	—	—	—	—	94	—	—	—
2	80	57	101	104	—	—	—	99	—
2½	—	—	—	—	—	—	100	—	—
3	72	51	109	103	—	—	110	119	—
3½	—	—	—	—	—	92	—	—	72
5	—	—	—	—	101	—	—	—	—
22	—	—	—	—	68	—	—	—	70

[a] Patton et al., 1948.
[b] Minutes in centrifuge. Prothrombin determined on oxalated samples served as control, and this control was considered to have a prothrombin concentration of 100%.
[c] F = percent fibrinogen.

8) was brought down to 50 seconds with a concentrate of platelet factor 3 (Seegers et al., 1959). With a platelet cofactor preparation the clotting time was reduced to 30 seconds. The latter, when added to the platelet factor 3 preparation, was no more effective than either one alone except with extensively diluted mixtures of the procoagulants. I emphasize that these experiments were done in nonsiliconed glass test tubes since many authors have presented evidence that glass surfaces activate material important for platelet utilization. Presumably this would be Hageman factor, functioning in the role of a platelet cofactor.

The injection of platelet extracts intravenously into rabbits did not produce demonstrable intravascular clotting (Epstein and Quick, 1953) even though the amounts exceeded that of the total circulating platelets. Hageman protein most likely remained inactive, and the reticuloendothelial system rapidly cleared the plasma of platelet products. Blocking this system left the animal vulnerable to clotting and disseminated intravascular clotting

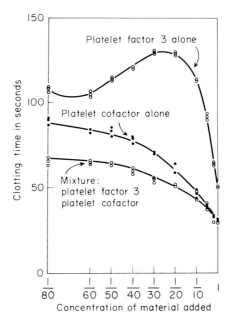

Fig. 8. The clotting time of mixed oxalated plasma from 6 different cows was determined by mixing 0.1 ml of plasma with 0.1 ml of procoagulant and 0.1 ml of 0.02 M CaCl$_2$ in imidazole buffered saline (pH 7.2) at 37°C. Without procoagulant added, the clotting time was 150 seconds. The procoagulants were: platelet factor 3 (top curve); platelet cofactor (middle curve); equal volumes of above two procoagulants mixed (lower curve). The numerals on abscissa designate the relative concentration of platelet factor 3 or platelet cofactor. The original concentration was 500 U/ml of platelet factor 3 and 600 U/ml of platelet cofactor. Example: at 1/40 the concentration was 12.5 U/ml platelet factor 3, 15 U/ml platelet cofactor, and the mixture contained, respectively, 6.25 + 7.5 units (Seegers *et al.*, 1959).

(Rodriguez-Erdmann, 1965, 1969). In another study frozen-thawed homologous platelet products were infused into rabbits (Evensen and Jeremic, 1969), with the conclusion that platelets contain weak procoagulant activity which is effectively cleared by the reticuloendothelial system. Evidently platelet products in portions of the circulation where blood flow is retarded or stopped are hazardous, because there is no clearing or other inactivating mechanism and clotting follows. The plasma lipids are poor procoagulants. Even the intravenous injection of appreciable quantities of purified autoprothrombin C was tolerated, but not when the animal had also been given phospholipids or platelet materials (Marciniak *et al.*, 1962a). In contrast to the ineffective plasma lipids those from the platelets functioned with autoprothrombin C.

IV. ROLE OF PLATELETS IN ACCELERATING THE FORMATION OF AUTOPROTHROMBIN C

It was found (Seegers, 1968; Seegers *et al.*, 1968) that the conversion of purified autoprothrombin III to autoprothrombin C takes place in the presence of calcium ions, phospholipid, and platelet cofactor (Fig. 9). A discussion of trypsin does not belong in this study (Marciniak *et al.*, 1962b). In the presence of the platelet cofactor preparation alone some autoprothrombin C formed, but the rate of formation and the yield was increased tremendously when phospholipid lipid activator, "cephalin," was also added. In place of the latter platelet homogenates or platelet factor 3 preparations were also effective.

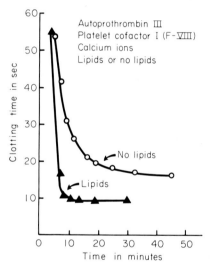

Fig. 9. Purified autoprothrombin III in the unmodified form was converted to auto-prothrombin C with purified platelet cofactor and calcium ions or with purified platelet cofactor and calcium ions and lipids (platelet lipids). The purified autoprothrombin III was used at a concentration which would make it convenient to follow the generation of autoprothrombin C. The reaction mixture was used in place of thromboplastin in the one-stage prothrombin time method. More autoprothrombin C (short clotting time) generated in presence of lipids than in their absence (Seegers *et al.*, 1968).

The platelet cofactor preparation used in the experiments was not a single component, but discounting the possibility of a second effective substance I can go on to say that one function of platelets serves to accelerate the formation of autoprothrombin C and platelet cofactor supports this. Keeping in mind that autoprothrombin C forms autocatalytically in 25%

sodium citrate I can suppose that platelets and platelet cofactor supply conditions for accelerating the spontaneous formation of autoprothrombin C. This conclusion presents a distinct perspective and by contrast there is no clarification of the role of platelets in the formation of autoprothrombin C in a recent consideration of the biochemical aspects of blood coagulation (Esnouf, 1969). It is interesting in this connection that the molecular size of autoprothrombin III was reduced when the zymogen was activated (Papahadjopoulos *et al.*, 1964). This preliminary suggestion was further explored in this laboratory. It was found that the amino acid composition of purified autoprothrombin III is similar to that of autoprothrombin C (Seegers *et al.*, 1969b). It can thus be concluded that activation involves a reduction in molecular size and that this is promoted by platelets and platelet cofactor.

Recently I had an opportunity to perform some experiments with purified autoprothrombin III and purified Hageman factor. The latter, with calcium ions, slowly produced a little autoprothrombin C. Purified platelet factor 3, with calcium ions, produced even more significant amounts of the enzyme. With Hageman factor and platelet factor 3 together about 20% of the autoprothrombin III became active at room temperature in 24 hours. In the control there was no spontaneous formation of autoprothrombin C. It is thus clear that platelet factor 3 and active Hageman factor each alone contribute to autoprothrombin C formation, and if the two are together this is appreciable, but still limited. These facts about platelets and Hageman factor were not taken notice of before.

V. ROLE OF PLATELETS IN ACCELERATING THE FORMATION OF THROMBIN

The formation of thrombin by autoprothrombin C is accelerated by Ac-globulin, calcium ions and platelets in the form of platelet homogenates or as isolated phospholipids or lipoprotein complexes. These accessories were already referred to before autoprothrombin C was isolated (Milstone, 1952c, 1955). On a w/w basis trypsin was about as effective as purified autoprothrombin C (Seegers and Marciniak, 1965). When the accessories were added, acceleration of autoprothrombin C activity was so extensive that the effectiveness of trypsin was comparatively feeble (Seegers *et al.*, 1963b; Papahadjopoulos *et al.*, 1964; Barton *et al.*, 1967; Baker and Seegers, 1967). The explosive effect of lipids under suitable conditions thus contrasts dramatically with the poor showing of lipids in earlier work (Chargaff *et al.*, 1936; Seegers *et al.*, 1938) or with their rather unimpressive effect in plasma or in blood.

In a systematic quantitative study (Baker and Seegers, 1967) of the complicated combinations of autoprothrombin C + Ac-globulin + phospholipid + calcium ions, it was found that a low concentration of one factor may be compensated for by a high concentration of another. Reducing either autoprothrombin C, Ac-globulin, phospholipid, or calcium ions toward zero concentration decreased the rate and yield of thrombin generation. "In association with rapid thrombin generation Ac-globulin and

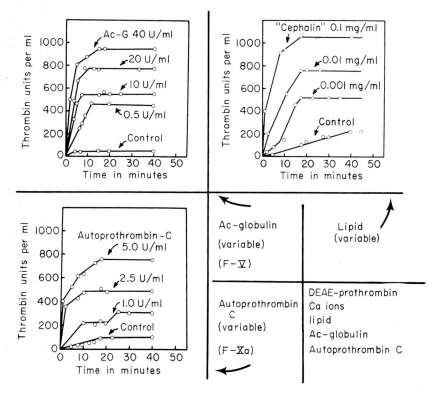

FIG. 10. Composite for data on the activation of DEAE-prothrombin at a substrate concentration of 1000 U/ml as measured by two-stage analysis. Activation with purified Ac-globulin (Aoki *et al.*, 1963), "cephalin" (from platelets, platelet factor 3 or brain), calcium ions, and purified autoprothrombin C (Seegers *et al.*, 1963a). Note that each accessory was in optimum concentration (top lines), when the yield of thrombin was reduced. Compare also the use of prethrombin as substrate (Baker and Seegers, 1967) and the different requirements for different zymogen substrates (Table II). Certain bile salts can be substituted for "cephalin." Test does not distinguish between platelet factor 3 (lipoprotein) or the lipid portion of platelet factor 3 (Barthels and Seegers, 1969).

autoprothrombin C were represented in approximately a 1:1 molar ratio. In that combination of Ac-globulin and autoprothrombin C the Michaelis constant for autoprothrombin C with prethrombin as a substrate was $3.14 \times 10^{-6} M$." As a first approximation it was concluded that the enzyme functions best when one mole is associated with one mole of Ac-globulin, with lipids in vastly higher concentration. Stable complexes between autoprothrombin C and phospholipids formed only when calcium ions were present (Papahadjopoulos et al., 1964). The work of Baker and Seegers (1967) was developed further with the use of DEAE-prothrombin in place of prethrombin (Barthels and Seegers, 1969). Thrombin formation from DEAE-prothrombin was so rapid that it was not possible to get satisfactory data for calculating the Michaelis constant. The relationships are shown (Fig. 10).

Furthermore, Barthels and Seegers (1969) found that bile salts were effective substitutes for lipids in a concentration where micelles form (Fig. 11). The approximate effectiveness from highest to lowest was: conjugated sodium salt of taurocholic acid, sodium cholate, sodium deoxycholate. Sodium dehydrocholate was ineffective. Autoprothrombin C is the enzyme for thrombin formation. For accelerating its activity, best results were obtained with the simultaneous presence of optimal concentrations of calcium ions, Ac-globulin, and lipids or bile salts. Reducing any one of the three to zero concentration decreased the rate and yield of thrombin generation.

The form in which the zymogen was used was found to be important. Prothrombin complex, DEAE-prothrombin, and prethrombin each had its peculiar requirements for yielding thrombin (Table II). Prothrombin complex and DEAE-prothrombin activated far more rapidly and required 10 times less autoprothrombin C than prethrombin. The yield of thrombin from these substrates was also higher than from prethrombin. DEAE-prothrombin required the least amount of lipid. For the bile salts the required concentrations were nearly always the same from one substrate to another. To a certain extent Benadryl could also be substituted for lipids.

In association with rapid thrombin generation from DEAE-prothrombin the Ac-globulin and autoprothrombin C were represented in approximately a 6:1 molar ratio. This was intended as a preliminary estimate. The results with bile salts uphold previous ideas about the surfaces furnished by micelles, a negative charge at the surface in the form of phosphate, and arrangement of the charge (Wallach et al., 1959; Silver et al., 1963; Kazal, 1964–1965; Daemen et al., 1965; Gobbi et al., 1967). Ac-globulin is a cofactor, and we

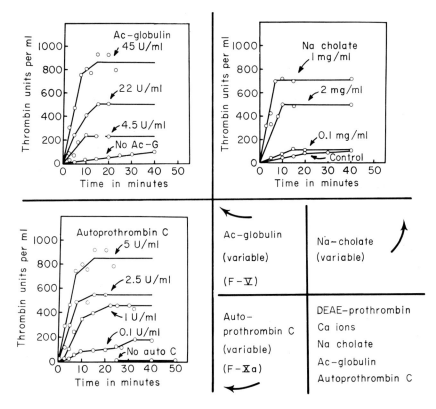

FIG. 11. Composite results with the activation of DEAE-prothrombin at a substrate concentration of 1000 U/ml as measured by two-stage analysis. Reagents used were purified Ac-globulin (Aoki *et al.*, 1963), sodium cholate, calcium ions, and purified autoprothrombin C (Seegers *et al.*, 1963a). Each variable could be reduced to limit the thrombin yield. Na taurocholate serves as a substitute for the function of platelet lipids. Compare also the use of prethrombin as a substrate (Baker and Seegers, 1967) and the different quantities of accessories needed for different thrombin zymogens (Table II). Data of Barthels and Seegers (1969).

may suppose that it helps bind the enzyme to the substrate, and that the surface on which the reacting molecules orient themselves is supplied by phospholipids.

It is by no means certain whether or not all of the potential thrombin in prothrombin is converted to thrombin. Under special conditions, with trypsin, for example, twice the ordinary amount of thrombin activity is obtained. There is inconclusive evidence (Seegers *et al.*, 1969b) that thrombin occurs twice in the prothrombin molecule. By assuming that some activa-

TABLE II

QUANTITY OF PROCOAGULANT NEEDED FOR VARIOUS THROMBIN ZYMOGENS[a]

Substrate	Ac-G[b]	Auto-C[c]	Lipids[d]	Bile salt[e]
Prothrombin complex	45	5	1.0	1.0
DEAE–prothrombin	45	5	0.1	1.0[f]
Prethrombin	45	50	1.0	1.0

[a] Barthels and Seegers, 1969.
[b] Ac-G = Ac-globulin (F-V) in units/ml.
[c] Auto-C = autoprothrombin C (F-X_a) in units/ml.
[d] Lipids = phospholipids.
[e] Bile salt = Na cholate or taurocholate in mg/ml.
[f] At this point 0.1 mg dihydroxycholic acid was found to be optimum.

tions bring out the full activity from each molecule, while other activations do not, one can account for the variable specific activity of purified prothrombin.

VI. TWO-STAGE REAGENT REFRACTORY STATE

In pioneer work the two-stage reagents for the quantitative analysis of prothrombin were introduced (Warner et al., 1936) and later modified to include Ac-globulin (Ware and Seegers, 1949). This procedure has found wide acceptance. Prothrombin readily becomes refractory to these reagents. In other words, the prothrombin becomes modified so that it does not readily transform to thrombin. The refractory state was first produced with thrombin (Mertz et al., 1939). Since that time many other conditions have been found for producing the effect and it occurs spontaneously (Cho and Seegers, 1958). The spontaneous development of the refractory state did not involve the appearance of new N-terminal amino acids (Seegers et al., 1970). By contrast, with calcium ions and platelets or platelet factor 3 (Fig. 12) the refractory state developed rapidly (Seegers, 1951–1952) and new N-terminal amino acids were found to appear (Seegers et al., 1970). Platelets by themselves thus induce a profound change in prothrombin. In some unknown way proteolysis occurs in the presence of platelets whether one works with prothrombin complex or with DEAE-prothrombin. Also

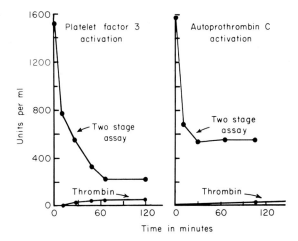

FIG. 12. Purified prothrombin complex was made refractory to two-stage analytical reagents (left), with optimum concentration of purified platelet factor 3 at pH 7.2, 28°C, and 0.008 M calcium chloride. Samples for N-terminal analysis for the activated prothrombin were taken at 120 minutes. In the other experiment the same purified prothrombin complex (1600 U/ml) was activated with purified autoprothrombin C (23 U/ml) at pH 7.2 and 28°C samples for N-terminal analysis at 105 minutes. Note that more thrombin formed with platelet factor 3 than with the autoprothrombin C. In both activations there was proteolysis. In both cases N-terminal alanine and glycine were found in equal proportions. Serine was also found. Glutamic and aspartic acids were present in small quantities. Alanine belongs to the original N-terminal of prothrombin (Seegers et al., 1970).

a little thrombin forms in either case. Recently I found that purified Hageman factor produces the refractory state with very little formation of thrombin, and this may be another way in which Hageman factor functions.

With DEAE-prothrombin, combinations of sodium cholate and phosphatidyl serine were also effective in producing the refractory state but either one alone was not. We thus see a great difference between platelet factor 3 (lipoprotein complex) and the phospholipid by itself (Alkjaersig et al., 1955b; Penner et al., 1956). With my colleagues, I have written on the subject of the two-stage refractory state many times during the past 30 years, and do not recall seeing new experiments on the subject from another laboratory. This is, however, an important aspect of blood coagulation. It may be that a certain unspecified portion of prothrombin invariably becomes two-stage refractory while some becomes thrombin, and still another portion is converted to an inhibitor. Furthermore, the composition of thrombin itself needs further clarification, because 3.7 S thrombin is different from 3.2 S thrombin.

VII. THE PLATELET COFACTOR ASSAY

A. Introduction

From an inspection of Fig. 10 it is self-evident that conditions are fulfilled for the assay of Ac-globulin, autoprothrombin C, platelet factor 3, prothrombin, and even calcium ions. When all accessories are there under optimum conditions, the reduction of any one component reduces the thrombin yield. Consequently, the yield of thrombin becomes a quantitative measure of any one component which is alone varied (Johnson *et al.*, 1952b). The availability of purified prothrombin complex at the mid century period made assays possible which were not restricted to deficiency plasmas. It was at this time that irregular clotting was being studied with intense interest and often without simultaneous testing with purified components. As a consequence, conflicting conclusions were recorded and defended as long as possible.

A typical example of divergent views occurred in the cases of hemophilia A and hemophilia B. The latter disease was discovered (Aggeler *et al.*, 1952; Biggs *et al.*, 1952) in the same year that platelet cofactor II was found (Johnson *et al.*, 1952a). The clinician's approach was to say the disease is due to factor IX deficiency while the other avenue of development stressed the evidence for an abnormal prothrombin molecule. Autoprothrombin II activity was found to develop normally during clotting, and was derived from purified prothrombin complex. In the case of hemophilia A, work with the abnormal plasma (except work of Tocantins) brought forth the conclusion that hemophilia A lacks platelet cofactor, while work with prothrombin complex as a basis for assay brought evidence that platelet cofactor is present in the plasma and that an inhibitor accounts for the poor clotting of hemophilia A blood. Evidence on these points has been summarized (Mammen, 1963; E. Hecht, 1966a,b). The deficiency hypothesis is evidently not accurate without modification.

B. The Platelet Cofactor Assay Mechanics

The platelet cofactor assay depends on the use of purified prothrombin complex as a substrate. Ac-globulin is added in standardized amounts. Platelet homogenate or purified platelet factor 3 fulfill the platelet requirement. The test material with platelet cofactor activity is placed in the mixture and completes conditions for accelerating the generation of thrombin. The following reactions take place:

$$
\begin{array}{c}
\text{Calcium ions} \\
\text{Platelet cofactor} \\
\text{Platelet factor 3}
\end{array}
$$

Autoprothrombin III $------------\rightarrow$ Autoprothrombin C

$$
\begin{array}{c}
\text{Calcium ions} \\
\text{Ac-globulin} \\
\text{Platelet factor 3} \\
\text{Autoprothrombin C}
\end{array}
$$

Prothrombin $------------\rightarrow$ Thrombin

The thrombin concentration is determined repeatedly over a period of 2 hours. The higher the potency of the platelet cofactor the greater is the yield of thrombin until the predetermined quantity of thrombin zymogen is consumed (converted to thrombin). The arrangement of reagents is as follows:

Prothrombin complex (3000 U/ml with Ac-G)	1.0 ml
Platelets or platelet factor 3 (about 80 U/ml)	0.5 ml
Calcium ions (0.16 M) in imidazole buffer	0.5 ml
Cofactor supplied by: plasma, diluted plasma or serum, or other preparations	1.0 ml

The above system was varied as a matter of convenience from year to year, but not with respect to the principle that one measures a cofactor of platelets—material which gives response with platelets. One variation was either to use barium carbonate adsorbed bovine serum as a source of Ac-globulin or to use purified Ac-globulin. In some work a small amount of purified thrombin was added at zero time. In contrast to the thromboplastin generation test (Bell and Alton, 1954), it is not satisfactory to replace platelets or platelet factor 3 with lipid activator. In the first stage the analysis depends upon the formation of autoprothrombin C followed by the formation of thrombin. In the second stage the thrombin concentration is actually measured. This is done repeatedly and reflects the amount of autoprothrombin C which forms.

Under the right conditions some substances with platelet cofactor activity alone convert purified autoprothrombin III to autoprothrombin C. For example, the procoagulant fraction from urine functions as a platelet cofactor (Fig. 13) and the activity can very nicely be measured in the platelet cofactor assay (Caldwell et al., 1963). This fraction also functions

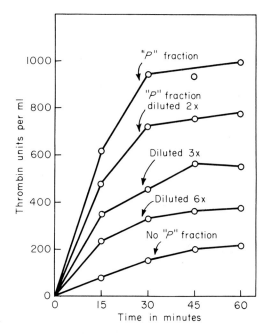

FIG. 13. When purified prothrombin complex was activated to thrombin, the amount of thrombin formed depended on the concentration of P fraction. The activation mixture contained: CaCl₂ 0.32 M one part; platelets two parts; diluted serum Ac-globulin three parts; P fraction (6 mg/ml) two parts; and prothrombin 3000 U/ml four parts. Complete activation of prothrombin to thrombin was obtained when the activation mixture contained 1 mg/ml of P fraction. This amount of P fraction was then diluted 2, 3, and 6 times. The amount of thrombin formed was decreased in direct relationship to the decreased amount of P fraction present (Caldwell *et al.*, 1963).

by converting autoprothrombin III to autoprothrombin C (Fig. 14) as was demonstrated with the use of purified autoprothrombin III (Seegers *et al.*, 1969a), It is thus likely that the platelet cofactor assay depends upon suitable conditions for the generation of autoprothrombin C and upon suitable conditions, *in the same reaction mixture*, for this enzyme to produce thrombin in quantities proportional to the amount of autoprothrombin C developed. In the platelet cofactor assay it is thus important for the prothrombin complex (prothrombin and autoprothrombin III) to be a standardized product as well as the Ac-globulin. It is interesting that the incorporation of purified autoprothrombin III in the first stage promotes the formation of thrombin, but relatively large amounts are needed.

In the assay one invariably finds that platelets or platelet factor 3 alone form about 200 units of thrombin rapidly and then no more forms. This

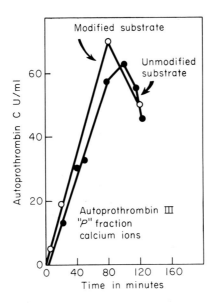

Fig. 14. Purified autoprothrombin III conversion to autoprothrombin C with the procoagulant fraction from urine. Both forms of autoprothrombin III, the unmodified and modified, were used (250–270 U/ml). Procoagulant fraction was at 130 U/ml (von Kaulla's units) and calcium chloride at 0.025 M concentration. Lipids, as used under the form of platelet factor 3, were not essential for the reaction. The procoagulant did not discriminate between the modified and unmodified substrate of autoprothrombin III (Seegers *et al.*, 1969a).

implies that platelet factor 3 promotes limited autoprothrombin C generation. To test this I made some purified autoprothrombin III and added some purified platelet factor 3 and found that platelet material did indeed promote the activation of autoprothrombin III. Although it was a weak procoagulant, this must be recognized as a function of platelets. Furthermore, Hageman factor functions as a platelet cofactor (Mammen and Grammens, 1967). Consequently, any stimulus which simultaneously activates Hageman factor and the platelets (release reaction or even VM) might be expected to yield appreciable amounts of autoprothrombin C and hence accelerate blood coagulation. This is not in the sense of the "cascade" or "waterfall" concept with a series of prior reactions, *but specifically I mean a direct generation of autoprothrombin C from its precursor.* An example would be the fatty acids (Hoak *et al.*, 1967). They initiate blood coagulation, by activating Hageman factor and aggregating platelets. In other words, it seems to me this implies that Hageman factor acts as a cofactor with platelet factor 3 and there is *direct* activation of autoprothrombin III.

C. Platelet Cofactor Assay in Hemophilia A and B

1. Two Platelet Cofactors

The assay was applied in many ways (Table III). At the beginning it was found (Fig. 13) that two cofactors exist (Johnson *et al.*, 1952a). Platelet cofactor I (now called platelet cofactor) was not found in serum while another one *was* (platelet cofactor II, later called autoprothrombin II). The antihemophilic factor was at that time considered to be missing in hemophilia A plasma and found to be absent from serum (Graham *et al.*, 1951). Likewise, platelet cofactor activity measured under entirely different test conditions was not found in hemophilia A plasma or serum. So it seemed evident that the platelet cofactor activity measured with purified

TABLE III

Activation of Prothrombin Substrate in Platelet Cofactor Assay

Rapid and complete with	Retarded and incomplete with
1. Thromboplastin	1. Normal serum
2. Normal plasma	2. Hemophilic plasma
3. Hemophilic plasma ether treated	3. Hemophilic serum
4. Hemophilic serum ether treated	4. PTA plasma
5. Normal serum ether extracted	5. PTA serum
6. PTC plasma ether extracted[a]	6. PTA plasma ether extracted
7. PTC serum ether extracted[a]	7. PTA serum ether extracted
8. Procoagulant from urine	8. PTC plasma ether extracted
9. Fibrinogen split products[b]	9. PTC serum ether extracted
10. Purified Hageman factor	10. Serum barium carbonate adsorbed
11. Antihistamine compounds[c]	11. Dicumarol serum
12. Autoprothrombin II preparations	12. Inhibition produced with dextran
	13. Inhibition produced with top layer of high speed centrifuged plasma[d]
	14. Inhibition produced with inhibitor from hemophilia A plasma
	15. Platelet factor 3 alone

[a] Variable from one patient to another.

[b] Used in high concentration.

[c] Not especially effective, but depends upon concentration.

[d] Top layer contained very little platelet cofactor activity; bottom layer had very much (Johnson *et al.*, 1954).

reagents and F-VIII, measured with "deficient plasma," could be considered identical. The other cofactor was discovered in serum (Fig. 15, 16, and 17) with the use of the platelet cofactor assay. It was then shown to be related to the irregularity in hemophilia B (Johnson and Seegers, 1954a,b).

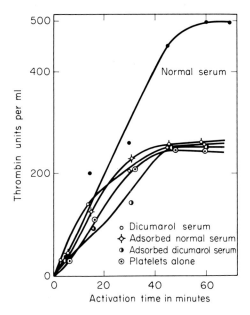

FIG. 15. Normal serum generated limited amount of thrombin in platelet cofactor assay. The thrombin generation which occurred was due to autoprothrombin II (platelet cofactor II). This can be adsorbed on barium carbonate. With such adsorbed serum no more thrombin was generated than with platelet factor 3 alone. Autoprothrombin II is not found in Dicumarol serum. None of the serums contain platelet cofactor I (Johnson and Seegers, 1956).

In further work from this laboratory a low concentration of both platelet cofactor I and platelet cofactor II was found in the plasma from the original plasma thromboplastin antecedent (PTA) case which was reported (Johnson et al., 1955). Why would the platelet cofactor assay give such a result when both platelet cofactor and platelet cofactor II are found in this plasma by other tests? It may be that some hypothetical substance such as the PTA factor (F-XI) is needed for the plasma to develop cofactor activity in the test. Cofactor I becomes inactivated when blood clots, while by contrast platelet cofactor II activity develops when blood clots and it is derived from the prothrombin complex. In siliconed glassware the hemophilia B correcting properties did not develop from the purified prothrombin

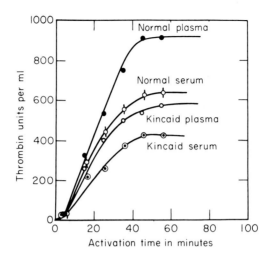

Fig. 16. Analysis for platelet cofactor activity (platelet cofactors I and II in plasma and platelet cofactor II in serum) in blood of patient Kincaid. Note plasma–serum difference in amount of thrombin generated resembles that found in normal blood. Like normal blood, Kincaid blood had platelet cofactor I in plasma but not in serum. The platelet cofactor II activity in Kincaid serum was less than in normal serum. With platelets alone, thrombin yield was about 225 U/ml (analysis by Shirley A. Johnson). Kincaid was one of original hemophilia B cases discovered.

complex (Schröer *et al.*, 1965). Platelet cofactor II (F-IX, autoprothrombin II) did not form readily from the prothrombin complex obtained as a concentrate from hemophilia B plasma (Seegers *et al.*, 1965). We thus see that platelet cofactor II has special requirements for its formation, but much more data is needed regarding its chemical nature, mechanisms of its function, and what the alteration is in hemophilia B. Recently it was demonstrated that purified Hageman factor can increase the yield of autoprothrombin II (platelet cofactor II) in serum (Grammens, 1969).

2. Platelet Cofactor II

Platelet cofactor II (autoprothrombin II) activity was obtained from purified prothrombin complex (Seegers and Johnson, 1956; Mammen *et al.*, 1960a), by digesting the prothrombin complex with thrombin (Mammen *et al.*, 1960b). This preparation substituted nicely for serum in the thromboplastin generation test (Ulutin *et al.*, 1961a,b) and some physical chemical properties were described (Harmison and Seegers, 1962). The molecular weight was found to be in the 50,000 range with $s_{20,w} = 4.3$. When Dicumarol

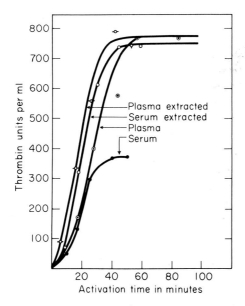

FIG. 17. Analysis for platelet cofactor activity in blood of Stephen Christmas. With plasma and plasma first extracted with ether practically all the substrate converted to thrombin. With serum much less thrombin generated, and plasma-serum difference was unusually high. Platelet cofactor I concentration was high. This activity was easily recovered by ether extraction of serum. With platelets alone about 225 U/ml thrombin generated; consequently, higher amount with serum indicates significant amounts of autoprothrombin II in serum (analysis by Shirley A. Johnson). Christmas disease named after person who donated the blood for our experiment, later also called hemophilia B.

was given the capacity of blood to develop autoprothrombin II activity diminished to a very low level (Fig. 16) (Johnson and Seegers, 1956; Johnson *et al.*, 1957).

Antibodies to purified platelet cofactor II were readily produced (Barnhart, 1967), and were studied by immunoelectrophoresis with the conclusion that the autoprothrombin II preparation had one more antigenic determinant group than the prothrombin complex from which it was derived. The results were as follows:

Antibody + prothrombin complex = one fast mobility arc

Antibody + autoprothrombin II   = one slow mobility arc

Antibody + plasma   = one slow mobility arc
                                  and one fast mobility arc

The autoprothrombin II antibody probably reacted with two substances in plasma. One could have been the prothrombin complex while the other might have been a prothrombin complex derivative such as prethrombin or autoprothrombin II. The prothrombin complex from which the autoprothrombin II was obtained by digestion and purification also produced antibody, but it gave *only one* precipitation band with plasma (fast mobility arc). The digestion of the prothrombin complex with thrombin evidently uncovered a new antigenic determinant group hidden in the original prothrombin complex. Other authors have also found prothrombin complex derivatives (Soulier *et al.*, 1968; Prou-Wartelle *et al.*, 1968; Josso *et al.*, 1968).

It still remains to be determined how much autoprothrombin III is in the best platelet cofactor II preparations, and to what extent that could influence the platelet cofactor assay and the correction of hemophilia B prothrombin consumption. The activity might be due only to a digestion product of prothrombin, or due to such a product functioning as a carrier of autoprothrombin III. The autoprothrombin II is a procoagulant in the platelet cofactor assay in which the substrate is the prothrombin complex from which the autorprothrombin II is derived.

3. PLATELET COFACTOR I (PLATELET COFACTOR)

With hemophilia A plasma, a low concentration of platelet cofactor was found (Johnson *et al.*, 1952a). Extraction with ether developed the activity. It was then concluded that the cofactor is actually present in hemophilia A and that the abnormality is due to an inhibitor (Johnson, 1953; Seegers, 1954). The cofactor activity was made to disappear from plasma by adding purified thrombin and subsequently ether extraction restored the activity (Johnson and Seegers, 1954b). Consequently, it was evident that thrombin required some kind of inhibitor source material to make the cofactor activity disappear. Partially purified cofactor was not inactivated with thrombin unless some of the inhibitor source material was also present. In attempts to uphold the deficiency theory in hemophilia it was suggested that platelet cofactor might be different from AHF (Graham and Barrow, 1957; Brinkhous, 1958), but this is not a satisfactory way to account for the facts (Mammen, 1963). It does, however, seem likely that the postulated inhibitor in hemophilia A is a protein (Mammen, 1963).

4. PLATELET COFACTOR AND SPHINGOSINE

The platelet cofactor assay was found useful for following the fractionation of plasma for the purpose of obtaining concentrates of the platelet cofactor. Additionally it was possible to study the effects of an inhibitor such as sphingosine (E. Hecht *et al.*, 1957). Small amounts proved to have a procoagulant effect while large amounts depressed the generation of thrombin (Fig. 18). This kind of approach to problems in blood coagulation thus makes it possible to quantitate the effects of procoagulants as well as anticoagulants. It remains to be determined what the specific role of sphingosine is. Since the compound also retards the effects of tissue thromboplastin the effect must be on some common product, and the most likely one is autoprothrombin C. Sphingosine might be a substrate for the enzyme.

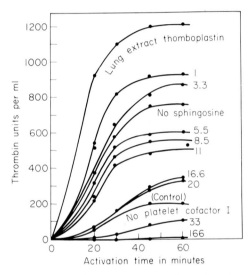

FIG. 18. Platelet cofactor assay in which a potent plasma fraction of platelet cofactor was inhibited with sphingosine. The amount of synthetic sphingosine in each reaction mixture is indicated on each curve in terms of γ per ml. In low concentration the yield of thrombin was increased. Thromboplastin was used to establish the maximum thrombin potential in the preparation of prothrombin complex. If the "no sphingosine" control had gone to the top, it would not have been possible to demonstrate the procoagulant effects of small amounts of sphingosine. This control was thus carefully selected.

D. Platelets Supplement Tissue Thromboplastin

It was shown that platelets contain material which made tissue thromboplastin more effective (Lee *et al.*, 1957). It was called platelet cothromboplastin and was considered to be a distinct component of platelets different from all others. Although concentrates of platelet factor 3 were available (Alkjaersig *et al.*, 1955c), no one tested them for cothromboplastin activity. Recently it was found, however, that platelet factor 3 and tissue thrombo-

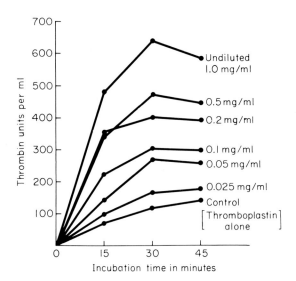

Fɪɢ. 19. The activation of prothrombin to thrombin with brain extract thrombo-plastin and various concentrations of platelet factor 3. Each incubation mixture contained a final concentration of 1000 U/ml prothrombin, 0.033 mg/ml brain extract thrombo-plastin, 0.004 *M* calcium chloride solution, and a constant quantity of barium carbonate adsorbed serum (the source of Ac-globulin). The bottom curve represents the thrombin formed when these reagents were incubated for 15, 30, or 45 minutes at 28°C. The other curves represent the thrombin formed when platelet factor 3 was also present in the incubation mixtures. The platelet factor 3 preparation used for these analyses contained 1.0 mg/ml protein (biuret). The concentrations of platelet factor 3 shown beside each curve were obtained by diluting the stock preparation with physiological saline solution before addition to the incubation mixture. Thus, the undiluted (1.0 mg/ml) platelet factor 3 used to obtain the thrombin shown in the top curve represents a final concentration of 0.166 mg/ml platelet factor 3 in the incubation mixture. (From Wayne State University, Thesis of Ruth A. Davis, 1969.)

plastin can complement each other (Fig. 19) in the cofactor assay (Davis, 1969). Since the function of thromboplastin is to generate autoprothrombin C, and platelet factor 3 does this to a lesser degree, it is easy to see that the two procoagulants function together. The "intrinsic" and "extrinsic" procoagulant systems thus supplement each other.

Platelets and platelet materials may have procoagulant or anticoagulant effects, and depending upon conditions, these may be weak or powerful. In the absence of tissue materials, platelets are virtually essential for blood clotting. Failure to emphasize this is one of the weak points in the "cascade" or "waterfall" diagrams (Davie and Ratnoff, 1964; Macfarlane, 1964). Their procoagulant properties can be supplemented by materials from tis-sues. Just as platelet substances can be released we can imagine that the cells of the blood vessel wall and perhaps those beyond the lining of the vessel wall can release compounds in a manner yet to be discovered. For example, there is a compensatory response to brain cortex anoxic anoxia which is retarded if intravascular red cell aggregation is induced (Bicher and Knisely, 1970). Perhaps such stimuli to the tissues are associated with release of procoagulant materials that can function with the platelet, and thus promote blood coagulation. The release reaction applies generally to endocrine mechanisms, and now that it applies to platelets (Stormorken, 1969) we can imagine that other tissues are not necessarily dormant, and that might include the cells of blood vessels.

E. Platelet Cofactor Activity and Dextran

Dextran was found to inhibit the generation of thrombin in the platelet cofactor assay (Seegers et al., 1955b). The effect involved both cofactors; namely, platelet cofactor I and platelet cofactor II (autoprothrombin II). Dextrans of low molecular (mol. wt. = 64,000) weight were more effective than those of higher weight (mol. wt. = 74,000). They were effective in concentrations that might be used in blood plasma volume expander work. Related substances like avocado gum, okra mucilage, alfalfa gum, corn fiber gum, and alginic acid were also effective. Low molecular weight dextran inhibited platelet activation on formvar films observed with the electron microscope (Barnhart and Quintana, 1967). It also inhibited platelet activation with thrombin. The effects of dextran on platelet function are now well recognized and being applied to clinical problems. One example is mentioned.

Intravenous use of low molecular weight dextran reduced the tendency of platelet aggregation and decreased blood viscosity. In acute cerebral ischemia platelets were found to be hypersensitive to spreading on formvar films as observed with the electron microscope. Dendritic and spread forms were more abundant than with normal persons. Dextran tended to restore the patient's platelets to normal. The clinical data provided evidence for a beneficial effect of the dextran for the patient. This is an instance of correlation of laboratory findings and clinical results (Gilroy et al., 1970).

F. Platelet Cofactor Activity and Lysed Fibrinogen

There is much evidence to support the view that the conversion of auto-prothrombin III to autoprothrombin C can be spontaneous; hence, a variety of conditions can promote it, and the cofactor assay is subject to nonspecific influences. A good example is the effectiveness of lysed fibrinogen (Triantaphyllopoulos and Triantaphyllopoulos, 1967).

The cofactor activity was found in chromatographic components A, D (α-derivative) and E (β-derivative). The activity was also found in preparations heated at 60°C for 15 minutes and in derivatives of fibrinogen obtained from hemophilia A blood (Triantaphyllopoulos *et al.*, 1970). Large quantities of the lysed fibrinogen had to be used, but probably platelet cofactor was ruled out and the effect was indeed due to the fibrinogen derivatives. The fact that the fibrinogen split products from hemophilia A were active could still be due to platelet cofactor, because such plasma contains it.

VIII. SOME PLATELET COMPONENTS OF SPECIAL RELEVANCE IN BLOOD CLOTTING

A. Introduction to Platelet Factors

Platelet constituents have been studied by the same technical approaches as those in plasma. Ac-globulin activity and something that would shorten the clotting time of fibrinogen was found in platelets (Ware *et al.*, 1948). Not knowing what these effects were due to they were regarded as an activity and given arabic numbers; namely, platelet factor 1 and 2, and later numbers were again assigned when other factors were recognized. A procoagulant and antiheparin activity was ascribed to platelet derived material (van Creveld and Paulssen, 1951, 1952) and called platelet factor 3. This was divided into procoagulant factor 3 and the antiheparin factor number 4 (Jürgens, 1952, 1954; Deutsch *et al.*, 1955). The coaguable material (Ware *et al.*, 1948) was called factor 5. Still continuing in my laboratory a method for the large scale production of bovine platelets was developed (Seegers *et al.*, 1954), and attempts were made to find out whether the clottable component was identical to fibrinogen. Concentrates were found to resist lysis (Johnson and Schneider, 1953). This was due to an inhibitor of fibrinolysis, or platelet factor 6. Plasma Ac-globulin was found to be more stable in platelet-poor plasma (Fahey *et al.*, 1948), and the addition of a platelet extract to decalcified human plasma decreased the plasma Ac-globulin stability. No special substance was postulated for this activity and, hence, no new number was needed. It may be that designations by arabic numbers will naturally get lost. Serotonin of platelets needs no number and I have seen reference to 28 enzymes of platelets where the list gave the trivial name as well as the systematic name and EC number.

B. Components of Special Interest

1. PLATELET AC-GLOBULIN

The Ac-globulin activity of platelets could be handled differently in laboratory procedures from the Ac-globulin in plasma (Ware *et al.*, 1948). It was easily sedimented by centrifugation at 32,000 *g*. In kinetic studies the activity resembled that of serum Ac-globulin rather than plasma Ac-globulin

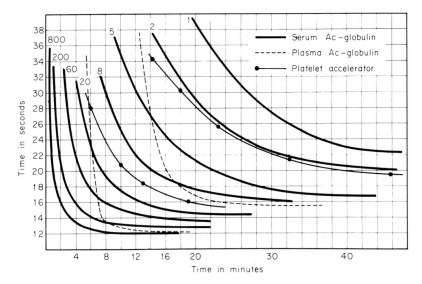

FIG. 20. Acceleration of thrombin formation by varying concentrations of serum Ac-globulin, plasma Ac-globulin, and platelet accelerator. The heavy continuous lines represent prothrombin activation curves obtained by incubating graded amounts of serum Ac-globulin with constant amounts of purified prothrombin (1.34 U/ml), thromboplastin, and calcium ions for varying lengths of time (abscissa) under the conditions specified by the two-stage procedure for prothrombin analysis. The thrombin formed in this reaction was measured by adding fibrinogen and recording the clotting time (ordinate). The prothrombin and thromboplastin were essentially free of accelerator. Concentrations of serum Ac-globulin (U/ml × 1000) are represented by the large numbers at the tops of the curves.

The two broken lines represent prothrombin activation curves obtained by the same method of analysis but with two different concentrations of plasma Ac-globulin instead of serum Ac-globulin. The slopes of these curves are not the same as the curves for serum Ac-globulin. The slopes of these curves are not the same as the curves for serum Ac-globulin because the inactive plasma Ac-globulin is being changed to active serum Ac-globulin during the period of incubation. The two light continuous lines represent prothrombin activation curves obtained by the same method of analysis but with two different concentrations of platelet accelerator. The slopes of these curves are identical with those for serum Ac-globulin (Ware *et al.*, 1948).

(Fig. 20). In plasma the effect of accelerator activity is a little delayed as compared with serum or platelet Ac-G. This was nicely demonstrated in bovine serum where, in contrast to human serum, Ac-globulin activity remains (Murphy and Seegers, 1948). Thrombin produces the change from plasma Ac-globulin to serum Ac-globulin (Ware and Seegers, 1948), and in disseminated intravascular coagulation associated with placenta abruptio we actually found serum Ac-globulin in the circulation (J. F. Johnson et al., 1952).

A new aspect was introduced with the observation that platelets from parahemophilia have very little Ac-globulin, but acquire this when incubated with normal platelet poor plasma (Hjort et al., 1955a,b). This raised the possibility that the Ac-globulin of platelets is nothing more than an adsorption phenomenon, or part of the "plasmatic atmosphere" of platelets. This idea gained momentum to such an extent that some authors regarded other platelet factors in that same light. By the very nature of the experiment (Hjort et al., 1955a,b) it was not possible to test whether the "adsorbed" Ac-globulin was serum Ac-globulin. Further attention to this resulted in the failure to dissociate the activity from particles and the making of a concentrate (Fell and Seegers, 1958). Platelet Ac-globulin is not a simple adsorption product and the activity may also be associated with granules in the platelets (Schulz and Hiepler, 1959). It seems to me that magic is implied when speaking about "plasmatic atmosphere" of platelets. A well-washed platelet will no longer be covered with plasma. What remains? I like to say it is the platelet, taking into account how extensive or thorough the washing procedure was, and then proceeding to demonstrate how and what can be obtained from the washed platelet. Additionally one has to keep in mind that the pressure of centrifugation on platelets also has an effect.

2. FIBRINOPLASTIC ACTIVITY

In the initial experiments a certain thrombin solution clotted purified fibrinogen in 15.8 seconds. Pretreatment of the fibrinogen with a platelet extract reduced the clotting time with the same thrombin to 11 seconds (Ware et al., 1948). The material located in the hyalomer of platelets (Schulz and Hiepler, 1959) was stable 30 minutes at 53°C, precipitated by half saturation with ammonium sulfate, adsorbed on magnesium hydroxide and barium sulfate, and eluted with sodium citrate solution. Presumably an enzyme is involved, and is concerned with the polymerization phase of fibrin formation (Lüscher, 1959).

The factor was purified (Niewiarowski *et al.*, 1967, 1968) and easily precipitated by zinc ions. It was called a "fibrinogen activating factor" because purified fibrinogen was made more sensitive to thrombin, by producing trichloroacetic acid soluble material. The product tended to destroy antithrombin III activity, and was a weak platelet aggregating agent.

3. PLATELET FACTOR 3

The procoagulant activity of platelets is referred to in the literature from divergent views, from which it is hard to synthesize or abstract the gem worth the center of attention. The phospholipids of platelets have procoagulant characteristics. When these are isolated they do not have distinguishing characteristics with which to regard them as different from what can be isolated from various sources such as brain, spinal cord, plant sources or the lard barrel (E. R. Hecht, 1965; Marcus and Zucker, 1965). That much seems to be clear from the very substantial efforts of contemporary contributors (Wallach *et al.*, 1959; Silver *et al.*, 1963; Kazal, 1964-1965; Daemen *et al.*, 1965). In pioneer work (Chargaff *et al.*, 1936) the platelet phosphatides reduced the clotting time of chicken plasma from 100 to 15 minutes—not seconds! In my early work with prothrombin preparations it was remarked that "...with cephalin the conversion of prothrombin into thrombin is usually incomplete, and always requires many hours..." (Seegers *et al.*, 1938). However, under the correct conditions (Fig. 10) the lipids produce the same dramatic results as an enzyme such as autoprothrombin C. It is indeed an outstanding example of a function of lipids which, for its impact on the imagination, is unsurpassed by other examples of lipid function in biology.

More is needed than phospholipid and the extra seems to be protein material. The "platelet factor 3" prepared in this laboratory was one of the first (Alkjaersig *et al.*, 1955c) and contains lipoprotein, cholesterol, and perhaps other material (Penner *et al.*, 1956). For convenience it can be called lipoprotein and converting it to the "protein" and phospholipid components destroys some of its procoagulant properties. The lipoproteins of erythrocytes resemble those of platelets in this respect (Shinowara, 1951, 1957). He used the term "thromboplastic cell component." Phospholipids are not distinguished from platelets in an activity analysis such as presented by means of Fig. 10 where lipids function with Ac-globulin, autoprothrombin C, and calcium ions in the formation of thrombin. The conditions described (Fig. 10 and 11) fulfill the requirements for the quantitative determination of platelet factor 3.

Phospholipids do not make purified prothrombin complex refractory to the two-stage analytical reagents (Fig. 12) whereas platelet factor 3 readily did this. One could say that *if purified prothrombin is not made refractory, the substance cannot properly be called platelet factor* 3. In that frame of reference a Russell's viper venom test is not a test for platelet factor 3 because phospholipid suffices to make that test positive. Nor is a method based on an adaptation of the one-stage prothrombin time sufficient (Egli, 1961) for it measures what is defined in another way. Generally just a procoagulant activity is measured (Inceman and Tangün, 1969). It is interesting that a substitute for platelets (Bell and Alton, 1954), in the form of phospholipid, was generally used in the thromboplastin generation test (Biggs and Douglas, 1953). However, this test also requires platelet factor 3 if purified autoprothrombin II is used in place of serum (Ulutin *et al.*, 1961a,b; Seegers and Ulutin, 1961). Sometime it might be interesting and rewarding to find out why this test functions with phospholipid when serum is used but fails when purified autoprothrombin II (factor IX?) is used.

With the emphasis on lipoprotein complex the analogy with tissue thromboplastin is evident. The latter material consists of phospholipid complexes and a small amount of "protein" (Deutsch *et al.*, 1964; Irsigler 1964; Nemerson, 1968; E. Hecht and Wijngaards, 1969a,b). Separation was achieved with the use of pyridine and recombination of lipid and "protein" occurred with pyridine. The latter was evaporated and the aqueous emulsion made from the residue was active as thromboplastin. To restore the original thromboplastin activity, it was possible to use another phospholipid besides the original. Many years ago I made a summary (Seegers, 1956) which gives some characteristics of platelet factor 3 and thromboplastin (Table IV). It might be well to adopt the meanings I have ascribed to the terms thromboplastin, platelet factor 3, and lipid activator. The latter would be the phospholipid procoagulants.

The platelet factor 3 preparation which originated in this laboratory has proved to be very useful (Alkjaersig *et al.*, 1955c). To make the preparation, packed platelets are suspended in water. They are frozen and thawed to break up the platelet, and the process is carried further with ultrasonic waves. Clottable factor is removed with the use of thrombin. Kaolin is used to remove undesired components including PF-1 and PF-4. Charcoal adsorption, as included in the original method, is not employed any longer. The activity is then sedimented in a preparative ultracentrifuge and taken up in the desired solvent. Such preparations can be frozen and preserved for a long period of time. In the original platelets, platelet factor 3 is not very stable. At refrigerator temperature half the activity was gone in 4 days

TABLE IV

SOME CHARACTERISTICS OF THROMBOPLASTIN AND PLATELET FACTOR 3[a]

Name	Constituents	Cofactors
Thromboplastin[b]	Protein[c], lipid[d]	Cothromboplastin (F-VII), (species aspects) important
Platelet factor 3[b]	Protein[c], lipid[d]	Platelet cofactor (F-VIII), platelet cofactor II (F-IX?), certain nonspecific substances

[a] Adapted and modified (Seergers, 1956).

[b] Lipids in these lipoproteins before or after separation from their "protein(s)" can function with Ac-globulin, autoprothrombin C and calcium ions to generate thrombin activity from its zymogen.

[c] Inert unless combined with lipid.

[d] Used in partial thromboplastin test, lipid from PF-3 or lipid from thromboplastin can be combined in special way to give thromboplastin activity in generation of auto-prothrombin C activity (Deutsch *et al.*, 1964; E. Hecht and Wijngaards, 1969b). The lipid alone does not convert autoprothrombin III to autoprothrombin C.

(Deutsch *et al.*, 1955). By contrast, purified platelet factor 3 is more stable and can be preserved for years in the frozen state. Freeze drying has thus far not been possible.

4. ANTIHEPARIN SUBSTANCE

Platelet-poor plasma is more sensitive to the anticoagulant effects of heparin than platelet-rich plasma (Waugh and Ruddick, 1944; Conley *et al.*, 1948, 1949). The first fractions of platelets obtained with antiheparin activity also had platelet factor 3 (van Creveld and Paulssen, 1952). The two were separated (Jürgens, 1952, 1954; S. A. Johnson *et al.*, 1954; Deutsch *et al.*, 1955; Deutsch, 1955).

At a concentration of 10^7 intact normal platelets neutralized 0.02–0.04 units of heparin, but if homogenized, up to 0.06 units were neutralized. The activity was easily soluble in buffered saline, but not in organic solvents. It was stable at —20°C for at least one year; and stable at 100°C for 10 minutes after purification. It was concentrated 100-fold with the use of DEAE-cellulose chromatography. The activity was found in brain extracts and erythrocytes and may thus be a regular cell component (Deutsch and Kain, 1961). It was finally purified from platelets and found to be a protein

(Niewiarowski *et al.*, 1967). It neutralized heparin activity, and the antithrombin activity of fibrinogen breakdown products.

Antiheparin material is reduced or missing in certain types of thrombopathy, and also in patients under anticoagulant treatment, and with cirrhosis of the liver and chronic uremia (Deutsch and Kain, 1961). Some release from platelets occurs upon inducing aggregation with ADP (Niewiarowski and Thomas, 1969), and this release was inhibited with aspirin (Youssef and Barkhan, 1969). Aspirin and other antiinflammatory agents probably function by stabilizing cell membranes (O'Brien *et al.*, 1970b). The material with the activity seems to be in three forms; namely, (1) inactive in the platelet surface, (2) active at the platelet surface, and (3) in a soluble form after the "release reaction" (O'Brien *et al.*, 1970a). In contrast to ADP aggregation, that with adrenalin was not associated with platelet release (Niewiarowski *et al.*, 1968). A further discussion of the release of antiheparin activity has appeared (O'Brien *et al.*, 1970b,c).

5. PLATELET FIBRINOGEN

The amebocyte of invertebrates naturally comes to mind in any discussion of thrombocytes and a recent review is most helpful (Levin, 1967). The blood of *Limulus* contains the amebocyte as the only cell. Cell-free plasma is incoaguable, but cell lysate was gelled by endotoxin. Amebocytes play a role in the initial stages of coagulation, and endotoxins from pathogens can produce amebocytopenia, intravascular clotting, subsequent incoaguable blood, and death. This sequence is similar to that of disseminated intravascular coagulation in man and animals. Fortunately death need not follow in man, and fibrinolysis is a defensive mechanism. Lobsters also have amebocytes and a plasma protein similar to mammalian protein or fibrinogen. The latter is clotted by plasma transglutaminase instead of thrombin (Lorand, 1965). Evidently thrombin developed rather late in evolution.

One might suppose evolutionary progression. Clottable protein is in the amebocyte as well as platelets. First, there was probably complete reliance on the cell for clotting. Then the cell and plasma were the source of the clot produced by a transglutaminase enzyme. In the mammal the plasma continued to be the main source of clottable protein, but the enzyme thrombin prepared the protein for polymerization and subsequent cross-linking by plasma transglutaminase. The latter is incidentally in platelets and activated by thrombin (Lüscher, 1957; Buluk *et al.*, 1961).

Clottable protein was found in the mammalian platelet (Roskam, 1923;

Ware *et al.*, 1948). Many attempts were made to establish identity between clottable protein and fibrinogen. It was found in low concentration in afibrinogenemia. It was purified with methods used for obtaining fibrinogen from plasma (Solum and Lopaciuk, 1969a). The platelet clottable protein is indeed fibrinogen. However, there were certain interesting differences (Solum and Lopaciuk, 1969b). These were in intrinsic viscosity, carbohydrate, and sialic acid content. With the platelet fibrinogen there was a slower polymerization rate of the fibrinogen monomer.

IX. SUMMARY

In paraffin or silicone-lined glassware platelet-poor plasma clots very slowly if at all, and very little prothrombin is consumed. The addition of platelets or platelet homogenates accelerates this clotting, but even then the time required is about a minute as compared with seconds if thromboplastin is added. Intravenously infused platelet homogenates do not produce extensive disseminated intravascular clotting unless the reticuloendothelial system is blocked.

There are three basic chemical reactions which account for the coagulation of blood; namely, (1) formation of autoprothrombin C, (2) formation of thrombin, and (3) formation of fibrin.

Only thrombin is needed for the formation of fibrin from fibrinogen, and only autoprothrombin C is required for the formation of thrombin from prothrombin; autoprothrombin C can form spontaneously. Thrombin as well as autoprothrombin C produces autocatalytic responses. The three basic reactions must be accelerated to be of value in our regular physiology. *Platelets and/or their breakdown products participate in accelerating all three basic reactions.*

The formation of autoprothrombin C from its precursor, autoprothrombin III, is accelerated by such enzymes as trypsin, cathepsin, papain, and an enzyme in Russell's viper venom. It is accelerated with calcium ions and a fraction obtained from urine. It is also accelerated by calcium ions and thromboplastin, and the latter seems to be "activated" by cothromboplastin. Platelet factor 3 functions synergistically with thromboplastin.

The conversion of autoprothrombin III to autoprothrombin C is also accelerated in the presence of calcium ions and platelet factor 3. With the further addition of platelet cofactor the rate is increased, but still the activation tends to be slower and less complete than with tissue thromboplastin. With the use of the platelet cofactor assay it was demonstrated that platelet cofactor II and other substances function as cofactors with platelet factor 3. Included is Hageman protein. Platelet factor 3 and Hageman factor together produce appreciable amounts of active autoprothrombin C from its precursor, but not as much as with thromboplastin. When Hageman factor and platelets are simultaneously "activated" an appreciable procoagulant effect is produced in circulating blood. Under those conditions the platelets have a direct role in autoprothrombin C formation; and, therefore, also in thrombin formation. Their participation induces relatively slow reactions, and hence, areas of slow blood flow or stasis favor clotting. Furthermore, under those conditions, the reticuloendothelial system does not remove platelet materials or other procoagulants. Dextran and sphingosine inhibit the procoagulant function of platelets, as demonstrated with the platelet cofactor assay. This assay made it possible to make valuable quantitative determinations, without having to resort to "deficiency" plasmas obtained from patients. Examples given are work on the analysis of hemophilia A and B plasmas, and the effects of inhibitors.

The formation of thrombin by autoprothrombin C, in the presence of calcium ions, is accelerated in a spectacular manner by the *simultaneous* presence of plasma Ac-globulin and platelet factor 3. Here the lipid portion of platelet factor 3 is also sufficient, or also the lipid portion of thromboplastin. Moreover, certain bile salts can replace the function of the lipid or lipoprotein from platelets. Like bile salts the platelets supply micelles for the required surface on which the enzyme, autoprothrombin C, and the Ac-globulin "coenzyme" function. Prothrombin complex, DEAE-prothrombin, and prethrombin each have peculiar requirements for being converted to thrombin.

Platelet factor 3 readily produces the two-stage reagent refractory state in prothrombin. The lipid portion of platelet factor 3 does not have this capacity.

Platelets contain substances of special interest in blood coagulation. These include an enzyme that alters fibrinogen in some unknown way with the result that clotting with thrombin is facilitated. Platelets also contain platelet Ac-globulin, antiheparin material, platelet fibrinogen, and the fibrin stabilizing enzyme.

ACKNOWLEDGMENTS

This work was aided by grants HE 03424 and HE 05141 from the National Heart Institute, National Institutes of Health, U.S. Public Health Service. My thanks are expressed to Dr. R. J. Broersma, Jr., for helping me arrange the references, and to Miss Cheri Emery for typing the manuscript.

REFERENCES

Aggeler, P. M., White, S. G., Glendening, M. B., Page, E. W., Leake, T. B., and Bates, G. (1952). *Proc. Soc. Exp. Biol. Med.* **79**, 692.

Alkjaersig, N., Deutsch, E., and Seegers, W. H. (1955a). *Amer. J. Physiol.* **180**, 367.

Alkjaersig, N., Abe, T., Johnson, S. A., and Seegers, W. H. (1955b). *Amer. J. Physiol.* **182**, 443.

Alkjaersig, N., Abe, T., and Seegers, W. H. (1955c). *Amer. J. Physiol.* **181**, 304.

Aoki, N., Harmison, C. R., and Seegers, W. H. (1963). *Can. J. Biochem. Physiol.* **41**, 2409.

Apitz, K. (1943). *Ergeb. Inn. Med. Kinderheilk.* **63**, 1.

Astrup, T. (1939). *Nature (London)* **144**, 76.

Astrup, T. (1941). *Enzymologia* **9**, 337.

Astrup, T. (1944). *Acta Physiol. Scand.* **7**, Suppl. 21.

Astrup, T. (1950). *Advan. Enzymol.* **10**, 1.

Astrup, T. (1957). *Dan. Med. Bull.* **4**, 160.

Baker, W. J., and Seegers, W. H. (1967). *Thromb. Diath. Haemorrh.* **22**, 205.

Barnhart, M. I. (1967). *In* "Blood Clotting Enzymology" (W. H. Seegers, ed.), pp. 217–277. Academic Press, New York.

Barnhart, M. I., and Quintana, C. (1967). *Blood* **30**, 541.

Barnhart, M. I., and Riddle, J. M. (1967). *Thromb. Diath. Haemorrh.* Suppl. 26, 87.

Barthels, M., and Seegers, W. H. (1969). *Thromb. Diath. Haemorrh.* **22**, 13.

Barton, P. G., Jackson, C. M., and Hanahan, D. J. (1967). *Nature (London)* **214**, 923.

Bell, W. N., and Alton, H. G. (1954). *Nature (London)* **174**, 880.

Bessis, M. (1956). "Cytology of the Blood and Blood-Forming Organs" (translated by E. Ponder). Grune & Stratton, New York.

Bicher, H. I., and Knisely, M. H. (1970). *J. Appl. Physiol.* (in press).

Biggs, R., and Douglas, A. S. (1953). *J. Clin. Pathol.* **6**, 23.

Biggs, R., Douglas, A. S., Macfarlane, R. G., Dacie, J. V., Pitney, W. R., Merskey, C., and O'Brien, J. R. (1952). *Brit. Med. J.* **2**, 1378.

Brinkhous, K. M. (1947). *Proc. Soc. Exp. Biol. Med.* **66**, 117.

Brinkhous, K. M. (1958). *Acta Haematol.* **20**, 125.

Budtz–Olsen, O. E. (1951). "Clot Retraction." Thomas, Springfield, Illinois.

Buluk, K., Januszko, T., and Olbromski, J. (1961). *Nature (London)* **191**, 1093.

Caldwell, M. J., von Kaulla, K. N., von Kaulla, E., and Seegers, W. H. (1963). *Thromb. Diath. Haemorrh.* **9**, 53.

Chargaff, E., Bancroft, F. W., and Stanely–Brown, M. (1936). *J. Biol. Chem.* **116**, 237.

Chen, R., and Doolittle, R. F. (1969). *Proc. Nat. Acad. Sci. U.S.* **63**, 420.

Cho, M. H., and Seegers, W. H. (1958). *Proc. Soc. Exp. Biol. Med.* **97**, 642.

Conley, C. L., Hartmann, R. C., and Lalley, J. S. (1948). *Proc. Soc. Exp. Biol. Med.* **69**, 284.

Conley, C. L., Hartmann, R. C., and Morse, W. I. (1949). *J. Clin. Invest.* **28**, 340.

Daemen, F. J. M., van Arkel, C., Hart, H. C., van der Drift, C., and van Deenen, L. L. (1965). *Thromb. Diath. Haemorrh.* **13**, 194.

Davey, M. G., and Lüscher, E. F. (1963). *Semin. Hematol.* **5**, 5.

Davie, E. W., and Ratnoff, O. D. (1964). *Science* **145**, 1310.

Davis, R. A. (1969). Ph.D. Thesis, Wayne State University, Detroit, Michigan.

DeRobertis, E., Paseyro, P., and Reissig, M. (1953). *Blood* **8**, 587.

Deutsch, E. (1955). "Blutgerinnungsfaktoren." Deuticke, Vienna.

Deutsch, E., and Kain, W. (1961). *In* "Blood Platelets" (S. A. Johnson *et al.*, eds.), pp. 337–345. Little, Brown, Boston, Massachusetts.

Deutsch, E., Johnson, S. A., and Seegers, W. H. (1955). *Circ. Res.* **3**, 110.

Deutsch, E., Irsigler, K., and Lomoschitz, H. (1964). *Thromb. Diath. Haemorrh.* **12**, 12.

Egli, H. (1961). *Thromb. Diath. Haemorrh.* **6**, 533.

Epstein, E., and Quick, A. J. (1953). *Proc. Soc. Exp. Biol. Med.* **83**, 453.

Esnouf, M. P. (1969). *Proc. Roy. Soc.* **173**, 269.

Evensen, S. A., and Jeremic, M. (1969). *5th Congr. Asian Pac. Soc. Haematol.*, 1969, Abstracts.

Fahey, J. L., Ware, A. G., and Seegers, W. H. (1948). *Amer. J. Physiol.* **154**, 122.

Fell, C., and Seegers, W. H. (1958). *Can. J. Biochem. Physiol.* **36**, 645.

Ferguson, J. H. (1960). "Lipoids and Blood Platelets." Univ. of North Carolina Press, Chapel Hill, North Carolina.

Fukutake, K., Cho, M. H., and Seegers, W. H. (1958). *Amer. J. Physiol.* **194**, 280.

Gilroy, J., Barnhart, M. I., and Meyer, J. S. (1970). *J. Amer. Med. Ass.* (in press).

Gobbi, F., Barbieri, U., and Ascari, E. (1967). *Thromb. Diath. Haemorrh.* **17**, 495.

Graham, J. B., and Barrow, E. M. (1957). *J. Exp. Med.* **106**, 273.

Graham, J. B., Penick, G. D., and Brinkhous, K. M. (1951). *Amer. J. Physiol.* **164**, 710.

Grammens, G. L. (1969). Ph.D. Thesis, Wayne State University, Detroit, Michigan.

Hagen, E., Wechsler, W., Zilliken, F., Hannen, C., and Jürgens, J. (1968). *Exp. Biol. Med.* **3**.

Hampton, J. R. (1967). *J. Atheroscler. Res.* **7**, 729.

Harmison, C. R., and Seegers, W. H. (1962). *J. Biol. Chem.* **237**, 3074.

Hecht, E. (1966a). *Med. Welt.* **17**, 2139.

Hecht, E. (1966b). *Klin. Wochenschr.* **14**, 797.

Hecht, E., and Wijngaards, G. (1969a). *Thromb. Diath. Haemorrh.* **21**, 534.

Hecht, E., and Wijngaards, G. (1969b). *Thromb. Diath. Haemorrh.* **21**, 546.

Hecht, E., Landaburu, R. H., and Seegers, W. H. (1957). *Amer. J. Physiol.* **189**, 203.

Hecht, E. R. (1965). "Lipids in Blood Clotting." Thomas, Springfield, Illinois.

Henry, R. L., and Steiman, R. H. (1968). *Microvascular Res.* **1**, 68.

Hjort, P., Rapaport, J. S., and Owren, P. A. (1955a). *Scand. J. Clin. Lab. Invest.* **7**, 97.

Hjort, P., Rapaport, J. S., and Owren, P. A. (1955b). *Blood* **10**, 1139.

Hoak, J. C., Warner, E. D., and Connor, W. E. (1967). *Circ. Res.* **20**, 11.

Inceman, S., and Tangün, Y. (1969). *J. Lab. Clin. Med.* **74**, 1969.

Irsigler, K. (1964). *Thromb. Diath. Haemorrh.* **13**, 433.

Jackson, C. M., and Hanahan, D. J. (1968). *Biochemistry* **7**, 4506.

Jaques, L. B. (1967). *Progr. Med. Chem.* **5**, 139.

Jaques, L. B., Fidlar, E., Feldsted, E. T., and MacDonald, A. S. (1946). *Can. Med. Ass. J.* **55**, 26.

Johnson, J. F., Seegers, W. H., and Braden, R. G. (1952). *Amer. J. Clin. Pathol.* **22**, 322.

Johnson, S. A. (1953). *Amer. J. Clin. Pathol.* **23**, 875.

Johnson, S. A., and Greenwalt, T. J. (1965). "Coagulation and Transfusion in Clinical Medicine." Little, Brown, Boston, Massachusetts.

Johnson, S. A., and Guest, M. M., eds. (1969). "Dynamics of Thrombus Formation and Dissolution." Lippincott, Philadelphia, Pennsylvania.

Johnson, S. A., and Schneider, C. L. (1953). *Science* **117**, 229.

Johnson, S. A., and Seegers, W. H. (1954a). *J. Appl. Physiol.* **6**, 429.

Johnson, S. A., and Seegers, W. H. (1954b). *Rev. Hematol.* **9**, 529.

Johnson, S. A., and Seegers, W. H. (1956). *Circ. Res.* **4**, 182.

Johnson, S. A., and Seegers, W. H., eds. (1966). "Physiology of Hemostasis and Thrombosis." Thomas, Springfield, Illinois.

Johnson, S. A., Rutsky, J., Schneider, C. L., and Seegers, W. H. (1952a). *Proc. 4th Int. Congr. Int. Soc. Hematol.*, 1952, p. 373.

Johnson, S. A., Smathers, W. M., and Schneider, C. L. (1952b). *Amer. J. Physiol.* **170**, 631.

Johnson, S. A., Deutsch, E., and Seegers, W. H. (1954). *Amer. J. Physiol.* **179**, 149.

Johnson, S. A., McClaughry, R. I., and Seegers, W. H. (1955). *J. Mich. State Med. Soc.* **54**, 797.

Johnson, S. A., Seegers, W. H., Koppel, J. L., and Olwin, J. H. (1957). *Thromb. Diath. Haemorrh.* **1**, 158.

Johnson, S. A., Sturrock, R. M., and Rebuck, J. W. (1959). *Proc. 4th Int. Congr. Biochem.*, 1958, Vol. 10, p. 105.

Johnson, S. A., Monto, R. W., Rebuck, J. W., and Horn, R. C., eds. (1961). "Blood Platelets." Little, Brown, Boston, Massachusetts.

Josso, F., Lavergne, J. M., Gouault, M., and Soulier, J. P. (1968). *Thromb. Diath. Haemorrh.* **20**, 88.

Jürgens, R. (1952). *Deut. Med. Wochenschr.* **77**, 1265.

Jürgens, R. (1954). *Arch. Exp. Pathol. Pharmakol.* **222**, 107.

Kazal, L. A. (1964–1965). *Trans. N.Y. Acad. Sci.* [2] **27**, 613.

Kipfer, R., and Seegers, W. H. (1968). *Thromb. Diath. Haemorrh.* **19**, 204.

Kowalski, E., and Niewiarowski, S. (1967). "Biochemistry of Blood Platelets." Academic Press, New York.

Laki, K. (1943). *Stud. Inst. Med. Chem., Univ. Szeged* **3**, 5.

Laki, K. (1968). "Fibrinogen." Marcel Dekker, New York.

Langdell, R. D., Graham, J. B., and Brinkhous, K. M. (1950). *Proc. Soc. Exp. Biol. Med.* **74**, 424.

Lechner, K., and Deutsch, E. (1965). *Thromb. Diath. Haemorrh.* **13**, 314.

Lee, P., Johnson, S. A., and Seegers, W. H. (1957). *Thromb. Diath. Haemorrh.* **1**, 16.

Lenggenhager, K. (1949). "Weitere Fortschritte In der Blutgerinnungslehre." Thieme, Stuttgart.

Levin, J. (1967). *Fed. Proc., Fed. Amer. Soc. Exp. Biol.* **26**, 1707.

Lister, J. (1863). *Lancet* **2**, 149.

Lorand, L. (1965). *Fed. Proc., Fed. Amer. Soc. Exp. Biol.* **24**, 784.

Lorand, L., Chenoweth, D., and Domanik, R. A. (1969). *Biochem. Biophys. Res. Commun.* **37**, 219.

Lüscher, E. F. (1957). *Schweiz. Med. Wochenschr.* **87**, 1220.

Lüscher, E. F. (1959). *Ergeb. Physiol., Biol. Chem. Exp. Pharmakol.* **50**, 1.

McClaughry, R. I., and Seegers, W. H. (1952). *Proc. Soc. Exp. Biol. Med.* **80**, 372.

Macfarlane, R. G. (1964). *Nature (London)* **202**, 498.

Macfarlane, R. G. (1969). *Proc. Roy. Soc., Ser. B* **173**, 261.

Macfarlane, R. G., and Ash, B. J. (1964). *Brit. J. Haematol.* **10**, 217.

Mammen, E. F. (1963). *Thromb. Diath. Haemorrh.* **9**, 30.

Mammen, E. F., and Grammens, G. (1967). *Thromb. Diath. Haemorrh.* **18**, 306.

Mammen, E. F., Yoshinari, M., and Seegers, W. H. (1960a). *Thromb. Diath. Haemorrh.* **5**, 38.

Mammen, E. F., Thomas, W. R., and Seegers, W. H. (1960b). *Thromb. Diath. Haemorrh.* **5**, 218.

Marciniak, E., and Seegers, W. H. (1962). *Can. J. Biochem. Physiol.* **40**, 597.

Marciniak, E., and Seegers, W. H. (1965). *New Istanbul Contrib. Clin. Sci.* **8**, 117.

Marciniak, E., Rodriguez–Erdmann, F., and Seegers, W. H. (1962a). *Science* **137**, 421.

Marciniak, E., Cole, E. R., and Seegers, W. H. (1962b). *Thromb. Diath. Haemorrh.* **8**, 425.

Marcus, A. J. (1969). *N. Engl. J. Med.* **280**, 1330.

Marcus, A. J., and Zucker, M. B. (1965). "The Physiology of Blood Platelets." Grune & Stratton, New York.

Mertz, E. T., Seegers, W. H., and Smith, H. P. (1939). *Proc. Soc. Exp. Biol. Med.* **41**, 657.

Michal, F., and Firkin, B. G. (1969). *Annu. Rev. Pharmacol.* **9**, 95.

Milstone, J. H. (1947). *Science* **106**, 546.

Milstone, J. H. (1948a). *J. Gen. Physiol.* **31**, 301.

Milstone, J. H. (1948b). *Proc. Soc. Exp. Biol. Med.* **68**, 225.

Milstone, J. H. (1949). *Blood* **4**, 1290.

Milstone, J. H. (1951). *J. Gen. Physiol.* **35**, 1.

Milstone, J. H. (1952a). *Yale J. Biol. Med.* **25**, 19.

Milstone, J. H. (1952b). *Yale J. Biol. Med.* **25**, 173.

Milstone, J. H. (1952c). *Medicine (Baltimore)* **31**, 411.

Milstone, J. H. (1955). *J. Gen. Physiol.* **38**, 757.

Milstone, J. H. (1964). *Fed. Proc., Fed. Amer. Soc. Exp. Biol.* **23**, 742.

Morawitz, P. (1904). *Beitr. Chem. Physiol. Pathol.* **5**, 133.

Murphy, R. C., and Seegers, W. H. (1948). *Amer. J. Physiol.* **154**, 134.

Mustard, J. F. (1967). *Exp. Mol. Pathol.* **7**, 366.

Nemerson, Y. (1968). *J. Clin. Invest.* **47**, 72.

Niewiarowski, S., and Thomas, D. P. (1969). *Nature (London)* **222**, 1269.

Niewiarowski, S., Farbiszewski, R., and Poplawski, A. (1967). *In* "Biochemistry of Blood Platelets" (E. Kowalski and S. Niewiarowski, eds.), pp. 35–45. Academic Press, New York.

Niewiarowski, S., Poplawski, A., Lipinski, B., and Farbiszewski, R. (1968). *Exp. Biol. Med.* **3**, 121.

Nossel, H. L. (1964). "The Contact Phase of Blood Coagulation." Davis, Philadelphia, Pennsylvania.

O'Brien, J. R., Finch, W., and Clark, E. (1970a). *Nature (London)* (in press).

O'Brien, J. R., Finch, W., and Clark, E. (1970b). *Lancet* (in press).

O'Brien, J. R., Shoobridge, S., and Finch, W. (1970c). *Thromb. Diath. Haemorrh.* (in press).

Papahadjopoulos, D., Yin, E. T., and Hanahan, D. J. (1964). *Biochemistry* **3**, 1931.

Patton, T. B., Ware, A. G., and Seegers, W. H. (1948). *Blood* **3**, 656.

Penner, J. A., Duckert, F., Johnson, S. A., and Seegers, W. H. (1956). *Can. J. Biochem. Physiol.* **34**, 1199.

Prou-Wartelle, O., Soulier, J. P., and Hallé, L. (1968). *Thromb. Diath. Haemorrh.* **20**, 99.

Quick, A. J. (1951). "The Physiology and Pathology of Hemostasis." Lea & Febiger, Philadelphia, Pennsylvania.

Quick, A. J. (1957). "Hemorrhagic Diseases." Lea & Febiger, Philadelphia, Pennsylvania.

Quick, A. J. (1966a). "Hemorrhagic Diseases and Thrombosis." Lea & Febiger, Philadelphia, Pennsylvania.
Quick, A. J. (1966b). *Thromb. Diath. Haemorrh.* **16**, 318.
Reno, R. S., and Seegers, W. H. (1967). *Thromb. Diath. Haemorrh.* **23**, 198.
Rodriguez–Erdmann, F. (1965). *Blood* **26**, 541.
Rodriguez–Erdmann, F. (1969). *Thromb. Diath. Haemorrh.* Suppl. 36, 63.
Roskam, J. (1923). *Arch. Int. Physiol.* **20**, 241.
Schröer, H., Heene, D. L., and Seegers, W. H. (1965). *Thromb. Diath. Haemorrh.* **13**, 266.
Schulz, H., and Hiepler, E. (1959). *Klin. Wochenschr.* **37**, 237.
Seegers, W. H. (1949). *Proc. Soc. Exp. Biol. Med.* **72**, 677.
Seegers, W. H. (1951). *Enzymes* **2**, 1106.
Seegers, W. H. (1951–1952). *Harvey Lect.* **47**, 180.
Seegers, W. H. (1954). *Schweiz. Med. Wochenschr.* **29**, 781.
Seegers, W. H. (1956). *Proc. 6th Int. Congr. Int. Soc. Hematol.*, 1956, p. 469.
Seegers, W. H. (1962). "Prothrombin." Harvard Univ. Press, Cambridge, Massachusetts.
Seegers, W. H., ed. (1967a). "Blood Clotting Enzymology." Academic Press, New York.
Seegers, W. H. (1967b). "Prothrombin In Enzymology, Thrombosis and Hemophilia." Thomas, Springfield, Illinois.
Seegers, W. H. (1968). *Pfluegers Arch. Ges. Physiol. Menschen Tiere* **299**, 226.
Seegers, W. H., and Johnson, S. A. (1956). *Amer. J. Physiol.* **184**, 259.
Seegers, W. H., and Kagami, M. (1964). *Can. J. Biochem.* **42**, 1249.
Seegers, W. H., and Marciniak, E. (1965). *Life Sci.* **4**, 1721.
Seegers, W. H., and Marciniak, E. (1970). *In* "Hemophilias" (K. M. Brinkhous, ed.), pp. 43–53. Univ. of North Carolina Press, Chapel Hill, North Carolina.
Seegers, W. H., and Ulutin, O. N. (1961). *Thromb. Diath. Haemorrh.* **6**, 270.
Seegers, W. H., Brinkhous, K. M., Smith, H. P., and Warner, E. D. (1938). *J. Biol. Chem.* **126**, 91.
Seegers, W. H., McClaughry, R. I., and Fahey, J. L. (1950). *Blood* **5**, 421.
Seegers, W. H., Johnson, S. A., Fell, C., and Alkjaersig, N. (1954). *Amer. J. Physiol.* **178**, 1.
Seegers, W. H., Alkjaersig, N., and Johnson, S. A. (1955a). *Amer. J. Physiol.* **181**, 589.
Seegers, W. H., Levine, W. G., and Johnson, S. A. (1955b). *J. Appl. Physiol.* **7**, 617.
Seegers, W. H., Mammen, E. F., Lee, J. M., Landaburu, R. H., Cho, M. H., Baker, W. J., and Shepard, R. S. (1959). *In* "Hemophilia and Other Hemorrhagic States" (K. M. Brinkhous, ed.), pp. 38–46. Univ. of North Carolina Press, Chapel Hill, North Carolina.
Seegers, W. H., Aoki, N., and Marciniak, E. (1962). *New Istanbul Contrib. Clin. Sci.* **5**, 170.
Seegers, W. H., Cole, E. R., Harmison, C. R., and Marciniak, E. (1963a). *Can. J. Biochem. Physiol.* **41**, 1047.
Seegers, W. H., Cole, E. R., and Aoki, N. (1963b). *Can. J. Biochem. Physiol.* **41**, 2441.
Seegers, W. H., Cole, E. R., Aoki, N., and Harmison, C. R. (1964). *Can. J. Biochem.* **42**, 229.
Seegers, W. H., Marciniak, E., and Heene, D. (1965). *Tex. Rep. Biol. Med.* **23**, 675.
Seegers, W. H., Heene, D. L., and Marciniak, E. (1966). *Thromb. Diath. Haemorrh.* **15**, 1.
Seegers, W. H., Marciniak, E., Kipfer, R. K., and Yasunaga, K. (1967). *Arch. Biochem. Biophys.* **121**, 372.
Seegers, W. H., McCoy, L., and Marciniak, E. (1968). *Clin. Chem.* **14**, 97.

Seegers, W. H., McCoy, L., Marciniak, E., and Murano, G. (1969a). *Thromb. Diath. Haemorrh.* Suppl. 36, 239.

Seegers, W. H., Murano, G., McCoy, L., and Marciniak, E. (1969b). *Life Sci.* 8, 925.

Seegers, W. H., Murano, G., and McCoy, L. (1970). *Thromb. Diath. Haemorrh.* 23, 26.

Shinowara, G. Y. (1951). *J. Lab. Clin. Med.* 38, 11.

Shinowara, G. Y. (1957). *J. Biol. Chem.* 225, 63.

Silver, M. J., Turner, D. L., Rodalewicz, I., Giordano, N., Holburn, R., Herb, S. F., and Luddy, F. E. (1963). *Thromb. Diath. Haemorrh.* 10, 164.

Solum, N. O., and Lopaciuk, S. (1969a). *Thromb. Diath. Haemorrh.* 21, 419.

Solum, N. O., and Lopaciuk, S. (1969b). *Thromb. Diath. Haemorrh.* 21, 428.

Soulier, J. P., Hallé, L., and Prou–Wartelle, O. (1968). *Thromb. Diath. Haemorrh.* 20, 121.

Stormorken, H. (1969). *Scand. J. Haematol.* Suppl. 9E 1541, 3.

Tocantins, L. M. (1938). *Medicine (Baltimore)* 17, 156.

Tocantins, L. M. (1948). *Blood* 3, 1073.

Triantaphyllopoulos, D. C., and Triantaphyllopoulos, E. (1967). *Life Sci.* 6, 601.

Triantaphyllopoulos, D. C., Brunetti, A. J., and Triantaphyllopoulos, E. (1970). *Brit. J. Haematol.* 18, 127.

Tullis, J. (1953). *Amer. J. Med. Sci.* 226, 191.

Ulutin, O. N., Mammen, E. F., and Seegers, W. H. (1961a). *Thromb. Diath. Haemorrh.* 5, 456.

Ulutin, O. N., Johnson, J. F., and Seegers, W. H. (1961b). *Amer. J. Physiol.* 201, 660.

van Creveld, S., and Mastenbroek, G. G. A. (1946). *Nature (London)* 158, 447.

van Creveld, S., and Paulssen, M. M. P. (1951). *Lancet* 2, 242.

van Creveld, S., and Paulssen, M. M. P. (1952). *Lancet* 1, 23.

Vroman, L. (1967). *In* "Blood Clotting Enzymology" (W. H. Seegers, ed.), pp. 279–322. Academic Press, New York.

Wallach, D. F. H., Maurice, P. A., Steele, B. B., and Surgenor, D. M. (1959). *J. Biol. Chem.* 234, 2829.

Ware, A. G., and Seegers, W. H. (1948). *Amer. J. Physiol.* 152, 567.

Ware, A. G., and Seegers, W. H. (1949). *Amer. J. Clin. Pathol.* 19, 471.

Ware, A. G., Fahey, J. L., and Seegers, W. H. (1948). *Amer. J. Physiol.* 154, 140.

Warner, E. D., Brinkhous, K. M., and Smith, H. P. (1936). *Amer. J. Physiol.* 114, 667.

Waugh, T. R., and Ruddick, D. W. (1944). *Can. Med. Ass. J.* 50, 547.

Weidenbauer, F., and Reichel, C. (1942). *Biochem. Z.* 311, 307.

Williams, W. J. (1969). *In* "Thrombosis" (S. Sherry *et al.*, eds.), pp. 345–354. Natl. Acad. Sci., Washington, D. C.

Youssef, A. H., and Barkhan, P. (1969). *Brit. Med. J.* 1, 394.

12

PLATELETS IN HEMOSTASIS AND THROMBOSIS*

SHIRLEY A. JOHNSON

* Supported by USPHS Project Grant HE 12121-02 and the Veterans Administration.

I. INTRODUCTION

In 1852 Jones watching "granular lymph material" collect at the site of an injury recorded this phenomenon as thrombus formation. Although Donné (1842) and Zimmerman (1845) had independently described platelets, Jones did not associate his "granular lymph material" with these bodies. It was Bizzozero (1882) who demonstrated that the deposit formed from blood at the site of the injury was made up of platelets. Hayem (1877) showed that the same type of collection of platelets formed a plug to arrest bleeding in hemostasis. It has remained for this present decade with its refined tools and techniques to describe the subtle differences between these two related phenomena, hemostasis and thrombosis. Lubnitsky (1885) by studying histological sections of developing hemostatic plugs observed single platelets cohering to each other to form irreversible aggregates. Eberth and Schimmelbusch (1886a,b) extended these studies in other mammalian species and in a wide variety of different vessels. Welch (1887) continued recording observations of these phenomena and by the end of that decade the picture of thrombus formation was complete but without detail. More meaningful data were not recorded until the elaborate and varied tools of this century came into common use in investigative laboratories. These nineteenth century investigators must have wished for the time when these phenomena would be well enough understood to be controlled.

II. INITIATION OF CHANGES IN ENVIRONMENT IN WHICH PLATELETS CIRCULATE, i.e., CHANGES IN VESSEL WALL

Under ordinary conditions platelets suspended in whole blood in a milieu of plasma, red blood cells, and white cells are not attracted to each other nor to the endothelial cells lining the blood vessels. The vascular tree is an open conducting tube with no serious obstructions. Changes in this environment cause the platelets to cohere to each other and adhere to the endothelial cells, if they are altered or injured, and to any connective tissue that may be exposed to the flowing blood. Marked atherosclerosis causes extensive changes to take place in the vessel wall. It exposes basement membrane, elastin, and collagen to elements in blood leading to formation of many platelet aggregates composed of varying amounts of fibrin and varying numbers of red and white blood cells which attach to the exposed tissue. While thrombi and hemostatic plugs are formed from constituents of the blood, the initial cause of platelet aggregation must come from changes in the vessel wall.

This is not to say that hypercoagulability brought about by elevated levels of any of the plasma procoagulants or by a decrease of the activity of the fibrinolytic mechanism does not play a part in thrombus formation. This hypercoagulability may make it possible for thrombi to form more readily, but it is most likely that changes in the endothelial cells are essential to initiate aggregation of platelets and attachment of these aggregates to the vessel wall.

Probably a smaller change in the endothelium will cause thrombi to form if the blood is hypercoagulable but the hypercoagulability alone is not likely to produce platelet aggregation. Discussions concerning the possibility that hypercoagulability alone initiates thrombosis are largely hypothetical for some atherosclerotic changes are always observed in the vessel wall in man at ages prior to those in which thrombosis is prevalent. Wessler and Yin (1969) have shown that injection of nonactivated factor X was not thrombogenic while injection of one-tenth that amount of activated factor X was thrombogenic. Probably plasma coagulation factors are activated when changes in the endothelial cells occur.

The pattern of deposition from flowing blood at orifices and bifurcations has been studied in swine by Mustard *et al.* (1961) by use of artificial systems inserted into the circulation in the carotid artery and jugular vein. The models represented an aneurysm, vessel bifurcations, and a vessel with a right-angled branch. Using these shunts it was shown that slowing or whirling and eddying of the flowing blood favors formation of platelet deposits.

Although the nature of venous thrombosis in man differs very much from arterial thrombosis, our experimental studies of ultrastructure of thrombi formed in guinea pigs due to obstruction show that small platelet aggregates form on either altered venous or arterial endothelium 4 minutes after obstructing the flow of blood. This is in agreement with Bizzozero (1882) and Wessler and Yin (1969). The dissimilarities in these two types of thrombosis are due to differences in rate of blood flow and composition of the vessel wall, not due to differences in the endothelial cells. The experimental venous thrombosis in rats produced by Ashford (1969) results in more fibrin than we see in studies on experimental arterial thrombosis which may be related to venous stasis.

It appears to us that the vessel wall must change at least enough to result in deterioration of the luminal membrane of the endothelial cells for an obstructing thrombus to form. Although some investigators believe that thrombi can form without endothelial damage, we have never observed it experimentally. Our *in vivo* experiments would lead one to believe that obstructing thrombi found in parts of blood vessels where the endothelium is normal are caused by relocation of original thrombi or by embolization.

If the changes in the vessel wall are sufficient to produce large enough platelet aggregates to obstruct the flow of blood but do not cause external bleeding, the obstruction is called a thrombus. If a gap occurs in the vessel wall so that bleeding occurs, the arrest of this bleeding by platelet aggregation is called hemostasis. Hemostasis and thrombosis are achieved by the interrelation of mechanisms of blood coagulation, platelet aggregation, accumulation of white blood cells, and clumping and hemolysis of red blood cells. Hemostasis is a physiological process of tremendous importance and thrombosis is the accidental expression of this process. The two differ in the proportion of each of these mechanisms involved and we think should not be considered to be equivalent.

Great strides have been made in our knowledge of compounds which either augment or inhibit platelet aggregation *in vitro* due to "the state of the art" in the form of the aggregometer which makes it possible to record aggregation. This instrument consists of a cuvette through which a beam of light passes and changes in the optical density can be recorded. When addition of adenosine diphosphate (ADP) to a sample of platelet-rich plasma in the cuvette brings about the aggregation of platelets, the plasma becomes clearer with large platelet clumps being moved by the stirrer and the optical density decreases. By using the instrument large numbers of compounds affecting platelet aggregation have been selected.

Unfortunately extrapolation from aggregation in citrated platelet-rich plasma to that in flowing blood *in vivo* has not been carried out with as much enthusiasm or discernment and at this time it is difficult to estimate the value of the data accumulated by the use of the aggregometer. The interaction and influence of one of the formed elements with the others in thrombus formation is very dramatic and impresses anyone studying *in vivo* thrombus formation with an electron microscope. Studies on platelet-rich plasma throw no light on this type of interaction.

On the other hand, our understanding of the surface of the luminal membrane of the healthy endothelium lining the vessels in animals and human beings has been hampered by "the state of the art." Chemists do know a great deal about nonwettable surfaces, but the gap between this knowledge and that of the lining endothelium is enormous and is still difficult to bridge. A few meaningful studies are being made (Vroman, 1967) but it is true that the contribution to be made by understanding nonwettable surfaces lies ahead of us.

The development of satisfactory artificial organs is one of the important areas in medicine hampered by our lack of basic knowledge of surfaces. Among the several approaches tried, the Dutton chamber is probably the best. This device allows the fresh unaltered blood *in vivo* to reach the foreign surface under observation. A changeable plate which constitutes part of the wall of the chamber can be removed and examined at designated intervals, to show how deposits of blood elements are built into a thrombus. When Epon plates were used it was possible to view the ultrastructure of the thrombi deposited. A granular, noncellular material which could be fibrinogen, a fibrin fragment or some unknown blood constituent always covered the surface of the Epon before platelets adhered and was considered to be the first step in thrombogenesis. Platelets deposited on top of the layer singly became aggregates and contained considerable fibrin. Fibrin strands were seen to arise from the noncellular layer and later a fibrin network formed which trapped blood cells in a fashion similar to a blood clot. The granular, noncellular layer was 200 Å thick following 2 minutes of blood flow, 400 Å thick at 8 minutes and was *necessary* for platelet adherence. Possibly adsorption of this film or layer renders the surface wettable (Dutton *et al.*, 1969).

We have known for sometime that contact with wettable surfaces initiates some platelet activities and more recently that it activates factors XI and XII (Ratnoff and Miles, 1964). It is most surprising that the only work linking contact activation of factor XII and platelets is that of Seegers *et al.* (see Chapter 11). Very little more is known about the nature of surfaces to which platelets will stick than was known 20 years ago.

III. PLATELET AGGREGATION

A. Sources of Adenosine Diphosphate Available to Bring About Aggregation of Platelets

Although many compounds may bring about platelet aggregation, components in two different vital processes, ADP and thrombin, are considered to be prime initiators. Adenosine diphosphate has been shown to be formed and released from injured endothelium, red blood cells, and the platelets themselves.

1. Release of Adenosine Diphosphate from Injured Endothelium

Honour and Mitchell (1964) suggested that the formation of "white bodies" presumed to be platelet aggregates resulting from injury to vessels on the surface of the brain in rabbits was due to release of a substance like ADP from the injured endothelium or smooth muscle. For this substance to come from the smooth muscle cells and to exert an effect on the lumen, it must have passed through or between the injured endothelium. These investigators had shown earlier that the external application of ADP to vessels which had undergone only minor injury produced platelet clumps of similar size and stability indicating that ADP could pass through the slightly injured vessel wall as well.

We chose to study thrombus formation in small (80–150 μ) mesenteric arterioles in guinea pigs under as physiological conditions as could be arranged. The vessels were pinched for 1 minute with a pair of fine forceps and the area of vessel 2 mm in length proximal to the traumatized section was studied. The injury inflicted was to the endothelium only, as not even ultrastructural changes to underlying elastin or smooth muscle cells were ever detected. The injury was not inflicted by the forceps per se but probably by the turbulent currents as blood flowed back to the bifurcations (Sawyer et al., 1953) since the vessel did not become patent again.

Four minutes following injury, ultrastructural examination revealed platelet aggregates adhering to damaged endothelial cells. The aggregates may have formed in the lumen of the vessel and then attached to the injured endothelial cells, but the platelets probably adhered individually and built up a mural thrombus in situ on the wall. Single separated platelets were observed collecting near the endothelium while free aggregates were never seen in the lumen of the vessel. Much of the endothelial cell was sloughed in 4 minutes usually leaving a thin layer of amorphous endothelium against which the platelets adhered. The elastic layer was always continuous and undisturbed and identifiable collagen has never been observed exposed to the lumen of the arteriole. Although a few fibrin fibers could be seen in each platelet aggregate there was no evidence that enough thrombin had formed to account for the many aggregated platelets observed.

We observed the proportion of adenine nucleotides to change in whole blood samples aspirated by hypodermic syringe from the thrombosing area (normal vessel ATP 0.9 μmole/ml, ADP 0.1 μmole/ml, thrombosing vessel ATP 0.5 μmole/ml, ADP 0.5 μmole/ml). To determine how ADP could be released from injured endothelial cells (Johnson, 1968) the method that Marchesi and Barrnett (1964) had used to locate ATPase activity in blood vessels performing different functions was employed. We observed the ATPase activity to be in the vesicles of the abluminal membrane of the endothelial cells in small normal mesenteric arteries. This membrane remained attached to the elastica when the endothelial cell was injured and the nucleus sloughed (Johnson *et al.*, 1969). The sloughing of a portion of the cell left these enzyme sites exposed so ATP could be broken down to ADP to initiate thrombus formation. We consider this ADP released by the injured endothelial cell to be the initiating mechanism for formation of the thrombi we have observed. This ATPase may be substrate inhibited, for when the platelets aggregate covering the injured endothelial cells no ATPase activity can be observed in these sites.

2. Release of Adenosine Diphosphate from Red Blood Cells in Hemostasis and Thrombosis

In 1960 Hellem found that adhesion of platelets to glass beads followed by aggregation of platelets as whole citrated blood was passed over a glass bead column was due to a substance "factor R" released from the red blood cells. Gaarder *et al.* (1961) showed that "factor R" was ADP. The greater part of adenine nucleotides and potential reservoir of ADP in whole blood resides in the red blood cells. In his test system Hellem found no evidence of release of ADP from the *platelets*, for passage of platelet-rich plasma over the glass bead column resulted in very little platelet adherence. Hellem *et al.* (1961) postulated that microhemolysis might be the mechanism which which provided the ADP *in vivo* in hemostasis and thrombosis.

Marr and associates (1965) identified fibrin fibers in ultrastructure in close proximity to red blood cells 15–20 seconds after transection of small mesenteric arterioles in guinea pigs. Well-developed loci of fibrin fibers were identified by the characteristic periodicity of 240 Å 30 seconds after transection of the vessel and were seen also near extravascular collagen fibers (Fig. 1).

Marr and associates also found that about 50% of the total blood ATP was broken down to ADP in the blood shed 20 seconds after transection of mesenteric arterioles in guinea pigs. The ADP appears to accumulate in shed blood for no evidence of adenosine monophosphate or adenosine was observed. The total amounts of ATP and ADP remained constant in the blood collected at different times during bleeding. These experiments show that *in vivo* under physiological conditions both ADP and thrombin appear simultaneously in the early stages of hemostasis.

We have not been able to show that adenine nucleotides (Marr *et al.*,

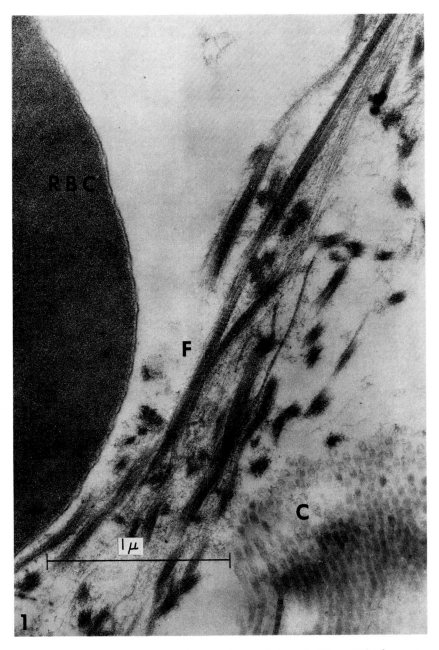

FIG. 1. Fibers of fibrin (F) showing the characteristic periodicity of 220 Å can be seen adjacent to a red blood cell (RBC) and collagen (C) 30 seconds after bleeding began in mesenteric arteriole of a guinea pig. Fixed in osmium. 52,000×.

1965) are added to the shed blood from the damaged vessel wall as was suggested by Born (1962). No difference was found between the total amount of adenine nucleotides in the plasma of shed blood in comparison with the total amount in the plasma of circulating blood sampled by heart puncture.

The quantity of ADP observed in whole shed blood exceeded that obtainable from platelets, with the result that we concluded that much of it must be of red blood cell origin. We considered it of great significance that most of the fibrin observed in the early stages of hemostasis was in close proximity to red blood cells. On the basis of these two observations, we postulated that both the newly evolved ADP and the partial thromboplastin of red blood cells may contribute substantially to the initiation of hemostasis. The known physiologic mechanism that could most likely account for the release of these two substances from red blood cells was hemolysis.

Some red blood cells in an *in vivo* hemostatic plug fixed 1 minute after transection of a small mesenteric arteriole in a guinea pig were found to display reduced electron density when they were compared with normal circulating red blood cells (Table I). Hemolysis was quantitated biochemically in circulating blood drawn by heart puncture (hemoglobin, mean 5.1 ± 1.1 mg/100 ml) and in blood shed (hemoglobin, mean 11.4 ± 4.6 mg/100 ml) from transected mesenteric arterioles, and it was established that hemoglobin was higher in the plasma of shed blood (Fig. 2). Since hemolysis does occur it probably is the mechanism whereby both ADP and partial thromboplastin are released from red blood cells in the initial stages of hemostasis (Pederson *et al.*, 1967).

Rorvick *et al.* (1968) showed that the adenine nucleotides released in the blood after passing through the glass bead column were related to hemolysis of the red blood cells.

TABLE I

NUMBER OF HEMOLYZED RED BLOOD CELLS COUNTED WITH THE ELECTRON MICROSCOPE

Type of red blood cell specimen	No. counted	No. hemolyzed	Hemolysis (%)
In vivo plug	1073	1059	98.69
In 0.35% saline	1145	1122	97.99
In 0.9% saline	1371	21	1.53

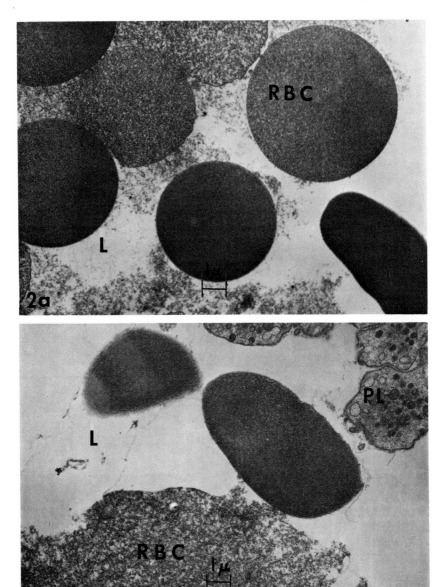

FIG. 2. (a) Swelling and reduction of electron density of red blood cells (RBC) shows hemolysis has taken place one minute after bleeding began within the lumen (L) of a mesenteric vessel in a guinea pig. Fixed in osmium. 6620×. (b) Two intact red blood cells approaching hemolyzed red blood cells (RBC). A platelet (PL) aggregate can also be seen. Fixed in osmium. 7100×.

Throughout the remainder of this chapter the ADP released from the vessel wall and from red blood cells shall be called exogenous ADP.

Harrison and Mitchell (1966) showed that platelet adhesiveness as measured by the rotating-glass-bulb method depends upon the liberation of ADP from mechanically damaged erythrocytes. When ADP was removed by enzymic phosphorylation the level of whole blood adhesiveness was reduced to that of platelet-rich plasma. Mechanically damaged red cells produce a greater increase in platelet adhesiveness measured in platelet-rich citrated plasma than do quantities of intact erythrocytes. The mechanical damage the erythrocytes underwent was evaluated by measurement of the rise of plasma potassium during rotation of whole blood in the glass flasks.

3. Release of Adenosine Diphosphate from Platelets in Hemostasis and Thrombosis

In 1966 Macmillan showed that small amounts of exogenous ADP aggregated a few of the platelets in a specimen of platelet-rich plasma. Sometime later the remainder of the platelets clumped. This secondary wave of clumping was considered to be due to release of what we call endogenous ADP from the few platelets which aggregated initially. Addition to platelet-rich plasma of adrenalin and thrombin in low concentrations also produced secondary aggregation (O'Brien, 1966).

The details of platelet aggregation are discussed in Chapter 6 by Nachman, but the relationships of the sources on ADP will be dealt with here. Although the ADP of platelets must play a significant role in hemostasis and thrombosis our present knowledge indicates that it cannot be responsible for the initiation of aggregation. Clearly some platelets must aggregate before ADP is released. Endogenous ADP cannot initiate thrombus formation. Some inhibitors of platelet aggregation are effective against both exogenous and endogenous ADP such as pyridazine, an antiinflammatory agent, while others, of which acetylsalicylic acid is an example, inhibit only release of endogenous ADP. Many *in vivo* animal experiments must be done before it can be established which type of inhibitor is the most effective antithrombotic agent.

B. Platelet Aggregation Brought About by Thrombin

It has been known since 1956 that platelets aggregate when in contact with thrombin (Lüscher, 1956b; Bounameaux, 1956). These investigators continued to use an historic term, viscous metamorphosis, to describe the whole process of platelet aggregation, disintegration, and clot retraction. The term viscous metamorphosis had a use when these processes were viewed as a whole either by the naked eye or the light microscope. Our knowledge of biochemistry and of electron microscopy has made it possible to describe platelet aggregation in much greater detail and has expanded our knowledge of these processes enormously so the term viscous metamorphosis no longer has meaning and is better forgotten. While once aggregation and retraction were considered under this all encompassing heading we now feel that platelet aggregation is a necessary preliminary step to clot retraction and that studies of one usually shed little light on the other. What was once a single mechanism has expanded into at least twenty separate areas such as platelet membrane changes, energy relationships of ADP, platelet degranulation, and evolution of thrombin.

In 1959 M. B. Zucker and Borrelli expanded the studies on the role of thrombin in platelet aggregation. Mustard *et al.* (1964) found that addition of 3 units/ml of thrombin to platelet-rich plasma caused platelet aggregation *several minutes* after addition of thrombin. Gross coagulation took place later. This thrombin was a commercial product containing many impurities. We have observed (Webber and Johnson, 1970) that changes in the platelets take place 3 *seconds* after addition of purified thrombin (courtesy of Seegers) to human platelet-rich plasma (Figs. 3–6). Ultrastructural examination of the platelets at this time shows formation and extrusion of membranes which have formed from electron dense α granules. These same changes are observed *in vivo* in platelets approaching a hemostatic area in a bleeding blood vessel and are discussed at some length elsewhere in this chapter (see Section III,C). Fibrin can also be seen in this area 1 minute after bleeding begins. One important characteristic of platelet aggregation induced by thrombin is its irreversibility (Roskam, 1963; Johnson *et al.*, 1965).

In 1966 Marr *et al.* showed that degradation of ATP to ADP in whole blood initiated by the injured arterial wall is completely inhibited when the mechanisms of coagulation are depressed by EDTA or heparin. In a different experimental model, Horowitz and Papayoanou (1968) presented some evidence that ADP brought about activation of platelet factor 3. It does not appear to be possible to explore this relationship between activation of the coagulation mechanisms and breakdown of ATP further at this stage of our knowledge but the two processes seem to be connected.

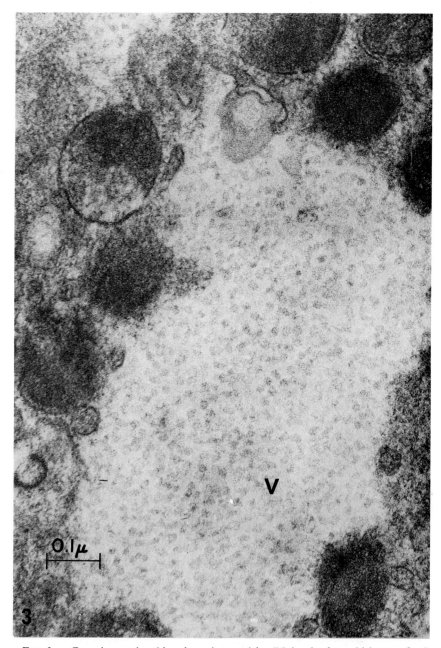

FIG. 3. *a* Granules are breaking down into vesicles (V) in platelets which were fixed with glutaraldehyde 3 seconds after the addition of thrombin. No aggregation has taken place in this platelet-rich plasma which was being stirred in the aggregometer. This is the *first stage* in release of platelet factor 3. 150,000×.

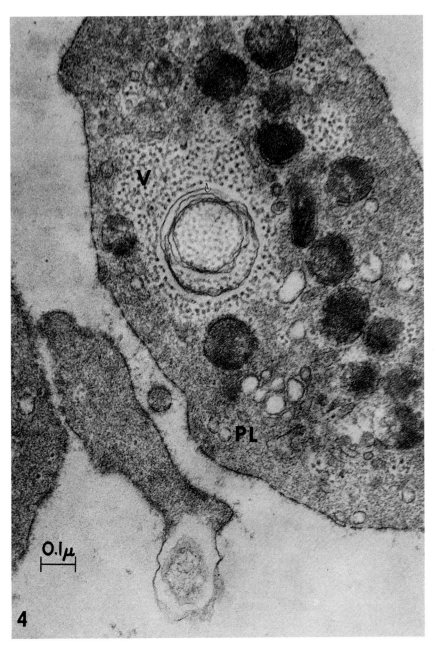

FIG. 4. Concentric rings of membrane form from vesicles (V) in the *second stage* in plaelets (PL) *in vitro*. The platelet-rich plasma was fixed with glutaraldehyde 3 seconds after the addition of thrombin. No aggregation had taken place. 110,000×.

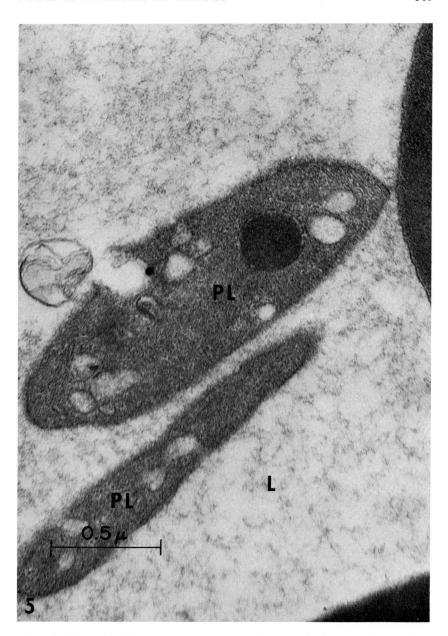

Fɪɢ. 5. The vesicle filled area becomes a vacuole bounded with a membrane. Then the membrane complex moves to surface and is extruded in *stage three*. This electron micrograph is taken from a section of mesenteric arteriole fixed with glutaraldehyde 1 minute after bleeding began. These platelets (PL) are approaching the hemostatic area but have not aggregated. L, lumen. 60,000×.

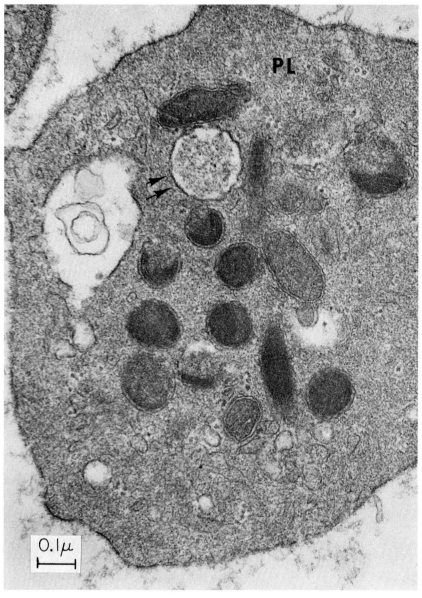

FIG. 6. The vacuoles refill from platelet cytoplasm (see arrows) becoming α granules which are regenerated in *stage four*. By this mechanism, platelet factor 3 can be released without apparent loss of α granules. The freshly aggregated platelets contain the same number of α granules that circulating platelets possess. The platelet (PL) was fixed with glutaraldehyde 3 seconds after thrombin was added *in vitro*. Addition of ADP does not produce any more membrane mechanisms than stirring alone. 75,000×.

C. Inhibitors of Platelet Aggregation

Much work has been carried out testing inhibitors of platelet aggregation induced by ADP in platelet-rich plasma or washed platelets *in vitro*. Very little has been done to ascertain whether or not these same inhibitors are effective antithrombogenic agents *in vivo*. Born (1964) evaluated 2-chloro-adenosine in an ideal experimental design involving *in vitro* and *in vivo* experiments. While this drug prevented aggregation of platelets by ADP it was extremely toxic.

IV. ACTIVATION OF PLASMA PROTHROMBIN

A. Release of Tissue Thromboplastin to Participate in Coagulation Mechanisms

We have observed much more fibrin in hemostatic plugs when all the layers in the vessel wall have been transected than in experimental thrombi resulting from injury to the endothelium only. Other investigators (H. D. Zucker, 1949; Hovig, 1963; Mustard *et al.*, 1967) have not seen fibrin fibers so early in hemostatic plugs but in their experiments the bleeding end of the vessel has been washed with Ringer's solution removing or diluting the thrombin as it is formed. Small fibrin fibers probably were rinsed away as soon as they formed as well as thrombin. To prevent excessive dehydration, since the bleeding vessels were not immersed in solution in our experiments, we used lower illumination of the experimental area which made it necessary to select larger vessels (80–150 μ in diameter). When smaller vessels (30–50 μ) were selected for study (Hovig, 1963) the hemostatic plug was observed to be composed of platelet aggregates primarily, while in the larger vessels studied in our laboratory, fibrin, red blood cells, and platelet aggregates combine to achieve hemostasis.

The fact that more fibrin is found in hemostatic plugs when all layers of the vessel wall were exposed (Marr *et al.*, 1965) than when only the endothelial cells were damaged (Johnson, 1966) raises the possibility that the layers of the wall external to endothelium contained more thromboplastin activity. Kwaan (1969) using fluorescein-tagged antihuman fibrinogen serum was able to show, in human blood vessels collected at autopsy examination within 6 hours of death, that the smooth muscle cells in the arterial wall contain more thromboplastin activity than other vascular tissue. This work shows that one can expect to find less fibrin in platelet aggregates

when the smooth muscle layer of the vessel wall remains intact and un-
exposed to flowing blood. We have no evidence that thromboplastic materials penetrate intact endothelium to enter the lumen.

B. Appearance of Partial Thromboplastin

We had observed that the electron density of the red blood cells varied
enormously in hemostatic areas (Johnson et al., 1965) and had shown that
these cells were hemolyzing. Much earlier Shinowara (1951) had described
the thromboplastin cell component (TCC) of erythrocytes, later called
erythrocytin by Quick et al. (1954) as a partial thromboplastin which with
the antihemophilic factor is a potent activator of prothrombin to thrombin.
Release of this material by hemolyzing red blood cells in vivo would result
in precipitous activation of the coagulation mechanisms.

Our work suggests that both ADP and the partial thromboplastin of red
cells are released in quantity as the red blood cells hemolyze. The fact that
the fibrin fibers observed early in hemostatic plug formation were long,
individual unattached fibers located near red blood cells lends credence to
these findings. This fibrin, which was found immediately adjacent to the
red blood cells was probably formed by activation of prothrombin to
thrombin by the released partial thromboplastin. When the rate of thrombin
formation was sufficiently rapid to overwhelm the antithrombins plasma
fibrinogen could be converted to fibrin locally.

C. Release of Platelet Factor 3

Proximal to the hemostatic area many single platelets are seen collected
in the lumen. Many of these platelets possess a structure of concentric
membranes extruding from the platelet into the plasma. The α granules so
labeled by Schulz et al. (1958) and Rodman et al. (1962) can be seen
disintegrating into a collection of vesicles often mistaken for storage
glycogen. The vesicles then form the membranous structure which is
released (Figs. 3–6). This membrane release, although it does take place
in some platelets in aggregates, is maximal in the platelets approaching
the hemostatic area. Apparently enough thrombin can accumulate in the
vessel proximal to the injury to initiate release of platelet material and to
convert fibrinogen to fibrin. This membrane formation resembles what is
seen when purified thrombin (courtesy of Seegers) is added to a suspension
of platelet-rich plasma in vitro. Addition of ADP does not result in any
more membrane formation than stirring alone. We believe that this release

of membranes formed from the α granules represents release of platelet factor 3. White and Krivit (1966) showed release of lipid micelles from platelets in platelet-rich plasma which probably represents one stage of this release of membranes.

Because freshly aggregated platelets contain many granules, organelles and vesicles which disappear later we have always considered that the α granules containing platelet factor 3 were released after aggregation (Fig. 7). Other workers studying the release phenomenon (release of serotonin, ADP, and platelet factor 3) have agreed. We have recently shown (Webber and Johnson, 1970) that the α granules are reproduced in the empty vacuoles. The cytoplasmic material increases in electron density until the α granules are completed. There is no evidence that α granules in platelets decrease markedly in number until some seconds after aggregation so these granules must be regenerated constantly. The number at any given moment represents a balance between those α granules forming membranes and those new ones being created rather than the original complement of granules enclosed in the platelet as it left the megakaryocyte. This new concept emphasizes the activity which is going on in the circulating platelet. A platelet can no longer be considered to be a static cell circulating unchanged until it performs its prime function once but rather a dynamic structure able to regenerate some of the hemostatic materials from within itself.

After aggregation, degranulation continues and the limiting membranes disintegrate and disappear (Fig. 8). By the time the bleeding has stopped we estimate that more than half the platelets which were involved in the hemostatic process have contributed their contents and disappeared. The remaining ones have been built into the hemostatic plug. Whether a particular population of platelets, such as the old ones, disintegrates, or whether the disintegration is a random process determined by the location of the circulating platelet near the hemostatic plug is not known.

Castaldi et al. (1962) observed bridgelike processes crossing the interval between adjacent platelets in aggregates formed by adding calcium to platelet-rich plasma. Johnson et al. (1965) noted that the spaces between platelets are not consistently empty in hemostatic plugs formed during 1 minute of bleeding after transection of a mesenteric vessel in a guinea pig (Fig. 9). They also noted alternate areas of electron density between the platelets and suggest that they represent an early stage in fibrin formation, for by 3 minutes these areas contain fibrin. Hovig (1969), and independently Shirasawa and Chandler (1969), describe the same bridgelike processes in platelet aggregates induced by addition of ADP to native blood. Hovig likens them to aggregation of polystyrene particles suspended in fibrinogen.

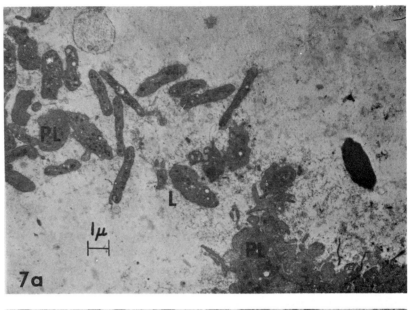

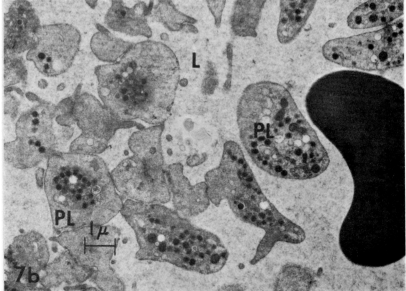

FIG. 7. (a) Platelets (PL). The shape of the platelets can be seen to change from discoid to spherical as they approach the hemostatic plug in a mesenteric arteriole. Fixed with glutaraldehyde 1 minute after bleeding began. L, lumen. 6000×. (b) Early aggregation of platelets can be seen in a mesenteric vessel fixed with glutaraldehyde 1 minute after bleeding began. 8600×.

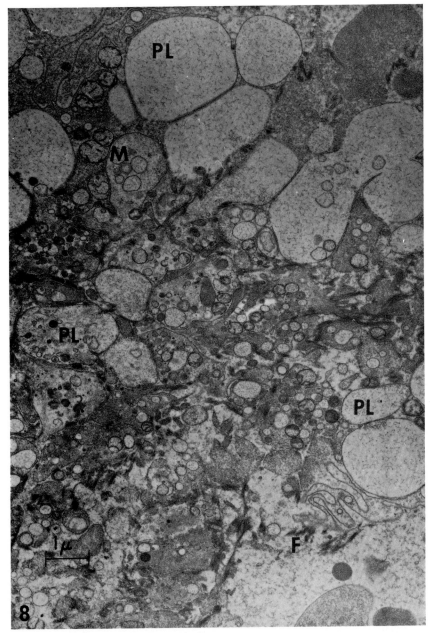

FIG. 8. Platelet aggregate showing many empty platelets (PL) with disintegrated membranes (M) in a part of the hemostatic plug where platelets have been aggregated longest. This mesenteric arteriole in the guinea pig was fixed with glutaraldehyde 1 minute after bleeding began. F, fibrin. 12,000×.

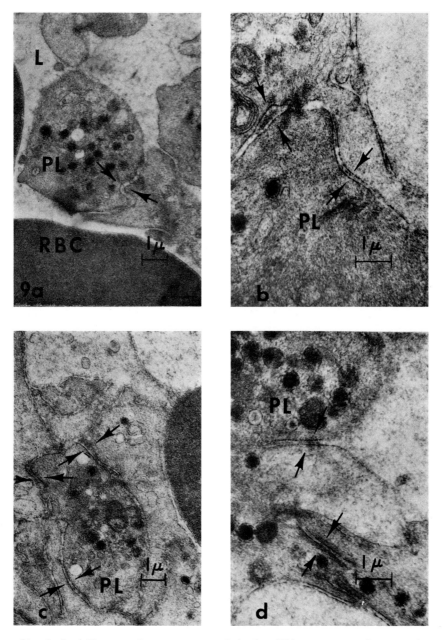

FIG. 9. (a–c) The spaces between aggregated platelets (PL) are not empty (see arrows). The material seen does not usually exhibit the periodicity of fibrin although it probably is fibrin. (d) However, shows characteristic periodicity of fibrin (see arrows). L, lumen (a) 700 × ; (b) 9500 × ; (c) 7000 × ; (d) 9500 × .

A material coating the particles appears to bridge the gap between aggregated particles. All evidence points to the possibility of a product of the blood coagulation mechanisms located in the space between platelets in aggregates.

Clinical observations of patients have led to some general evaluations of bleeding. Any one of the clotting factors or the number of platelets can be reduced to about 50% of the normal without obvious impairment of hemostatic efficiency even after major injury. At 25% of the normal the individual would not be expected to show signs of abnormal bleeding from minor injuries, but extensive trauma or major surgery might lead to serious bleeding. At 10% of the normal, trouble from even minor injuries is likely to occur. The effect of two or more deficiencies combined is much greater than the effect of a deficiency of similar magnitude of one alone (Jaques, 1962).

D. Dissolution of Platelet Thrombi

When aggregation of platelets is induced by ADP *only*, disaggregation may follow. Some years ago we observed a much greater drop in platelet count in rabbits and guinea pigs when infusion of ADP was carried out than when physiological saline was given. After the infusion was discontinued the platelet count returned to normal over a 2-hour period (Johnson, 1965). We concluded that the infusion of ADP resulted in formation of platelet aggregates which were sequestered in the capillary bed. Chandler and Nordoy (1964) showed that on infusion of low concentrations of ADP in the rat, thrombi found on autopsy in capillaries and arterioles of the lung were unstable. It is now clear that aggregation of platelets induced by ADP alone is reversible. Platelet aggregation induced by thrombin is always irreversible. It has been our observation that *in vivo* aggregation of platelets in hemostasis is induced by both ADP and thrombin at the same time, so disaggregation probably is not important. When platelet thrombi are formed, much less fibrin is seen if only the endothelium is damaged so here disaggregation may take place. We have always found at least one fibrin fiber in each small thrombus indicating that some thrombin was formed rapidly as the platelets aggregated.

E. Clot Retraction *in Vivo*

Bettex-Galland and Lüscher in 1959 discovered that platelets contain a contractile protein (thrombosthenin) with activity related to the breakdown of ATP by ADP (Waller *et al.*, 1959). Clot retraction is dependent on glycolytic activity (Lüscher, 1956a; Bettex-Galland and Lüscher, 1959) and the initiation of the mechanism appears to depend on platelet aggregation which in the physiological state is probably triggered by thrombin. As might be expected, clot retraction is inhibited by agents that poison or inhibit platelet aggregation. Although something is known of how clot retraction takes place *in vitro* in platelet-rich plasma, no one has attempted to apply these findings to *in vivo* hemostasis or thrombosis.

V. DESCRIPTION OF CHANGES IN THE VESSEL WALL THAT INITIATE PLATELET AGGREGATION

A. Injured Endothelium

While the blood cells play vital roles in thrombus formation because of their large numbers and proximity to the prethrombotic area, they cannot be responsible for the initial change in the environment. This change must come from the vessel wall (Johnson, 1966). Thrombi formed 4 minutes after slight injury to the endothelium caused by turbulent blood flow do contain a few fibrin fibers but not enough to suggest that much thrombin has formed from plasma prothrombin to be responsible for the platelet aggregation (Johnson, 1968). Much less thrombin is required to aggregate platelets than to convert fibrinogen to fibrin, but the presence of much thrombin in the plasma as thrombi form would result in considerable fibrin formation which is easily identifiable in ultrastructure.

Even very serious efforts by Altschul (1954) revealed little evidence that the proliferation of endothelial cells lining the blood vessels took place in the adult. This means that extensive damage to the endothelial cells caused by turbulent blood or trauma could only be repaired with difficulty. This is probably the main reason why thrombosis is such a problem today, since man's life-span has been extended so dramatically. Perhaps some genetic change will take place to meet the extended longevity resulting in an increase in the rate of reproduction of endothelial cells. The large number of vitally important functions performed by the vascular endothelium have been described by Majno (1965). Of these our work shows that the endothelial supportive function of platelets whereby platelets interact with the endothelial cells is the main source of nourishment for endothelial cells thus contributing enormously to their health and extended life (Johnson *et al.*, 1964; Van Horn and Johnson, 1966, 1968; Wojcik *et al.* 1970).

On injury much of the endothelial cell can be sloughed without exposing basement membrane, elastin, or collagen fibers to the blood. We (1966) have observed mural platelet thrombi to form on the injured endothelium within several minutes of the injury. Poole *et al.* (1963) also observed this in one of the most thoughtful investigations of thrombus formation carried out using modern techniques. MacFarlane (1968) lists surfaces such as glass, metals, fabrics, bacteria, particles of carbon, latex, damaged endothelium, and connective tissue to which platelets will adhere. An amorphous area of cytoplasm is usually what remains of the endothelial cell after part is sloughed. Such injury produced experimentally or pathologically results in marked loss of cellular detail of the cell when observed in ultrastructure. Although most published electron micrographs of injured blood vessels show much less detail than normal tissue amorphous endothelial cytoplasm is usually visible.

Baumgartner *et al.* (1967) interpreting their own electron micrographs state that there is no evidence of any part of endothelial cells remaining after the injury as the endothelial cells migrate from their moorings. They feel that the basement membrane is always exposed and that the platelets will adhere only to the basement membrane and not to injured endothelial cells. The free endothelial cells observed in the plasma by Spaet and Gaynor (1970) are not intact and no membranes are visible so it is difficult to determine whether the abluminal membrane of the endothelial cell remains adhering to the basement membrane or is a part of the detached endothelial cell.

Tranzer and Baumgartner (1967) stretched blood vessels producing gaps between the endothelial cells which were filled by single platelets adhering to the basement membrane. These platelets remain unchanged morphologically: No degranulation or platelet membrane disintegration is observed, as is characteristic of platelet aggregation in thrombi. When the vessel resumed its normal size the adherence was reversible and the platelet moved back into the circulating plasma. Spaet and Gaynor (1970) state that platelets adhering to basement membrane never degranulate. When all the evidence is weighed we believe that platelets will adhere and aggregate on injured endothelium and on all types of connective tissue in the vessel wall.

B. Basement Membrane

Basement membrane, consisting of a subendothelial layer, the *lamina rara*, an adjacent layer, the *lamina densa*, and a fuzzy outer layer, the *zona diffusa*, was shown by Lazarow and Speidel (1964) to have collagen as its principal protein. They observed that collagenase hydrolyzed glomerular basement membrane completely and that tritium-labeled proline was incorporated into basement membrane of the glomerulus in amounts equivalent to that incorporated into collagen fibers. Dische (1964) showed that the lens capsule, much of which is basement membrane, is made up of 80% dry weight of a collagenlike protein which is linked to a glycan consisting of glucose and galactose but not hexosamine. Compared to the other types of connective tissues, basement membrane is characterized by a lower degree of organization. From our ultrastructural investigation of exposure of vascular connective tissue to formed elements of the blood we conclude that basement membrane is less thrombogenic than other connective tissue.

C. Location of Synthesis of Connective Tissue

Fibroblasts synthesize only collagen and elastin. The polyribosomes of the rough endoplasmic reticulum furnish the site of synthesis and sequestration of exportable proteins in these cells. The proteins complexed with the polysaccharide as in cartilage are passed to the Golgi region while the collagen proteins move directly out of the cell either by release from vesicles or from spaces communicating with the rough endoplasmic reticulum. Once outside the fibroblast, collagen or elastin molecules aggregate into fibrils, so the smaller fibrils are considered to be most recently extruded (Ross, 1967). Collagen is the component of connective tissue most readily identified in ultrastructure by the characteristic periodicity of 640 Å. According to Ross and Benditt (1965) extracellular collagen fibrils must be more than 100 Å in diameter to display this periodicity.

It has been suggested that smooth muscle cells are also associated with formation of collagen, elastic fibers, and basement membrane for in the blood vessel wall these connective tissues surround smooth muscle cells. The vascular endothelium is also implicated in basement membrane synthesis, largely on the basis of proximity.

D. Collagen

1. RELATIONSHIP TO PLATELETS

It was Hugues (1960) who first suggested that platelets adhere to connective tissue. M. B. Zucker and Borrelli (1962) described the aggregating effect of suspensions of connective tissues on platelets *in vitro*. Hovig using electron microscopy identified the particles in the suspensions of connective tissue responsible for platelet adherence to be collagen fibrils on the basis of the characteristic periodicity. These observations have been interpreted to mean that platelets adhere specifically to collagen. Of the components of vascular connective tissue striated collagen is especially easy to identify in ultrastructure on the basis of the periodicity in contrast to structureless components such as elastin and basement membrane. We have observed platelets to adhere to striated collagen as well as to these other not easily identifiable components of connective tissues. It is impossible to identify and locate elastin and basement membrane in the vessel wall once they are dislocated either by injury, disease, or by migrating red and white blood cells.

Collagenase is often used to establish the specificity of the protein collagen in any component of connective tissue and its specificity is dependent on a peptide structure with proline as the imine and one of several other amino acids providing the carboxyl group (Eastoe, 1967).

Although investigators of the mechanisms of hemostasis and thrombosis are extremely interested in the relationship of platelets to connective tissue, the literature on connective tissue contains no references to this phenomenon (Ramachandran, 1967). Eastoe (1967) states that the protein collagen is made up largely of glycine, alanine, proline, and hydroxyproline; the presence in quantity of the latter two amino acids being characteristic of all connective tissue (Juva, 1967). Collagen fibers contain essentially no carbohydrate. However, Luft (1965) has found a thin layer of acid mucopolysaccharide around collagen fibrils *in vivo* exhibiting an intimate relationship between proteins, polysaccharides and fibrous proteins. It is possible that all living cells are surrounded by this layer so platelet adherence to a structure may be due to an interruption in the acid mucopolysaccharide layer rather than to particular characteristics of the individual components. The proteins making up elastin, collagen, and basement membrane have essentially the same composition.

Mustard *et al.* (1967) observed that a group of compounds with anti-inflammatory action (pyrazole compounds such as butazolidin and anturan) prolonged platelet survival, reduced platelet turnover by 50%, and suppressed the platelet–collagen reaction when given to humans and animals. These compounds did not inhibit aggregation of platelets by ADP.

In addition to attraction for platelets, collagen initiates blood coagulation by activation of factor XII (Niewiarowski, 1967). When in contact with red blood cells, collagen acts as a foreign surface bringing about hemolysis facilitating the release of ADP and partial thromboplastin from the red blood cells into the hemostatic and thrombosing areas (Johnson, 1966).

Elastins (Eastoe, 1967) contain less hydroxyproline, are very different in ultrastructure with globular units of 200 Å in diameter containing lucent centers, and possess remarkable hydrothermal stability.

There is a complete disassociation between the particular groups on collagen that affect platelet aggregation and Hageman factor. For activation of Hageman factor the negatively charged acidic groups such as carboxyl groups of glutamic and aspartic acids are critical but do not seem to be involved in platelet aggregation. The positively charged ε amino groups of lysine appear to be necessary for platelets to aggregate on collagen but they do not influence Hageman factor activation (Wilner et al., 1968).

2. Relation and Content of Hydroxyproline in Collagen, Elastin, and Basement Membrane in Walls of Blood Vessels

Although there is conclusive evidence to show that platelets adhere to all components of connective tissue when they escape through breaks in the endothelial barrier, it is not known what characteristic of connective tissue attracts platelets. Because of the problem of harvesting large enough quantities of basement membrane, elastin, and collagen from the walls of arterioles and venules, we carried out quantitative chemical studies on extravascular connective tissue. To compare the uptake and oxidation of proline to hydroxyproline in collagen fibers, elastin fibers, and basement membrane located in the walls of blood vessels, we injected tritium-labeled proline intraperitoneally into 10-day-old guinea pigs (Johnson et al., 1969). It is believed by Juva (1967) that the peptide-bound proline is hydroxylated sequentially at suitable sites when the peptide chain grows to sufficient length. It is necessary to inject labeled proline and not hydroxyproline because free hydroxyproline is not incorporated into the collagen protein.

Animals were sacrificed 24 hours, 3, 6, and 9 days later and electron autoradiographs (Kopriwa, 1967) of ultrathin sections of mesenteric vessels were prepared.

On the basis of geometry of the preparation and the range distribution of tritium particles, Caro (1964) predicts that 90% of the tracks will be located on the labeled tissue or within 0.13 μ of it. We were able to confirm the findings of Lazarow and Speidel (1964) locating the tracks in basement membrane, epithelium, and lumen of capillaries in the glomeruli.

The number of tracks in blood vessels should be reported per unit area because the area of basement membrane, elastin, and collagen vary so much. After these areas were measured by planimetry, we decided it was impossible to separate basement membrane in blood vessels from elastin accurately so we used the term elastin complex to include both elastin and basement membrane. Statistical analyses show that the number of tracks was significantly higher in the elastin complex, 31.7, than in the adjacent structures of endothelium, 12.3, or smooth muscle, 8.1. The label is clearly concentrated in the elastin complex and in collagen fibers. The number of grains was just significantly higher in the elastin complex, 31.7, than in identifiable striated collagen, 24.3 ($P < 0.05$). If the property of collagen fibers, which is responsible for platelet adherence, is the characterizing protein-containing hydroxyproline, then platelets may be expected to adhere to exposed elastin and basement membrane as readily as they adhere to collagen fibers.

The data both in the literature and in our study point to the striking similarity in location of synthesis of hydroxyproline and in the chemistry of collagen, elastin fibers, and basement membrane. Our own observations in hemostasis and thrombosis *in vivo* are in agreement with this for we observe platelets to adhere to any component of exposed connective tissue as well as to injured endothelium when they come in contact with them (Fig. 10).

VI. SEQUENCE OF EVENTS

A. Hemostasis

By definition hemostasis is the arrest of bleeding when all cellular layers of the vessel wall are ruptured and blood escapes from the lumen through the gap to the interstitial spaces. The formed elements, red and white blood cells and platelets brush against tissue not normally exposed to them such as connective tissue (basement membrane, elastin, and collagen) and materials such as thromboplastins normally held within the tissue cells. By the time these formed elements have been shed outside the vessel wall they have come in contact with the changed surfaces classically called foreign surfaces and the hemostatic mechanisms are activated.

Fifteen seconds after bleeding begins we have identified (Fig. 1) in ultrastructure long fibrin fibers on the basis of the characteristic periodicity of 240 Å. Because this early fibrin is always seen adjacent to red blood cells we have concluded that when these cells contact the changed surface of the injured vessel hemolysis takes place. This hemolysis could release the ADP which was converted from triphosphate and the partial thromboplastin of the erythrocyte.

The hemophilic factors in plasma interact with the partial thromboplastin

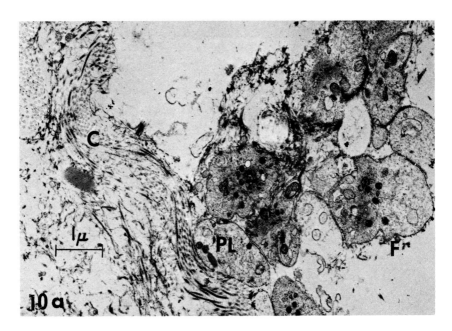

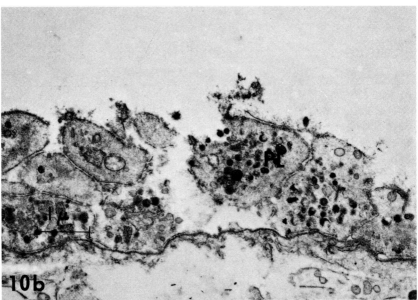

FIG. 10. (a) Platelets (PL) can be seen aggregating against collagen (C) 20 seconds after the vessel was transected. Fibrin (F) is visible intermixed with platelets. 12,500×. (b) Platelets (PL) aggregating against a structure that does not appear to be collagen outside the vessel. 15,400×.

to activate plasma prothrombin to thrombin responsible for the conversion of the fibrinogen to fibrin adjacent to red blood cells.

The concentration of the released ADP and newly formed thrombin both of which bring about aggregation of platelets is built up steadily. Platelets flow into this area and aggregation begins. The first aggregates to form are small and some attach to the damaged lip of the vessel while some are free in the lumen as the concentration of these aggregating agents increases in the plasma. These platelets in newly formed aggregates contain many granules. The space between the platelets seems clear and empty with little or no evidence of fibrin between the platelets.

By 20 *seconds* about half the total ATP of whole blood has been changed to ADP (Marr *et al.*, 1965). Since these determinations of adenine nucleotides were carried out on native whole blood we do not know whether the ADP is of red blood cell or platelet origin. We showed (Johnson *et al.*, 1967) that 90% of the adenine nucleotides of whole blood is in the red blood cells.

Thirty seconds after bleeding begins very extensive platelet aggregation has taken place. The hemostatic area has a high concentration of ADP and thrombin and all of the platelets flowing into this turbulent area are drawn into aggregates.

Much more fibrin is seen due to release of tissue thromboplastin from the exposed smooth muscle as Kwaan (1969) has shown. Interstitial collagen fibers are exposed and dislocated and are frequently seen adjacent to fibrin fibers. The plasma prothrombin was probably activated to thrombin by the changes in plasma factor XII as it came in contact with collagen as Niewiarowski suggested (1967).

After 1 *minute* of bleeding, confluence of many of the fibrin loci has taken place. The rate of thrombin formation must have been high to convert so much fibrinogen to fibrin. Many red blood cells have clumped against the external aspects of the vessel wall, the cells are swollen and spherical, and have little electron density indicating that much of the hemoglobin has been lost by hemolysis.

The space between the aggregated platelets is no longer empty; opaque areas have appeared that are probably fibrin although no characterizing periodicity is seen (Fig. 9). The platelet aggregates are very large and fall into two different types, the random type and rosette type. The random type of aggregate is made up of platelets with and without granules arranged in a random fashion. It has been stated by Hovig (1963) that ADP-induced aggregation is followed immediately by degranulation. Our observations have led us to conclude that degranulation is a function of time and that *in vivo* aggregates observed 1 minute after bleeding begins contain many degranulated platelets while those seen 15 seconds after contain very few.

The second type of aggregate is the rosette form. The platelets in the center of the rosette are intact, containing α granules and are surrounded by concentric rings of empty platelets. It is not known what stimulus is present on the periphery of the aggregate. Perhaps the aggregates form so fast that those platelets at the center are isolated very rapidly from the environment as others surround them (Johnson *et al.*, 1967) before degranulation is complete.

By 3 minutes when bleeding stops and hemostasis has been achieved, the hemostatic capsule consisting mostly of platelets in capillaries but of platelets, fibrin, and red blood cells in small arterioles has completely sealed the gap in the wall of the vessel. The events described above lead to the arrest of bleeding in 3–5 minutes and give a progressive picture of the dynamics of the conventional bleeding time test.

FORMATION OF THE FIBRIN NETWORK

The first fibrin fibers identified in the hemostatic area are unattached to any cells or formed elements, but after 1 minute of bleeding fibrin fibers emanate from platelet aggregates to ensnare red blood cells. By 3 minutes the fibrin fibers have come together in cords made up of several fibers and form a network which entraps red blood cells. Many platelets in aggregates have disintegrated but some remain as a nucleus or focal point for the fibrin network (Johnson *et al.*, 1967). This platelet, fibrin, and red blood cell structure is firmly attached to the outside of the arterial wall to encapsulate the severed end of the vessel and appears to be the mechanism whereby hemostasis was achieved in bleeding arterioles varying from 80–150 μ in diameter. The forces and controls that cause the isolated fibrin fibers to form a network have not been studied and the uncovering of them may lead to our understanding of what appear today to be nonspecific bleeding disorders due to weak fibrin clots (Fig. 11). A schema summarizing the hemostatic mechanisms appears in Fig. 12.

B. Thrombosis

How the traumatized cells in the vessel wall transfer the stimuli to the lumen of the vessel thus altering the formed elements and plasma to form thrombi is not known. Shimamoto and Ishioka (1963) describe how adrenaline triggers release of tissue thromboplastic activity into the lumen of

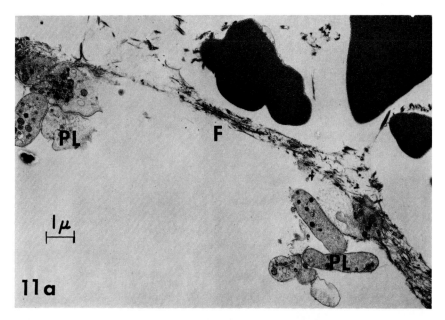

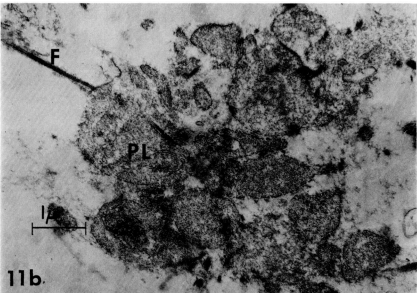

FIG. 11. (a) Fibrin (F) network beginning to form in hemostatic plug 20–40 seconds after initiation of bleeding. The fibrin cords are emanating from small platelet (PL) aggregates which later comprise a network to entrap red blood cells. 7300×. (b) Fibrin (F) fiber emanating from platelet (PL) aggregate 1 minute after bleeding began. Note periodicity of fibrin. 14,500×.

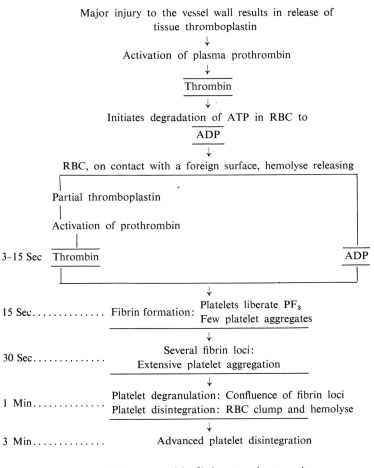

Major injury to the vessel wall results in release of
tissue thromboplastin
↓
Activation of plasma prothrombin
↓
Thrombin
↓
Initiates degradation of ATP in RBC to
ADP
↓
RBC, on contact with a foreign surface, hemolyse releasing

Partial thromboplastin

Activation of prothrombin

3–15 Sec   Thrombin   ADP

↓

15 Sec.............. Fibrin formation: Platelets liberate PF₃
                                       Few platelet aggregates

↓

30 Sec..............   Several fibrin loci:
                     Extensive platelet aggregation

↓

1 Min.............. Platelet degranulation: Confluence of fibrin loci
                     Platelet disintegration: RBC clump and hemolyse

↓

3 Min..............   Advanced platelet disintegration

RBC entrapped in fibrin network emanating
from platelet aggregates

FIG. 12. Scheme of hemostasis.

vessels in rabbits causing swelling of the extracellular spaces which result
in herniation of intimal cells into the plasma. Sawyer *et al.* (1953) found that
sufficient injury to the vessel wall created a positive current which could
attract negatively charged red blood cells, white cells, and platelets creating
a prethrombotic area. A negative current provided protection against
collection of formed elements. These workers, and independently Schwartz
(1965) observed a lack of correlation between the extent of the thrombosis
and cellular damage to the vessel wall but a positive correlation between

location of thrombus and injury to wall. They felt that their experiments supported the concept that thrombosis was due to electrostatic attraction of the negatively charged surface of the formed elements to the positively charged injured vessel wall.

The mechanisms of blood coagulation, formation, and release of ADP from ATP, liberation of material from vessel wall and blood cells into the lumen of the vessel, platelet aggregation, and finally arrest of blood flow are evoked in both hemostasis and thrombosis. We consider that these mechanisms are functioning normally when bleeding is followed by establishment of a hemostatic plug in 3–5 minutes.

When these mechanisms are initiated without external bleeding the abnormal situation of thrombosis occurs and the normal flow of blood is obstructed. Both hemostasis and thrombosis are initiated by injury to or disease in the vascular wall. The nature of the changes in the vessel wall are very different in these two processes. All cellular layers must be severed in hemostasis for external bleeding to occur so that endothelial and smooth muscle cells are ruptured and contribute material to the blood. Connective tissue, including basement membrane, elastin, and collagen is also exposed. In simple thrombosis, such as we have created only the endothelial cells are altered to release enzymes and other cell contents in the plasma to bring about changes in the red blood cells, white blood cells, and platelets.

Atherosclerosis which leads to much clinical thrombosis does damage layers deep in the vessel wall so thromboplastin may be released and connective tissue exposed thus mimicking the conditions leading to hemostasis (Duff and McMillan, 1951).

1. Changes in Endothelium

Edwards and Burchell (1958) showed that the endothelium is easily damaged by turbulent currents of blood and Mustard *et al.* (1961) by inserting a shunt in the aorta of pigs beautifully demonstrated the location of cellular deposits at bifurcations which lead to rapid build-up of small thrombi. Four minutes after a small constriction had been briefly applied, we observed sufficient changes in the fine structure of the endothelial cells. Small mural thrombi which later developed into occluding thrombi had resulted from this short period of trauma.

When the endothelium was injured slightly, Branemark and Eckholm (1968) saw erythrocytes adhering to pointlike areas of the endothelium. Passing red cells showed no tendency to adhere to these attached cells. The red blood cell was anchored on the vessel wall by an offshoot, projecting through a discontinuity in the endothelium, such as we have seen red blood cells put forth as they begin to pass through the wall of capillaries in thrombocytopenia (Van Horn and Johnson, 1966).

Branemark and Ekholm saw no evidence of red blood cells passing through junctions when the vascular endothelium was injured, however. In this study the red blood cells did not pass on through the wall but after a time moved away from the vessel wall and into the lumen again.

2. Movement of White Blood Cells

Microscopic examination of damaged vessels shows that white blood cells collect where the endothelial injury is most severe. The neutrophils migrate through the endothelial layer causing disorganization of the vessel wall (Johnson, 1968). The changes in the vessel wall brought about by disease processes must be greatly augmented by this disrupted migration of white and red blood cells.

3. Red Blood Cells

Red blood cells are seen near the thrombosing area, entrapped within the platelet aggregates. Many of them are seen hemolyzing, releasing partial thromboplastin and ADP which brings about platelet aggregation and thrombin formation soon after the endothelium is injured.

4. Platelet Aggregation

The first ADP released into plasma comes from the abluminal membrane of the endothelial cells exposed when the parts of the cells are sloughed. This release of ADP must be one of the resulting changes taking place in vascular endothelium as it changes from a nonwettable to a wettable surface *in vivo*. Small mural thrombi are observed 4 minutes after the constriction occurs, adhering to the damaged endothelial cytoplasm. These thrombi consist of from 2 to 16 platelets with one or more fibrin fibers inside. The platelets seem to adhere singly to the vessel wall as a number of individual platelets are seen collected near the injured cell. Small platelet aggregates are not seen free in the plasma. The thrombi are considerably larger by 20 minutes, and by 1 hour an obstructing thrombus has formed ensnaring many white and red blood cells.

By 1 hour much platelet disintegration has taken place, most of the platelets have lost their organelles and much membrane damage has occurred. A great deal of cellular debris is evident.

The white blood cells are rich in lysosomes and the eosinophils in particular have been shown by Barnhart and Riddle (1963) to contain profibrinolysin. These cells when caught in thrombi, disintegrate (Johnson, 1966, 1968) and digest aggregates of platelets, fibrin, and red blood cells. The debris seen is probably undigested portions of these blood cells.

Much fibrin is seen between the platelets and undoubtedly much has been lysed. Kwaan (1969) has shown that the vascular endothelial cells are rich in fibrinolysin which is released when the cells are injured and could also contribute to removal of fibrin.

REFERENCES

Altschul, R. (1954). "Endothelium," pp. 50–70. Macmillan, New York.

Ashford, S. P. (1969). *In* "Thrombosis" (S. Sherry *et al.*, eds.) pp. 447–460. Natl. Acad. Sci., Washington, D.C.

Barnhart, M. I., and Riddle, J. M. (1963). *Blood* **21**, 306.

Baumgartner, H. R., Tranzer, J. P., and Studer, A. (1967). *Thromb. Diath. Haemorrh.* **18**, 592.

Bettex–Galland, M., and Lüscher, E. F. (1959). *Nature (London)* **184**, 276.

Bizzozero, J. (1882). *Virchows Arch. Pathol. Anat. Physiol.* **90**, 261.

Born, G. V. R. (1962). *Nature (London)* **194**, 927.

Born, G. V. R. (1964). *Nature (London)* **202**, 95.

Bounameaux, Y. (1956). *Experientia* **12**, 355.

Branemark, P. I., and Eckholm, R. (1968). *Blut* **16**, 274.

Caro, L. G. (1964). *Methods Cell Physiol.* **1**, 327–363.

Castaldi, P. A., Firkin, B. G., Blackwell, P. M., and Clifford, K. I. (1962). *Blood* **20**, 567.

Chandler, A. B., and Nordoy, A. (1964). *Scand. J. Haematol.* **1**, 91.

Dische, Z. (1964). *In* "Small Blood Vessel Involvement in Diabetes Mellitus" (M. D. Siperstein, A. R. Colwell, and K. M. Meyer, eds.), pp. 201–213. Am. Inst. Biol. Sci., Washington, D.C.

Donné, A. (1842). *C. R. Acad. Sci.* **14**, 366.

Duff, G. L., and McMillan, G. C. (1951). *Amer. J. Med.* **11**, 92.

Dutton, R. C., Webber, A. J., Johnson, S. A., and Baier, R. E. (1969). *J. Biomed. Mater. Res.* **3**, 13.

Eastoe, J. E. (1967). *In* "Treatise on Collagen" (G. N. Ramachandran, ed.), Vol. 1, pp. 1–72. Academic Press, New York.

Eberth, J. C., and Schimmeibusch, C. (1886a). *Virchows Arch. Pathol. Anat. Physiol.* **103**, 39.

Eberth, J. C., and Schimmelbusch, C. (1886b). *Virchows Arch. Pathol. Anat. Physiol.* **105**, 331.

Edwards, J. E., and Burchell, H. B. (1958). *Circulation* **18**, 946.

Gaarder, A., Jonson, J., Laland, S., Hellem, A., and Owren, P. A. (1961). *Nature (London)* **192**, 531.

Harrison, M. J. G., and Mitchell, J. R. A. (1966). *Lancet* **2**, 1163.

Hayem, G. (1877). *C. R. Acad. Sci.* **95**, 18.

Hellem, A. J. (1960). *Scand. J. Clin. Lab. Invest.* **12**, Suppl. 51.

Hellem, A. J., Borchgrevink, C. F., and Ames, S. B. (1961). *Brit. J. Haematol.* **7**, 42.

Honour, A. J., and Mitchell, J. R. A. (1964). *Brit. J. Exp. Pathol.* **45**, 75.

Horowitz, H. I., and Papayoanou, M. F. (1968). *Thromb. Diath. Haemorrh.* **19**, 18.

Hovig, T. (1963). *Thromb. Diath. Haemorrh.* **9**, 248.

Hovig, T. (1969). *In* "Thrombosis" (S. Sherry *et al.*, eds.), pp. 374–391. Natl. Acad. Sci., Washington, D.C.

Hugues, J. (1960). *C. R. Soc. Biol.* **154**, 866.

Jaques, L. B. (1962). *Circulation* **25**, 130.

Johnson, S. A. (1965). Unpublished results.

Johnson, S. A. (1966). *Proc. 11th Congr. Int. Soc. Hematol.*, Plenary Sessions. N.S.W. Gov. Printer, Sydney, Australia.

Johnson, S. A. (1968). *Thromb. Diath. Haemorrh.* Suppl. 28, 65.

Johnson, S. A., Balboa, R. S., Dessel, B. H., Monto, R. W., Siegesmund, K. A., and Greenwalt, T. J. (1964). *Exp. Mol. Pathol.* **3**, 115.

Johnson, S. A., Balboa, R. S., Pederson, H. J., and Buckley, M. (1965). *Thromb. Diath. Haemorrh.* **13**, 65.

Johnson, S. A., Fredell, L., Shepard, J. A., Tebo, T. H., Chang, C., Pederson, H. J., and Van Horn, D. L. (1967). *In* "Physiology of Hemostasis and Thrombosis" (S. A. Johnson and W. H. Seegers, eds.), p. 44. Thomas, Springfield, Illinois.

Johnson, S. A., Webber, A. J., Wojcik, J. D., and Yun, J. (1969). *In* "Dynamics of Thrombus Formation and Dissolution" (S. A. Johnson and M. M. Guest, eds.), pp. 72–94. Lippincott, Philadelphia, Pennsylvania.

Jones, T. W. (1852). *Phil. Trans. Roy. Soc. London* **142**, 131.

Juva, K. (1967). *Scand. J. Clin. Lab. Invest.* **41**. Suppl. 19, 1.

Kopriwa, B. M. (1967). *J. Histochem. Cytochem.* **15**, 501.

Kwaan, H. C. (1969). *In* "Dynamics of Thrombus Formation and Dissolution" (S. A. Johnson and M. M. Guest, eds.), pp. 114–120. Lippincott, Philadelphia, Pennsylvania.

Lazarow, A., and Speidel, E. (1964). *In* "Small Blood Vessel Involvement in Diabetes Mellitus" (M. D. Siperstein, A. R. Colwell, and K. M. Meyer, eds.), pp. 127–150. Am. Inst. Biol. Sci., Washington, D.C.

Lubnitsky, S. (1885). *Arch. Exp. Pathol. Pharmakol.* **19**, 185.

Luft, J. H. (1965). *J. Cell Biol.* **27**, 118.

Lüscher, E. F. (1956a). *Experientia* **12**, 294.

Lüscher, E. F. (1956b). *Vox Sang.* **1**, 133.

Macfarlane, R. G. (1968). *Int. Rev. Exp. Pathol.* **6**, 55–133.

Macmillan, D. C. (1966). *Nature (London)* **211**, 140.

Majno, G. (1965). *In* "Handbook of Physiology" (Am. Physiol. Soc., J. Field, ed.). Sect. 2, Vol. III, pp. 2293–2375. Williams & Wilkins, Baltimore, Maryland.

Marchesi, V. T., and Barrnett, R. J. (1964). *J. Ultrastruct. Res.* **10**, 103.

Marr, J., Barboriak, J. J., and Johnson, S. A. (1965). *Nature (London)* **205**, 259.

Marr, J., Tebo, T. H., and Johnson, S. A. (1966). *Nature (London)* **211**, 1306.

Mustard, J. F., Downie, H. G., Murphy, E. A., and Rowsell, H. C. (1961). *In* "Blood Platelets" (S. A. Johnson *et al.*, eds.), pp. 191–204. Little, Brown, Boston, Massachusetts.

Mustard, J. F., Hegardt, B., Rowsell, H. C., and Macmillan, R. L. (1964). *J. Lab. Clin. Med.* **64**, 548.

Mustard, J. F., Glynn, M. F., Hovig, T., Jorgensen, L., Packham, M. A., Nishizawa, E., and Rowsell, H. C. (1967). *In* "Physiology of Hemostasis and Thrombosis" (S. A. Johnson and W. H. Seegers, eds.), pp. 288–326. Thomas, Springfield, Illinois.

Niewiarowski, S. (1967). *In* "Physiology of Hemostasis and Thrombosis" (S. A. Johnson and W. H. Seegers, eds.), pp. 71–73. Thomas, Springfield, Illinois.

O'Brien, J. R. (1966). *Proc. 11th Congr. Intern. Soc. Haematol.*, N.S.W. ïGov. Printer, Sydney, Australia.

Pederson, H. J., Tebo, T. H., and Johnson, S. A. (1967). *Amer. J. Clin. Pathol.* **48**, 62.

Poole, J. C. F., French, J. E., and Cliff, W. J. (1963). *J. Clin. Pathol.* **16**, 523.

Quick, A. J., Georgatos, J. G., and Hussey, C. V. (1954). *Amer. J. Med. Sci.* **228**, 207.

Ramachandran, G. N. (1967). *In* "Treatise on Collagen" (G. N. Ramachandran, ed.), Vol. 1. Academic Press, New York.

Ratnoff, D. D., and Miles, A. A. (1964). *Brit. J. Exp. Pathol.* **45**, 328.

Rodman, N. F., Mason, R. S., Devitt, N. B., and Brinkhous, K. M. (1962). *Amer. J. Pathol.* **40**, 271.

Rorvick, T. O., Holmsen, I., and Stormorken, H. (1968). *Thromb. Diath. Haemorrh.* **19**, 77.

Roskam, J. (1963). *Thromb. Diath. Haemorrh.* **10**, 253.

Ross, R. (1967). *In* "Treatise on Collagen" (B. S. Gould, ed.), Vol. 2, Part A, pp. 1–82. Academic Press, New York.

Ross, R., and Benditt, E. P. (1965). *J. Cell Biol.* **27**, 83.

Sawyer, P. N., Pate, J. W., and Weldon, C. S. (1953). *Amer. J. Physiol.* **175**, 108.

Schulz, H., Jurgens, R., and Hiepler, E. (1958). *Thromb. Diath. Haemorrh.* **2**, 300.

Schwartz, S. I. (1965). *Monogr. Surg.* **2**, 159.

Shimamoto, T., and Ishioka, T. (1963). *Circ. Res.* **12**, 138.

Shinowara, G. Y. (1951). *J. Lab. Clin. Med.* **38**, 11.

Shirasawa, K., and Chandler, A. B. (1969). *Amer. J. Pathol.* **57**, 127.

Spaet, T. H., and Gaynor, E. (1970). *Thromb. Diath. Haemorrh.* Suppl. (to be published).

Tranzer, J. P., and Baumgartner, H. R. (1967). *Nature (London)* **216**, 1126.

Van Horn, D. L., and Johnson, S. A. (1966). *Amer. J. Clin. Pathol.* **46**, 204.

Van Horn, D. L., and Johnson, S. A. (1968). *J. Lab. Clin. Med.* **71**, 301.

Vroman, L. (1967). *In* "Blood Clotting Enzymology" (W. H. Seegers, ed.), pp. 279–322. Academic Press, New York.

Waller, M. D., Lohr, G. W., Grignoni, F., and Gross, R. (1959). *Thromb. Diath. Haemorrh.* **3**, 520.

Webber, A. J., and Johnson, S. A. (1970). *Amer. J. Pathol.* **60**, 19.

Welch, W. H. (1887). "William Henry Welch Papers and Addresses," Vol. I, pp. 47–65. Johns Hopkins Press, Baltimore, Maryland (reprinted, 1920).

Wessler, S., and Yin, E. T. (1969). *Progr. Hematol.* **6**, 201–232.

White, J. G., and Krivit, W. (1966). *Blood* **27**, 167.

Wilner, G. D., Nossel, H. L., and LeRoy, E. C. (1968). *J. Clin. Invest.* **47**, 2616.

Wojcik, J. D., Van Horn, D. L., Webber, A. J., and Johnson, S. A. (1969). *Transfusion (Philadelphia)* **9**, 324.

Zimmerman, G. (1845). *Arch. Physiol. Heilk.* **4**, 65.

Zucker, H. D. (1949). *Blood* **4**, 631.

Zucker, M. B., and Borrelli, J. (1959). *J. Appl. Physiol.* **14**, 575.

Zucker, M. B., and Borrelli, J. (1962). *Proc. Soc. Exp. Biol. Med.* **109**, 779.

13

_____

ROLE OF PLATELETS IN FIBRINOLYSIS

HAU C. KWAAN

I. INTRODUCTION

In the normal process of hemostasis, the fibrin clot formed is removed from the body by the proteolytic action primarily of the fibrinolytic enzyme plasmin, and to a lesser extent, of other but nonspecific proteases. The platelet, while contributing to the different phases of hemostasis also is involved in this process of fibrin resolution. The platelet not only contains various inhibitors of fibrinolysis, but also may indirectly influence the plasma fibrinolytic activity by the stimulation of the endothelial release of plasminogen activator. This could be mediated through the platelet amine contents, such as serotonin and histamine. On the other hand, products of fibrinolysis and fibrinogen degradation may exert a profound influence on platelet adhesiveness and aggregability. Thus, a complex interrelationship exists between the platelet and the fibrinolytic system.

II. THE FIBRINOLYTIC SYSTEM

A clear understanding of this interrelationship is aided by the recent knowledge gained through extensive studies made in the field of fibrinolysis. Detailed description of this system can be found in many excellent reviews on the subject (Astrup, 1956a,b; Sherry *et al.*, 1959; von Kaulla, 1963; Sherry, 1968). However, the following resumé will be helpful to a discussion of the fibrinolytic system in relationship to the platelet. The proteolytic enzyme responsible for fibrinolysis is plasmin. It is derived from the activation of its inactive precursor, plasminogen. A scheme showing the various factors that participate in the physiological activation of plasminogen proposed in 1956 by Astrup (1956a) (Fig. 1) is still applicable as a working concept today.

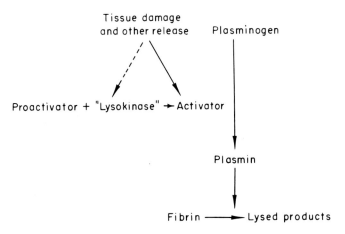

Fig. 1. A scheme for the activation of the fibrinolytic system (Astrup, 1956a). The interrupted line indicates a hypothetical pathway involving a proactivator–activator system.

Plasminogen is a β-globulin (Robbins and Summaria, 1963), with molecular weight of approximately 89,000 (Davies and Englert, 1960), and is widely distributed in the body in plasma, transudates, and other body fluids. It is present in the euglobulin fraction of plasma and is, therefore, included in the commonly used test for fibrinolytic activity, the euglobulin lysis time. The plasminogen activator is believed to originate from the intima of blood vessels (Mole, 1948; Kwaan and McFadzean, 1956) and is released by a variety of stimuli such as ischemia, epinephrine, histamine, and serotonin (Kwaan *et al.*, 1957a,b, 1958a,b). Histochemical studies revealed its localization in endothelial cells (Todd, 1959; Warren, 1963; Kwaan and Astrup, 1963; Kwaan, 1966) (Fig. 2). Biochemical assays showed that it is present in blood and in a number of biological fluids such as lacrimal fluid, milk, saliva, seminal fluid, and urine (Albrechtsen *et al.*, 1958).

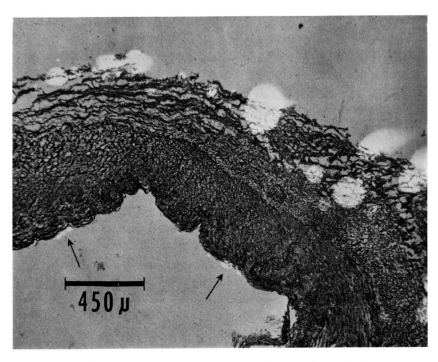

FIG. 2. The histochemical demonstration of plasminogen activator in a human coronary artery using the fibrin slide method (Kwaan and Astrup, 1967). The white zones indicate sites with plasminogen activator. It can be seen in the vasa vasorum in the adventitia and to a small degree in the endothelium of the intima (arrows). Harris' alum hematoxylin stain.

Astrup (1956a) postulated that the plasminogen activator is formed from another precursor in plasma he termed "proactivator." The activation is accomplished in the body by a "lysokinase" and *in vitro* by streptokinase, an enzyme in the filtrate of hemolytic streptococcus cultures. The existence of this "proactivator," however, is in doubt. Evidence for and against the two-step activation of plasmin, namely from "proactivator" to "activator" and from "plasminogen" to "plasmin," will be discussed in a later section.

A number of inhibitors in plasma keep the fibrinolytic activity at a low physiological level and maintain an equilibrium with the activators (Norman and Hill, 1958; Brakman and Astrup, 1963; Bernik and Kwaan, 1969). There are sufficient amounts of antiplasmin in normal blood so that plasmin cannot be detected by the usual methods. However, the plasminogen activator can be measured. It varies from a low level at rest to a high level under conditions such as exercise or an increase in sympathetic activity. The fluctuation is increased markedly in certain diseases such as cirrhosis of the liver (Ratnoff, 1949; Kwaan et al., 1956), surgical stress (Macfarlane, 1937, acute leukemia (Jürgens, 1963), disseminated carcinoma of the prostate (Ratnoff, 1952), and in conditions associated with severe anoxia (Tagnon et al., 1946). It also may be increased in response to any widespread intravascular clotting, such as that seen in the recently recognized syndrome of disseminated intravascular coagulation or defibrination syndrome (Kowalski et al., 1965; Rodriguez-Erdmann, 1965).

The physiological role of fibrinolysis is best understood by looking at its local action in the prevention of a sustained thrombus formation. The fibrinolytic mechanism is activated when fibrin deposition takes place on a vessel wall. A number of hypotheses have been advanced to explain the actual mechanism by which the fibrinolytic system works to resolve or lyse such fibrin deposits. These include: (1) The fibrin clot preferentially adsorbs plasminogen activator and plasmin due to a greater affinity for these enzymes than that for the corresponding inhibitors (Mullertz, 1956, 1957); (2) the fibrin deposits activate a release mechanism locally, so that a larger concentration of plasminogen activator is available at the site of fibrin deposition; (3) the hypothesis of Sherry et al. (1959) that plasminogen exists in vivo as a "two-phase" system. This includes a soluble-phase form in the body fluids ("plasma plasminogen"), and a gel-phase form in the fibrin deposits and in thrombi ("clot plasminogen"). They postulated that activation of the plasma plasminogen is minor and slow, due to the intermixture of this soluble phase with the inhibitors. However, a rapid activation of the gel phase or clot plasminogen takes place in the thrombus (Fig. 3).

Whichever working concept one adopts for the activation of plasminogen activator, the ultimate result of these reactions is fibrin resolution. This will be achieved most efficiently if the fibrin formation takes place within an undamaged vessel wall (Kwaan and Astrup, 1965). However, if fibrinolytic activity is deficient at the site of fibrin formation, such as due to local injury of the vessel involved, fibrin resolution will be greatly hindered. In support of this concept is the fact that a sustained thrombus in a blood vessel is difficult to produce experimentally unless the vessel wall is first

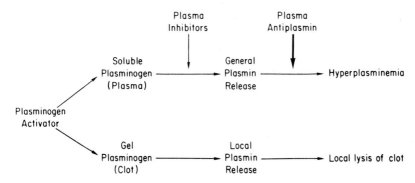

FIG. 3. The hypothesis of the "two-phase" system of plasminogen activation, explaining why it is easier to produce local lysis of the clot than to produce hyperplasminemia when plasminogen activator is released. The plasma inhibitors of fibrinolysis further impair the production of any significant plasmin activity in the circulating blood. The heavier arrow indicates a stronger antiplasmin effect.

damaged mechanically or chemically by a sclerosing agent (Kwaan and Astrup, 1965).

The fate of a thrombus also depends to a great extent on its content, especially of platelets. For example, a platelet-rich clot is more difficult to lyse than a platelet-poor clot (Hume, 1958, Alkjaersig, 1961). Thus, any effects of the platelets on the fibrinolytic system will have a direct bearing on the fate of the thrombus and deserve detailed consideration.

III. "PROACTIVATOR" AND ACTIVATOR OF FIBRINOLYSIS IN PLATELETS

The early concept of the fibrinolytic system was based on a number of observations of the *in vitro* activation of plasminogen by an enzyme streptokinase in the filtrate of hemolytic streptococci (Christensen and MacLeod, 1945). Later, it was found that certain animal plasminogens, including bovine plasminogen, could not be activated by streptokinase. Mullertz and Lassen (1953) later found that bovine plasminogen could be activated by streptokinase if a small amount of normal human plasma globulin was added to the mixture. This was the basis for the hypothetical "proactivator," which is converted to "activator" by streptokinase, which in turn would activate bovine plasminogen (Fig. 4). This concept was subsequently incorporated into Astrup's scheme of 1956 (1956a) (Fig. 1) for the activation of the fibrinolytic system. However, a different interpretation of the sequence of reaction was offered by Kline and Fishman in 1961. They suggested that variations in plasminogen reactivities with streptokinase in different animal species were responsible. They observed that while bovine plasminogen does not react to streptokinase, a streptokinase–plasmin complex is a potent activator for plasminogen of this species. The activation of bovine plasminogen after the addition of small amounts of human plasma then could be explained by the activation of streptokinase of the human plasminogen thereby producing the streptokinase–plasmin complex, which then activates the bovine plasminogen autocatalytically (Kline and Fishman, 1966). A number of previously reported "proactivators" present

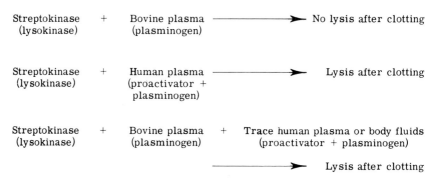

Fig. 4. The reactions between streptokinase and different forms of plasma. This is the basis for the "proactivator–activator" system postulated by Mullertz and Lassen (1953).

in various human body fluids and tissues could thus be explained by the presence of traces of contaminant human plasminogen. In the case of human platelets, plasminogen has been identified by immunologic techniques to be present in well-washed platelets (Nachman, 1965). This may account for the action of a "streptokinase cofactor" reported earlier by Lewis et al. (1962). On the other hand, certain other observations of a proactivator in platelets could not be explained in this fashion, such as those of Holemans and Gross (1961). This proactivator can be rapidly removed from the platelet by repeated washings. It reacts only with streptokinase and not with urokinase, a plasminogen activator, thus indicating that it cannot be a plasminogen. This work was subsequently confirmed by Larrieu (1965). Much of these findings can be interpreted only with difficulty in view of the inhibitors of fibrinolysis present in the platelets. These inhibitors may explain in part some of the results.

While it is not possible to tell if the platelet does contain this hypothetical "proactivator," the presence of plasminogen in the platelet is firmly established. Using ultrasound sonicated human platelets previously washed ten times as antigenic material, Nachman (1965) demonstrated a substance immunologically identical to plasminogen. In addition to plasminogen, platelets also contain a plasminogen activator (Reid and Silver, 1964). This activator is released from the platelets only after the appearance of viscous metamorphosis. Other nonspecific proteases also were found in platelets, notably Cathepsin A which is obtained from the intracellular granules of platelets separated by ultracentrification (Nachman and Ferris, 1968). These enzymes are fibrinogenolytic and are distinct from plasmin. They are released when intracellular granule lysis occurs in the platelet upon the formation of platelet thrombi. Probably the action of these proteases is limited to fibrinogenolysis and confined to the fibrinogen present within the platelets (first shown by Johnson et al., 1952), and to the fibrin interstices of the platelet thrombus. They appear to be a supplementary lytic enzyme to the more potent action of plasmin, and are unlikely to contribute significantly to the resolution of the fibrin network surrounding the platelet thrombus. The same can be said of all other components of the fibrinolytic system described above. In this respect, the platelet is similar to the leukocyte, which also contains nonspecific fibrin-digesting enzyme (Rulot, 1904), "leukoprotease" (Opie, 1907), as well as plasminogen (Henry, 1965). Yet the leukocyte differs by its mobility with which it may infiltrate a thrombus after its formation carrying with it a plasminogen content. It also differs from the platelet by its ability to phagocytose fibrin particles, which had been shown by electron microscopy to be present inside the polymorphonuclear neutrophils (Riddle and Barnhart, 1964).

IV. PLATELETS AS RELEASING AGENT OF ENDOTHELIAL PLASMINOGEN ACTIVATOR

Plasminogen activator is the prime physiological component of the fibrinolytic system. The role played by the platelets will be minimal if their contribution is confined to the release of their content of the various fibrinolytic components discussed above. Platelets, therefore, must exert their major effect on the fibrinolytic system through some indirect means. Since plasminogen activator can be released from the vessel wall by various vasoactive agents locally (Kwaan et al., 1957a,b, 1958a,b) and systemically (Holemans, 1963, 1965), yet another role of the various amines present within the platelets should be sought. The amines in platelets are vasoactive including serotonin, which is by far the most extensively studied and perhaps the most important one, and also histamine, epinephrine, and norepinephrine. In human subjects as well as in rabbits and in rats, the local actions of these amines were investigated in relationship to their ability in the release of fibrinolytic activity from the vessel wall. In normal human subjects an intravenous or a paravenous injection of epinephrine, norepinephrine, serotonin, or histamine produced a rapid increase in the fibrinolytic activity in blood from the stimulated segment of the vessel. The increase in fibrinolytic activity was not limited locally to the site of injection. Increased fibrinolytic activity also developed proximally as well as distally in the veins of the same limb that was stimulated, and in some subjects in the veins of the contralateral limb. This development of increased fibrinolytic activity could be blocked by a prior local injection of atropine. These observations led to the conclusion that release of fibrinolytic activity from the veins is the result of the stimulation of a cholinergic effector mechanism. A similar mechanism also was observed in arteries (Kwaan et al., 1958b). By producing thrombi in the marginal veins of rabbit's ears, the plasminogen activator releasing mechanism of the vein wall was

TABLE I

INFLUENCE OF VASOACTIVE AMINES ON RATE OF THROMBOLYSIS[a]

Type of experiment	Lysis time of thrombi in hours[b]
Control rabbits	20.0 ± 7.0
Serotonin 3.0 μg intravenously	2.9 ± 1.7
Serotonin 0.3 μg intravenously	4.5 ± 1.7
Serotonin 0.03 μg intravenously	23.0 ± 9.0
Serotonin 0.1 μg paravenously	Lysis within 15 min
Thrombocytopenia	63.0 ± 15.6
Thrombocytopenia + 0.3 μg serotonin	2.4 ± 1.4
Reserpine	No lysis in 4 animals 14–18 in remainder
Serotonin inhibitor	No lysis
Monoamine oxidase inhibitor	5
Epinephrine intravenously	6.3 ± 2.0

[a] A summary of the findings of Kwaan et al. (1958a) showing the influence of the various vasoactive amines and of platelets on the rate of thrombolysis of experimentally produced thrombi in rabbit ear veins.

[b] Mean $\pm$ SD.

investigated by observing the rate of lysis of the thrombi. Because serotonin in blood is primarily carried in platelets, this amine was given particular attention in this study. While in control thrombi, the mean lysis time was 20 hours, the local injection of 0.3 μg of serotonin (5 hydroxytryptamine) creatinine sulphate resulted in the acceleration of this lysis to a mean of 2.9 hours (Table I). This accelerated lysis of the thrombi by the injection of serotonin was dose related. Animals given 0.03 μg locally did not show significantly accelerated thrombolysis.

The rate of clot lysis was much more rapid and required smaller amounts of serotonin if the serotonin was applied paravenously. When as little as 0.1 μg of serotonin was given paravenously, the fibrinolytic activity produced was so intense that the fibrin lysed as rapidly as it was formed. In the same manner, the rate of thrombolysis also could be altered by varying the amount of endogenous (i.e., platelet) serotonin available at the site of the clot. Following the production of a moderate thrombocytopenia by anti-platelet serum, with a platelet count of less than 30,000/mm^3, the time of lysis was greatly delayed (mean of 63 hours). Some of the thrombosed venous segments in such rabbits did not resolve by lysis, but underwent organization. Impaired thrombolysis in thrombocytopenic rabbits could be reversed by adding exogenous serotonin to the thrombus. The lowering of the serotonin content of the platelets by the administration of reserpine to the rabbits for a period of 10 days resulted in a similar impairment of thrombolysis. The same effect also was achieved by pharmacological agents antagonistic to serotonin while the opposite was obtained when synergistic agents such as monoamine oxidase inhibitors were locally applied. These findings established the important role played by serotonin in local throm-bolysis, and confirmed the earlier hypothesis based on studies on human veins that a major function of the serotonin liberated from disintegrating platelets *in vivo* is the stimulation of fibrinolytic activity. Although epi-nephrine, norepinephrine, and histamine, either mixed in the clot or injected paravenously, will produce accelerated lysis in experimental thrombi, the role played by the catecholamines and histamine of the platelets is a relatively minor one. Furthermore, due to species difference in the relative contents of these amines, there is little catecholamines and even less histamine in human platelets.

The release of plasminogen activator from endothelium in experimentally produced thrombi can be demonstrated by histochemical technique using a modified fibrin slide method (Kwaan and Astrup, 1967) (Figs. 5 and 6). However, plasminogen activator is a characteristic of normal vascular endothelium. Thus, the degree of increase in its activity in the presence of

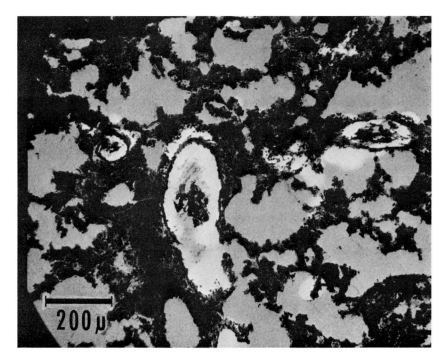

FIG. 5. Fibrin thrombi in pulmonary vessels after intravenous thrombin injection, seen in a frozen section of lung prepared by the fibrin slide method. The white areas represent sites of plasminogen activator activity, which can be seen to surround the thrombi. Harris' alum hematoxylin stain (Kwaan *et al.*, 1967).

a locally formed thrombus is difficult to assess. If platelets do play a part in releasing plasminogen activator, several situations must be present locally before this release mechanism can be brought into maximal function. First, in the process of thrombus formation, the intimal lining must not be injured to the degree that fibrinolytic activity is abolished. Second, platelets must be present locally in such concentration that their serotonin content can be released in sufficient quantities. An effective way to accomplish this would be the trapping of disintegrating platelets by the fibrin meshwork in the thrombus, so that the released serotonin would not be washed away by circulating blood. Third, such actions of the serotonin is short-lived, since it is rapidly inactivated by monamine oxidase present in normal blood.

Any fibrin formation accompanied by platelet deposition would be lysed more effectively when a high concentration of platelets were present. This will account for the lack of fibrin in the neighborhood of a platelet thrombus.

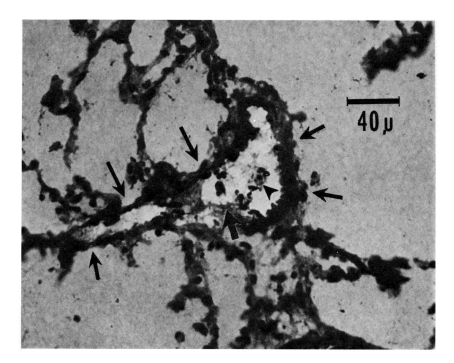

FIG. 6. Frozen section of lung prepared by the fibrin slide method. The specimen was taken from a rat after the intravenous injection of homologous platelet aggregates produced *in vitro* by ADP. The platelet embolus (arrowhead) can be seen partially occluding the lumen of a small pulmonary artery surrounded by a pale zone (arrows) indicating release of plasminogen activator. Harris' alum hematoxylin stain.

On the other hand, it has been shown recently that other factors may release plasminogen activator locally from the vascular endothelium. Bernik and Kwaan (1970), in their study on living human tissue cell cultures, observed that cultures from human blood vessels produce more plasminogen activator in the presence of a fibrin clot undergoing lysis than in its absence. Thus, the platelet may be important but are not the only factors that control the release mechanism of plasminogen activator from the vascular endothelium.

V. INHIBITORS OF FIBRINOLYSIS IN PLATELETS

Different inhibitors of the fibrinolytic system have been described. They may be directed against plasmin or individually against various kinds of plasminogen activators. A selective inhibition of some of the plasminogen activators has been observed in various physiological and pathological conditions. Saline extracts of tumor tissues and serum from patients with primary carcinoma of the liver contain an inhibitor against the plasma plasminogen activator of healthy subjects obtained after stimulation with vasoactive agents (Kwaan et al., 1959). A urokinase inhibitor was reported in pregnancy (Brakman and Astrup, 1963), and an inhibitor against tissue activator of plasminogen was found in the blood of patients with multiple myeloma (Mohler et al., 1967). In tissue cultures, certain cells also produced antiplasmin as well as a urokinase inhibitor (Bernik and Kwaan, 1969). In platelets, an antiplasmin activity was first described by Johnson and Schneider in 1953, which later was confirmed by others (Stefanini and Murphy, 1956; Alkjaersig, 1961; Holemans and Gross, 1961). This platelet inhibitor of plasmin was investigated in detail by Alkjaersig (1961), who showed that it is distinct from the antiplasmin found in plasma, and that it cannot be removed from the platelets by repeated washings. Using the caseinolytic method of assay on reaction mixtures of lyophylized platelets and plasmin, she clearly showed that the platelet inhibitor inhibits plasmin at different concentrations in a linear fashion and at a rapid rate in contrast to a nonlinear relationship and a slower rate of reaction of the plasma plasmin inhibitor. She believed that this platelet inhibitor is an important component of the total plasma antiplasmin content.

Holemans and Gross (1961) first noted that in addition to the inhibitory effect on plasmin, platelets also inhibit urokinase-induced lysis of bovine or human fibrin. They suggested that platelets may contain both antiplasmin and antiurokinase. However, they could not establish with certainty that the antiurokinase effect was due to antiplasmin activity. Den Ottolander et al. (1967, 1969a,b) confirmed the antiurokinase activity of platelets and furthermore showed with a tube lysis method the presence of antistreptokinase, antitissue (porcine heart) activator, and antiblood activator. Antiurokinase activity was by far the most potent of the antiactivators.

Recently, using the method described by Brakman and Astrup (1963), we have found (Kwaan and Suwanwela, 1970), in a reaction mixture where no antiplasmin activity is present to interfere with the fibrin plate assay, that washed human platelets definitely contain selective inhibitors against three kinds of plasminogen activators: human urokinase; plasma plasminogen activator after stimulation with vasoactive agents; and tissue plasminogen activator extracted from human heart. Although the activity was not marked, inhibition against urokinase was greatest. The results of this study are outlined in Table II. Using the caseinolytic assay method, the presence of antiplasmin was confirmed. Platelets from patients with throm-

TABLE II

PLATELET INHIBITORS OF FIBRINOLYSIS[a]

		Human urokinase (CTA Units)	Human plasma plasminogen activator (CTA Units)	Human heart plasminogen activator (CTA Units)
Healthy control	mean	3.40	1.78	2.18
(10 subjects)	range	1.11–7.52	0.48–3.67	0.09–7.0
Thrombocytosis	mean	4.35	2.31	1.44
(7 patients)	range	0.92–8.63	1.25–3.95	0.62–3.20
Polycythemia vera (1 patient) mean of two determinations		17.99	5.29	5.59

[a] The results of inhibitory activity of washed human platelet suspensions on the various plasminogen activators at concentrations where the antiplasmin activity is so low that it will not interfere with the test. The units expressed in each case is the amount of plasminogen activator activity that was inhibited by 10^9 platelets. (CTA = Committee on Thrombolytic Agents, National Heart Institute.)

bocytosis also were studied. Included were patients with polycythemia vera and thrombocytosis secondary to bronchogenic carcinoma. Seven of these patients showed inhibitory activities of their platelets similar to those of the healthy subjects. The exception was seen in one patient with polycythemia vera who had an unusually high degree of inhibitory activity against all the plasminogen activators, especially urokinase. He did not show, however, any clinical signs or symptoms of thrombosis, nor did the other coagulation studies done on his blood samples reveal any changes suggestive of a hypercoagulable state. The presence of fibrinolytic inhibitors in human platelets against human urokinase, porcine tissue activator extracted from ovary and from heart, and human plasmin was also reported by Thorsen et al. (1970).

VI. CLINICAL SIGNIFICANCE OF ROLE OF PLATELETS IN FIBRINOLYSIS

Much of the work on the relationship between platelets and the fibrinolytic system was prompted by the clinical observations of two groups of disease entities, one with thrombocytopenia, and the other with grossly excessive platelet counts, both of which are associated with hemorrhagic manifestations accompanied by increased fibrinolytic activity. This intriguing relationship led to the studies showing that both activators and inhibitors of the fibrinolytic system are present in the platelets as described above. Excess or deficiency of the platelets thus could lead to bleeding if other physiological components of the hemostatic mechanism are also altered by the disease process.

The group of clinical conditions with thrombocytopenia is associated with increased fibrinolysis most commonly in acute leukemia and aplastic anemia (Giraud et al., 1954; Pisciotta et al., 1955; Stefanini and Murphy, 1956). From the evidence presented in the section on platelet inhibitors of fibrinolysis, one would conclude that clots in these patients, made up with very few platelets, would be relatively more susceptible to lysis. However, this deficit is counterbalanced by the diminished release of serotonin resulting in less stimulation of local fibrinolytic activity at the site of the hemostatic clot.

The second group of conditions is generally referred to as thrombocythemia. Hemorrhagic complications are frequently encountered in an uncommon disease entity in this group known as "primary hemorrhagic thrombocythemia." Bleeding also may be seen rarely in the course of polycythemia vera, secondary thrombocythemia in chronic myelogenous leukemia, and agnogenic myeloid metaplasia. In these conditions, the mechanism of bleeding is not well understood. Although some clotting factors and thromboplastin generation tests were shown to be deficient, no conclusive mechanism has been found to account for the bleeding. Pertinent to the present discussion is the report of increase in fibrinolytic activity in one of these conditions, namely, chronic myelogenous leukemia with thrombocytosis (Webb et al., 1963), when there is bleeding and thrombocytosis. Although no direct correlation between the platelet count and fibrinolytic activity was observed, the bleeding and the excessive fibrinolytic activity disappeared after treatment with busulfan, which also brought the platelet count to normal. Van Creveld and Mochtar (1960) also described a case of acute leukemia in which a rebound thrombocytosis during remission was associated with an increased fibrinolytic activity. However, the role of platelets in the increase in fibrinolytic activity in this group of conditions is generally believed to be minor.

Of perhaps greater clinical significance is the role of platelets in thrombosis. Since thromboembolic complications are much more frequent than bleeding manifestations in thrombocytosis, and since studies of platelet function in the fibrinolytic system indicate a more inhibitory than activator effect on the balance, the dissolution of a platelet-rich thrombus deserves some attention. Platelet-rich clots lyse more slowly than platelet-poor clots *in vitro* (Hume, 1958; Alkjaersig, 1961). Using a histological fibrin "autograph" technique, Todd (1969) produced beautiful "autographs" clearly showing that in arterial and ventricular mural thrombi, where the greatest concentrations of platelets occur, such as along the lines of Zahn, fibrinolytic activity was completely absent. It also has been the author's experience with urokinase therapy on arterial thrombosis that arterial mural thrombi, being richer in platelet contents, are generally more difficult to lyse than venous thrombi. Possibly a high local concentration of platelets in such situations would carry with it large amounts of inhibitors of fibrinolysis. This amount could be sufficient to outweigh any benefits obtained from the platelet function of releasing fibrinolytic activity from the vessel wall.

VII. INFLUENCE OF FIBRINOLYSIS ON PLATELET FUNCTIONS

No discussion on the relationship between the platelets and the fibrinolytic system would be complete without reference to the changes of platelet function produced by excessive fibrinolytic activity. One platelet function which is affected by fibrinolysis is that of clot retraction. Rapid lysis of fibrin strands will interfere with the retraction process.

Another more significant effect on platelet function is an indirect one. Excessive fibrinolysis is associated with the release of fibrinogen degradation products (FDP) as a result of proteolysis of fibrinogen. Kowalski *et al.* (1964) first reported on an inhibition of platelet aggregation and "viscous metamorphosis" by FDP. Subsequent work by others confirmed the inhibition of FDP on platelet aggregation. This may be of clinical significance in situations where the hemostatic mechanism is already impaired by the increased fibrinolytic activity. Thomas *et al.* (1967) reported excessive fibrinolysis, high FDP levels, and impaired ADP-induced platelet aggregation in patients with cirrhosis of the liver who were bleeding at multiple sites. Niewiarowski *et al.* (1970) found that low molecular weight FDP formed by plasmin action inhibits both the first and second phases of platelet aggregation. Details on this phenomenon will be found in the chapter on platelet aggregation (Chapter 9 by Aledort).

The findings of von Kaulla and Thilo (1970) that the synthetic fibrinolytic agents also inhibit ADP- and thrombin-induced platelet aggregation opens up an exciting possibility that a drug might be designed with a dual action, namely, prevention of thrombus formation and induction of thrombolysis.

VIII. CONCLUSION

In conclusion, the mass of evidence presented in the above sections has indicated that the platelet plays a multitude of roles in fibrinolysis. On one hand, the platelet supplies plasminogen, activator, and vasoactive amines that are potent releasing agents for fibrinolytic activity from the vessel wall. On the other hand, the platelet carries with it strong inhibitors of fibrinolysis. Histochemical studies showed beyond doubt that when high concentrations of platelets occur in a thrombus, lysis fails to occur (Todd, 1969). These findings cast a new light on our concept of the hemostatic mechanism. If one considers that the aim in hemostasis is to arrest bleeding without producing massive thrombosis, then the autocatalytic chain reaction of clotting set off by the injury must be checked early in the process. In addition, the fibrin barrier would have to be removed by fibrinolysis soon after bleeding is arrested. Perhaps a more efficient way in accomplishing this dual objective is the formation of a platelet thrombus. By the intriguing design described here, the platelet possesses both these capabilities. In the event of an injury to a blood vessel, the platelet would be the "first line" defense in securing hemostasis and fibrin formation; the platelet plug will strengthen this function. This fibrin network within the platelet plug will not lyse due to the high content of inhibitors of fibrinolysis. Yet the platelet thrombus would bring serotonin in contact with the vessel wall, resulting in the production of an intense fibrinolytic activity in the immediate vicinity of such a thrombus. We have no knowledge of how intense this may be in humans, but in the rat and rabbit, we have evidence that it may be such as to cause the removal of fibrin as rapidly as it is formed in the process of coagulation (Kwaan et al., 1958a). Together with the reflex release of fibrinolytic activity in the adjacent segments of the injured vessel (Kwaan et al., 1957a), the combined fibrinolytic activity can remove the fibrin clot surrounding the original nidus of platelet plug and to restrict extension of the thrombus. The possible applications, both physiological and clinical, of this concept are clear.

IX. SUMMARY

It is common knowledge that the platelet is an important component of the hemostatic mechanism. But its role in the fibrinolytic system has received much less attention. The fibrinolytic system consists of a proteolytic enzyme, plasmin, with its precursor plasminogen, and the plasminogen activator.

A proactivator–activator system in addition has been postulated. The platelet contains in varying proportions the different components of the activator system. It also releases fibrinolytic activity from a blood vessel wall mediated through its content of serotonin, catecholamines, and histamine. The platelets themselves contain at the same time substantial amounts of inhibitors of fibrinolysis of different types. The significance of these findings is discussed with reference to the new understanding of the ideal hemostatic mechanism. This mechanism is one that should accomplish its prime mission of arresting bleeding without causing thrombosis. New evidence provided by the use of a histochemical technique for demonstration of fibrinolytic activity also are presented showing the relationship of the platelets in a thrombus to thrombolysis.

REFERENCES

Albrechtsen, O. K., Storm, O., and Claassen, M. (1958). *Scand. J. Clin. Lab. Invest.* **10**, 310.

Alkjaersig, N. (1961). *In* "Blood Platelets" (S. A. Johnson J. W. Rebuck, and R. C. Horn, Jr., eds.), p. 329. Little, Brown, Boston, Massachusetts.

Astrup, T. (1956a). *Lancet* **2**, 565.

Astrup, T. (1956b). *Blood* **11**, 781.

Bernik, M. B., and Kwaan, H. C. (1969). *Fed. Proc., Fed. Amer. Soc. Exp. Biol.* **28**, 510.

Bernik, M. B., and Kwaan, H. C. (1970). *Clin. Res.* **18**, 398.

Brakman, P., and Astrup, T. (1963). *Scand. J. Clin. Lab. Invest.* **15**, 603.

Christensen, L. R., and MacLeod, C. M. (1945). *J. Gen. Physiol.* **28**, 559.

Davies, M. C., and Englert, M. E. (1960). *J. Biol. Chem.* **235**, 1011.

Den Ottolander, G. J. H., Leijnse, B., and Cremer–Elfrink, H. M. J. (1967). *Thromb. Diath. Haemorrh.* **18**, 405.

Den Ottolander, G. J. H., Leijnse, B., and Cremer–Elfrink, H. M. J. (1969a). *Thromb. Diath. Haemorrh.* **21**, 28.

Den Ottolander, G. J. H., Leijnse, B., and Cremer–Elfrink, H. M. J. (1969b). *Thromb. Diath. Haemorrh.* **21**, 35.

Giraud, G., Cazal, P., Latour, H., Izarn, P., Levy, A., Puech, P., Barjon, P., and Ribstein, M. (1954). *Montpellier Med.* **46**, 687.

Henry, R. L. (1965). *Thromb. Diath. Haemorrh.* **8**, 35.

Holemans, R. (1963). *Lancet* **2**, 364.

Holemans, R. (1965). *Amer. J. Physiol.* **208**, 511.

Holemans, R., and Gross, R. (1961). *Thromb. Diath. Haemorrh.* **6**, 196.

Hume, R. (1958). *Scot. Med. J.* **3**, 479.

Johnson, S. A., and Schneider, C. L. (1953). *Science* **117**, 229.

Johnson, S. A., Smathers, W. M., and Schneider, D. L. (1952). *Amer. J. Physiol.* **170**, 631.

Jürgens, J. (1963). *Folia Haematol. (Frankfurt am Main)* **8**, 52.

Kline, D. L., and Fishman, J. B. (1961). *J. Biol. Chem.* **236**, 2807.

Kline, D. L., and Fishman, J. B. (1966). *Proc. Soc. Exp. Biol. Med.* **121**, 184.

Kowalski, E., Kopec, M., and Wegrzynowicz, Z. (1964). *Thromb. Diath. Haemorrh.* **10**, 406.

Kowalski, E., Budzynski, A. Z., Kopec, M., Latallo, Z., Lipinski, B., and Wegrznowicz, Z. (1965). *Thromb. Diath. Haemorrh.* **13**, 12.

Kwaan, H. C. (1966). *Fed. Proc., Fed. Amer. Soc. Exp. Biol.* **25**, 52.

Kwaan, H. C., and Astrup, T. (1963). *Arch. Pathol.* **76**, 595.

Kwaan, H. C., and Astrup, T. (1965). *Circ. Res.* **17**, 477.

Kwaan, H. C., and Astrup, T. (1967). *Lab. Invest.* **17**, 140.

Kwaan, H. C., and McFadzean, A. J. S. (1956). *Clin. Sci.* **15**, 245.

Kwaan, H. C., and Suwanwela, N. (1970). To be published.

Kwaan, H. C., McFadzean, A. J. S., and Cook, J. (1956). *Lancet* **1**, 132.

Kwaan, H. C., Lo, R., and McFadzean, A. J. S. (1957a). *Clin. Sci.* **16**, 241.

Kwaan, H. C., Lo, R., and McFadzean, A. J. S. (1957b). *Clin. Sci.* **16**, 255.

Kwaan, H. C., Lo, R., and McFadzean, A. J. S. (1958a). *Brit. J. Haematol.* **4**, 51.

Kwaan, H. C., Lo, R., and McFadzean, A. J. S. (1958b). *Clin. Sci.* **17**, 361.

Kwaan, H. C., Lo, R., and McFadzean, A. J. S. (1959). *Clin. Sci.* **18**, 251.

Kwaan, H. C., Coccheri, S., and Astrup, T. (1967). *Proc. 1st Int. Symp. Tissue Factors, 1967*, p. 165.

Larrieu, M. J. (1965). *Nouv. Rev. Fr. Hematol.* **5**, 261.

Lewis, J. H., Wilson, J. H., and Merchant, W. R. (1962). *Proc. Soc. Exp. Biol. Med.* **109**, 248.

Macfarlane, R. G. (1937). *Lancet* **1**, 10.

Mohler, E. R., Kennedy, J. N., and Brakman, P. (1967). *Amer. J. Med. Sci.* **253**, 325.

Mole, R. H. (1948). *J. Pathol. Bacteriol.* **60**, 413.

Mullertz, S. (1956). *Acta Physiol. Scand.* **38**, Suppl. 130.

Mullertz, S. (1957). *Ann. N. Y. Acad. Sci.* **68**(1), 38.

Mullertz, S., and Lassen, M. (1953). *Proc. Soc. Exp. Biol. Med.* **82**, 264.

Nachman, R. L. (1965). *Blood* **25**, 703.

Nachman, R. L., and Ferris, B. (1968). *J. Clin. Invest.* **47**, 2530.

Niewiarowski, S., Ream, V. J., and Thomas, D. P. (1970). *Proc. 18th Annu. Symp. Blood, 1970*, p. 12.

Norman, P. S., and Hill, B. M. (1958). *J. Exp. Med.* **108**, 639.

Opie, E. L. (1907). *J. Exp. Med.* **9**, 391.

Pisciotta, A. V., Hinz, J. E., and Schulz, E. G. (1955). *Clin. Res.* **3**, 9.

Ratnoff, O. D. (1949). *Bull. Johns Hopkins Hosp.* **84**, 29.

Ratnoff, O. D. (1952). *J. Clin. Invest.* **31**, 521.

Reid, W. O., and Silver, M. J. (1964). *Amer. J. Physiol.* **206**, 1255.

Riddle, J. M., and Barnhart, M. I. (1964). *Amer. J. Pathol.* **45**, 805.

Robbins, K. C., and Summaria, L. (1963). *J. Biol. Chem.* **238**, 952.

Rodriguez–Erdmann, F. (1965). *N. Engl. J. Med.* **273**, 1370.

Rulot, H. (1904). *Arch. Int. Physiol.* **1**, 152.

Sherry, S. (1968). *Annu. Rev. Med.* **19**, 247.

Sherry, S., Fletcher, A. P., and Alkjaersig, N. (1959). *Physiol. Rev.* **39**, 343.

Stefanini, M., and Murphy, I. S. (1956). *J. Clin. Invest.* **35**, 355.

Tagnon, H. J., Levenson, S. M., Davidson, C. S., and Taylor, F. H. L. (1946). *Amer. J. Med. Sci.* **211**, 88.

Thomas, D. P., Ream, V. J., and Stuart, R. K. (1967). *N. Engl. J. Med.* **276**, 1344.

Thorsen, S., Brakman, P., and Astrup, T. (1970). Personal communication.

Todd, A. S. (1959). *J. Pathol. Bacteriol.* **78**, 281.

Todd, A. S. (1969). *In* "Dynamics of Thrombus Formation and Dissolution" (S. A. Johnson and M. M. Guest, eds.), p. 321. Lippincott, Philadelphia, Pennsylvania.

Van Creveld, S., and Mochtar, I. A. (1960). *Ann. Paediat.* **194**, 65.

von Kaulla, K. N. (1963). "Chemistry of Thrombolysis: Human Fibrinolytic Enzymes." Thomas, Springfield, Illinois.

von Kaulla, K. N., and Thilo, D. (1970). *J. Med. Chem.* (in press).

Warren, B. A. (1963). *Brit. J. Exp. Pathol.* **44**, 365.

Webb, A. T., Meyer, F. L., and Lanser, E. R. (1963). *Arch. Intern. Med.* **111**, 280.

14

IMMUNOLOGICAL REACTIONS INVOLVING PLATELETS*

ROGER M. DES PREZ and SAMUEL R. MARNEY, Jr.

* Supported by Research Grant HE-08399 from the National Institutes of Health, and a Veterans Administration Training Grant in infectious diseases.

I. INTRODUCTION

The subject of platelet injury by immunologic means is at present receiving much attention, in part because of current interest in the broader subject of immunologically-induced cell injury, but also because of increasing awareness of the wide variety of experimental and clinical situations in which platelet damage by, or in the course of, immune reactions seems likely to play an important pathogenic role. Histologic studies over several decades have suggested that platelets may be involved in the pathogenesis of the Arthus phenomenon, the general and local Shwartzman reactions, and anaphylactic states. The phenomenon of intravascular coagulation, an important pathophysiologic mechanism in a number of infectious and allergic illnesses, has focused attention on the role of damaged platelets in the development of this abnormality. There is firm evidence that some drug induced and posttransfusion purpuras are due to platelet injury by antigen–antibody complexes, and suggestive evidence that idiopathic thrombocytopenic purpura (ITP) and postinfectious purpura may be based on similar mechanisms. Finally, some forms of acute rejection of transplanted organs involve platelet injury, at least in part.

In spite of studies spanning more than three decades, however, the subject of immune injury to platelets remains a confused one. There is, for instance, no agreement on the roles of complement and divalent cations in its production, the similarities and differences of platelet injury to immune hemolysis are not clearly understood, the importance of platelet phagocytosis, if any remains unclear and there is disagreement as to whether or not platelet aggregation invariably accompanies immune injury and to the role of platelet nucleotides therein. This confusion seems to be due primarily to three considerations which it would be useful to introduce at the onset. *First, several experimental models have been categorized together as examples of immune platelet injury without sufficient attention to some critical operational differences.* The type of antibody, whether the antigen is a portion of the platelet membrane or unrelated to it, the ratio of antigen and antibody, the size of the challenge, the type of anticoagulant used, and whether or not an agitated system is employed all may critically modify the results observed. *Second, indexes used to demonstrate that immune injury to platelets has occurred are complex, varied, and incompletely understood.* The erythrocyte is a fairly simple cell and the endpoints used to discern immune injury are standardized and relatively straightforward. In comparison, the platelet is more complex, with subcellular compartments, contractile proteins, and a number of biologically active intracellular components, all of which have been utilized in a variety of ways as indexes of immune injury in *in vitro* studies. *Third, there are critical species differencies which make it difficult to apply results obtained in one animal system to another.*

A. Different Types of Immune Injury to Platelets

In 1905, Marino demonstrated that *heterologous antisera specific for platelet antigens* produced platelet agglutination. Several years later, Achard and Aynaud (1909) observed the still poorly understood phenomenon that *platelets also aggregate in the presence of antigen–antibody reactions unrelated to platelet antigens.* Katz and associates (1940a,b, 1949, 1950), and McIntire *et al.* (1949) extended these observations, demonstrating that release of platelet histamine also occurred after *addition of antigen to the blood of animals immunized with that antigen,* and that this reaction was not a consequence of blood coagulation. Humphrey and Jaques (1955) in a modification of the previously used experimental models, *added both antigen and antibody to nonimmune rabbit blood.* This important publication demonstrated a requirement for divalent cation and a plasma factor with the heat lability of serum complement, confirmed the fact that thrombin was not the agent producing platelet injury, and demonstrated similar injury of homologous platelets by antigen–antibody reactions in human, dog, and guinea pig plasmas as well. In a little noted section of that publication, they demonstrated that activation of plasma with agar or with chloroform, maneuvers known to generate anaphylatoxin, produced a similar form of platelet injury. They proposed that a proteolytic activity was generated, probably through the complement system, which then acted upon the platelet membrane. They were unable, however, to conclusively demonstrate such activity in a fluid phase separate from antigen and antibody. These conclusions have largely stood the test of time.

In 1961, Barbaro took direct issue with the notion that complement was involved in platelet injury by unrelated antigen–antibody reactions (1961a,b). He demonstrated that platelet injury by unrelated antigen and antibody was greatest when antibody was present in excess and lacking entirely in antigen excess, whereas complement fixation is maximum in the area of antigen–antibody equivalence. He also reported that inactivation of complement by a variety of methods did not entirely abolish the ability of plasma to support platelet injury. He concluded that the heat-labile plasma factor required was other than complement. The critical difference between these studies and previous ones with which they disagreed was *the use of preformed immune precipitates as the challenge*. It now is clear that platelet injury by preformed immune precipitates, while probably mediated in part by complement in plasma milieux permitting complement activity, may also be due to complement-independent mechanisms (Des Prez and Bryant, 1969). Movat *et al.* (1965a,b) regard the interaction of platelets and preformed immune precipitates as *an example of platelet phagocytosis*, a complement-independent phenomenon requiring a heat-labile γ-globulin unrelated to the complement system.

The above mentioned studies did agree on the requirement for calcium ion and a heat labile plasma factor. In contrast, Miescher and Cooper (1960) reported that immune complexes fixed onto platelets and caused platelet aggregation in the presence of large concentrations of sodium EDTA. Also in contrast to Barbaro's studies, Miescher found that antigen–antibody ratios in antigen excess were optimum. The critical difference again had to do with the details of the challenge, which in these experiments consisted of *extremely large concentrations of antigen and antibody, mixed together to form soluble complexes prior to addition to blood*. An absolute requirement for heat-labile plasma factors was also questioned by Barbaro and Zvaifler (1966) and subsequently by Henson and Cochrane (1969b) who indicated that some, though not all, rabbits after certain specific forms of immunization transiently produce *homocytotropic antibody which has the property of fixing onto platelets and other tissues and causing cell injury after combination with antigen in the absence of plasma*. Last, studies of Schoenbechler *et al.* have demonstrated that *combination of antigen with sensitized lymphocytes results in platelet injury, presumably due to a lymphocyte toxic factor* injurious to the platelet membrane (Schoenbechler and Sadun, 1968; Schoenbechler and Barbaro, 1968). This reaction is also presumed to be independent of plasma factors.

B. Endpoints Used to Demonstrate Immune Injury to Platelets

1. PLATELET AGGREGATION

Historically, platelet aggregation was the first index used to demonstrate immunologic platelet injury. This has proved to be a complex and often unreliable endpoint. Shulman has described incomplete antibodies to platelet antigens, which neither aggregate platelets nor fix complement and are detectable only by competitive inhibition of complement fixing antibodies with the same specificity (Shulman et al., 1962). These antibodies may be responsible, nevertheless, for marked thrombocytopenic states in vivo. Thus, certain important antibodies may not be detectable by aggregation studies. Moreover, platelet aggregation may be produced by several quite different mechanisms. Antibodies to platelet antigens may produce aggregation without the participation of complement or divalent cation. Platelet phagocytosis results in release of ADP and aggregation, partially but not entirely due to the effects of the nucleotide. Reactions involving complement cause platelet aggregation and release of ADP, but in proper experimental circumstances C_3'-dependent, ADP-independent aggregation can be clearly demonstrated (Section II,A,5). Platelet aggregation has been shown to be an unreliable test to detect platelet antibodies in idiopathic thrombocytopenic purpura, as in many instances aggregation has been found to be actually due to thrombin remaining in the serum of blood clotted in the presence of suboptimal numbers of platelets (Jackson et al., 1963).

2. RELEASE OF INTRACELLULAR PLATELET COMPONENTS

Release of normally intracellular platelet constituents into the surrounding medium has been the most frequently employed index of immunologically-induced platelet injury. However, this phenomenon is also quite complex. The constituents most frequently measured are histamine and serotonin. Platelet nucleotides, potassium, platelet amino acids, and radio-labeled rubidium (as an index of potassium) have also been employed. Studies by Buckingham and Maynert (1964) have shown that these various constituents have different subcellular locations and their release may accordingly represent different forms or levels of cell injury. Potassium and amino acids not incorporated into protein are present free in the cytoplasm and might be expected to leak out of the platelet when the membrane has been made more permeable for any reason. In contrast, serotonin, histamine, and that portion of ADP which is released are granule-associated at least for the most part (Wurzel *et al.*, 1965; Holmsen and Day, 1968). Buckingham and Maynert (1964) demonstrated that parachloromercuribenzoate appeared to cause increased permeability of the platelet membrane followed by increased permeability of the granule membrane. Incubation with parachloromercuribenzoate resulted in prompt loss of potassium and amino acids from the platelet followed by a much smaller loss of serotonin. This effect was seen even when isotonic sucrose was employed as the suspending medium and so could not have been caused by an initial influx of sodium or calcium. In contrast, trypsin and thrombin cause an initial burst of serotonin (and histamine) release followed by progressive reaccumulation of the amines in the platelet during the course of prolonged incubation (Des Prez, 1964; Buckingham and Maynert, 1964). Trypsin produces little loss of cytoplasmic amino acids; accordingly its effect must be more complicated than simply production of membrane permeability. The concept of the *platelet release reaction* evolved from the observation that removal of calcium ion (by chelation) prevented release of platelet nucleotides by trypsin and thrombin, but when excess calcium ion was restored to the platelet–enzyme mixture, release was then observed (Grette, 1962). Grette emphasized the presence of contractile proteins in platelets and suggested that the release reaction was dependent on the appearance of intracellular calcium which in some way triggered a muscle-like contraction causing extrusion of intracellular components. Others have proposed that release actually represents extrusion of platelet granules. Enzyme studies have demonstrated that some but not all of the enzymes associated with platelet granules appear in the supernate during release reactions; therefore, it is possible that some granules with a specific makeup are extruded and others are not. Analogies have been drawn between platelet release reactions and both muscle contraction and the activity of neurosecretory granules (Holmsen and Day, 1968).

Release of platelet components by immune reactions requires calcium (and magnesium) ion and in that sense is analogous to the release reactions. However, in contrast to the effects of thrombin and trypsin, immune release of amines is delayed, progressive, and not associated with reaccumulation of amines in the platelets over the course of prolonged incubation (Gocke and Osler, 1965). Release of granule associated constituents is preceded by a loss of cytoplasmic components, and so some permeability of the membrane is likely (Siraganian *et al.*, 1968a). Whether the divalent cation is necessary for the initial membrane injury, for intracellular events secondary to that injury as a result of ion influx, or both, is not known.

Release of platelet components following phagocytosis of particles (Movat *et al.*, 1965a,b) is probably a quite different phenomenon from release due to immune reactions or to enzymes, such as thrombin or trypsin.

3. OTHER ENDPOINTS

Other studies of immune platelet injury have utilized inhibition of clot retraction, inhibition of thromboplastin formation, and complement fixation as endpoints. The relation of these phenomena to platelet aggregation and to release of intracellular components is not known.

C. Species Differences

The aggregation of blood cells in the presence of antigen (unrelated to the cell), antibody, and the first four components of complement has been termed immune adherence. Receptors mediating immune adherence are present on platelets in nonprimate species, but in primates the erythrocyte is the reactive cell. As will be discussed, there are many similarities between immune adherence and rabbit platelet injury by soluble antigen and antibody (Siqueira and Nelson, 1961) (Section II,A,9). Henson's recent studies of leukocyte aggregation in the presence of particulate antigen, antibody, and complement also emphasize species differences (Henson, 1969). He indicated that platelets from all species tested failed to adhere to erythrocytes coated with antibody and complement when the antibody species was γG (EA$^{\gamma G}$C$'$), whereas leukocytes were aggregated by this complex. In contrast, when an γM antibody was used (EA$^{\gamma M}$C$'$), platelets from cat, horse, mouse, rat, and rabbit adhered to the sensitized cell, but platelets from pig, ox, sheep, goat, man, and baboon did not. It is of note that this species grouping is not the same as that reported for the immune adherence phenomena. Moreover, the activity of γM and lack of activity of γG with respect to platelet injury is at variance with other studies of immune platelet injury in which the opposite was found to be the case. Species variation is also emphasized by the interaction between platelets and bacterial endotoxin. In the rabbit, platelet injury by bacterial endotoxin can be easily demonstrated both *in vivo* and *in vitro*. In man there is much to suggest that *in vivo* platelet–endotoxin interactions do occur, but this has been difficult to demonstrate in *in vitro* studies (see Section H). These several illustrations of important species variation in models of platelet injury illustrate that it is difficult and usually impossible to make generalizations from specific experimental results.

II. IMMUNE INJURY TO RABBIT PLATELETS

Immune platelet injury has been more thoroughly investigated in the rabbit than in any other species. This is in part due to precedent, in part to easy availability, and probably in part due to the large size and rich amine content of rabbit platelets which make them quite easy to work with. As mentioned, there are peculiarities which make comparison between the rabbit and other species very difficult. Nevertheless, the rabbit platelet will receive more than perhaps its fair share of attention in this chapter, principally because of the large amount of detailed information available concerning this species.

A. Platelet Injury by Soluble Antigen and Antibody

1. GENERAL DESCRIPTION

Addition of soluble antigen and antibody to lightly heparinized (50 μg heparin/ml) nonimmune rabbit platelet-rich plasma (R-PRP) results in a progressive release of histamine, serotonin (Gocke and Osler, 1965), and platelet nucleotides into plasma. This reaction takes place in either static or rotated systems, although it is somewhat enhanced in the latter (Marney and Des Prez, 1969). Siraganian et al. (1968a) have demonstrated that a lag period of 2–5 minutes occurs after addition of the reagents before release of histamine begins. Release of serotonin and histamine occur together. Labeled rubidium, which is thought to be distributed and transported in the same manner as potassium, is released a minute or two prior to release of histamine (Siraganian et al., 1968a). The exact timing of nucleotide (ADP) release in comparison to release of cytoplasmic (potassium, rubidium) or granule associated (histamine, serotonin) components has not been established with certainty, but it is very probable that it occurs with the granule-associated amines. The rate and extent of release depends in a rough way on the challenge dosage, increases for 10–20 minutes, and levels off at about 30 minutes, progressing only slightly for the next hour. This is in clear contrast to amine release produced by thrombin or trypsin, which is nearly maximum after 1 minute, is nonprogressive, and is followed by reaccumulation of amines by the platelets (Des Prez, 1964; Buckingham and Maynert, 1964). In rotated systems containing a sufficient concentration of platelets (100,000/mm^3), aggregation occurs and precedes release of amines by 1 or 2 minutes (Des Prez and Marney, 1969). Aggregation is

also observed in static systems when the concentration of platelets is sufficiently large. Others have observed platelet surface stickiness (Humphrey
and Jaques, 1955) and swelling (Gocke and Osler, 1965). Release of serotonin and other granule-associated platelet constituents is temperature-
dependent, requires divalent cation, is inhibited by citrate by mechanisms
more complex than simple divalent ion chelation (Section II,A,2), and
requires a plasma factor which is destroyed by heating at 56°C for 30
minutes. Coagulation is accelerated during the course of the reaction. This
can be observed in noncoagulated whole blood (Robbins and Stetson, 1959),
or in rabbit platelet-rich plasma anticoagulated with small (4 µg/ml) concentrations of heparin (Shore et al., 1962). Although most studies have
emphasized the role of the platelet in coagulation acceleration by soluble
antigen and antibody, an effect independent of blood cells, possibly relating
to Hageman factor activation, has also been reported (McKay et al.,
1958).

It is clear from the work of several investigators that the initial reaction
does not require prior fixation of either antibody or antigen on the platelet
membrane (Gocke and Osler, 1965; Siraganian et al., 1968c), suggesting
that the initial reaction occurs in the fluid phase. However, efforts to
establish the existence of a fluid phase reactant separate from the antigen–
antibody complex have not been successful.

Preincubation of antigen and antibody in the absence of platelets causes
a progressive decrement in the extent of amine release which occurs after
readdition of platelets (Henson and Cochrane, 1969b; Gocke and Osler,
1965). It has been repeatedly demonstrated that complexes formed at
antibody excess are more active with respect to platelet injury (Gocke and
Osler, 1965; Barbaro, 1961b; Siraganian et al., 1968a). Henson and Cochrane (1969b) observed that preincubation of antigen and excess antibody
in the absence of plasma resulted in decrease in histamine-releasing ability
to levels observed with mixtures of antigen and antibody at equivalence.
They postulated that preincubation allowed a rearrangement of the complex
toward a configuration resembling complexes formed at equivalence. In
the presence of plasma, however, they demonstrated another type of inhibition of histamine releasing ability not based on rearrangement of the
complex since it was observed when antigen–antibody ratios were maintained
at equivalence. To explain this effect, they postulated a second mechanism
involving generation of an inhibitory factor from plasma which suppressed
histamine release by complexes formed at equivalence as well as by those
formed at antibody excess. They further demonstrated that evolution of this
inhibitor was temperature dependent (did not develop at 0°C), required

divalent cation, and was enhanced in plasma lacking the sixth component of complement. In this regard, it is of note that Humphrey and Jaques (1955) found that hyperimmune plasmas did not sustain antigen-induced histamine release and postulated generation of an inhibitor substance.

2. Divalent Cation Requirements; Effect of Chelators

Chelators have been extensively employed as a means of estimating the divalent ion requirements of different forms of platelet injury. The data in Table I have been calculated using standard values for rabbit plasma calcium and magnesium concentrations. These calculations have not taken into account second-order chelation and the weak chelating properties of proteins and so are only approximations. The following points seem worth emphasizing.

(1) *The relation of chelator concentration to total divalent ion concentration is critically important.* With respect to EDTA, three very different circumstances can be defined. First, when the concentration of EDTA is less than that of calcium ion, some calcium is not bound. Second, when the concentration of EDTA is greater than the *combined* concentrations of calcium and magnesium, very little of either ion remains in ionized form (illustrated by column under 0.17% EDTA). Third, when the concentration of EDTA is *greater than that of calcium but less than calcium plus magnesium* (illustrated in column under 0.1% EDTA), the total unbound cation is distributed between calcium and magnesium roughly according to the ratio of their respective association constants. This provides substantial concentrations of both cations.

(2) *Magnesium salts of EDTA or EGTA always contain unbound cation.* The use of a magnesium salt of a chelator by definition provides more divalent cation than chelator. Thus the concentration of ionized calcium in the presence of MgEDTA or MgEGTA is always manyfold greater than would be the case in the presence of excess concentrations of sodium EDTA or sodium EGTA.

Sodium EDTA in concentrations exceeding the combined concentrations of Mg^{2+} and Ca^{2+} in the platelet–plasma–buffer mixture completely inhibits release of serotonin and histamine by soluble antigen and antibody (Table II). It is of some importance that plasma obtained from blood anticoagulated with 1% EDTA is often reactive, presumably due to the larger concentrations of cation which may be provided in this concentration of ligand (Table I). Siraganian *et al.* (1968b) have reported that the reaction

TABLE I

APPROXIMATE CONCENTRATIONS OF UNIONIZED DIVALENT CATIONS IN RABBIT PLASMA CONTAINING VARIOUS ANTICOAGULANTS

	Heparin	Na citrate (0.38%)	NaEDTA (0.17%)	NaEDTA (0.1%)	MgEDTA	NaEGTA	MgEGTA
Concentration in whole blood	30–100 μg/ml	12.9 mM	4.5 mM	2.7 mM	4.5 mM	4.5 mM	4.5 mM
Concentration in plasma[a]	50–166 μg/ml	21.5 mM	7.5 mM	4.5 mM	7.5 mM	7.5 mM	7.5 mM
pK calcium[b]	—	3.22	10.59	10.59	10.59	10.9	10.9
Plasma ionized calcium[c]	3.8 mM[d]	0.1 mM	$<1 \times 10^{-8}$ mM	3×10^{-3} mM	5×10^{-2} mM	1.2×10^{-8} mM	1×10^{-5} mM
pK magnesium[b]	—	3.20	8.69	8.69	8.69	5.2	5.2
Plasma ionized magnesium[c]	1.2 mM[d]	0.1 mM	$<1 \times 10^{-6}$ mM	0.5 mM	5 mM	8×10^{-5} mM	5 mM

[a] Calculated assuming hematocrit of 40%.

[b] Chaberek and Martell, 1959.

[c] Calculated using stated concentrations and dissociation constants.

[d] Mean values for rabbit calcium and magnesium (Dittmer, 1961).

TABLE II

EFFECTS OF CHELATORS ON RELEASE OF SEROTONIN FROM RABBIT PLATELETS BY SOLUBLE
ANTIGEN AND ANTIBODY

Plasma concentration of chelators (mM)	Effects
21.5 citrate	Inhibitory only if added prior to interaction of antigen, antibody, and C
4.5 NaEDTA	Variable depending on whether Mg^{2+} plus Ca^{2+} is more or less than chelator
7.5 NaEDTA	Inhibitory
7.5 MgEDTA	Noninhibitory
7.5 NaEGTA	Inhibitory
7.5 MgEGTA	Inhibitory

is Mg^{2+}-dependent and Ca^{2+}-independent, a notion which implies that the action of complement in mediating platelet injury is fundamentally different from that subserving immune hemolysis. While it appears certain that EAC' hemolysis and complement mediated platelet damage proceed somewhat by different mechanisms, the evidence offered does not substantiate the notion that only Mg^{2+} and not Ca^{2+} is required. These authors demonstrated that this form of platelet injury takes place in MgEDTA. However, Bryant and Jenkins (1968) have reported that human EAC' hemolysis also takes place in the presence of this chelator. Siraganian *et al.* (1968b) also has stated that the reaction is not inhibited in MgEGTA, a chelator which, by virtue of the large difference in its avidity for Ca^{2+} and Mg^{2+}, does not have the disadvantage of EDTA (Hovig, 1964). In contrast, studies in the writers' laboratory have demonstrated that 7.5 m/moles MgEGTA does inhibit platelet injury by soluble antigen and antibody, although smaller concentrations of this chelator (4.5 mM) produce variable results. Moreover, it is perhaps relevant to emphasize that MgEGTA has different effects on complement activity in human and in rabbit plasma when hemolysis rather than platelet injury is the endpoint observed. As illustrated in Fig. 1, EAC' hemolysis in rabbit serum takes place in the presence of MgEGTA, whereas human EAC' hemolysis does not (Marney and Des Prez, 1969), implying that the calcium ion requirement for hemolytic complement activity in rabbit systems is less than in human systems. Thus, interpretation of chelator experiments requires precise knowledge of the concentration of the ligand, the concentrations of the ions which it binds, the characteristics of the reaction being investigated, and realization that subtle species differences may exist.

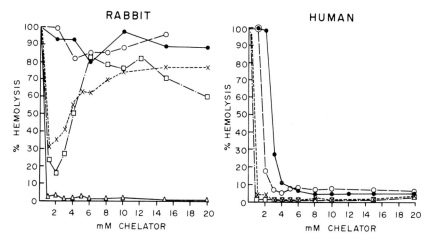

FIG. 1. *Effect of MgEGTA on EAC hemolysis in rabbit and human serum.* Data represent whole serum (filled circles), 50% serum (open circles), 20% serum (x's), 10% serum (open squares), and 4% serum (open triangles). (Marney and Des Prez, 1969, The Williams & Wilkins Co., Baltimore, Maryland.)

Henson and Cochrane (1969b) in experiments utilizing MgEGTA, reduced plasma concentrations (4%) and added calcium or magnesium, have provided evidence that antigen–antibody induced release of platelet histamine does *have an absolute requirement not only for Mg^{2+} but also for Ca^{2+}* in a concentration slightly larger than that required for EAC' hemolysis in rabbit systems (Table III). This slight difference in Ca^{2+} requirement for immune platelet injury as compared to EAC' hemolysis in rabbit serum may indicate that the calcium ion requirement for internal platelet changes resulting in release of granule associated components is slightly larger than that needed for complement activity with respect to membrane damage.

The effect of citrate appears to be unique and may provide some insight into basic mechanisms. Rabbit platelet-rich plasma prepared from blood anticoagulated with a final concentration of 0.38% citrate does not demonstrate release of amines when challenged with soluble antigen and antibody (Humphrey and Jaques, 1955; Haining, 1956b; McIntire *et al.*, 1949; Des Prez and Bryant, 1966), although platelet aggregation is seen (Section

TABLE III

CATION REQUIREMENTS FOR HISTAMINE RELEASE[a]

Plasma	Molarity $\times 10^{-4b}$		Hemolysis (%)	Platelet clumping	Histamine release (%)
	Ca^{2+}	Mg^{2+}			
4% plasma + 4 × $10^{-4}M$	—	—	0	0	0
EGTA	12	—	100	+	30
	—	12	35	0	0
	8	4	100	+	60
10% plasma + 5 × $10^{-4}M$	—	—	0	0	0
EGTA	10	—	100	+	48
	—	10	60	+	28
	6.6	3.3	100	+	60

[a] Histamine release from 2.5 × 10^8 platelets was produced by addition of 10 μg Ab N and 0.1 μg Ag N in the presence of 4 or 10% rabbit plasma. Platelet clumping was observed microscopically. Duplicate tubes contained 2.5 × 10^7 sensitized sheep erythrocytes instead of platelets (from Henson and Cochran, 1969b).

[b] Final molar concentration in the reaction mixture.

II,A,5). However, as demonstrated in Fig. 2, if antigen, antibody, and heparinized platelet-poor plasma are allowed to react in the absence of citrate, an activity is generated which then causes release of platelet amines when first citrate and then platelets are readded (Des Prez and Bryant, 1966). This was initially interpreted to indicate that the initial phase of the reaction involved the divalent cation-dependent steps of complement activation and that these were inhibited by citrate; the later stages of the platelet injury reaction were regarded as divalent cation independent as is known to be the case with the later stages of immune hemolysis. However, this interpretation is no longer tenable for two reasons. First, inhibition of platelet injury by citrate is not reversible by readdition of divalent cations (Humphrey and Jaques, 1955; Haining, 1956b; McIntire et al., 1949). Second, citrate does not abolish EAC' hemolysis in systems employing undiluted rabbit or human plasma. The inhibition of reactivity when citrate is present from the outset but not when it is added after initial interaction of antigen, antibody, and plasma is suggestively similar to generation of anaphylatoxin by agar in rat serum: formation of anaphylatoxin is prevented by citrate, but its activity, once formed, is not (Rocha e Silva, 1952). The mechanism of citrate inhibition of platelet injury by soluble antigen

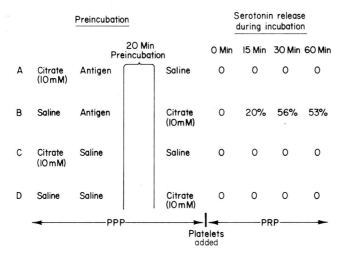

| | Preincubation | | | Serotonin release during incubation | | | |
				O Min	15 Min	30 Min	60 Min
			20 Min Preincubation				
A	Citrate (10 mM)	Antigen	Saline	O	O	O	O
B	Saline	Antigen	Citrate (10 mM)	O	20%	56%	53%
C	Citrate (10 mM)	Saline	Saline	O	O	O	O
D	Saline	Saline	Citrate (10 mM)	O	O	O	O

←————————PPP————————→ | ←————PRP————→

Platelets
added

FIG. 2. *Effect of addition of citrate before and after antigen–antibody interaction on release of serotonin from subsequently added platelets.* Heparinized platelet-rich plasma was prepared using blood of an immunized rabbit, divided into 4 aliquots, platelets separated from each by centrifugation, and the platelet buttons set aside. Citrate was added to 2 aliquots (A and C) and a control amount of saline to the other two (B and D) prior to addition of egg albumin (A and B) or control saline challenge (C and D). All samples were then preincubated for 20 minutes, following which citrate (to B and D) and saline (to A and C) were added in reverse order. Platelet buttons were then resuspended in each sample, incubation and rotation carried out, and release of serotonin measured over a further 60-minute period of incubation. Platelet-rich plasma, PRP; and platelet-poor plasma, PPP. (Des Prez and Bryant, 1966, The Rockefeller University Press, New York, New York).

and antibody remains unexplained but is difficult to attribute to its activity as a chelator of divalent cations.

As mentioned above, in contrast to most other studies, Miescher and Cooper (1960) reported that NaEDTA did not inhibit platelet aggregation by immune complexes. Using large concentrations of soluble complexes prepared in antigen excess, they demonstrated rabbit platelet aggregation in the presence of NaEDTA in a final concentration of 13 mmoles. Moreover, they demonstrated fixation of the complexes onto the platelets by fluorescent staining techniques. Amine release was not measured in these experiments. Complexes prepared at equivalence or antibody excess were much less active in producing these changes, in clear contrast to release of amines by antigen and antibody. The experimental details of these studies were so different from most referred to above that comparison is difficult. However, they make it quite clear that attachment of soluble immune complexes to platelets may occur in the absence of divalent cation or complement; release of platelet amines and other granule associated substances probably does not occur under these circumstances.

3. Nature of Plasma Cofactors

All investigators agree that release of amines from rabbit platelets by soluble antigen and antibody requires a plasma factor with the heat lability of complement. A mixture containing 10% plasma in buffer provides optimum activity and larger concentrations of plasma are slightly inhibitory (Gocke and Osler, 1965; Siraganian et al., 1968a). Initially disagreement existed as to whether or not this plasma factor was complement (Barbaro, 1961b; Gocke, 1965). This confusion now appears to be due to the fact that two different experimental systems, platelet injury by soluble antigen and antibody, on the one hand, and by preformed immune precipitates, on the other, were regarded as the same (Section II,C) (Des Prez and Bryant, 1966). Studies by Gocke (1965) and Henson and Cochrane (1969a,b) have established the identity of the heat labile plasma factor as complement beyond reasonable doubt. The latter authors used plasma depleted of C_3' by treatment with cobra factor and plasma congenitally lacking C_6' to establish that both of these complement components were required in the release of platelet amines by soluble antigen and antibody.

The involvement of the complement system in platelet amine release and the fact that complement-derived anaphylatoxins cause vascular permeability and release of amines from mast cells led naturally to the notion that the platelet injury might be due to anaphylatoxin as well. The demonstration that agar-treated rabbit plasma released platelet amines was consistent with this notion (Humphrey and Jaques, 1955). However, Miescher and Gorstein (1961) reported that generation of anaphylatoxin in rabbit blood by immune precipitates did not produce a fluid phase platelet amine releasing capacity; Henson and Cochrane (1969b) have reported similar results using rabbit anaphylatoxin generated with cobra factor. The question remains an open one, however, since platelet injury may require anaphylatoxin or a similar activity in intimate contact with the platelet membrane rather than in the fluid phase. Rabbit anaphylatoxin is, moreover, a weaker reactant in biologic systems measuring anaphylatoxin activity (rat uterus bioassay, histamine release from mast cells) than is anaphylatoxin generated from the plasma of other species (Haining, 1956b).

A requirement for a plasma factor or factors in addition to complement is possible, but there is no evidence bearing directly on this point.

4. Effect of Antigen–Antibody Ratio and Antigen Dose

It seems clear that amine release by soluble antigen and antibody can be mediated by γG since methods used to prepare antibody excluded γM and γA (Des Prez and Bryant, 1966). Sera for preparation of the antibody were obtained after prolonged immunization, making the existence of contaminating homocytotropic antibody unlikely. The Fc fragment of the γG molecule is essential, since its prior removal by pepsin digestion eliminates its ability to produce amine release (Gocke and Osler, 1965; Des Prez and Bryant, 1969). The reactivity of purified γM antibody in amine release by soluble antigen and antibody has not been rigorously studied.

Several groups are in agreement that an antigen–antibody ratio in antibody excess is most efficient in producing release of amines by soluble antigen and antibody. Siraganian and associates' careful studies (1968a) established that an Ab/Ag ratio of 20:1 (by weight) was most efficient, ratios of 40:1 and 50:1 were slightly less so, a 10:1 ratio (equivalence with respect to the precipitin reaction in the ovalbumen–antiovalbumen system studied) was distinctly less active, and ratios of 5:1 and 2.5:1 were inactive. The reason that antigen–antibody interactions at antibody excess are more efficient in producing complement mediated platelet damage remains unclear.

Several observations apparently contradict this emphasis on antibody excess. As previously mentioned, Miescher and Cooper (1960) found that platelet aggregation by soluble immune complexes was maximum with complexes prepared in antigen excess. However, the experimental details were quite different from studies focused on amine release. The platelet–plasma mixture contained EDTA in a concentration sufficient to eliminate complement activity (13 mmoles final concentration), and the challenge was extremely large concentrations of soluble complexes formed at antigen excess. In contrast, Ishizaka and Ishizaka (1962) found that soluble complexes prepared in antigen excess did not produce platelet aggregation. These discrepancies emphasize the importance of superficially minor differences in experimental details.

5. Aggregation: Effects of ADP and Cobra Factor

Siraganian and associates (1968c) state that release of platelet amines by antigen–antibody reactions is not associated with platelet aggregation and is not modified by platelet nucleotides. These authors utilized a platelet concentration of $20,000/mm^3$ and a static system. Recently completed studies in the writers' laboratories using both agitated and nonagitated systems and a somewhat greater platelet concentration have indicated that platelets do aggregate during the course of injury by soluble antigen and antibody and that platelet ADP does play a role (Marney and Des Prez, 1969). In aggregometer studies (Chronolog Aggregometer) addition of soluble antigen (ovalbumen) and antibody in a 20:1 Ab/Ag ratio caused aggregation with an onset in 2 minutes. At threshold dosage a biphasic wave of aggregation was seen with the second wave occurring about 3 minutes after challenge (Fig. 3). The first wave of aggregation was indifferent

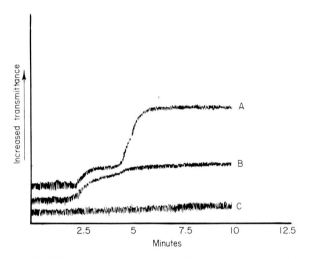

FIG. 3. *Effect of AMP and cobra factor on platelet aggregation by soluble antigen and antibody in heparinized plasma.* The above are superimposed reproductions of traces transcribed with an aggregometer (Chronolog Corporation) which measures increased light transmittance through a *cuvette* containing stirred platelet-rich plasma as an index of aggregation. Trace A was obtained by adding egg albumin (0.5 μg N) and anti-EA γ-globulin (10 μg N) to PRP in the *cuvette*. Trace B was obtained in a similar fashion, but AMP (10 μM/ml final concentration) had been added prior to challenge with antigen and antibody. Trace C was also obtained in like manner except that cobra factor in concentration sufficient to inactivate C_3 was added 3 minutes prior to challenge with antigen and antibody.

to the presence of AMP in the mixture, but the second was eliminated thereby. This is consistent with the notion of an initial membrane change favoring platelet-to-platelet adhesion and a second phase of ADP release which accentuates the aggregation process. It is noteworthy that the initial phase of aggregation precedes platelet amine release and probably platelet ADP release as well. In a general way, the data regarding antibody–antigen ratios were applicable to this index of platelet injury as well as to amine release: At threshold dosage Ab/Ag ratios in antigen excess were inactive and a 20:1 ratio was optimum. Mixtures in antigen excess produced aggregation only at large challenge dosage. Studies of platelet adhesion to glass bead columns indicated that the early aggregation phenomenon was associated with increased platelet stickiness. Pretreatment of plasma with very small concentrations of cobra factor (C_3' depletion) eliminated aggregation entirely. Most interestingly, citrate, which entirely prevents amine release by soluble antigen and antibody, did not prevent platelet aggregation although the second wave of aggregation, thought to represent ADP release, was not seen. However, aggregation in citrated plasma was entirely eliminated by cobra factor treatment (Fig. 4). Thus, antigen–antibody

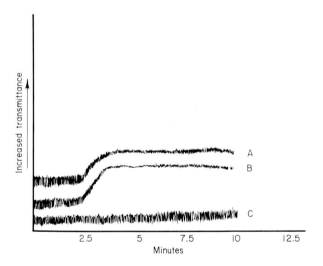

Fig. 4. *Effect of AMP and cobra factor on rabbit platelet aggregation by soluble antigen and antibody in citrated plasma.* The data were obtained as described in Fig. 3 excepting that citrated plasma was employed. Note that there is no biphasic aspect to trace A (antigen and antibody) and that inclusion of AMP (trace B) is without effect. Inclusion of cobra factor so as to inactivate complement (trace C) prevented aggregation entirely,

complexes can fix onto platelets and cause aggregation without producing amine release. Inhibition of this reaction by cobra factor indicates that at least the first four components of complement are required for this aggregation even in circumstances (citrated plasma) in which amine release does not occur.

Platelet aggregation by soluble antigen and antibody may thus proceed by several mechanisms or stages, all of which may contribute to the end result: First, fixation of C_3' on the membrane produces platelet-to-platelet adhesion; second, complement mediated membrane damage may produce ADP release with further aggregation; third, release of platelet serotonin, which lowers the threshold for ADP-induced aggregation may cause further enhancement; fourth, in nonanticoagulated systems thrombin would produce further aggregation.

It is of note that details of platelet aggregation by preformed immune precipitates are quite different from those described above (Section II,C).

6. Relationship to Coagulation Changes

Since thrombin produces release of platelet amines, it was reasonable to suggest that histamine release by antigen and antibody might be due to thrombin formation. This possibility has been excluded by several lines of evidence: (1) Hypoprothrombinemia, induced by either prior dicoumerol therapy or barium sulfate adsorption of plasma, does not inhibit amine release; (2) soy bean trypsin inhibitor, a potent inhibitor of prothrombin conversion, is also without effect; (3) the concentration of heparin or hirudin required to inhibit antigen–antibody-induced histamine release is several orders of magnitude larger than that required to inhibit the effects of thrombin either on platelets or on fibrinogen polymerization; (4) amine release by thrombin is immediate and reverses with continuing incubation whereas that due to antigen–antibody interactions is progressive and irreversible (McIntire et al., 1949; Des Prez, 1964; Shore et al., 1962; Tidball and Shore, 1962).

Although antigen-induced amine release is not due to thrombin, the type of platelet injury which results in amine release also accelerates blood coagulation. Robbins and Stetson (1959) observed that the silicone clotting time was accelerated when antigen and antibody were added to whole blood and that platelets were necessary for this effect. Horowitz et al. (1962), using an assay system sensitive to platelet factor 3 (Stypven time), indicated that this coagulation acceleration was due to platelet injury which increased the availability of platelet factor 3 for thromboplastin formation. Although antigen–antibody reactions have been reported to accelerate coagulation in platelet-free systems, it seems likely that for the most part clotting is accelerated through platelet injury (McKay et al., 1958). It has been suggested that platelets injured or altered in a number of ways may serve as a "foreign surface" causing activation of Hageman factor (Fergusen, 1967), and it seems likely that immune injury produces the same effect. Shore et al. (1962) have reported that coagulation acceleration and histamine release are inhibited in parallel fashion by tolsoyl-arginine-methyl-ester (TAME), whereas lysine-ethylester (LEE) is without effect. They postulated development of a complement-mediated TAME sensitive enzyme activity which either possessed thromboplastic activity itself or acted on platelets to produce blood thromboplastin. The latter seems the more likely explanation.

7. INHIBITORS OF THE REACTION

A variety of inhibitory substances have been employed in an attempt to better understand release of platelet amines by soluble antigen and antibody. As mentioned above, citrate and oxalate inhibit amine release. It perhaps merits repeating that citrate is inhibitory only if added before interaction of antigen, antibody, and complement, and that citrate does *not* prevent complement-dependent immune hemolysis in rabbit plasma. In contrast to citrate, TAME and acetyl-tyrosine-ethyl-ester (AcTEE) inhibit amine release by soluble antigen and antibody whether added from the start or after initial interaction of antigen, antibody, and complement. Both of these substances are inhibitors of C_1'-esterase. However, with respect to platelet injury by soluble antigen and antibody, it seems likely that they also act at some other esterolytic step, since preincubation of antigen, antibody, and complement should provide opportunity for the complement sequence to proceed beyond the C_1' step. Lysine-ethyl-ester (LEE) is not inhibitory (Shore *et al.*, 1962), and soy bean trypsin inhibitor (SBTI), which also inhibits the plasminogen system as well as prothrombin conversion, has no effect (McIntire *et al.*, 1949). Experiments with other esterase inhibitors are reported as in progress at the time of this writing (Henson and Cochrane, 1969b).

Heparin in high concentration was found to be inhibitory by one group. However, studies from our laboratories have demonstrated that as little as 120 μg/ml of heparin is inhibitory when a small challenge concentration of antigen and antibody is employed (Des Prez and Bryant, 1966). It seems likely that the concentration of heparin required for inhibition varies depending on challenge dosage; in all instances, however, the required heparin concentration was much greater than that needed to inhibit the action of thrombin either on platelets or on fibrinogen. Hirudin is not inhibitory in concentrations much greater than those required for its antithrombin activity (Henson and Cochrane, 1969b).

Haining (1956b) demonstrated inhibition by sodium chloride in slightly greater than physiologic concentration, by smaller concentrations of sodium salicylate and sodium benzoate, and by very small (10 mmole) concentrations of 3-hydroxy-2-phenyl cinchoninic acid (HPCA). These authors discussed this inhibition in terms of parallel effects on anaphylatoxin activity. In contrast to citrate, which prevents the formation but not the action of anaphylatoxins, salicylate and 3-hydroxy-2-phenyl cinchoninic acid were felt to interfere with the formation but not the action of this activity once formed.

Gocke (1965) demonstrated that classic methods used to inactivate complement components inhibit antigen–antibody-induced histamine release in parallel fashion. More recently, Henson and Cochrane (1969b) have demonstrated that neither plasma previously treated with cobra factor so as to inactivate C_3', nor plasma from rabbits congenitally deficient in C_6' supports this form of platelet damage.

A variety of other substances such as n-ethyl maleimid, ninhydrin, allicin, and phenol have been reported as inhibitory (Mueller-Eckhardt and Lüscher, 1968b; Westerholm, 1965). A detailed study of inhibitor patterns will probably provide useful information as to basic mechanisms.

8. Nature of the Injury

It is apparent that soluble antigen and antibody can cause several different types or levels of platelet injury depending on the experimental conditions employed.

(1) *As demonstrated by Miescher, very large concentrates of soluble complexes prepared in antigen excess can cause platelet aggregation in the presence of high concentrations of EDTA* (Miescher and Cooper, 1960). Although measurements were not made, it seems very likely that amine release would not occur in such systems. Involvement of complement was excluded by the presence of NaEDTA. The results suggest direct attachment of antibody to the platelet.

(2) *In properly selected experimental circumstances, complement dependent aggregation can be dissociated from complement-dependent amine release.* The data in Fig. 4 (Section II,A,5) demonstrate platelet aggregation by soluble antigen and antibody in citrated platelet-rich plasma (in which circumstance, amine release does not occur) and inhibition of this aggregation by depletion of C_3' (using cobra factor).

(3) *In heparinized plasma, antigen, antibody, and complement produce not only platelet aggregation but also release of both cytoplasmic and granule associated intracellular materials.* The leaking of cytoplasmic materials is

most probably due to a complement mediated cytotoxic effect with resulting loss of membrane integrity. As mentioned, Siraganian and associates (1969b) demonstrated that loss of cytoplasmic materials, once initiated at 37°C, continued at a slower rate at 4°C, whereas loss of histamine was arrested at the lower temperature. Also, addition of NaEDTA interrupts histamine loss. The nature of the membrane injury is unknown, but the inhibitory effect of citrate when present from the outset but not when added after initial interaction of antigen, antibody, and complement suggests that it is different from that subserving immune (EAC′) hemolysis at least in part, since this is not inhibited by citrate in rabbit plasma. The different effects of citrate depending on time of addition are very suggestive of anaphylatoxin activity. Inhibition by TAME and other synthetic esters supports the notion that an esterase is involved, perhaps located on the platelet membrane. It is the writers' present hypothesis that membrane injury is due to a proteolytic byproduct of the complement system, resembling anaphylatoxin, but differing in that there is an additional requirement for close juxtaposition of the proteolytic activity to the platelet membrane, perhaps by location on an antigen–antibody–complement complex which itself fixes onto the platelet membrane. The mechanism of this attachment remains unknown, although there is much to suggest that the Fc fragment of γ-globulin, when altered so as to fix complement, also may attach directly to the platelet membrane.

In contrast to release of platelet cytoplasmic constituents, membrane injury is a necessary but not sufficient condition for release of granule associated amines and ADP. This requires both membrane injury and divalent cations in concentrations greater than those provided in NaEDTA plasma and a temperature greater than 4°C. How much calcium ion is required for intracellular events associated with loss of granule associated constituents is not known. The data illustrated in Table III (Henson and Cochrane, 1969b) suggest that it is larger than that required for EAC′ hemolysis in rabbit plasma.

9. Relationship to Immune Adherence

Particulate antigens treated with antibody and complement cause aggregation of primate erythrocytes and of nonprimate platelets. Siqueira and Nelson have reported many similarities between this phenomenon of immune adherence (IA) and the aggregation of rabbit platelets by soluble antigen and antibody, and have suggested that the mechanisms involved might be the same (Siqueira and Nelson, 1961). They described two phases in platelet aggregation by soluble antigen and antibody. The first was dependent on heat labile plasma factors, took place in the temporary absence of platelets, and was inhibited by minor increases in ionic strength or by citrate; the second phase was not inhibited by citrate or by large increases in ionic strength, and the activity had acquired considerable heat stability. The similarities of these features to those described above for amine release by soluble antigen and antibody are impressive.

The central problem in attributing platelet injury by soluble antigen and antibody entirely to the IA mechanism is raised by the fact that platelet injury as manifested by amine release is observed in species not having IA receptor sites on platelets (Humphrey and Jaques, 1955). A second difficulty is raised by the demonstration that not only C_3' but also C_6' is required for amine release by soluble antigen and antibody, whereas only the first four components of complement are required for IA (Henson and Cochrane, 1969b; Siqueira and Nelson, 1961). It should be emphasized that the endpoint utilized in immune adherence studies was platelet aggregation rather than release of amines. Nevertheless, with regard to the rabbit at least, a role of IA in immunologic platelet injury by soluble antigen and antibody remains likely.

B. Platelet Injury by Particulate Antigens and Complement

Release of amines from rabbit platelets by glycogen has been discussed by Waalkes and Coburn (1959a,b). These and other studies have demonstrated many similarities between amine release by soluble antigen and antibody and by glycogen, suggesting that similar mechanisms are involved. Westerholm (1965), in a detailed comparison of these two systems of platelet injury, indicated that both required heat-labile plasma factors and divalent cations and demonstrated similar time courses of amine release, and the effects of several inhibitors were shown to be the same. The only difference noted concerned the effect of increased plasma ionic strength: amine release by soluble antigen and antibody was inhibited by minor increases in salt concentration, whereas release by glycogen was not.

Henson and Cochrane (1969b) have documented a further difference in platelet injury by particulate antigen as compared to soluble antigen and antibody. The particulate antigen studied was zymosan. Both types of challenge were inhibited by treatment of plasma with cobra factor so as to inactivate C_3', but only the soluble system required C_6' (demonstrated by the use of plasma from rabbits congenitally deficient in C_6'). There are some peculiarities of the interaction of particulate antigens and antibody with the complement system which may contribute to this particular form of platelet injury. Gewurz and associates (1968) have shown that bacterial endotoxin, a particulate antigen, produces fixation of the six terminal complement components (C_3' and beyond) with very little fixation of the first three components, and that soluble antigen and antibody, in contrast, produce fixation of the first three components and much less depletion of C_3' and subsequently acting components. Preformed immune precipitates produced efficient fixation of all. The same authors (Shin *et al.*, 1969) showed that this effect of endotoxin was not a direct one on isolated C_3' but rather required prior fixation of serum factors and presumably the first three complement components on the endotoxin surface. Earlier literature concerning the properdin controversy also suggested that zymosan, in combination with small concentrations of C_1', C_4', and C_2', forms a very efficient C_3' converting activity (Nelson, 1958). It has been postulated that the efficiency of C_3' conversion is greatly enhanced if the C_{142} complex is located on a surface.

As mentioned, the phenomenon of immune adherence requires only the first four components of complement and is mediated in part by receptor sites for fixed C_3' on the membranes of nonprimate platelets. It seems reasonable to postulate that fixation of a particulate antigen coated with large quantities of C_3' onto the platelet might then cause changes resembling the platelet-surface reaction or platelet phagocytosis. However, this is speculation, to date not supported by experimental data.

C. Platelet Injury by Preformed Immune Precipitate

1. General Description

Preformed immune precipitate (PIP) mixed with rabbit platelet-rich plasma produces release of platelet amines, release of ADP, and platelet aggregation. In contrast to platelet injury by soluble antigen and antibody, amine release is slower, often requiring as much as 10–15 minutes to commence. It then progresses over a 30–60-minute period. In clear contrast to the soluble system, citrate does not inhibit amine release by preformed immune precipitate (Des Prez and Bryant, 1966). Heat-labile plasma factors only enhance this form of platelet injury, but appreciable amine release occurs in the presence of plasma heated so as to inactivate complement (56°C, 30 minutes) (Barbaro, 1961b). The dosage of preformed immune precipitate required is quite large, as much as 10 mg precipitate nitrogen/ml of platelet-rich plasma being necessary. Precipitates made with antibody previously subjected to pepsin digestion so as to remove Fc fragment are as active as precipitates made with nondigested antibody, again in contrast to platelet injury by soluble antigen and antibody (Des Prez and Bryant, 1969). Agitation is required, little release or aggregation being noted in static systems.

2. DIVALENT CATION REQUIREMENT

In clear contrast to the soluble system, citrate and oxalate do not prevent this form of platelet injury. NaEDTA in concentration equal to or exceeding the combined concentrations of Ca^{2+} and Mg^{2+} is completely inhibitory. Lower concentrations of EDTA (0.1% in whole blood or 4.5 mM in plasma) which are sufficient to prevent coagulation often are not inhibitory. The effects of MgEDTA and MgEGTA on release of amines by preformed immune precipitate have not been studied, but both of these chelators themselves produce platelet aggregation of a type unrelated to ADP and not associated with amine release, thought to be due to the large concentration of magnesium ion present in plasma containing these chelators (Des Prez et al., 1967).

3. NATURE OF THE PLASMA REQUIREMENT

A plasma factor with the heat lability of complement facilitates interaction of platelets and PIP. A buffer mixture containing 10% plasma is optimum, and larger plasma concentrations are slightly inhibitory (Barbaro, 1961b). As mentioned above, Barbaro (1961b) demonstrated that heating plasma to 56°C for 30 minutes, so as to produce total inactivation of complement, only reduced platelet release by preformed immune precipitate to about 50% of control (nonheated plasma). This observation led to a detailed analysis of the role of complement, which demonstrated that other modes of C′ inactivation, such as pretreatment of plasma with zymosan or salicyl-aldoxime, also reduced but did not eliminate release of platelet amines by preformed immune precipitate. On this and other grounds, he concluded that the plasma factor involved was not complement. Movat and associates also concluded that complement was not required for the preformed immune precipitate–platelet interaction (Movat et al., 1965a,b), and have suggested that the required plasma factor is a γ-globulin. Evidence against a role for C′ has also been offered by Mueller-Eckhardt and Lüscher (1968a).

4. Effects of Antigen–Antibody Ratio and Antibody Class

Barbaro has demonstrated that at threshold dosage, preformed immune precipitate prepared in antibody excess is most active in producing platelet damage, and preformed immune precipitate prepared in antigen excess is least active (Barbaro, 1961a). The importance of antigen–antibody ratios is not so great at larger dosage. This difference between efficiency in the production of platelet damage (maximum at antibody excess) and complement fixation (maximum near equivalence) was used as further evidence against a role for complement (Barbaro, 1961b). As mentioned, pepsin digestion of antibody prior to the formation of preformed immune precipitate, a maneuver which eliminates the ability of antibody to fix complement, does not abolish the ability of the preformed immune precipitate to produce platelet injury. The importance of antibody class, specifically the activity of precipitates formed with γM, has not been determined.

5. Inhibitors of the Reaction

Quantitative data concerning inhibitors of the preformed immune precipitate–platelet interaction are sparse. Inhibition by iodoacetate and by phenyl butazone has been reported by Mustard and associates (Mustard *et al.*, 1967; Movat *et al.*, 1965a). Heparin is inhibitory only in concentrations much larger than required for inhibition of the soluble system, and the reaction is not abolished by increases in plasma ionic strength to anticomplementary levels (Des Prez and Bryant, 1969).

6. Aggregation: Effects of AMP and Cobra Factor

In heparinized platelet-rich plasma, the preformed immune precipitate–platelet interaction produces large platelet aggregates and positive aggregometer traces (Fig. 5). In contrast to platelet injury by soluble antigen and antibody, the onset of aggregation is delayed for 5–10 minutes and the tracing is not biphasic. The effects of AMP and of cobra factor in this system have not been completely investigated. In citrated platelet-rich plasma, small platelet aggregates are seen on microscopy, but the extent of the aggregation is not sufficient to produce increased light transmission in the aggregometer.

7. Nature of Injury

Table IV summarizes some differences between platelet injury by soluble antigen and antibody and by preformed immune precipitate. Movat,

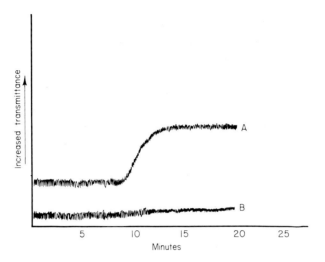

FIG. 5. *Aggregation of rabbit platelets by preformed immune precipitates (PIP) in heparinized and in citrated plasma.* Heparinized platelet-rich plasma was challenged with PIP prepared at equivalence in a concentration of 100 μg precipitate N/ml of plasma (trace A). Note that aggregation did not commence for 10 minutes. In citrated plasma (trace B) the very small aggregates formed did not produce much deflection of the aggregometer trace but did cause narrowing of the oscillations.

TABLE IV

SUMMARY OF DIFFERENCES BETWEEN PLATELET INJURY BY SOLUBLE ANTIGEN AND ANTIBODY AND PLATELET INJURY BY IMMUNE PRECIPITATES[a]

Differentiating feature	Soluble system	Precipitate system
Activity in citrated plasma	Inhibited	Not inhibited
Heparin concentration effecting complete inhibition	120 μg/ml	>1000 μg/ml
Ionic strength (conductivity-mMho) effecting complete inhibition	20–24[b]	>30[c]
Pepsin-digested antibody	Inactive[b]	Active[c]

[a] From Des Prez and Bryant, 1969.
[b] In heparinized plasma.
[c] In citrated plasma.

Mustard, and associates (Movat *et al.*, 1965a,b; Mustard, 1967) have demonstrated phagocytosis of preformed immune precipitate by platelets and regard this as a special example of the interaction between platelets and a variety of foreign surfaces to which platelets either adhere or, when the surfaces exist as sufficiently small particles, they ingest (Mustard *et al.*, 1967). The platelet surface reaction is not inhibited by citrate, requires plasma factors other than complement, and is associated with release of platelet constituents including serotonin, histamine, and ADP, the latter resulting in platelet aggregation. Thus, it seems likely that the reaction between platelets and preformed immune precipitate may proceed both by complement-independent mechanisms in experimental conditions inhibiting complement and by complement-dependent mechanisms in circumstances in which complement is present and not inhibited, and that separation of these two mechanisms of platelet damage may be quite difficult.

D. Platelet Injury by Homocytotropic Antibody

It is well established that polymorphonuclear leukocytes may become coated with a certain species of antibody which has the property of producing cell injury upon combination with antigen in the absence of plasma cofactors (Lichtenstein and Osler, 1964). Barbaro and Zvaifler (1966) were the first to report that a similar form of complement independent immune injury due to so-called *homocytotropic antibody* (cytotropic for homologous tissues) could be demonstrated with rabbit platelets as well. This species of antibody, which has also been referred to as homologous passive cutaneous anaphylaxis (PCA)-mediating antibody and as non-C′-dependent passive cutaneous anaphylaxis-mediating antibody, is thought to be present transiently in the circulation in some, but not all, animals during the first 2 weeks following immunization with antigen in complete adjuvant (Zvaifler and Becker, 1966; Onoue *et al.*, 1966; Henson and Cochrane, 1969b).

Subsequently, Schoenbechler and Barbaro (1968) have reported that the platelet injury, which Barbaro had attributed to this mechanism, was actually due to platelet toxins elaborated by sensitized lymphocytes contaminating the platelet suspension (*vide infra*). In like manner Siraganian *et al.* (1968c) were unable to demonstrate platelet injury in the absence of plasma in circumstances in which homocytotropic antibody could be presumed to be present. However, Henson and Cochrane (1969b) believe that the mechanism initially postulated by Barbaro and Zvaifler does produce platelet injury in the rabbit. The critical evidence bearing on this point was their ability to produce deposition of immune complexes in the vascular endothelium, a phenomenon they regard as dependent on platelet injury, in rabbits depleted of C_3' by treatment with cobra factor. The experimental conditions of these studies were complex, and whether or not platelets can be injured by the interaction of antigen and this special category of cell-fixed antibody in the absence of complement remains a matter of disagreement (Siraganian and Oliveira, 1968).

E. Platelet Injury by Products of Leukocytes

As mentioned above, Schoenbechler and associates have demonstrated that rabbit platelets can be injured during the course of interaction of antigen and lymphocytes obtained from animals sensitized with the antigen (Shoenbechler and Sadun, 1968; Schoenbechler and Barbaro, 1968). The studies documenting this opinion were performed in animals infected with Schistosoma mansoni and used Schistosomal products as the antigen. The interaction was not dependent on plasma cofactors and was not seen when phagocytes were substituted for lymphocytes. However, they suggested that in some circumstances the presence of phagocytes enhanced the degree of platelet injury. The basic mechanism of this form of platelet injury was not defined, although it was suggested that this might represent another manifestation of the cytopathic properties of the products of stimulated or transformed lymphocytes. The suggestion that platelets may be involved in reactions based on cellular immune mechanisms in addition to those based on humoral mechanisms is new and exciting.

F. Platelet Injury by Heterologous Antiplatelet Antibodies

This simplest form of immune platelet injury has surprisingly received relatively little experimental attention in the rabbit. The early experimental data has been reviewed by Miescher and Gorstein (1961). Guinea pig antirabbit platelet antibody was shown to produce aggregation of platelets and, in the presence of complement, lysis. The details of complement action, however, have not been investigated. Clot retraction is also inhibited by such heterorologous antibodies, and some antibody coated platelets may be ingested by phagocytes.

III. PLATELET INJURY BY BACTERIAL ENDOTOXIN

Radio-labeled endotoxin injected into rabbits promptly fixes onto white blood cells; serial samples of blood obtained immediately after such injections and centrifuged revealed almost all of the radioactivity in the buffy coat (Braude *et al.*, 1955). Herring *et al.* (1963) were able to separate leukocytes and platelets by special centrifugation techniques and found that it was the platelet component of the buffy coat to which endotoxin immediately became fixed. The label was next detected in the reticuloendothelial system (Braude *et al.*, 1955) and at no time circulated in plasma separate from cells to any appreciable extent. Such endotoxin injections cause immediate platelet aggregation and sequestration of these aggregates in capillary beds; during the first minute following relatively large (100 μg) dosage platelets virtually disappear from the circulation and return gradually over the following hour. A similar sequence of events is seen after injection of other particles such as india ink (Salvidio and Crosby, 1960; Cohen *et al.*, 1965). Platelet aggregates have been observed in pulmonary capillaries following intravenous administration of meningococcal toxin (Stetson, 1951), and both serotonin and substances with platelet aggregating properties have been detected in cell-free plasma following endotoxin injection (Shimamoto *et al.*, 1958; Davis *et al.*, 1960). Observations using the rabbit ear chamber have demonstrated that platelet aggregation is the first observable effect of endotoxin injection in the contralateral ear, and that platelet thrombi often result, in which leukocytes appear to be involved in a secondary fashion (Silver and Stehbens, 1965). These observations all suggest that the platelet is involved, either primarily or secondarily, in the earliest phases of bloodstream clearance of endotoxin and possibly of other particles as well, and in the production of the biologic effects of endotoxin.

Incubation of rabbit platelets with endotoxin *in vitro* produces platelet aggregation and progressive release of platelet amines (Davis *et al.*, 1961; Des Prez *et al.*, 1961). This platelet endotoxin interaction is temperature dependent, is inhibited by NaEDTA in concentrations exceeding the combined concentrations of magnesium and calcium ion, is not inhibited by citrate, requires a plasma factor with the heat lability of complement, and is observed only in rotated systems suggesting a requirement for cell–particle contact (Des Prez *et al.*, 1961). Coagulation is enhanced during such incubations, due principally to platelet injury resulting in increased availability of platelet factor 3 for thromboplastin formation, although effects due to Hageman factor activation have also been postulated (Horowitz *et al.*, 1962; McKay *et al.*, 1969). Although thrombin is generated at accelerated rates in blood–endotoxin mixtures not containing anticoagulants, it is clear that the effect of endotoxin on platelets is not mediated by thrombin since concentrations of heparin as great as 1 mg/ml are not inhibitory (Des Prez, 1964). Electron microscopic studies during the course of incubation of endotoxin with citrated rabbit platelet-rich plasma have demonstrated platelet degranulation, loss of membrane integrity, swelling, and some phagocytosis of endotoxin by the platelets (Davis, 1966; Spielvogel, 1967).

The parallels between the effects of endotoxin and of immunologic reactions on platelets is obvious, and it has been assumed by many that the endotoxin effect is basically due to reaction with antibody. Macroglobulin antibodies reactive with polysaccharide determinants of endotoxins of gram-negative bacteria exist in all species virtually from birth. Boyden has discussed these so-called natural antibodies as primitive "recognition factors" which exist prior to antigenic stimulation, and, by virtue of their reactivity with polysaccharide determinants widely distributed in nature, may provide the initial steps in the recognition of foreign particulate antigens (Boyden, 1966). While not rigorously established, it seems likely that endotoxins react with relatively primitive antibodies of this sort.

The role of complement in mediating the biologic effects of endotoxin is not entirely clear. Reduction of serum complement after endotoxin injection in rabbits has been demonstrated (Gilbert and Braude, 1962), and Spink and Vick (1961) have shown that a heat-labile plasma factor is necessary for the production of endotoxin shock in dogs. An interaction between endotoxin and the complement system has been clearly demonstrated by Gewurz *et al.* (1968) as discussed in Section II,B. Spielvogel's electron microscopic studies demonstrated that measures known to inactivate complement also inhibited rabbit platelet degranulation by endotoxin in citrated platelet-rich plasma. Further, he demonstrated that platelet degranulation was associated with adherence of endotoxin particles to the platelet membrane and that in primate blood (in which immune adherence receptor sites are on the erythrocytes rather than the platelets) platelet damage was not observed and endotoxin adhered to erythrocyte surfaces. He concluded that the effects of endotoxin on rabbit platelets *in vitro* were due to the immune adherence phenomenon and that the required heat-labile plasma factor was complement.

These studies make it very likely that complement is involved in both the production of endotoxin effects *in vivo* and the platelet–endotoxin interaction *in vitro*. However, two studies from the writers' laboratories suggest that heat-labile factors other than complement may be involved, and that noncomplement-dependent mechanisms of platelet injury may also be demonstrated under certain specific experimental conditions. The first demonstrated that adsorption of plasma with zymosan under conditions (16°C in the presence of NaEDTA) which do not allow complement fixation removed a heat-labile plasma factor necessary for platelet–endotoxin interactions in citrated plasma. It was postulated that this heat-labile factor was an antibodylike material with reactivity to endotoxin (Des Prez, 1967). The second demonstrated that pretreatment of rabbit plasma with cobra factor in a concentration eightfold greater than that required to eliminate EAC' hemolysis did not substantially decrease platelet amine release by endotoxin (Marney and Des Prez, 1969). Further, it has been demonstrated that very large heparin concentrations do not abolish the platelet–endotoxin interaction. Thus it seems likely that although complement clearly may enhance the rabbit platelet–endotoxin interaction, possibly by means of the immune adherence mechanism, other complement-independent mechanisms can also be demonstrated, possibly involving natural antibodies and the platelet-surface reaction (Section II,C,7) and representing an immune mechanism for particle clearance of less specificity and phylogenetically more primitive than those which are amplified by the complement system.

It should be mentioned that although rabbit platelet injury by endotoxin is well established, there is disagreement as to whether human platelets are similarly affected. Ream and associates (1965) report that human platelets are aggregated by endotoxin. Corn (1966), Mueller-Eckhardt and Lüscher (1968c), and Spielvogel (1967) indicate that primate platelets are not affected by endotoxin, which would seem to be at variance with clear evidence that endotoxin injections produce thrombocytopenia both in humans (Bennett and Cluff, 1957) and in baboons (Sutton et al., 1969). The in vitro studies of Corn and Upshaw, Mueller-Eckhardt and Lüscher, and Spielvogel, however, were all carried out in citrated plasma; unpublished studies in the writers' laboratory have shown that human platelets are aggregated by bacterial endotoxin when heparinized, rather than citrated, platelet-rich plasma is employed.

IV. OTHER EXPERIMENTAL MODELS OF RABBIT PLATELET INJURY

A number of other agents mixed with rabbit blood or platelet-rich plasma produce platelet aggregation, release of platelet components, or both. Although none of these systems has been exhaustively analyzed, all have features suggesting that the underlying mechanisms are similar in some ways to those underlying immunologically induced platelet injury.

A. Glycogen and Zymosan

As discussed above (Section II,B), rabbit platelet injury by glycogen was investigated by Waalkes and Coburn (1959a,b) and Westerholm (1965); Henson and Cochrane (1969b) have reported similar studies using zymosan. All of these reports emphasize the similarity of the pattern of platelet injury produced by these materials to that produced by antigen–antibody reactions. Further, Henson and Cochrane demonstrated that the first three components of complement were required for platelet injury by zymosan. The nature of the antibody itself is not clear, but it is assumed that it is a natural antibody reactive with polysaccharide determinants.

B. Agar

Humphrey and Jaques (1955) demonstrated that activation of plasma with agar produced release of histamine from rabbit blood. Detailed analysis of this system has not been published. Studies in progress in the writers' laboratory indicate that NaEDTA is inhibitory and citrate prevents the reaction if present from the outset, but not when addition of citrate is delayed. A plasma factor with the heat lability of complement facilitates the reaction, but the actual role of complement has not yet been analyzed.

C. Polyinosinic Acid

Yachnin has demonstrated that polyinosinic acid (poly I) interacts with the first component of complement in such a fashion that activation and utilization of complement are produced. He has also demonstrated that erythrocytes from patients with paroxysmal nocturnal hemoglobinuria, which are very sensitive to the lytic action of complement, are lysed in the presence of polyinosinic acid during the course of complement inactivation (Yachnin and Ruthenberg, 1965). Unpublished studies from the writers' laboratory have demonstrated that polyinosinic acid also produces platelet aggregation and release of platelet amines. The reaction appears to require cell particle contact, since agitation of the system is necessary for platelet injury to be produced. This is in contrast to platelet injury by soluble antigen and antibody, which occurs both in rotated and in static systems. Moreover, heat inactivation of plasma (56°C for 30 minutes) does not eliminate the reactivity of the system. Whether or not polyinosinic acid reacts directly with C'_{1q}, with γ-globulin so as to produce complement activation, or directly with receptor sites on the platelet membrane has not been determined.

D. Dextrans

Haining (1955, 1956a) reported detailed studies on the release of histamine from rabbit platelets by dextrans and dextran sulfate. Histamine release was found to be dependent on molecular weight; dextrans with molecular weights between 22,000 and 1,000,000 were effective whereas those with molecular weights below 14,000 were not. Sulfated dextrans were more active than dextrans and differed in that an optimum concentration was required to produce maximum histamine release, both larger and smaller concentrations being less effective. Sodium oxalate inhibited the platelet dextran interaction. The role of complement was not determined.

E. Aggregated γ-Globulin

Ishizaka and Ishizaka (1962) first demonstrated aggregation of rabbit platelets by heat-aggregated human γ-globulin (AGG). The system employed visual aggregation after 60 minutes as an endpoint. The reaction mixture contained a platelet suspension, a small amount of guinea pig serum as a complement source, and aggregated γ-globulin precipitates prepared by heat treatment and then centrifugation. The supernates from this treatment contained soluble aggregates which fixed complement but did not produce platelet aggregation. Complement enhanced but was not necessary for production of platelet aggregation by aggregated γ-globulin precipitates. Of particular interest, aggregation was produced by aggregated γ-globulin precipitates even in the presence of 10 mM NaEDTA, a finding suggestively similar to the report by Miescher and Cooper that large concentrations of soluble immune complexes produced aggregation of platelets in the presence of NaEDTA (Sections II,A,2 and II,A,8).

Aggregometer traces obtained during incubation of platelet-rich plasma with aggregated γ-globulin were reported by Davis and Holtz (1969). These demonstrated aggregation occurring in two waves, only the second of which was inhibitable by AMP. This is similar both in contour and in the effect of AMP to the aggregometer trace produced by soluble antigen and antibody as demonstrated in Fig. 3. Interestingly, both serotonin and epinephrine enhanced platelet aggregation by aggregated γ-globulin.

Mueller-Eckhardt and Lüscher (1968a) studied release of ADP from platelets by aggregated γ-globulin. They stated that complement was not required in the system they employed, but measures which diminished the ability of the aggregates to fix complement also diminished their ability to produce ADP release.

From the above studies the suggestion emerges that when γ-globulin is structurally altered in a manner so as to favor interaction with complement, it also acquires the ability to fix onto platelets. The notion that the platelet has membrane sites reactive with such altered γ-globulin is an attractive one.

V. PLATELET PARTICIPATION IN SOME MODELS OF IMMUNOLOGICALLY INDUCED TISSUE INJURY

The several models of immunologically induced tissue injury discussed below have all been extensively analyzed, and it is beyond the competence of the writers to attempt similar reviews. These models, however, are of interest to those concerned with platelet physiology since all are characterized by platelet–leukocyte thrombi, platelet aggregates, and alteration of the coagulation mechanism in some combination.

A. Generalized Anaphylaxis

Anaphylaxis is thought to be caused by chemical mediators released from target cells injured during the course of several different types of immunologic reactions. These mediators, which include serotonin, histamine, slow reacting substance of anaphylaxis (SRS-A), and bradykinin, all have profound effects on smooth muscle and vascular permeability. The target cell altered or injured by the immune reaction and the specific mediator or mediators vary between species, and only in the rabbit is platelet injury regarded as critical (Austen, 1965). In the rabbit, circulating immune complexes, resulting either from intravenous injection of antigen in a previously sensitized animal or from injection of antigen–antibody complexes themselves, produce platelet aggregation, thrombocytopenia, and at times fibrin thrombi, principally in the lungs but also in other organs. The associated bronchospam and hyperinflation of the lungs have been attributed to release of platelet histamine and possibly platelet serotonin as well (Waalkes and Coburn, 1959a,b). It is of interest that considerable protection is provided by prior heparinization in dosage too low to have an anticomplementary effect (Johansson, 1960), indicating that coagulation acceleration and thrombin evolution enhance the severity of anaphylaxis, possibly in part by producing further platelet injury. Whether or not complement is required for the platelet injury observed during anaphylaxis is not clear, but complement dependent reactions certainly at least enhance the end result. In other species, the critical cells mediating systemic anaphylaxis are other than the platelet. However, transient hypercoagulability and thrombocytopenia occur in all.

B. Passive Cutaneous Anaphylaxis (PCA)

The term passive cutaneous anaphylaxis designates the local inflammatory reaction induced by intracutaneous administration of antibody followed after an interval by intravenous administration of antigen. The histopathologic features are capillary permeability with transudation of fluid, platelet and leukocyte aggregates, some tendency to small vessel thrombosis, and some intimal necrosis. Such reactions may be produced by very small concentrations of antibody. Passive cutaneous anaphylaxis is differentiated from the Arthus reaction, in which larger accumulations of antigen–antibody complexes produce complement-dependent leukocyte chemotaxis, phagocytosis of the complexes, leukocyte degranulation, and, in the skin at least, microvascular injury, thrombosis, and hemorrhagic necrosis, presumably resulting from leukocyte lysosomal hydrolytic enzymes.

Most passive cutaneous anaphylaxis reactions result from attachment of antibody to target cells in the area of the preparatory injection. This cell-associated antibody causes cell injury upon reaction with antigen without the participation of complement. In homologous passive cutaneous anaphylaxis reactions (antibody obtained and reaction elicited in the same species), the antibody involved is different from γG, does not fix complement, and is regarded as analogous to human reagin or γE (homocytotropic antibody) (Onoue et al., 1966; Zvaifler and Becker, 1966). However, the detailed studies of Henson and Cochrane (1969a) suggest that both complement-dependent and complement-independent mechanisms, both involving injury to platelets, mediate passive cutaneous anaphylaxis in rabbits. Complement independent homologous passive cutaneous anaphylaxis reactions were elicited only in some rabbits early after immunization with antigen in complete Freund's adjuvant. This reaction was not inhibited by cobra factor treatment (C_3' depletion) of the animal and was thought to be due to the transient appearance of homocytotropic antibody (see Section II,D). In most rabbits, in contrast, passive cutaneous anaphylaxis reactions were found to be due to combination of γG, antigen, and complement and were inhibited by cobra factor treatment (see Section II,A).

C. Serum Sickness

Serum sickness can be produced in rabbits by injection of large amounts of a soluble antigen such as bovine serum albumin. This results in widespread vascular injury due to deposition of antigen–antibody complexes in vascular walls and complement-dependent chemotaxis of leukocytes to the site of immune complex deposition. Kniker and Cochrane (1968) believe that the initial event leading to deposition of immune complexes in the vessel walls is platelet injury with release of platelet factors producing endothelial permeability (histamine, serotonin, and perhaps other permeability factors). Turbulent flow was also felt to favor immune complex deposition. The participation of the platelet was established by demonstrating that either prior platelet depletion or prior treatment with a combination of histamine and serotonin antagonists prevented immune complex deposition. Cobra factor treatment (C_3' depletion) of the test animal did not prevent the appearance of the complexes within vascular walls, but did eliminate the accumulation of leukocytes around the complexes (complement dependent leukocyte chemotaxis) (Henson and Cochrane, 1969c). These authors concluded that the initial interaction between platelets and immune complexes might be due to both complement-dependent and complement-independent mechanisms.

D. Vasculitis Due to Platelet Aggregation

Hughes and Tonks (1959, 1962) have postulated that platelet aggregates themselves produce vasculitis. They observed that introduction of autologous whole blood clot into the pulmonary veins of rabbits produced myocarditis of a type quite similar to that observed following systemic anaphylaxis. They subsequently observed the same type of lesion following pulmonary vein infusion with isolated, clumped platelets prepared from lightly heparinized blood. Interestingly, *citrated* platelet-rich plasma was used as a control and did not produce these lesions (see Sections II,A,2,7, and 8). The myocardial injury consisted of areas of cellular infiltrate with undamaged muscle, other areas demonstrating actual muscle necrosis, extension of the process to subendocardial and subepicardial areas, and in some instances evolution to granuloma formation with giant cells. These authors also demonstrated that injection of antigen in a sensitized animal so as to produce anaphylaxis resulted in the appearance of platelet clumps in the blood of both ventricles within minutes.

In support of the notion that platelet aggregates per se produce vascular lesions, Mustard (1967) demonstrated that infusion of ADP into the pulmonary artery produced myocarditis and, further, that renal arterial infusion of ADP resulted in hematuria, proteinuria, and cylindruria. The concept that platelet aggregation from whatever initial cause may produce vascular and tissue injury leads to endless speculation concerning the pathogenesis of myocardial and renal changes in the many infectious and allergic states characterized by thrombocytopenia as a consequence of platelet aggregation and sequestration.

E. The Generalized Shwartzman Reaction

The generalized Shwartzman reaction (GSR) is a laboratory model of tissue injury produced in rabbits and some other species by two intravenous injections of bacterial endotoxin spaced 12–24 hours apart and resulting in bilateral renal cortical necrosis. The first injection *prepares* the animal and the second *provokes* the development of uncontrolled intravascular coagulation. Histologically, fibrin thrombi can be demonstrated in the small blood vessels of the lung and other viscera, but the most characteristic finding is glomerular capillary thrombosis due to intravascular deposition of fibrin and partially polymerized fibrinogen. Some authorities feel that bilateral adrenal hemorrhagic necrosis (Waterhouse-Friderichsen syndrome) and pituitary ischemic necrosis are based on microvascular thrombosis and necrosis of these organs and may be associated with the generalized Shwartzman reaction (Hardaway, 1966; McKay, 1965). This laboratory artifact has counterparts in clinical medicine, as renal cortical necrosis and glomerular fibrin deposition may be seen in a variety of overwhelming bacterial infections with both gram-negative (endotoxin containing) and gram-positive organisms. Further, a similar histopathologic picture underlies some instances of acute rejection of renal transplants (Starzl *et al.*, 1968) and some instances of postinfectious purpura fulminans. It is also relevant to the broader subject of immunologically induced platelet injury since in properly prepared animals bilateral glomerular thrombosis can be produced by injection of antigen in a previously sensitized animal, by injection of antigen–antibody complexes in a nonimmune animal, or by injection of antiplatelet antiserum (Lee, 1963; Levin and Cluff, 1965).

It is clear that hypercoagulability is one underlying feature of the generalized Shwartzman reaction. However, controversy exists as to whether the initial change leading to hypercoagulability involves platelet damage, leukocyte damage, or other factors such as shock, acidosis, high levels of circulating catechol amines or Hageman factor activation. Horn and Collins (1968a,b) have reported that the basic cell–endotoxin interaction resulting in fibrin deposition involves the polymorphonuclear leukocyte. Injections of endotoxin were shown to produce pulmonary sequestration of large numbers of leukocytes which, upon the second injection of endotoxin, ruptured and released leukocyte granules thought to have thromboplastic activity. In support of this thesis, Niemetz (1969) has reported that leukocytes obtained from endotoxin treated (prepared) animals have considerably enhanced thromboplastic potency. On the other hand, McKay and associates believe that the platelet–endotoxin interaction is more important than leukocyte injury in inducing the generalized Shwartzman reaction, noting that platelet clumping is the first change in blood formed elements seen after intravenous injections of endotoxin (Herring *et al.*, 1963; McKay *et al.*, 1966; Silver and Stehbens, 1965). Levin and Cluff (1965) attempted to determine whether or not the platelet was required by inducing thrombocytopenia with antiplatelet antiserum. However, in animals prepared for the generalized Shwartzman reaction (single injection of endotoxin), the antiplatelet antiserum itself produced renal cortical necrosis. Margaretten and McKay (1969) employed heparinization to prevent the induction of the reaction by antiplatelet antiserum. In this manner they were able, after the effect of heparin had dissipated, to demonstrate that the generalized Shwartzman reaction could not be induced in these thrombocytopenic animals.

The pathogenesis of the generalized Shwartzman reaction is obviously complex and statements concerning critical trigger mechanisms are usually oversimplifications. Inhibition of fibrinolysis (McKay, 1966), β-adrenergic blockade (Müller-Berghaus *et al.*, 1967), acidosis (Hardaway, 1966), high levels of circulating catecholamines, and activation of Hageman factor may all play important roles both in preparation for the generalized Shwartzman reaction and in its induction (McKay *et al.*, 1969). However, the weight of present evidence suggests that platelet injury plays a role in the generalized Shwartzman reaction and in most clinical states characterized by diffuse intravascular coagulation and renal cortical necrosis.

VI. IMMUNOLOGICALLY INDUCED PLATELET INJURY IN MAN

A. Thrombocytopenia Due to Drug Allergy

A large number of drugs have been implicated in the induction of thrombocytopenia by allergic mechanisms. However, the following discussion will be confined to quinidine, sedormid, and digitoxin, since studies concerning these drugs have been most significant in understanding mechanisms involved.

Ackroyd's studies of sedormid purpura (Ackroyd, 1948, 1949a,b,c, 1951), which must stand as models of simplicity and insight, provided the first substantial understanding of thrombocytopenia due to drug allergy. He demonstrated that addition of sedormid to the blood of patients with a history of sedormid purpura produced platelet aggregation, platelet lysis, complement fixation, and inhibition of clot retraction. Using mixtures of platelets, plasma, sedormid, and a complement source, it was shown that the critical factor was present in plasma and presumably antibody. Platelet injury occurred when normal (nonsensitized) platelets were substituted for sensitized platelets, but, in contrast, a mixture of normal plasma, platelets from a sedormid sensitive patient, complement, and drug produced no effect. All four components of the system, sensitized plasma (antibody), sedormid (antigen), a complement source, and platelets (either normal or sensitized), were required; mixtures of drug, sensitive plasma, and complement in the absence of platelets did not result in complement fixation. From this he concluded that the drug and platelet must exist in a haptene-carrier protein relationship and that any platelet could serve as the carrier, and assumed that there was a nonimmunologic tendency for adsorption of drug onto the platelet. In heparinized blood, both platelet aggregation and lysis were observed; in citrated blood, aggregation took place but lysis did not. This observation concerning the effect of citrate in dissociating aggregation and platelet membrane injury anticipated those described in Sections II,A,2,5, and 7 by a decade. Application of a sedormid-saturated patch to the skin of an allergic patient produced local purpura without systemic thrombocytopenia, indicating to Ackroyd that endothelial cells might also serve as a carrier for the drug haptene and be injured directly upon contact with antibody. His conclusions concerning the haptene-carrier protein relationship of drug and platelet, and the notion of direct endothelial injury now appear to be in error (*vide infra*), but the remainder of his conclusions have been well confirmed and only slightly amplified during the intervening years.

A similarly distinguished series of investigations concerning quinidine purpura by Shulman (1958a,b,c) addressed directly the question raised by Ackroyd, using more quantitative and sophisticated techniques. He confirmed that complement fixation required the presence of platelets in addition to antigen (quinidine) and antibody (sensitized plasma). However, equilibrium dialysis studies failed to demonstrate any affinity of the drug for platelets in the absence of antibody, as postulated by Ackroyd. The question of direct endothelial cell injury was approached by substituting intact endothelial cells for platelets in quantitative complement fixation studies with negative results. It now seems likely that the positive patch test observed by Ackroyd may have been due to vascular injury produced by local platelet aggregates (Section V,D) rather than to direct endothelial injury. The endpoints of clot retraction inhibition and complement fixation were found to be dissociable from a quantitative point of view. Complement fixation was observed with concentrations of antibody insufficient to produce clot retraction inhibition. Moreover, *in vivo* studies indicated that systemic thrombocytopenia was an even more sensitive endpoint. Infusion of quinidine in sensitive individuals produced thrombocytopenia at (calculated) concentrations of drug far lower than that required to demonstrate complement fixation *in vitro*, suggesting that clinical allergic thrombocytopenia may be produced by complement-independent mechanisms.

Horowitz *et al.* demonstrated that reduction in the Stypven clotting time as a means of detecting platelet factor 3 activation was a more sensitive method for detecting antiquinidine antibodies, at least in some cases. Two of the six patients studied in this fashion demonstrated positive results with the Stypven time test and negative quantitative complement fixation studies. These authors also demonstrated that the active antibody was a 7 S globulin and the 19 S fraction of sensitized plasma was inactive (Horowitz *et al.*, 1965). The same group, in studies of a patient with thrombocytopenia due to digitoxin, demonstrated the association of (tritiated) digitoxin with the γ-globulin fraction of immune serum in the absence of platelets (Young *et al.*, 1966). In the presence of both immune serum and platelets, labeled drug was shown to concentrate about the platelet surfaces; in the presence of normal serum, no such concentration was noted, confirming Shulman's equilibrium dialysis studies discussed above. They concluded that interaction of drug and antibody occurred prior to localization of the immune complex on the platelet.

From all of the above reports, two unanswered and critical questions emerge. The first concerns the mode of attachment of the immune complex on the platelet membrane; the second concerns the reason that drug and antibody produce complement fixation only in the presence of platelets. Answers to these questions should provide insight into the unique phenomenon of platelet injury by antigen–antibody reactions unrelated to the platelet itself.

B. Posttransfusion Purpura

In 1961 Shulman and associates reported studies of two patients in whom severe thrombocytopenic purpura developed approximately 1 week after transfusion. After recovery, the patients' serum was demonstrated to contain an antibody reactive with the platelets of a majority of normal persons, though not with the patients' platelets. Panel studies using quantitative complement fixation techniques revealed that 74% of platelet samples tested with this antibody produced strong reactions, 24% produced intermediate reactions, and 2% did not react at all. From these data they postulated that the strong reactors were homozygous and the intermediate reactors heterozygous for a platelet antigen demonstrating an autosomal dominant pattern of inheritance, and that the 2% of the population which did not react, including the index case, did not possess this antigen on their platelets. They designated the antigen Pl and it is now referred to as Pl^{A1}. Subsequently, it has been shown to be the same as the Zw^a antigen described 2 years earlier by van Loghem *et al.* (1959). This blood group has now become well established. The first patient was treated with exchange transfusion since she had been shown to have a factor in high titre which fixed complement with normal platelets. This resulted in prompt cessation of bleeding even though the antibody titre remained quite high. Shulman pointed out the two central puzzles of this experience: *First, extensive thrombocytopenia had occurred even though the antibody was not reactive with the patients' own platelets; second, recovery occurred during exchange transfusion using blood containing platelets reactive with the antibody.* He also noted that this illness is much rarer than would be the case if all homozygous recessive patients (2% of the population) were so affected by transfusion with platelets containing the Pl^{A1} antigen (98% of the population). These considerations led him to postulate that this represented another example of platelet injury during the course of antigen–antibody reactions unrelated to the platelet itself, in this case a reaction between the transfused Pl^{A1} antigen and the patients' anti-Pl^{A1} antibody. He further speculated that the rarity of the syndrome suggested a requirement for the antigen in an unusual state, perhaps as a colloid separate from the platelets, so that it might circulate for prolonged periods. Baldini (1965) attempted to reproduce this clinical situation by recurrent injections of homologous platelets into dogs. Abrupt and transient thrombocytopenia ensued in only a few of the animals so treated. During the period of thrombocytopenia, the survival time of autologous as well as homologous platelets was greatly shortened, and recovery occurred in spite of persisting high titers of anti-homologous platelet antibody. In those animals which did respond with thrombocytopenia, repeat challenge produced less severe effects. He felt that a critical balance between antigen and antibody was necessary in order to produce the type of immune complex capable of injuring the circulating platelets of the recipient animals.

C. Neonatal Purpura

The delineation of the Pl^A blood group in his studies in posttransfusion purpura led Shulman to postulate that some instances of neonatal purpura might be due to *in utero* sensitization of a Pl^A-negative mother with Pl^A-positive fetal platelets in a manner analogous to the sequence of events known to underlie erythroblastosis foetalis. In 1962, Shulman *et al.* confirmed this prediction in a case of neonatal purpura in which tests with anti-Pl^{A1} antibody from his posttransfusion purpura cases showed the father to be homozygous Pl^A-positive, the mother negative, and the infant heterozygous with respect to this antigen. As was anticipated, the mother's serum contained an antibody similar to the known anti-Pl^{A1} antibody and reactive with the father's and infant's platelets *in vitro*. In a second case, the same platelet typing pattern was demonstrated (using anti-Pl^A antibody from the posttransfusion purpura cases), but the mother's serum did not react with the father's or infant's platelets. To explain this, the presence in the mother's blood of a noncomplement fixing, nonagglutinating antibody with anti-Pl^A specificity was postulated, and this was then demonstrated by competitive inhibition of the known complement fixing anti-Pl^{A1} antibody by the mother's serum. Two points were emphasized: First, detection of this blocking type of anti-Pl^A antibody was possible only because a complement-fixing antibody with identical specificity was available for competitive inhibition experiments; second, this blocking antibody, otherwise undetectable by *in vitro* techniques, was capable nevertheless of producing severe thrombocytopenia in the infant.

This same remarkable publication demonstrated a second platelet antigen system in two other families with neonatal purpura. In contrast to the Pl^A system, 2% of the population were found to be homozygous for this antigen, 37% were heterozygous, and 60% did not possess it. This second antigen system was initially referred to as Pl^B but has been subsequently designated as $PlG_RL_Y^B$ when it became apparent that this particular antigen, in contrast to the Pl^A system, was also present on the surface of granulocytes and lymphocytes.

Shulman and associates (1964) have subsequently accumulated data on 72 mothers of infants with neonatal purpura. Complement-fixing antibodies were demonstrable in 17%, agglutinating antibodies in 5%, blocking antibodies in 29%, and in 49% no antibodies were detectable. It was assumed that these negative reactors actually had blocking (non-C′ fixing and nonagglutinating) antibodies which were undetectable because of unavailability of complement fixing antibodies with similar specificity. The majority of the identifiable maternal antibodies were anti-Pl^{A1} in specificity and blocking in type. The prognosis and therapy of this condition are discussed in this review.

D. Platelet Antigens

As mentioned in the preceding two sections, some of the earliest information concerning platelet antigen systems was developed from Shulman's studies of posttransfusion purpura and neonatal thrombocytopenic purpura. The first platelet antigen he described (Pl^{A1}) was found to be present only on platelets and was subsequently demonstrated to be identical with an antigen described previously by van Loghem et al. (1959). The second antigen described ($PlG_RL_Y^{B1}$), however, was found to be present on granulocytes and lymphocytes as well as on platelets. It is now felt that, in contrast to platelet-specific antigens, those present on all leukocytes are also present on all other tissues as well and are histocompatibility antigens. The nomenclature in the field of leukocyte antigens is confusing and not standardized, and it is anticipated that many more remain to be described. Table V presents one fairly current list of platelet-specific and leukocyte–platelet antigens, largely following the nomenclature employed by Shulman. The interrelationships of the various nomenclatures and the histocompatibility aspects of these antigens are discussed in reviews by van Rood et al. (1966), Hiller and Shulman (1969), Colombani et al. (1967), Shulman et al. (1964, 1966) and Shulman (1966). It is of great interest that many of these antigens are shared by nonhuman primates and, to a lesser degree, by other mammals (Hiller and Shulman, 1969).

In addition to their importance in neonatal and posttransfusion purpura, platelet and platelet–leukocyte antigens may also cause isoimmunization in patients receiving multiple transfusions. Shulman (1966) estimates that

TABLE V

PERCENT OF POPULATION POSSESSING KNOWN PLATELET ANTIGENS[a]

Antigen[b]	% Positive	Cells possessing antigens
$Pl^{A_1}(Zw^a)$	97	Platelets
$Pl^{A_2}(Zw^b)$	26	Platelets
$PlGrLy^{B_1}$	46	Platelets, granulocytes, lymphocytes, *et al.*
$PlGrLy^{C_1}$	30	Platelets, granulocytes, lymphocytes, *et al.*
Pl^{E_1}	>99.9	Platelets
Pl^{E_2}	5	Platelets
$PlGrLy^{F_1}$	65	Platelets, granulocytes, lymphocytes, *et al.*
Ko^a	17	Platelets
DUZO	22	Platelets

[a] Compiled from Shulman (1966) and Hiller and Shulman (1969).

[b] Pl^{A_1} same as Zw^a; Pl^{A_2} same as Zw^b; Pl denotes platelets; Gr, granulocytes; and Ly, lymphocytes.

5% of persons receiving up to 10 transfusions, 37% of those transfused with between 50 and 100 units of blood, and 80% of those with over 100 transfusions will demonstrate platelet antibodies. He feels that it is likely that isoimmunization is actually much more frequent than these figures would indicate because many antibodies are of the blocking type, not demonstrable by *in vitro* testing unless an agglutinating or complement-fixing antibody of the same specificity happens to be available. Platelet isoimmunization is, however, usually not attended by clinical difficulties excepting in patients receiving multiple transfusions and then only if thrombocytopenia is a part of the problem. It is stated that even platelet transfusions may be successfully administered for weeks with success without determining platelet type. In an occasional patient, however, transfused platelets may become rapidly sequestered and serve no hemostatic function; in such, typing may become necessary in order to obtain surviving platelets. In neonatal purpura with severe thrombocytopenia, there would seem to be need for platelet typing. However, Adner *et al.* (1969) have suggested an intelligent manner in which to circumvent the problem by first carrying out exchange transfusions (to lessen antibody), and then administering a transfusion of maternal platelets washed in normal plasma (so as to remove contaminating antibody).

E. Idiopathic Thrombocytopenic Purpura (ITP)

The notion that ITP is an immunologic disease received its first support from Harrington's demonstration that serum or plasma from ITP patients produced thrombocytopenia in normal recipients (Harrington *et al.*, 1951). Subsequent studies have demonstrated that this factor is a 7 S γ-globulin (Shulman *et al.*, 1965a). Efforts to demonstrate this factor by *in vitro* testing have, in general, been much less successful than its detection by production of thrombocytopenia *in vivo*. Shulman feels that this is likely to be due to its being a blocking type of antibody analogous to those described in neonatal purpura. Recently Karpatkin and Siskind (1969) have carried out extensive studies on ITP factor, made possible by the development of a quite sensitive coagulation test to detect increased platelet procoagulant activity. Utilizing this method, they were able to demonstrate ITP factor *in vitro* in the serum of most clinically affected patients. They confirmed that it resided in the γG fraction of blood and showed by immunoelectrophoresis that it formed a strong line of precipitation with antihuman γG, a weak line of precipitation with antihuman γA, and none with anti-γM. However, studies to detect elimination of the platelet-injuring properties with anti-immunoglobulin antibodies indicated that its activity was prevented by rabbit antihuman γG, but not by anti-γA. The ITP factor was stable at 56°C for 30 minutes and could be adsorbed onto platelets. Most interestingly, a quite similar activity was obtained from the sera of patients with systemic lupus erythematosis. Some of the systemic lupus erythematosis patients did not have thrombocytopenia, but did have an increased percentage of large platelets, interpreted by the authors as young platelets present in the peripheral blood because of rapid platelet turnover, analogous to reticulocytes in hemolytic anemia. One impediment to identifying the ITP factor as a γG antibody reactive with platelets was the demonstration that its molecular weight, determined by column chromatography, was roughly 330,000. In contrast, in two of the four patients with systemic lupus erythematosis in whom this determination was made, the molecular weight appeared to be approximately that of γG, that is to say, about 150,000.

Implicit in Shulman's studies and those of Karpatkin and Siskind is the assumption that the ITP factor is antibody reactive with platelet antigens, noncomplement fixing and nonagglutinating in nature. Shulman has provided beautiful quantitative evidence for the similarity of ITP factor to such known antiplatelet blocking antibodies (Shulman *et al.*, 1965b). He demonstrated that complement fixation was not required for the thrombocytopenic effect of both ITP factor and known antiplatelet antibody, and that antibody-coated platelets were sequestered in the reticuloendothelial system rather than destroyed in the circulation. Platelets with a small or moderate antibody load were largely removed in the spleen; larger antibody loads altered the principal locus of sequestration to the liver. Steroid therapy was shown to ameliorate thrombocytopenia at those antibody loads usually associated with splenic sequestration, but not in the case of more heavily coated cells usually removed by the liver.

Recent studies by Myllyla *et al.* (1969) offer another attractive interpretation as to the probable identity of at least some ITP factors. These authors developed a sensitive platelet agglutination system and applied it to the investigation of postrubella thrombocytopenic purpura. The system they employed utilized a very small virus antigen, platelets, and heated plasma (no complement present). They found that when a specific form of rubella antigen was employed, the platelet agglutination test was more sensitive than hemagglutination inhibition or complement fixation to detect antirubella antibodies. Particular importance was attached to the physical state of the antigen. This was prepared by sonication of infected cells and subsequent removal of all larger particles by high speed centrifugation. Sucrose gradient studies confirmed the fact that the antigen was smaller than whole virus or those portions of disrupted virus demonstrating greatest activity in complement fixation or hemagglutination inhibition studies. They postulated that platelet agglutination was produced by a very small antigen particle in combination with (γG) antibody. Noting that up to 70% of ITP in childhood is thought to be of postinfectious origin, they implied that most instances of ITP factor might be in fact small antigen in combination with antibody forming a complex with the capacity to fix onto platelets so as to cause platelet aggregation and sequestration. In this regard, the molecular weight of ITP factor as determined by Karpatkin and Siskind is compatible with that which would result from two γG molecules attached to a small antigen.

F. Thrombotic Thrombocytopenic Purpura (TTP)

In 1925, Moschcowitz reported the index case of thrombotic thrombocytopenic purpura, a 16-year-old girl with a 14-day fatal illness characterized by fever, arthralgia, weakness, petechiae, pallor, anemia, focal neurologic abnormalities, pulmonary edema, and terminal coma. The distinctive clinical course and the autopsy demonstration of hyaline thrombi in terminal arterioles and capillaries of heart, spleen, and kidneys were recognized as representing a previously undescribed syndrome. The clinical course of thrombotic thrombocytopenic purpura has been recently reviewed by Amorosi and Ultmann (1966) and by Lerner et al. (1967). The hallmarks are fever, hemolytic anemia with erythrocyte distortion and fragmentation, purpura or other bleeding, transient or permanent neurological signs, renal abnormalities, and bilirubinemia. Thrombocytopenia was present in 96% of the cases reviewed by Amorosi and Ultmann (1966).

The nature of the disseminated hyaline microthrombi, of obvious importance in terms of understanding the pathogenesis of the disease, is a matter of controversy. Moschcowitz (1925) believed the thrombi were agglutinated red blood cells. Gore (1950) described noninflammatory superficial subendothelial "prethrombotic" lesions and felt that platelets comprised the thrombi. Orbison (1952) described focal amorphous lesions replacing normal endothelial wall components and aneurysmal deformation of the small arteries, supporting the concept that the primary abnormality occurs within the vascular wall. Recent immunohistochemical studies by Feldman et al. (1966) revealed fibrin and smaller amounts of γG deposited in the subendothelial space of small vessels but no demonstrable complement. In some instances this intramural clot appeared to reach the lumen and was associated with intraluminal platelet aggregation or a fully developed thrombus.

The pathophysiology of thrombotic thrombocytopenic purpura remains an open issue. On the one hand, Taub et al. (1964) emphasize the decreased platelet survival, the presence of thrombin activity in serum, decreased fibrinogen, and the absence of perivascular infiltration or fibrinoid necrosis and suggest that thrombotic thrombocytopenic purpura represents diffuse primary intravascular coagulation with secondary vascular injury. Lerner et al. (1967), in contrast, emphasize the vascular abnormalities demonstrated on histological examination, the finding of normal coagulation factors in their patient, the many reports of normal prothrombin times in patients with this illness, and the often equivocal response to heparin therapy to support the thesis that thrombotic thrombocytopenic purpura is primarily a disease of vascular injury. Whether the initial event occurs within the vascular lumen or in the wall, intravascular coagulation is a feature in virtually all cases. The studies of Brain et al. (1962), Baker et al. (1968), Rubenberg et al. (1968), and Bull et al. (1968) have established that microangiopathic hemolytic anemia, which is present in virtually all cases of thrombotic thrombocytopenic purpura, is due to erythrocyte distortion and shearing caused by passage through fibrin meshworks and accordingly usually represents intravascular coagulation.

The occurrence of thrombotic thrombocytopenic purpura during pregnancy (Castleman and McNeeley, 1966), and in cases of disseminated
carcinoma (Joseph et al., 1967; Castleman and McNeeley, 1968b) suggests
that, in some instances at least, the primary event may be intravascular
coagulation with secondary vascular injury, perhaps mediated by platelet
aggregates (see Section V,D). Further, its occurrence in a patient with
possible drug allergy (Castleman and McNeeley, 1968a) suggests that in
some instances thrombotic thrombocytopenic purpura may result from
immunologically-induced platelet injury. However, in contrast to ITP,
the case for being an instance of immunological injury to platelets is not
strong. Brittingham and Chaplin (1957) attempted to produce thrombocytopenia by infusion of a patient's blood into a normal volunteer with
well documented negative results. And, as mentioned, the available immuno-
histological studies indicate that the nature of the vascular intramural
deposit is predominantly fibrin with little demonstrable immunoglobulin
and no detectable complement.

G. The Hemolytic-Uremic Syndrome

The hemolytic-uremic syndrome, first described by Gasser et al. (1955),
consists of the triad of microangiopathic hemolytic anemia, thrombocytopenia, and acute renal failure, most frequently observed in children.
Typically the onset occurs during convalescence following a minor illness,
usually gastroenteritis or an upper respiratory infection, and is characterized by the development of pallor, severe malaise, and prostration. Fever,
hepatomegaly, edema, and a hemorrhagic diathesis occur in any combination in approximately half. The anemia is associated with red cell abnormalities characteristic of mechanical trauma (burr cells, helmet cells, spherocytes). Thrombocytopenia, azotemia, and anuria or urinary abnormalities
suggesting glomerulitis (proteinuria, granular and hyaline casts, hematuria,
and pyuria) are demonstrable in all. Histological examination has demonstrated focal or generalized glomerular lesions with some degree of endothelial proliferation and intracapillary hyaline thrombi, sometimes recognized as platelet thrombi. The kidneys at autopsy demonstrate either patchy
or diffuse cortical necrosis with fibrinoid necrosis of intralobular and afferent
arterioles, frequently extending into the glomerular tufts (Brain et al.,
1967; Shinton et al., 1964; Shumway and Terplan, 1964).
Regarding pathogenesis, Lieberman et al. (1966) state that on histologic
grounds the lesions of this syndrome are indistinguishable from those of
thrombotic thrombocytopenic purpura except that they are limited to the

kidney, but that the typical clinical picture, the distinctive distribution of the pathologic changes, the occurrence predominantly in children, and the much more favorable prognosis (30–60% recovery rate) warrant its designation as a separate clinical entity. Whether or not discussion of this illness is germane to the subject of this chapter is entirely speculative, but its occurrence in the convalescent phase of otherwise trivial infectious illnesses, such as is observed in some cases of ITP and in purpura fulminans, certainly suggests the possibility of an immunologic basis.

H. Hyperacute Rejection of Renal Homografts

The usual course of rejection of renal transplants involves a gradual deterioration in function over a period of months to years and is almost certainly based on cellular immune mechanisms. In contrast, a small group of cases have been described in which rejection begins within minutes and involves diffuse vascular injury and prominent renal capillary thrombosis, resembling in some cases the generalized Shwartzman reaction (Starzl *et al.*, 1968). Terasaki and colleagues (1968) have demonstrated antibodies cytotoxic for the donor's cells in all. They point out that, while most cases of immediate renal rejection have been attributable to major erythrocyte blood group (ABO) incompatibility or to technical failure, the cases reported by them appeared to represent rejection based on isoimmunization with leukocyte or leukocyte–platelet antigens; all persons so affected had either received multiple transfusions or had been pregnant, situations known to induce such antibodies (see Section VI,D). It is worth emphasis that antigens of the leukocyte–platelet group are thought also to be present on most or all other tissues including the kidney. The involvement of platelets in this form of acute rejection is conjectural, and in point of fact it is likely that several types of interactions between recipient antibody, raised in response to isoimmunizing transfusions or to sensitization by fetal cells, and renal cells containing the antigen in question might be expected to produce acute tissue injury. Nevertheless, the prominence of thrombosis in some instances of this phenomenon makes it reasonable to suspect that immunologic injury to recipient platelets, perhaps in the course of an antigen–antibody reaction between transplant cells and host isoantibody, might play a role at least in some.

I. Purpura in Infections

Over the past decade it has become apparent that virtually all infections may, when severe enough, cause thrombocytopenia with or without intra-

vascular coagulation (McKay, 1965; Hardaway, 1966). Septicemia, both
with endotoxin-containing gram-negative bacteria and with organisms not
ordinarily regarded as endotoxin-containing (for instance, the pneumo-
coccus) may produce the generalized Shwartzman reaction and the Waterhouse-Friderichsen syndrome and are almost invariably associated with
lesser indexes of intravascular coagulation. Thrombocytopenia has been
observed with frequency in subacute bacterial endocarditis (Rabinovich
et al., 1965) and may be important in the pathogenesis of acute diffuse
glomerulonephritis complicating this condition. Thrombocytopenia is invariably observed in malaria when sought for, even in the mildest cases
(Hill et al., 1964). Severe malaria may be principally characterized by extensive intravascular coagulation. A remarkable pathologic study of malaria
among British troops during the Salonika campaign in World War I (Dudgeon and Clark, 1917) emphasized the occurrence of extensive arterial
thrombosis in the adrenals, kidneys, brain, and other organs. Rickettsial
disease is similarly characterized by extensive intravascular coagulation.
In Rocky Mountain Spotted Fever particularly, fatal cases demonstrate
extensive thrombosis, not only of vital organs but also of the digits, the
nose, the scrotum, and other exposed parts (Schaffner et al., 1965).

In contrast to thrombocytopenia occurring during the course of blood
stream contamination, in which reactions between platelets and organisms
seem likely, perhaps as a part of blood stream clearance mechanisms, some
viral illnesses produce extensive thrombocytopenic purpura during convalescence. This is typically the case with postrubella purpura, but experience with the hemolytic-uremic syndrome, ITP, and purpura fulminans
indicates that probably many other trivial and perhaps asymptomatic
illnesses may produce a similar sequence of events. Purpura fulminans
typically occurs a week or two after an upper respiratory infection and
results in extensive defibrination, thrombocytopenia, and purpura often
progressing to gangrene (Hjort et al., 1964). This time sequence is very
suggestive of antigen–antibody induced platelet injury, demonstrating a
requirement for a particular antigen–antibody ratio and perhaps a particular
form of viral antigen as demonstrated by Myllyla et al. (1969). The occurrence of Henoch-Schoenlein purpura following smallpox vaccination has
similar implications (Casteels-Van Daele, 1969) and is of further interest
in view of the occurrence of arthritis, gastrointestinal lesions, myocarditis,
and serositis in such illnesses.

The number of possible mechanisms whereby blood stream contamination with infectious agents and the antibody response thereto might interact
with platelets, endothelium, and the coagulation mechanism is obviously

great, and understanding of the details of these mechanisms is only now beginning (McKay and Margaretten, 1967). The accumulating evidence that platelet-mediated reactions may play a role in so great an array of infectious and allergic states, and the implications of such phenomena both in understanding pathogenesis and possibly in designing therapy as well, provide ample justification for a continued interest in the details of their production.

REFERENCES

Achard, C., and Aynaud, M. (1909). *C. R. Soc. Biol.* **61**, 83.

Ackroyd, J. F. (1948). *Clin. Sci.* **7**, 249.

Ackroyd, J. F. (1949a). *Clin. Sci.* **8**, 235.

Ackroyd, J. F. (1949b). *Clin. Sci.* **8**, 269.

Ackroyd, J. F. (1949c). *Quart. J. Med.* **18**, 299.

Ackroyd, J. F. (1951). *Clin. Sci.* **10**, 185.

Adner, M. M., Fisch, G. R., Starobin, S. G., and Aster, R. H. (1969). *N. Engl. J. Med.* **280**, 244.

Amorosi, E. L., and Ultmann, J. E. (1966). *Medicine (Baltimore)* **45**, 139.

Austen, K. F. (1965). *In* "The Inflammatory Process" (B. W. Zweifach, L. Grant, and R. T. McCluskey, eds.), pp. 587–612. Academic Press, New York.

Baker, L. R. I., Rubenberg, M. L., Dacie, J. V., and Brain, M. C. (1968). *Brit. J. Haematol.* **14**, 617.

Baldini, M. (1965). *Ann. N. Y. Acad. Med.* **124**, 543.

Barbaro, J. F. (1961a). *J. Immunol.* **86**, 369.

Barbaro, J. F. (1961b). *J. Immunol.* **86**, 377.

Barbaro, J. F., and Zvaifler, N. J. (1966). *Proc. Soc. Exp. Biol. Med.* **122**, 1245.

Bennett, I. L., Jr., and Cluff, L. E. (1957). *Pharmacol. Rev.* **9**, 427.

Boyden, S. V. (1966). *Advan. Immunol.* **5**, 1.

Brain, M. C., Dacie, J. V., and Hourihane, D. O'B. (1962). *Brit. J. Haematol.* **8**, 358.

Brain, M. C., Baker, L. R. I., McBride, J. A., and Rubenberg, M. (1967). *Quart. J. Med.* **36**, 608.

Braude, A. I., Carey, F. K., and Zalesky, M. (1955). *J. Clin. Invest.* **34**, 858.

Brittingham, T. E., and Chaplin, H. (1957). *Blood* **12**, 480.

Bryant, R. E., and Jenkins, D. E., Jr. (1968). *J. Immunol.* **101**, 664.

Buckingham, S., and Maynert, E. W. (1964). *J. Pharmacol. Exp. Ther.* **143**, 332.

Bull, B. S., Rubenberg, M. L., Dacie, J. V., and Brain, M. C. (1968). *Brit. J. Haematol.* **14**, 643.

Casteels–Van Daele, M. (1969). *N. Engl. J. Med.* **280**, 781.

Castleman, B., and McNeeley, B. U. (1966). *N. Engl. J. Med.* **275**, 1125.

Castleman, B., and McNeeley, B. U. (1968a). *N. Engl. J. Med.* **278**, 36.

Castleman, B., and McNeeley, B. U. (1968b). *N. Engl. J. Med.* **278**, 1336.

Chaberek, S., and Martell, A. E. (1959). "Organic Sequestering Agents," pp. 514 and 572. Wiley, New York.

Cohen, P., Braunwald, J., and Gardner, F. H. (1965). *J. Lab. Clin. Med.* **66**, 263.

Colombani, J., Colombani, M., Benajam, A., and Dausset, J. (1967). *In* "Histocompatibility Testing" (E. Curtoni, P. Mattiuz, and R. Tosi, eds.), p. 413. Williams & Wilkins, Baltimore, Maryland.

Corn, M. (1966). *Nature (London)* **212**, 508.

Davis, R. B. (1966). *Exp. Mol. Pathol.* **5**, 559.

Davis, R. B., and Holtz, G. C. (1969). *Thromb. Diath. Haemorrh.* **21**, 65.

Davis, R. B., Meeker, W. R., and McQuarrie, D. C. (1960). *Surg. Forum* **10**, 401.

Davis, R. B., Meeker, W. R., and Bailey, W. L. (1961). *Proc. Soc. Exp. Biol. Med.* **108**, 774.

Des Prez, R. M. (1964). *J. Exp. Med.* **120**, 305.

Des Prez, R. M. (1967). *J. Immunol.* **99**, 966.

Des Prez, R. M., and Bryant, R. E. (1966). *J. Exp. Med.* **124**, 971.

Des Prez, R. M., and Bryant, R. E. (1969). *J. Immunol.* **102**, 241.

Des Prez, R. M., and Marney, S. R., Jr. (1969). Unpublished observations.

Des Prez, R. M., Horowitz, H. I., and Hook, E. W. (1961). *J. Exp. Med.* **114**, 857.

Des Prez, R. M., Bryant, R. E., Katz, J. A., and Brittingham, T. E. (1967). *Thromb. Diath. Haemorrh.* **17**, 516.

Dittmer, D. S. (1961). "Biologic Handbooks, Blood and Other Body Fluids," p. 35. Fed. Am. Soc. Exptl. Biol., Washington, D.C.

Dudgeon, L. S., and Clark, C. (1917). *Lancet* **2**, 153.

Feldman, J. D., Mardiney, M. R., Unanue, E. R., and Cutting, H. (1966). *Lab. Invest.* **15**, 927.

Ferguson, J. H., Iatridis, S. G., and Iatridis, P. G. (1967). *In* "Platelets. Their Role in Hemostasis and Thrombosis" (K. Brinkhous *et al.*, eds.), p. 117. F. K. Schattauer-Verlag, Stuttgart.

Gasser, C., Gautier, E., Steck, A., Siebenmann, R. E., and Dechslin, R. (1955). *Schweiz. Med. Wochenschr.* **85**, 905.

Gewurz, H., Shin, H. S., and Mergenhagen, S. E. (1968). *J. Exp. Med.* **128**, 1049.

Gilbert, V. E., and Braude, A. I. (1962). *J. Exp. Med.* **116**, 477.

Gocke, D. J. (1965). *J. Immunol.* **94**, 247.

Gocke, D. J., and Osler, A. G. (1965). *J. Immunol.* **94**, 236.

Gore, I. (1950). *Amer. J. Pathol.* **26**, 155.

Grette, K. (1962). *Acta Physiol. Scand.* **56**, Suppl. 195.

Haining, C. G. (1955). *Brit. J. Pharmacol.* **10**, 87.

Haining, C. G. (1956a). *Brit. J. Pharmacol.* **11**, 107.

Haining, C. G. (1956b). *Brit. J. Pharmacol.* **11**, 357.

Hardaway, R. N. (1966). "Syndromes of Intravascular Coagulation." Thomas, Springfield, Illinois.

Harrington, W. J., Hollingsworth, J. W., and Moore, C. V. (1951). *J. Lab. Clin. Med.* **38**, 1.

Henson, P. M. (1969). *Immunology* **16**, 107.

Henson, P. M., and Cochrane, C. G. (1969a). *J. Exp. Med.* **129**, 153.

Henson, P. M., and Cochrane, C. G. (1969b). *J. Exp. Med.* **129**, 167.

Henson, P. M., and Cochrane, C. G. (1969c). *Fed. Proc., Fed. Amer. Soc. Exp. Biol.* **28**, 312.

Herring, W. B., Herion, J. C., Walker, R. I., and Palmer, J. G. (1963). *J. Clin. Invest.* **42**, 79.

Hill, G. J., II, Knight, V., and Jeffery, G. J. (1964). *Lancet* **1**, 240.

Hiller, M. C., and Shulman, N. R. (1969). *Ann. N. Y. Acad. Sci.* **162**, 429.

Hjort, P. F., Rapaport, S. I., and Jorgensen, L. (1964). *Scand. J. Haematol.* **1**, 169.

Holmsen, H., and Day, H. J. (1968). *Nature (London)* **219**, 760.

Horn, R. G., and Collins, R. D. (1968a). *Lab. Invest.* **18**, 101.

Horn, R. G., and Collins, R. D. (1968b). *Lab. Invest.* **19**, 451.

Horowitz, H. I., Des Prez, R. M., and Hook, E. W. (1962). *J. Exp. Med.* **116**, 619.

Horowitz, H. I., Rappaport, H. I., Young, R. C., and Fujimoto, M. M. (1965). *Transfusion (Philadelphia)* **5**, 336.

Hovig, T. (1964). *Thromb. Diath. Haemorrh.* **12**, 179.

Hughes, A., and Tonks, R. S. (1959). *J. Pathol. Bacteriol.* **77**, 207.

Hughes, A., and Tonks, R. S. (1962). *J. Pathol. Bacteriol.* **84**, 379.

Humphrey, J. H., and Jaques, R. (1955). *J. Physiol. (London)* **128**, 9.

Ishizaka, T., and Ishizaka, K. (1962). *J. Immunol.* **89**, 709.

Jackson, D. P., Schmid, H. J., Zieve, P. D., Levin, J., and Conley, C. G. (1963). *J. Clin. Invest.* **42**, 383.

Johansson, S. A. (1960). *Acta Physiol. Scand.* **50**, 95.

Joseph, R. R., Day, H. J., Sherwin, R. M., and Schwartz, H. G. (1967). *Scand. J. Haemat.* **4**, 271.

Karpatkin, S., and Siskind, G. W. (1969). *Blood* **38**, 795.

Katz, G. (1940a). *Science* **91**, 221.

Katz, G. (1940b). *Science* **91**, 617.

Katz, G. (1949). *Amer. J. Physiol.* **159**, 332.

Katz, G. (1950). *Proc. Soc. Exp. Biol. Med.* **73**, 605.

Kniker, W. T., and Cochrane, C. G. (1968). *J. Exp. Med.* **127**, 119.

Lee, L. (1963). *J. Exp. Med.* **117**, 365.

Lerner, R. G., Rapaport, S. I., and Meltzer, J. (1967). *Ann. Intern. Med.* **66**, 1180.

Levin, J., and Cluff, L. E. (1965). *J. Exp. Med.* **121**, 235.

Lichtenstein, L. M., and Osler, A. G. (1964). *J. Exp. Med.* **120**, 507.

Lieberman, E., Heuser, E., Donnell, G. N., Landing, B. H., and Hammond, G. D. (1966). *N. Engl. J. Med.* **275**, 227.

McIntire, F. C., Roth, L. W., and Richards, R. K. (1949). *Amer. J. Physiol.* **195**, 332.

McKay, D. G. (1965). "Disseminated Intravascular Coagulation." Harper, New York.

McKay, D. G. (1966). *In* "Diffuse Intravascular Clotting" (K. Brinkhouse *et al.*, eds.), pp. 107–119. Schattauer, Stuttgart.

McKay, D. G., and Margaretten, W. (1967). *Arch. Intern. Med.* **120**, 129.

McKay, D. G., Shapiro, S. S., and Shanberge, J. N. (1958). *J. Exp. Med.* **107**, 369.

McKay, D. G., Margaretten, W., and Csavossy, I. (1966). *Lab. Invest.* **15**, 1815.

McKay, D. G., Müller–Berhaus, G., and Cruse, V. (1969). *Amer. J. Pathol.* **54**, 393.

Margaretten, W., and McKay, D. G. (1969). *J. Exp. Med.* **129**, 585.

Marino, M. F. (1905). *C. R. Soc. Biol.* **58**, 194.

Marney, S. R., Jr., and Des Prez, R. M. (1969). *J. Immunol.* **103**, 1044.

Marney, S. R., Jr., and Des Prez, R.M. (1969). Unpublished Studies.

Miescher, P., and Cooper, N. (1960). *Vox Sang.* **5**, 138.

Miescher, P. A., and Gorstein, F. (1961). *In* "Henry Ford Hospital International Symposium, Blood Platelets," (S. Johnson *et al.*, eds.), p. 671. Little, Brown, Boston, Massachusetts.

Moschcowitz, E. (1925). *Arch. Intern. Med.* **36**, 89.

Movat, H. Z., Mustard, J. F., Taichman, N. S., and Uriuhara, T. (1965a). *Proc. Soc. Exp. Biol. Med.* **120**, 232.

Movat, H. Z., Weiser, W. J., Glynn, M. F., and Mustard, J. F. (1965b). *J. Cell Biol.* **27**, 531.

Müller–Berghaus, G., Goldfinger, D., Margaretten, W., and McKay, D. G. (1967). *Thromb. Diath. Haemorrh.* **18**, 726.

Mueller–Eckhardt, C., and Lüscher, E. F. (1968a). *Thromb. Diath. Haemorrh.* **20**, 155.

Mueller–Eckhardt, C., and Lüscher, E. F. (1968b). *Thromb. Diath. Haemorrh.* **20**, 327.

Mueller–Eckhardt, C., and Lüscher, E. F. (1968c). *Thromb. Diath. Haemorrh.* **20**, 336.

Mustard, J. F. (1967). *Exp. Mol. Pathol.* **7**, 366.

Mustard, J. F., Glynn, M. F., Nishizawa, E. E., and Packham, M. A. (1967). *Fed. Proc., Fed. Amer. Soc. Exp. Biol.* **26**, 106.

Myllyla, G., Vaheri, A., Veskari, T., and Penttinen, K. (1969). *Clin. Exp. Immunol.* **4**, 323.

Nelson, R. A., Jr. (1958). *J. Exp. Med.* **108**, 515.

Niemetz, J. (1969). *Fed. Proc., Fed. Amer. Soc. Exp. Biol.* **28**, 442.

Onoue, K., Yagi, Y., and Pressman, D. (1966). *J. Exp. Med.* **123**, 173.

Orbison, J. L. (1952). *Amer. J. Pathol.* **28**, 129.

Rabinovich, S., Evans, J., Smith, I. M., and January, L. E. (1965). *Ann. Intern. Med.* **63**, 185.

Ream, V. J., Deykin, D., Gurewich, V., and Wessler, S. (1965). *J. Lab. Clin. Med.* **66**, 245.

Robbins, J., and Stetson, C. A., Jr. (1959). *J. Exp. Med.* **109**, 1.

Rocha e Silva, M. (1952). *Brit. Med. J.* **1**, 779.

Rubenberg, M. L., Regoeczi, E., Bull, B. S., Dacie, J. V., and Brain, M. C. (1968). *Brit. J. Haematol.* **14**, 627.

Salvidio, E., and Crosby, W. H. (1960). *J. Lab. Clin. Med.* **56**, 711.

Schaffner, W., McLeod, A. C., and Koenig, M. G. (1965). *Arch. Intern. Med.* **116**, 857.

Schoenbechler, M. J., and Barbaro, J. F. (1968). *Proc. Nat. Acad. Sci. U.S.* **60**, 1247.

Schoenbechler, M. J., and Sadun, E. H. (1968). *Proc. Soc. Exp. Biol. Med.* **127**, 601.

Shimamoto, T., Yamazaki, H., Sagawa, N., Iwahara, S., Konishi, R., and Maezawa, H. (1958). *Proc. Jap. Acad.* **34**, 450.

Shin, H. S., Snyderman, R., Friedman, E., and Mergenhagen, S. E. (1969). *Fed. Proc., Fed. Amer. Soc. Exp. Biol.* **28**, 485.

Shinton, N. K., Galpine, J. F., Kendall, A. C., and Williams, H. P. (1964). *Arch. Dis. Childhood* **39**, 455.

Shore, P. A., Alpers, H. S., and Tidball, M. E. (1962). *Life Sci.* **1**, 275.

Shulman, N. R. (1958a). *J. Exp. Med.* **107**, 665.

Shulman, N. R. (1958b). *J. Exp. Med.* **107**, 697.

Shulman, N. R. (1958c). *J. Exp. Med.* **107**, 711.

Shulman, N. R. (1966). *Transfusion (Philadelphia)* **6**, 39.

Shulman, N. R., Aster, R. H., Leitner, A., and Hiller, M. C. (1961). *J. Clin. Invest.* **40**, 1597.

Shulman, N. R., Aster, R. H., Pearson, H. A., and Hiller, M. C. (1962). *J. Clin. Invest.* **41**, 1049.

Shulman, N. R., Marder, V. J., Hiller, M. C., and Collier, E. M. (1964). *Progr. Hematol.* **4**, 222.

Shulman, N. R., Marder, V. J., and Weinrach, R. S. (1965a). *Ann. N. Y. Acad. Sci.* **124**, 499.

Shulman, N. R., Weinrach, R. S., Libre, E. P., and Andrews, H. L. (1965b). *Trans. Assoc. Amer. Physicians* **78**, 374.

Shulman, N. R., Moor–Jankowski, J., and Hiller, M. C. (1966). *In* "Histocompatibility Testing" (D. Amos and J. J. van Rood, eds.), p. 113. Williams & Wilkins, Baltimore, Maryland.

Shumway, C. N., and Terplan, K. L. (1964). *Pediat. Clin. N. Amer.* **11**, 577.

Silver, M. D., and Stehbens, W. E. (1965). *Quart. J. Exp. Physiol.* **50**, 241.

Siqueira, M., and Nelson, R. A., Jr. (1961). *J. Immunol.* **86**, 516.

Siraganian, R. P., and Oliveira, B. (1968). *Fed. Proc., Fed. Amer. Soc. Exp. Biol.* **27**, 315.

Siraganian, R. P., Secchi, A. G., and Osler, A. G. (1968a). *J. Immunol.* **101**, 1130.

Siraganian, R. P., Secchi, A. G., and Osler, A. G. (1968b). *J. Immunol.* **101**, 1140.

Siraganian, R. P., Secchi, A. G., and Osler, A. G. (1968c). *J. Immunol.* **101**, 1148.

Spielvogel, A. R. (1967). *J. Exp. Med.* **126**, 235.

Spink, W. W., and Vick, J. (1961). *J. Exp. Med.* **114**, 501.

Starzl, T. E., Lerner, R. A., Dixon, F. J., Groth, C. G., Brettschneider, L., and Terasaki, P. I. (1968). *N. Engl. J. Med.* **278** 642.

Stetson, C. A., Jr. (1951). *J. Exp. Med.* **93**, 489.

Sutton, D., Rao, P., and Bachmann, F. (1969). *Fed. Proc., Fed. Amer. Soc. Exp. Biol.* **28**, 510.

Taub, R. N., Rodriguez–Erdmann, F., and Dameshek, W. (1964). *Blood* **24**, 775.

Terasaki, P. I., Thrasher, D. L., and Hauber, T. H. (1968). *In* "Advance in Transplantation" (J. Dausset *et al.*, eds.), p. 225. Williams & Wilkins, Baltimore, Maryland.

Tidball, M. E., and Shore, P. A. (1962). *Amer. J. Physiol.* **202**, 265.

Van Loghem, J. J., Jr., Dorjmeijer, H., Van Der Hart, M., and Schreuder, F. (1959). *Vox Sang.* **4**, 161.

van Rood, J. J., Van Leeuwen, A., Bruning, J. W., and Eermisse, J. G. (1966). *Ann. N. Y. Acad. Sci.* **129**, 446.

Waalkes, T. P., and Coburn, H. (1959a). *J. Allergy* **30**, 394.

Waalkes, T. P., and Coburn, H. (1959b). *Proc. Soc. Exp. Biol. Med.* **101**, 122.

Westerholm, B. (1965). *Acta Physiol. Scand.* **63**, 257.

Wurzel, M., Marcus, A. J., and Zweifach, B. W. (1965). *Proc. Soc. Exp. Biol. Med.* **118**, 468.

Yachnin, S., and Ruthenberg, J. M. (1965). *J. Clin. Invest.* **44**, 518.

Young, R. C., Nachman, R. L., and Horowitz, H. I. (1966). *Amer. J. Med.* **41**, 605.

Zvaifler, N. J., and Becker, E. L. (1966). *J. Exp. Med.* **123**, 935.

15

CLINICAL DISORDERS RELATED TO BLOOD PLATELETS

E. J. WALTER BOWIE and CHARLES A. OWEN, JR.

The blood platelet is a small cellular particle which, as the preceding chapters have made clear, has an intricate ultrastructure and an active metabolism which equip it for its prime role in the complex sequences of the hemostatic mechanism (Owen *et al.*, 1969a). It is not surprising that a decrease in number of platelets or a pathologic alteration of their function will result in a hemorrhagic diathesis which may be severe enough to cause exsanguination.

A detailed history and a careful physical examination are essential to the diagnosis. It is only from the history that we know whether a patient is or is not a bleeder. The history should evaluate the type of bleeding, exposure to toxic substances (including ionizing radiation), exact details of drugs ingested, and information about previous blood transfusions. A family history should be taken because the qualitative platelet diseases may be inherited, and thrombocytopenia occasionally is familial.

The physical examination allows the nature and extent of the bleeding to be assessed. In addition, some other disease may be present to which the thrombocytopenia may be secondary. For example, a palpable spleen may suggest a blood dyscrasia, liver disease, or systemic lupus erythematosus.

Disorders of platelets give rise to a defect of primary hemostasis with bleeding of the capillary type, in contrast to bleeding into the deeper tissues and hemarthroses which are seen in coagulation factor deficiencies. Several types of bleeding are associated with platelet diseases. Petechiae, the pinpoint hemorrhages from capillary loops, are perhaps the most helpful signs because they are characteristic of platelet abnormalities. They may occur in any area of the skin or mucous membranes but are most numerous over the legs, at sites of pressure and bony prominences. In areas where petechiae are chronic or recurrent, the skin develops a bronze pigmentation due to deposits of hemosiderin. However, petechiae are not pathognomonic of platelet disease because they also may occur in vascular disorders. There usually is little difficulty in recognizing petechiae, but tiny dermal angiomata may be confused with them; the raised appearance of angiomata becomes obvious on close inspection of the skin.

Ecchymoses also are common, but this type of bleeding may be seen in any hemorrhagic diathesis and is not particularly helpful in the differential diagnosis. Bleeding from the mucous membranes also occurs and results in epistaxis, hematemesis, melena, hematuria, and menorrhagia. Menorrhagia indeed may be the presenting symptom of thrombocytopenia (Doan et al., 1960; Hirsch and Dameshek, 1951), and a platelet count should always be obtained in these cases. Hemarthoses are rarely seen with platelet diseases but, on the other hand, intracerebral bleeding is a significant hazard, particularly in thrombocytopenia. Thus, the clinical assessment of a patient is not diagnostic of a platelet disease although it may be suggestive. The final diagnosis will depend on the results of laboratory tests, and the most important single test is a platelet count, which should always be confirmed by a blood smear.

The classification of platelet diseases gives rise to some difficulties because the etiology is obscure in certain instances and in others the very existence

TABLE I

CLASSIFICATION OF CLINICAL DISORDERS RELATED TO BLOOD PLATELETS

Quantitative platelet disorders

I. Thrombocytopenia

  A. Increased removal (destruction, utilization, or sequestration) of platelets

    1. Immunologic

      a. Isoimmune thrombocytopenia

        (1) Platelet antibodies from transfusions

        (2) Posttransfusion purpura

        (3) Isoimmune neonatal thrombocytopenia

      b. Autoimmune thrombocytopenia

        (1) Idiopathic thrombocytopenic purpura (acute, chronic, or recurrent)

        (2) Secondary autoimmune thrombocytopenia (collagen diseases; lympho-proliferative diseases)

        (3) Drug-induced

    2. Hereditary thrombocytopenia with intrinsic platelet defect

    3. Massive blood transfusion

    4. Enlarged spleen syndromes

    5. Thrombotic thrombocytopenic purpura

    6. Intravascular coagulation–fibrinolysis syndrome

  B. Decreased production of platelets

    1. Megakaryocytes decreased

      a. Hypoplasia of bone marrow

        (1) Acquired hypoplastic anemia

        (2) Megakaryocytic hypoplasias, including Fanconi's anemia

      b. Infiltration of bone marrow

    2. Megakaryocytes present in normal numbers

      a. Inherited thrombocytopenia

        (1) Inherited thrombocytopenia without associated abnormalities

        (2) Hereditary thrombopathic thrombocytopenia

        (3) May-Hegglin anomaly

        (4) Aldrich syndrome

        (5) Congenital absence of "thrombopoietin"

      b. Megaloblastic anemia

II. Thrombocythemia

TABLE I (*Continued*)

Qualitative platelet disorders

I. Thrombopathy

    A. Deficit

        1. Congenital (primary)

        2. Acquired (secondary)

    B. Functional

        1. Congenital (primary)

        2. Acquired (secondary)

    C. Plasmatic type

    D. Macrothrombocytic thrombopathy

II. Thrombasthenia

III. Abnormalities of platelet aggregation

    A. Portsmouth syndrome

    B. Aspirin

IV. von Willebrand's disease

V. Compound platelet defects

of the entity has not been clearly established. Furthermore, if a classification is too rigid or comprehensive, there is overlap between the subgroups. The classification we have adopted is outlined in Table I.

I. THROMBOCYTOPENIA: GENERAL ASPECTS

The thrombocytopenias as a group are unquestionably the commonest of the hemorrhagic diatheses (Owen *et al.*, 1969a). It is not possible to say at what level of platelet count bleeding will occur; 50,000/mm³ is often stated to be this level (Doan *et al.*, 1960; Linman, 1966). However, platelet counts considerably less than 50,000/mm³ may be associated with no apparent hemostatic defect, and, on the other hand, hemorrhage may occur when the platelet count is above this level. If, as has been suggested (Hellem,

1960), only a certain proportion of the circulating platelets have adhesive properties, hemostasis will be related not to the total number of circulating platelets but to the number of circulating platelets which are adhesive. Therefore, it can be postulated that there will be certain cases of thrombocytopenia in which hemostasis is normal because most of the circulating platelets are adhesive.

The most important laboratory manifestation of thrombocytopenia is a decreased circulating platelet count. Patients also may have a prolonged bleeding time by the Duke and Ivy techniques, an abnormal prothrombin consumption test which is corrected by platelets or phospholipid substitutes for platelet factor 3 such as cephalin or Inosithin (Owen and Thompson, 1960), abnormal clot retraction, and increased capillary fragility. The partial thromboplastin time is normal because a substitute for platelet factor 3 is added to the patient's plasma in this test. However, it is of interest that the plasma clot time, a test in which no partial thromboplastin is added, is also characteristically normal in these patients although in an occasional patient the time is prolonged (Owen et al., 1969a). In our experience the patients who have prolonged plasma clot times have evidence of decreased platelet production (as in hypoplastic anemia) and it seems likely that the majority of patients in whom the plasma clot time is normal have peripheral platelet destruction with the release of enough platelet factor 3 into the plasma so that the clotting time is normal (Owen et al., 1969a).

Many classifications of the thrombocytopenias have been attempted but none is entirely satisfactory. An etiologic classification perhaps would be most desirable but it is currently not possible because the etiology of many of the conditions is unknown. Our classification of the thrombocytopenias considers the dynamics of production and destruction of platelets and divides these diseases according to decreased life-span or decreased production. In general, the former are associated with normal or increased numbers of megakaryocytes in the bone marrow (megakaryocytic thrombocytopenia).

In certain types of thrombocytopenia, platelet production is decreased because the number of megakaryocytes in the bone marrow is decreased, for example, in hypoplastic anemia, the leukemias, and marrow infiltration by multiple myeloma and metastatic carcinoma. On the other hand, thrombocytopenia can occur despite the fact that the number of megakaryocytes and the platelet life-span are normal, for example, in megaloblastic anemias, congenital absence of a factor necessary for platelet production, and Aldrich syndrome. In these situations it seems likely that platelet production is ineffective. Decreased production of platelets, from one cause or another, is the commonest type of thrombocytopenia.

Most of these diseases are acquired although a hereditary type occurs rarely. Furthermore, in nearly every case, other aspects of bone marrow function are affected and there is often an accompanying anemia and leukopenia.

The clinical observation that thrombocytopenia may occur within a few hours of exposure to certain drugs establishes quite clearly that the platelet count has been decreased as a result of increased destruction, because the life-span of normal platelets is several days. The first clear demonstration that an immunologic reaction could produce thrombocytopenia came from experiments in animals. It was shown that the injection of a potent, specific, heterologous antiserum against platelets could produce a fulminating thrombocytopenia which was of rapid onset and resembled in many ways the thrombocytopenia produced by certain drugs (Bedson, 1924; Ledingham and Bedson, 1915; Tocantins, 1936). The subsequent work on drug-induced thrombocytopenia was most important in establishing that clinical thrombocytopenia could be produced by an immune mechanism. Furthermore, the immunologic thrombocytopenias can be subdivided into (1) isoimmune and (2) autoimmune. The possibility that idiopathic thrombocytopenic purpura (ITP) was an autoimmune disease was suggested by the fact that the disease was occasionally associated with hemolytic anemia. In addition, babies of mothers with ITP were often born with thrombocytopenia, suggesting that the humoral antiplatelet factor could pass the placental barrier. The classic experiments by Harrington and associates established that there was indeed an antiplatelet factor circulating in the plasma of patients with ITP (Harrington *et al.*, 1951).

The difficulty in demonstrating an immunologic basis for certain types of thrombocytopenia is a technical one and arises from the difficulty of performing platelet agglutination tests. The problem is that platelets have a natural propensity to become sticky under a variety of circumstances (including the performance of platelet agglutination tests) and the resulting platelet clump is indistinguishable morphologically from the platelet clump produced by agglutination due to an antigen–antibody reaction. The whole problem is discussed in detail in a previous chapter.

II. ISOIMMUNE THROMBOCYTOPENIAS

The demonstration of platelet agglutinins in the serum of repeatedly transfused patients and in the serum of mothers whose infants had neonatal thrombocytopenia led to the suggestion that platelets had isoantigens which were distinct from erythrocyte isoantigens (Harrington *et al.*, 1953; Stefanini *et al.*, 1953). A number of clinical problems may result from immunization by platelet isoantigens. First, patients who have received a number of transfusions may become refractory to platelet transfusions. Second, a distinct form of purpura, known as "posttransfusion purpura," may arise from sensitization to a specific platelet antigen. Third, neonatal thrombocytopenia has been described as the result of transplacental passage of platelet antibodies from mother to fetus.

A. Platelet Isoantibodies from Transfusions

The development of platelet isoantibodies is related to the number of transfusions; after 50 transfusions, 25–50% of patients have demonstrable sensitization (Shulman *et al.*, 1964). Baldini and colleagues (1962) studied 10 normal persons and found, in all 10, shortened platelet survival times after weekly transfusions of platelets although they were unable to detect any isoantibodies. On the other hand, Freireich and associates (1963) found that children with acute leukemia did not become refractory to platelet transfusions. The explanation may lie in the immunosuppressive nature of the therapy for acute leukemia and also in the compatibility of the platelets transfused, which usually were obtained from one or another of the patient's parents.

B. Posttransfusion Purpura

This syndrome is a distinct and unusual entity in which sensitization to a transfused platelet isoantigen results in a sudden fulminating and severe thrombocytopenia which clinically and immunologically bears some resemblance to drug-induced purpura. Generally, these patients have had one or more transfusions of whole blood usually because of a recent operation. After about a week there is a sudden onset of fulminating purpura as the result of severe thrombocytopenia. There may be practically no circulating platelets.

The sera of these patients have been found to contain an antibody directed against an antigen on the donor platelets but not on the patient's platelets; four of the few cases reported have had the same antibody (Shulman *et al.*, 1964). The mechanism proposed by Shulman and associates supposes that the antigen is able to circulate in a free form in the patient's plasma. The antibody is unusually "avid" and thus antigen–antibody complexes are formed at low concentrations of antigen. These complexes are then secondarily adsorbed to the platelets and result in platelet destruction.

The disease is self-limited and the platelet count will eventually return to normal spontaneously. However, the purpura is severe and, because it may last as long as 4 weeks, treatment may be necessary. In the cases reported in the literature, adrenal corticosteroids have been of no help. One patient had a prompt remission of the thrombocytopenia after an exchange transfusion (Shulman *et al.*, 1961). There is no indication for splenectomy.

C. Isoimmune Neonatal Thrombocytopenia

Neonatal thrombocytopenia is not common but nevertheless it is potentially serious because approximately 14% of the reported infants have died (Pearson *et al.*, 1964; Shulman, 1963); the commonest cause of death was intracranial hemorrhage. Neonatal thrombocytopenia has many different causes. Some of the babies have thrombocytopenia associated with Fanconi's anemia or with bilateral absence of the radii, and, in rare instances, the thrombocytopenia is familial (Bithell *et al.*, 1965; Quick and Hussey, 1963). Thrombocytopenia also may form part of the May-Hegglin anomaly and the Aldrich syndrome. Some of the babies whose mothers have ITP are born with thrombocytopenia due to transplacental passage of the antiplatelet factor from the maternal circulation.

All these types of neonatal purpura must be distinguished from isoimmune thrombocytopenia of the newborn which comprises about 20 of the reported cases. There is no history of thrombocytopenia in the mother or in the family, but the mother may have given birth to infants who have been thrombocytopenic. The diagnosis of isoimmune neonatal thrombocytopenia depends on serologic tests. Isoantibodies can be demonstrated against specific antigens on the platelet of the infant and the father but are absent from the platelets of the mother. The mechanism is akin to the incompatibility of the erythrocyte antigens in erythroblastosis fetalis.

The infant usually is not severely thrombocytopenic at birth but becomes so within a few minutes or hours. Bone marrow examination shows normal or increased numbers of megakaryocytes but an occasional case has been reported in which megakaryocytes were decreased or absent. The mother may become sensitized during her first pregnancy.

If the hemorrhagic manifestations and thrombocytopenia are severe, an exchange transfusion should be performed. This form of therapy is generally completely successful. If the platelet count is greater than 50,000/

mm³ and hemorrhagic manifestations are not significant, the patient can be observed without treatment. There is some evidence that prophylactic antepartum therapy with corticosteroids may have had beneficial results for the infant. Corticosteroid therapy to the infant may shorten the duration of thrombocytopenia.

III. IDIOPATHIC THROMBOCYTOPENIC PURPURA (ITP)

ITP, an autoimmune condition, can be divided into acute and chronic types (Hirsch and Dameshek, 1951); these types probably have different causes. It usually is possible to categorize a case of ITP but sometimes the differentiation is uncertain and will now be discussed in detail. In recent years, recurrent ITP has been differentiated from the acute and chronic forms (Dameshek et al., 1963). Recurrent ITP differs from the chronic form in that there is complete remission between the episodes. Unlike the chronic form, in remission the platelet count and platelet life-span become normal. The acute episodes are often precipitated by an infection.

The diagnosis of acute, chronic, or recurrent ITP should be made with circumspection if the spleen is found to be enlarged. The incidence of splenomegaly in ITP varies in different series reported in the literature, from 2.6% (Doan et al., 1960) to 10% (Hirsch and Dameshek, 1951), but nevertheless all patients who have splenomegaly should be suspected of having some underlying disease to which the thrombocytopenia is secondary.

A. Clinical Picture

1. ACUTE ITP

Although the acute form commonly occurs at any age, it is much more usual in children than the chronic form. Both sexes are affected equally. In the acute form there is often a history of an antecedent infection a week or 10 days before the purpura starts. The disease has been reported after upper respiratory infections, infectious mononucleosis, rubella, chicken pox, measles, and other exanthemata (Ackroyd, 1949; Baldini, 1966; Doan et al., 1960; Hirsch and Dameshek, 1951). The onset of purpura is sudden and may be associated with hemorrhagic bullae on the buccal mucosa. The petechiae and ecchymoses often start on the legs and spread over the entire body. The purpura may become confluent over large areas. Epistaxis and gingival bleeding are common and may be associated with hematemesis, melena, and hematuria. Similar clinical manifestations, including hemorrhagic mucosal bullae, are associated with certain forms of drug-induced thrombocytopenia. Spontaneous remission usually occurs from within one to several weeks although occasionally the disease may last for several months. In approximately 10–20% of patients in whom the purpura has the typical acute onset, the thrombocytopenia may persist chronically (Baldini, 1966; Linman, 1966).

2. Chronic ITP

The chronic type is usually but not always seen in early adult life, and females are more commonly affected than males (Doan *et al.*, 1960; Hirsch and Dameshek, 1951). In most cases the disease has an insidious onset and the bleeding manifestations may be mild, consisting mainly of purpura. Occasional cases have been discovered accidentally when a platelet count or bleeding time has been determined before an operation. Many patients have had purpura for months to years before the disease is diagnosed (Hirsch and Dameshek, 1951). Menorrhagia is common and is the presenting symptom in about half the women. Epistaxis, gingival bleeding, hematemesis, and melena also may occur. Exacerbations of the disease may be associated with the menses (Pepper *et al.*, 1956) and with intercurrent infections. There is no way of predicting clinically which of the cases with explosive onset will progress to the chronic form and which of the cases with insidious onset will remit spontaneously. Chronic ITP may continue for years, and it has been suggested that spontaneous cure never occurs (Baldini, 1966).

B. Laboratory Findings

The platelet count is decreased and there may be a prolonged bleeding time, increased capillary fragility, and an abnormal prothrombin consumption test which is corrected with Inosithin or other substitutes for platelet factor 3. If the thrombocytopenia is severe enough, clot retraction will be impaired.

A bone marrow examination should be performed in all cases to exclude acute leukemia and aplastic anemia as well as other possible causes of thrombocytopenia. In ITP the megakaryocytes are present in normal or increased numbers and there is little evidence morphologically of platelet formation. Since Frank's description (1915) of the megakaryocytes in this disease, a number of morphologic studies have been made. Some workers think that the megakaryocytes are morphologically normal (Robson, 1949; Wiseman et al., 1940). We would concur with other workers who report that many megakaryocytes are immature and appear rounded with clearly demarcated edges (Diggs and Hewlett, 1948). Degenerative changes have been found in the nuclei and cytoplasm (Pisciotta et al., 1953). This appearance could be explained by rapid release and destruction of platelets. An alternative and more likely explanation is that thrombopoiesis is ineffective, and the suggestion has been made that the platelet antibody also inhibits megakaryocytes (McKenna and Pisciotta, 1962) because platelets and megakaryocytes have common antigens (Vazquez and Lewis, 1960).

The marrow also may show an increase in eosinophils and lymphocytes (Diggs and Hewlett, 1948; Hirsch and Dameshek, 1951). The eosinophilia may be related to bleeding into the skin (Linman, 1966). If there has been an acute hemorrhage, the peripheral blood will show evidence of erythrocyte regeneration including reticulocytosis and perhaps a leukoerythroblastic blood picture with an increased leukocyte count. If bleeding has been chronic, the peripheral blood picture will be that of iron-deficiency anemia. Serum acid phosphatase activity may be increased, presumably because this enzyme is released from the destroyed platelet. It has been reported that determinations of this enzyme in platelet-poor plasma will differentiate between decreased platelet production, in which the acid phosphatase value is low, and increased peripheral platelet destruction, in which the acid phosphatase value is high (Oski et al., 1963).

C. Diagnosis and Etiology

The diagnosis of ITP is really one of exclusion. It is reasonable to arrive at this diagnosis when there is thrombocytopenia with normal or increased numbers of megakaryocytes in the bone marrow but no disease to which the thrombocytopenia may be secondary.

The possibility that ITP may be due to an immunologic mechanism was suggested by two clinical observations. One was that infants born to mothers with ITP may themselves be thrombocytopenic; this suggested that a humoral factor passed from the mother to the fetus and caused the thrombocytopenia (Epstein et al., 1950; Robson and Davidson, 1950). The other observation was that thrombocytopenia was associated with acquired idiopathic hemolytic anemia (R. S. Evans and Duane, 1949; Fisher, 1947); therefore, it seemed possible that the thrombocytopenia might be produced by an antibody mechanism similar to that known to cause the hemolysis.

The experiments of Harrington and associates (1951) clearly demonstrated that the plasma of patients with ITP contains an antiplatelet factor. These workers showed that plasma or blood from patients with ITP produced severe thrombocytopenia when transfused into normal recipients. They also showed that the antiplatelet factor was a globulin and was stable for at least 9 days at 5°C and at least 8 days at 25°C. More recently, Shulman and colleagues (1965a) showed that the antiplatelet factor was a species-specific 7 S γ-globulin which was adsorbed by platelets and affected autologous as well as homologous platelets.

Although the evidence that the antiplatelet factor is an antibody is compelling, the fact remains that no direct antibody test has given consistent results in ITP (Bridges et al., 1963; Corn and Upshaw, 1962). Jackson and associates (1963) have shown that the presence of thrombin may cause platelet aggregation and that, when prothrombin is adsorbed from the serum, platelet agglutination tests revert to negative in many cases of ITP. Indirect tests for platelet antibodies have been described but have given conflicting results. Tullis (1962) reported positive results with a quantitative agglutination test, and Nachman and Engle (1963) reported promising results from incubations of a platelet suspension in thrombocytopenic serum and measurement of the increase in α-amino acid nitrogen. More recently, Karpatkin and Siskind (1969), using two new tests (the dextran platelet agglutination test and the platelet factor 3 test), found antibodies in 25 of 30 patients with ITP.

A number of workers have studied platelet kinetics in ITP, with results that are not entirely in agreement. In some patients there appears to be a combination of increased peripheral destruction and decreased production of platelets (Cohen et al., 1961). However, Baldini (1966) suggested that an increased destruction of platelets is present in all patients with ITP and that, in contrast to erythropoiesis, there is very little evidence of a compensatory production of platelets (that is, increased thrombopoiesis). Platelet survival is only a few hours in acute ITP whereas, in chronic ITP, platelets survive 1–3 days (Baldini, 1966).

D. Role of the Spleen

There have been many suggestions concerning the role of the spleen in ITP. The thrombocytopenia has been ascribed to the elaboration of a myelosuppressive humor (Dameshek and Estren, 1947) by the spleen and to the sequestration and destruction of platelets in the spleen. However, there has been no convincing evidence of myelosuppression by the spleen, and recent work using tritiated thymidine (Rolovic *et al.*, 1966) has failed to show an increase in megakaryocytopoiesis after splenectomy in rats.

There is no question that the spleen sequesters platelets, and the work that defined the splenic platelet pool strongly suggests that the spleen plays a passive role in ITP (Aster, 1964, 1965; Penny *et al.*, 1966). The evidence for this passive role is the demonstration that rat platelets sensitized with antibody are sequestered in the spleen. In parabiotic rats, antiplatelet serum failed to produce thrombocytopenia in the splenectomized partner although thrombocytopenia developed in the intact partner (Harrington *et al.*, 1956). Shulman and associates (1965a,b) have shown that human platelets lightly sensitized with antibody are selectively sequestered in the spleen, and there is evidence that such a mechanism occurs in ITP (Aster and Keene, 1969).

The spleen is an important site of antibody production and there is evidence to suggest (Baldini, 1966) that part of the beneficial effect of splenectomy in ITP is the removal of a large amount of antibody-producing tissue. In view of the fact that platelets and megakaryocytes have common antigens (Vazquez and Lewis, 1960), the platelet antibody also may inhibit the megakaryocytes (McKenna and Pisciotta, 1962). It is possible, therefore, to synthesize all the various theories of the role of the spleen in the production of ITP into a unified group of interacting mechanisms.

E. Treatment

For many years after the introduction of splenectomy by Kaznelson (1916), this operation was the only therapy for ITP. After adrenocortical steroids became available, the therapeutic spectrum was broadened and thus became the subject of debate (Dameshek, 1960). Perhaps the difficulty of clearly delineating the disease, the difficulty in separating with certainty the idiopathic from the secondary type, and the occasional difficulty in distinguishing the acute from the chronic type were some of the reasons for the differences of opinion regarding therapy.

At present, most clinicians would agree that splenectomy is rarely necessary in acute ITP and that both splenectomy and adrenocortical steroid therapy have roles in the treatment of chronic ITP, depending on the clinical situation. The opponents of splenectomy were concerned by the possibility of an increased susceptibility to infection because of the removal of such a large mass of antibody-producing tissue (Smith *et al.*, 1957). In an extensive review of 1313 children reported in the literature, together with 154 patients of their own, Erickson and associates (1968) showed that there was an increase in meningitis and sepsis in children less than 1 year old and that in older children, although the incidence of infection was not increased, the mortality from infection was high. It also was thought by at least one group that splenectomy resulted in the dissemination of previously latent lupus erythematosus (Dameshek and Reeves, 1956; Rabinowitz and Dameshek, 1960) and that there was high relapse rate after splenectomy (Dameshek et al., 1958). The proponents of splenectomy did not think that infections or the dissemination of lupus erythematosus occurred frequently enough to contraindicate the procedure (Bunting et al., 1961; Doan et al., 1960; Meyers, 1961). In our experience, splenectomy has never resulted in the production of lupus erythematosus, and most of the reported cases had symptoms suggestive of lupus erythematosus at the time the diagnosis of ITP was made. Furthermore, the administration of adrenocortical steroids for long periods is not without its hazards and will inevitably produce Cushing's syndrome, osteoporosis and probably crush fracture of the vertebrae, and diabetes.

Because the treatment of the chronic form of the disease seen in adults is so different from that of the acute form of the disease seen in children, these two categories will be considered separately.

1. CHRONIC ITP

Various treatments have been tried, including X ray, ultraviolet light, snake venom (moccasin), parathyroid extract, elimination diets, foreign protein injection, calcium gluconate, epinephrine, ascorbic acid, various vitamins, and thyrotropic hormone. None has been effective. When splenectomy was the only effective treatment available, a patient with acute, severe hemorrhage was often splenectomized as an emergency procedure. Currently, such emergency therapy is completely contraindicated and all patients should be treated with adrenocortical steroids. At the other end of the scale is the patient who is thrombocytopenic but has no hemorrhagic manifestations. Such a patient requires no treatment, and he may be observed for a while to see whether the platelet count increases spontaneously. Patients without bleeding usually have platelet counts in excess of $50,000/mm^3$, although we have seen an occasional patient whose platelet count has been as low as $10,000/mm^3$ with no significant hemorrhage.

Any patient who has bleeding should be treated, and it seems reasonable to begin treatment with adrenocortical steroids. Prednisone is a commonly used and effective medicament and should be given initially in a dosage of 15 mg every 6 hours. On this regimen, the bleeding will decrease in most patients and the platelet count will increase in about 50% of patients. It is of interest that in some patients the bleeding manifestations abate but the platelet count does not change significantly. If bleeding persists or becomes worse despite this dosage of prednisone, then the dosage should be increased, to as high as 100 mg every 6 hours. There is a report that high doses of steroids may cause thrombocytopenia (Cohen and Gardner, 1961) although we have never seen this complication. If there is a favorable response, the dosage of prednisone can be decreased after 2–3 weeks and gradually diminished to a maintenance level of 5–15 mg daily. Although prednisone is widely used, there is no convincing evidence that other preparations are inferior (Baldini, 1966; Meyers, 1961).

In one study, ACTH was thought to give the best results (Bonnin, 1961).

Corticosteroids produce their therapeutic effect in a number of ways. These drugs decrease antibody synthesis, and Harrington and associates (1956) showed that they decrease the amount of circulating antiplatelet factor in patients with ITP. There is also some evidence that they have a direct effect on the capillaries to increase capillary resistance (Robson and Duthie, 1950). Shulman and associates (1965a,b) have shown that the splenic reticuloendothelium is the most active site for the sequestration of platelets minimally sensitized by ITP factor, and they thought that the effectiveness of corticosteroid therapy can be attributed to the inhibition of splenic sequestration. Heavily sensitized platelets are distributed generally throughout the reticuloendothelial system, and steroids have little effect in inhibiting this process. The possibility of treating refractory ITP by blockade of the reticuloendothelial system merits further consideration.

In several series in the literature (Bunting et al., 1961; Doan et al., 1960; Meyers, 1961), the incidence of sustained and complete remission after steroid therapy was low, varying from 8 to 15%. In most patients, when the steroid dosage is decreased the platelet count also decreases and hemorrhage recurs. In view of the fact that, in chronic ITP, splenectomy results in a remission rate as high as 80% (Carpenter et al., 1959; Doan et al., 1960; Meyers, 1961), there seems to be no justification for withholding this operation in patients who have failed to respond to a trial of corticosteroid therapy. Indeed, it has been stated that splenectomy is eventually necessary in patients with chronic ITP (Baldini, 1966). At the moment there is no way of predicting which patients will obtain a favorable response to splenectomy. External scintillation counting over the liver and spleen has been attempted but has not proved very helpful in patient selection. Shulman and associates (1965b) thought that a favorable response to corticosteroids was associated with a favorable response to splenectomy.

Many patients who fail to respond to splenectomy or who have a relapse after an initial improvement in the platelet count will nevertheless have amelioration of their bleeding manifestations. In such patients no further treatment is necessary, and observation is all that is required. However, if bleeding manifestations continue to be troublesome, maintenance therapy with adrenocorticosteroids is indicated. Such maintenance therapy also is indicated in patients for whom splenectomy would be an unacceptable risk because of some other medical condition.

Although the life-span of platelets is shortened in both acute and chronic ITP, platelet transfusions may be helpful in controlling an acute episode of bleeding. Platelet transfusions also may be used in preparing the patients for splenectomy, although some surgeons think that such transfusions are not necessary because they have noticed that the bleeding diminishes dramatically after the splenic pedicle is clamped.

In the patients whose bleeding is not satisfactorily controlled with small doses of prednisone after splenectomy, consideration should be given to treatment with immunosuppressive drugs. There are several reports on the use of these drugs in autoimmune diseases including ITP (Dameshek, 1965; Dameshek and Schwartz, 1960). Azathioprine (Imuran), one of the more widely used immunosuppressive agents, has produced encouraging results in the treatment of refractory ITP. Bouroncle and Doan (1969) reported that azathioprine was effective in inducing complete hematologic and clinical remission in 12 patients and partial remission in 2 of the 17 ITP patients treated.

The possibility that failure to respond to splenectomy or the recurrence of thrombocytopenia after a period of remission is due to an accessory spleen deserves consideration, although the likelihood of such a finding should not be overrated. The likelihood of there being an accessory spleen is increased by the absence of Howell-Jolly bodies in the peripheral blood of the patient who has undergone splenectomy. In such a case, a splenic scan may show an accessory spleen.

ILLUSTRATIVE CASE: ITP WITH ACCESSORY SPLEEN. The patient was a 33-year-old woman. At age 11 years she had undergone splenectomy for thrombocytopenic purpura, and the platelet count had returned to normal. (The operative report confirmed that a 200-gm spleen had been removed.) She had had no problems until, at age 29, she had mumps after which purpura recurred and menorrhagia developed. The platelet count was low, and she was treated with prednisone and with norethynodrel and mestranol (Enovid) but this did not control the menstrual flow and hysterectomy was performed. In 1967, at age 33, she was unconscious for 3 days and had two generalized convulsions during that period; she was treated with diphenyl-hydantoin (Dilantin) and phenobarbital.

She was seen at the Mayo Clinic 2 months later, when physical examination showed several ecchymoses on the gluteal areas and right thigh and a few petechiae on the palate. Apart from the scars of her previous surgical procedures, physical findings were not remarkable. The platelet count was 22,000/mm³, hemoglobin 14 gm/100 ml, and leukocyte count 9400/mm³ with a normal differential count. The thrombocytopenia was confirmed by examination of a peripheral blood smear. The erythrocyte morphology was normal and no Howell-Jolly bodies were present. Because the smear showed none of the changes associated with splenectomy, the presence of an accessory spleen was suspected. A splenic scan using ⁵¹Cr-labeled heat-treated erythrocytes showed the presence of splenic tissue, measuring 9 by 9 cm, in the left upper quadrant of the abdomen. The accessory spleen was removed (weight, 110 gm). By the next day the platelet count had increased to 258,000/mm³ and continued to increase to a level of 1,510,000/mm³ 4 weeks later. Over the next 3 weeks the platelet count gradually decreased to normal (198,000/mm³) and has remained so since. She has not had any more hemorrhagic manifestations.

2. ACUTE ITP IN CHILDREN

There is little disagreement about the treatment of acute ITP in children. Splenectomy should be avoided because 80% of these patients undergo spontaneous remission in a few days to a few weeks. Corticosteroids should be administered in adequate dosage to control the bleeding and then tapered to maintenance levels and stopped. In 10–20% of these patients the ITP becomes chronic, but every effort should be made to avoid splenectomy until the thrombocytopenia has been present for 6–12 months.

IV. SECONDARY AUTOIMMUNE THROMBOCYTOPENIA

Thrombocytopenia may occur in association with a number of diseases, and in some of these instances it appears to be on an autoimmune basis. The diseases associated with such a thrombocytopenic mechanism include collagen diseases, particularly systemic lupus erythematosus, and the lymphoproliferative diseases, particularly chronic lymphocytic leukemia (Ebbe et al., 1962) and lymphocytic lymphoma. Thrombocytopenic purpura may be the initial manifestation of systemic lupus erythematosus (Rabinowitz and Dameshek, 1960). It has been suggested that splenectomy may accelerate the development of the disease (Dameshek and Reeves, 1956), but this view is controversial and many workers including ourselves fail to find an increased incidence of systemic lupus erythematosus after splenectomy (Bunting *et al.*, 1961; Doan *et al.*, 1960; Meyers, 1961).

A. Clinical Picture

The nature of the underlying disease is the most important determinant of the clinical picture, and this also is true of the hematologic and other laboratory findings. The usual features of thrombocytopenia may be present, including a prolonged bleeding time, impaired clot retraction, increased capillary fragility, and shortened prothrombin consumption test. Megakaryocytes will be present in normal or increased numbers unless the bone marrow has been infiltrated, as in chronic lymphocytic leukemia. There may be an associated hemolytic anemia or neutropenia. In systemic lupus erythematosus, other coagulation abnormalities may be found, particularly a thrombopathy resulting from circulating anticoagulant and an acceleration of thromboplastin generation (Bowie *et al.*, 1963). Despite the thrombocytopenia, bleeding manifestations are not common in systemic lupus erythematosus. In fact, in many patients, thromboembolic phenomena may occur despite the presence of a circulating anticoagulant (Bowie *et al.*, 1963).

B. Treatment

Therapy is directed toward the underlying disease. The thrombocytopenia often will respond satisfactorily to the administration of corticosteroids. Splenectomy is not indicated in patients who have a benign self-limiting disease such as infectious mononucleosis. However, in certain situations, such as the lymphoproliferative diseases, if the bleeding manifestations are difficult to control or if the treatment of the underlying disease or use of corticosteroid therapy fails, splenectomy may give gratifying results.

V. DRUG-INDUCED THROMBOCYTOPENIA

Drugs may produce purpura in a number of ways. The platelet count may be normal, in which case the purpura is due to a direct toxic effect on the capillaries. On the other hand, suppression of the bone marrow or an immune mechanism may result in increased platelet destruction and thrombocytopenia. In all cases of purpura it is important to make detailed inquiries regarding drug exposure. Specific inquiries should be made regarding the use of analgesics, laxatives, vitamin preparations, and sedatives because the use of these medicaments is so common that the patient often does not think of them as "drugs." It is particularly important to establish the time relationship between use of the drug and the onset of the purpura.

A. Clinical Features

Numerous drugs have been thought to cause thrombocytopenia but in most instances this association has been based on circumstantial evidence and not on specific immunologic studies. A list of drugs associated with thrombocytopenia is given in the Registry on Blood Dyscrasias by the Council on Drugs of the American Medical Association. Currently, quinidine is probably the drug most commonly associated with immunologic thrombocytopenia. In a patient who is sensitive to this drug, the onset of purpura may be explosive and thrombocytopenia may occur within half an hour of the ingestion. In some cases there may be prodromal symptoms including chills and pruritus. Hemorrhagic manifestations include petechiae and ecchymoses which may involve extensive areas of the trunk and limbs. Epistaxis, gingival bleeding, and hemorrhagic vesicles on the buccal mucous membranes also may occur. The purpura should subside and the platelet count should return to normal within a few days after withdrawal of the drug. In a patient with megakaryocytic thrombocytopenia who is ingesting a drug, it is often difficult to know whether the thrombocytopenia is due to drug sensitivity or is an unrelated type of thrombocytopenia such as ITP. If the thrombocytopenia persists for several weeks after the drug has been withdrawn, one can be quite sure that the decreased platelet count is not due to a drug-induced antibody.

There are a number of methods for the demonstration of antiplatelet factor in drug-induced thrombocytopenia. These tests include platelet agglutination or lysis, complement fixation, inhibition of clot retraction, and liberation of platelet factor 3 activity (Horowitz et al., 1962). The administration of a small amount of the suspected drug to the patient will bring about a prompt decrease in the platelet count. A test of this nature, although diagnostic, is obviously hazardous and is best avoided.

B. Pathophysiologic Mechanism

In 1934 there were separate reports that apronalide (Sedormid; allylisopropylacetylurea) and quinine produced thrombocytopenia (Loewy,

1934; Peshkin and Miller, 1934). Ackroyd (1960) showed that four factors are necessary for the production of thrombocytopenia by apronalide: serum from the drug-sensitive patient; the drug; normal platelets; and complement. It was also shown (Steinkamp et al., 1955) that, in a normal recipient who had taken quinine, thrombocytopenia could be induced by transfusion with plasma from a patient who had quinine sensitivity. Ackroyd (1960) proposed that the drug acted as a hapten, combining with a platelet protein and so forming an autoantibody. The resulting antigen–antibody reaction caused complement fixation and platelet lysis. More recently it was suggested (Shulman, 1963) that the drug combines with a plasma protein and that the subsequent antigen–antibody complex is secondarily adsorbed onto the platelet surface.

C. Treatment

The offending drug should be identified, and the patient should be instructed never to take it again. Splenectomy should never be advised. Corticosteroids are not contraindicated but there is no evidence that they have any beneficial effect in these situations.

VI. HEREDITARY THROMBOCYTOPENIA WITH INTRINSIC PLATELET DEFECT

By analogy with erythrocytes, it might have been surmised that thrombocytopenia could be caused by an intrinsic defect in platelet metabolism, and such a mechanism recently has been reported by Murphy and colleagues (1969a). These authors described five patients with thrombocytopenia who were in three different generations of one family. Although the clinical picture resembled that of ITP, the thrombocytokinetic studies were not consistent with this diagnosis. The patients' platelets showed decreased survival when labeled with ^{51}Cr and injected into the patients or into normal subjects, but normal platelets survived normally in the patients. On this evidence the authors suggested that the patients' platelets were destroyed as the result of an intrinsic defect and not because of some factor extrinsic to the platelet.

The platelets appeared normal morphologically. Clot retraction, aggregation with ADP, and platelet factor 3 activity were normal. No abnormality was found in the rate of glycolysis or level of ATP. Fourteen enzymes of the glycolytic and hexosemonophosphate shunt pathways were measured and found to be normal.

The platelet count increased in two patients who were splenectomized, but there was no improvement in the platelet survival times.

The same authors (Murphy *et al.*, 1969b) reported similar platelet survival studies in two brothers who had abnormally small platelets. Levels of hexokinase, phosphoglycerate mutase, enolase, and phosphoglycerate kinase were low, although no abnormality could be found in the parents' platelets.

VII. THROMBOCYTOPENIA FROM MASSIVE BLOOD TRANSFUSION

Blood transfusions may cause thrombocytopenia in a number of different ways. We have already discussed the interesting syndrome of posttransfusion purpura. Repeated transfusions will result in the production of platelet isoantibodies, and studies have shown extremely rapid disappearance of transfused platelets in multiply transfused patients (Baldini *et al.*, 1962; Shulman *et al.*, 1964). In patients who require large quantities of blood because of severe hemorrhage, thrombocytopenia may result because platelets are lost and platelet production is insufficient to meet the demand. The platelets in stored blood are poorly viable, and the transfusion causes further dilution of the already decreased numbers of circulating platelets. Other mechanisms also seem to be implicated because, in some instances, thrombocytopenia may persist for 3 or 4 days. It may be due to naturally occurring isoagglutinins or thrombocytopenic factors in the transfused blood (Stefanini and Chatterjea, 1952). In evaluating the clinical situation the possibility that the thrombocytopenia may be the cause rather than the result of the hemorrhage should always be considered.

In any patient who has been multiply transfused, there is always the question of whether hypocalcemia from the citrate in the administered blood may be causing or aggravating the hemorrhage. We have never seen such a situation and indeed have never seen a patient with tetany who has hemorrhagic manifestations. However, there is a well-documented report of hemorrhage on the basis of hypocalcemia after transfusion (Soulier, 1958). There is another report of hemorrhage associated with hypocalcemia after transfusion, but the authors did not think that the hypocalcemia was the cause of the hemorrhage (Aggeler *et al.*, 1967).

VIII. THROMBOCYTOPENIA WITH ENLARGED SPLEEN SYNDROMES

Thrombocytopenia may be found in a number of conditions which are associated with massive enlargement of the spleen, such as Gaucher's disease, portal hypotension with congestive splenomegaly, chronic infections (including kala-azar and tuberculosis), Felty's syndrome, sarcoidosis, and lymphoma. Studies in which surgically removed spleens were perfused have demonstrated the existence of a splenic platelet pool (Penny *et al.*, 1966). Experiments utilizing ^{51}Cr-labeled platelets also indicate the existence of a splenic reservoir of platelets proportional to the size of the organ. The platelets in the spleen exchange with platelets in the general circulation and there is evidence that, when the spleen is massively enlarged, up to 90% of the circulating platelets may be concentrated in this organ with a resultant peripheral thrombocytopenia (Aster, 1965). It also has been shown that splenomegaly will increase the platelet transfusion requirements threefold to sixfold (Aster, 1964). The patients with big spleens have abundant megakaryocytes in the bone marrow unless, as in the case of patients with lymphoma, infiltration of this organ has occurred.

IX. THROMBOTIC THROMBOCYTOPENIC PURPURA

In 1925, Moschcowitz reported the case of a 16-year-old girl in a paper entitled "An Acute Febrile Pleiochromic Anemia with Hyaline Thrombosis of the Terminal Arterioles and Capillaries: An Undescribed Disease." Since that time the disease has been referred to by a number of names including "thrombocytic acroangiothrombosis," "generalized capillary and arteriolar platelet thrombosis," "generalized platelet thrombosis," and "diffuse platelet thrombosis with thrombocytopenia and hemolytic anemia." There was no further report of the condition in the literature until 1936 when Baehr, Klemperer, and Schifrin reported four cases. Since that time, many cases have been described and, in 1947, Singer, Bornstein, and Wile proposed the term "thrombotic thrombocytopenic purpura."

A. Clinical Picture

The disease can occur at any time of life and is more common in females. The onset is usually fairly sudden with general malaise, headache, weakness, neurologic symptoms, and fever. The patient appears pale and exhibits purpura of varying severity. The course usually is acute and, in general, is fatal within a few weeks. The neurologic manifestations include an alteration of the state of consciousness, and the patient may be delirious or in coma. Motor paralyses, generalized convulsions, flaccid paraplegia, and varying disturbances of sensation including hemianesthesia have been described. In most cases the spleen and liver are not enlarged.

Laboratory findings include thrombocytopenia although in an occasional case the platelet count is normal. Fragmented erythrocytes (schistocytes) and, occasionally, spherocytes are seen. The reticulocyte count is increased and the bone marrow shows increased erythropoiesis with abundant megakaryocytes. The Coombs' test is usually negative.

The clinical manifestations of thrombotic thrombocytopenic purpura are due to thrombotic vascular lesions which occur in the capillaries and terminal arterioles of many organs, but their etiology remains uncertain. The characteristic lesion is a hyaline thrombus and it is uncertain whether this arises as the result of a primary vascular lesion with secondary thrombus formation or represents the equivalent of a generalized Shwartzman reaction with diffuse intravascular coagulation. Autopsy studies suggest that the initial lesion is a hyalinelike change in the walls of the small arteries and arterioles with encroachment on the lumen by protrusions of the mural lesion. A fibrin–platelet thrombus may be initiated at the site of the endothelial damage. Many vessels show saccular or fusiform aneurysmal dilatation (Cooper et al., 1952). The possibility of an autoimmune basis has been suggested but the studies by Brittingham and Chaplin (1957) contradict this hypothesis.

Lerner and colleagues (1967) performed extensive coagulation studies on a patient with thrombotic thrombocytopenic purpura and found no evidence of intravascular coagulation. In their review of the literature they noted that previous coagulation studies had been fragmentary and in the three cases of afibrinogenemia there was considerable doubt as to the accuracy of the diagnosis of thrombotic thrombocytopenic purpura. Detailed coagulation studies will have to be performed on many more patients before intravascular coagulation can really be excluded. The diagnosis is rarely made during life but in occasional cases the typical lesions have been found on biopsies of bone marrow (Cooper et al., 1952) and skin.

The hemolytic anemia often is attributed to the damage inflicted on erythrocytes as they pass through the distorted small vessels, and it has been suggested that thrombocytopenia may be due to the same mechanism (Baldini, 1966). Such a mechanism seems unlikely because motion-picture studies of the microcirculation show that erythrocytes and platelets can undergo marked distortion in their passage through capillaries and still recover their former shapes without apparent damage. A more likely explanation is that the fragmentation of erythrocytes is produced by passage through the fibrin network resulting from intravascular clotting (Bull *et al.*, 1968; Rubenberg *et al.*, 1968). In this case, the presence of fragmented erythrocytes would be consistent with the occurrence of intravascular coagulation in thrombotic thrombocytopenic purpura.

B. Treatment

A number of therapeutic regimens have been suggested for these patients, but none has very much to offer. Some patients seem to have been benefited by steroid therapy, and it would seem reasonable to give steroids to all patients. Splenectomy has been used in a number of cases, and it has been suggested that a combination of steroid therapy and splenectomy be used in all cases (Hill and Cooper, 1968).

It also would seem reasonable to use some type of therapy that would prevent the formation of the hyaline thrombi in small vessels, which are responsible for the clinical manifestations of the disease. If fibrinolytic therapy becomes more generally available, serious consideration should be given to this mode of treatment. There are conflicting reports on the use of heparin but some patients seem to have benefited from this therapy, and it would seem reasonable to use heparin in all cases of thrombotic thrombocytopenic purpura. Alternatively, agents which interfere with platelet aggregation, such as dipyridamole (Persantine) and acetylsalicylic acid, can be used, and there is an encouraging report on the use of clinical dextrans (Lerner *et al.*, 1967).

X. THROMBOCYTOPENIA IN THE INTRAVASCULAR COAGULATION– FIBRINOLYSIS SYNDROME

One of the more intriguing types of thrombocytopenia is that associated with lengthened prothrombin time and partial thromboplastin time, decreased plasmatic concentrations of fibrinogen and factors V and VIII, increased levels of split-products of fibrinogen and fibrin, and other evidence of active fibrinolysis. This bleeding syndrome has been called "afibrinogenemia" (Risak, 1935), "defibrination" (Lasch *et al.*, 1966; Soulier *et al.*, 1952), "consumption coagulopathy" (Lasch *et al.*, 1961), "disseminated intravascular coagulation" (Schneider, 1951), and, the term we prefer, "intravascular coagulation with fibrinolysis" or "ICF syndrome" (Owen *et al.*, 1969a).

When all manifestations of the ICF syndrome are present, as described above, the diagnosis is simple and the problem is whether to interfere with the intravascular clotting (heparin), the fibrinolysis (ε-aminocaproic acid [EACA]), both, or neither.

The diagnostic and therapeutic problems arise when not all the characteristics of the ICF syndrome are demonstrable, as often is true in the chronic form. When the course is chronic, the thrombocytopenia may be slight ($>100,000/mm^3$), the prothrombin time near normal, factors V and VIII only moderately decreased, and euglobulin lysis time normal, but the plasma fibrinogen level may be less than 100 mg/100 ml. Here, treatment is frustrating because the patient may be suffering from a bothersome but not life-threatening bleeding, prolonged administration of heparin is virtually impossible, and the improvement in *in vitro* test results often is not matched by any significant reduction in the bleeding tendency of the patient.

The principal problem in correlation of abnormal laboratory data with clinical bleeding tendencies is our ignorance of the turnover rates, pool sizes, and compensatory rates of synthesis of many of the clotting factors. Fibrinogen is the clotting factor that has been evaluated most carefully. From studies with radioactive fibrinogen it seems that, of the 300 mg of fibrinogen in each 100 ml of plasma, about 2 mg is being turned over hourly, that is, 2 mg is catabolized and replaced by 2 mg of new fibrinogen each hour (Amris and Amris, 1964; Christensen, 1958; Hammond and Verel, 1959; Owen *et al.*, 1969b; Takeda, 1966). Furthermore, about four-fifths of the body's fibrinogen is in the blood, the remainder being in lymph and other extravascular fluid spaces.

It is possible to calculate, using ^{131}I-labeled fibrinogen, the pool size and turnover rate of fibrinogen in a patient with the ICF syndrome and to compare these with normal. When this is done, surprising results often are encountered. A patient may have a normal level of fibrinogen in his blood, with increased, normal, or decreased turnover. Or, the plasma fibrinogen level may be decreased because of increased turnover or simply because of inability of the liver to synthesize fibrinogen rapidly enough, as in hepatic cirrhosis (Hollard and Kolodié, 1968; Tytgat *et al.*, 1968). As a matter of fact, from the scanty literature available, the highest rates of turnover of fibrinogen reported are not in patients with hypofibrinogenemia but in patients with malignancy and in those with increased fibrinogen levels in conditions such as active rheumatoid arthritis or glomerulonephritis.

It thus becomes apparent that the plasmatic level of any factor involved in the ICF syndrome depends on (1) its rate of degradation and (2) its rate of synthesis. If the liver is just able to keep up with the destruction of fibrinogen, as an example, the plasma concentration of this protein remains normal. When hepatic synthesis can no longer compensate, the plasma fibrinogen level decreases. In this case, when the accelerated degradation of fibrinogen is suddenly blocked by the administration of heparin, the plasma fibrinogen level may increase to or above normal. One can consider the patient to be compensated or decompensated, depending on whether or not he can synthesize the coagulation factor as fast as it is being destroyed.

When the ICF syndrome is examined in this light, one realizes that the body may be able to compensate for the destruction of one factor but not for the destruction of another. Thus, it is conceivable that the liver may be able to synthesize considerably more factor V, under stress, than the marrow can produce in the way of platelets. Such a patient could have a normal prothrombin time and a normal level of factor V at the same time that thrombocytopenia exists. Such is often seen, particularly in patients with the chronic form of the ICF syndrome.

To extend this line of reasoning, one might imagine that a chronic, smoldering ICF phenomenon actually could lead to increased levels of some of the factors involved because of persistent overcompensation. If one accepts this as a possibility, he is now confronted with the "hypercoagulability syndrome," namely, the patient with chronically increased level of factor VIII, for example. Because at least half of the patients with histories of thrombotic occlusion of arteries or veins (Pascuzzi et al., 1961; Spittell et al., 1960), as well as patients with metastatic malignancy (Amundsen et al., 1963) and normal persons postoperatively (Amundsen et al., 1963), have significantly increased levels of factor VIII, their basic pathophysiologic process actually may be a compensated form of the chronic ICF syndrome. In such cases the tendency toward thrombosis, notorious in the instances mentioned, may not be the result of the increased factor VIII level at all but the result of chronically accelerated intravascular coagulation. If this is so, the generalized ICF patterns and localized thrombotic phenomena may be variations of a common process.

A. Clinical and Laboratory Manifestations of ICF Syndrome

Although some think that primary fibrinolysis may occur clinically, the consensus, based on animal studies (Hardaway et al., 1960; Kowalski et al.,

1965), is that intravascular coagulation precedes and induces fibrinolysis. Oozing is noted from mucous surfaces and at sites of trauma such as along surgical incisions and through venipuncture holes. Large ecchymoses characterize the more serious cases.

The ICF syndrome is a serious, and at times fatal, complication of pregnancy (Ratnoff et al., 1955), notably in the presence of abruptio placentae (Bonnar and Crawford, 1965). When a dead fetus is retained (Pritchard and Ratnoff, 1955) or when there is retention of some placental fragments (Croizat and Favre-Gilly, 1949), bleeding may begin suddenly and without warning. Amniotic fluid embolism (P. Gross and Benz, 1947), eclampsia (Hjort and Rapaport, 1965), and criminal abortion (Gollub et al., 1959) also may be complicated by the ICF syndrome.

The acute ICF syndrome may accompany severe infections ("bacteremic shock," "purpura fulminans") (McKay et al., 1962), surgical trauma (Ulin and Gollub, 1966), incompatible blood transfusions (Krevans et al., 1957), snake bites (Ghitis and Bonelli, 1963; Reid et al., 1963), heat stroke (Delhaes et al., 1966), and acute injuries (Innes and Sevitt, 1964) particularly if associated with crushing and shock (Whitaker, 1967). Administration of meprobamate, sodium meralluride (Mercuhydrin), or diatrizoate sodium (Hypaque) has been reported to have induced the syndrome (Trinkner and Perkins, 1964).

Although cancer of any organ may be associated with intravascular clotting and chronic bleeding (Didisheim et al., 1969), prostatic malignancy (Rapaport and Chapman, 1959) is the one most regularly implicated. Other causes of the chronic ICF syndrome are giant hemangiomatosis (Blix and Aas, 1961; Hagedorn et al., 1969) and chronic liver disease (Johansson, 1964). The syndrome is undoubtedly related to the hemangiomatous condition because the clinical and laboratory abnormalities subside if the vascular tumor is excised or irradiated. The mechanism is not so clear in the case of liver disease because a decreased level of several clotting factors in the plasma could reflect impaired hepatic synthesis. However, evidence of fibrinolysis is more suggestive of intravascular clotting as the precipitating event. Rarer causes of the chronic ICF syndrome are dissecting aneurysm (Fine et al., 1967; Kazmier et al., 1969), cyanotic heart disease (Denis et al., 1967), allergic vasculitis (Gigon et al., 1964), sarcoidosis (Nilsson et al., 1957), amyloidosis (Bowie et al., 1969b; Redleaf et al., 1963), sickle cell anemia (Hilgartner et al., 1961), thalassemia (Soardi, 1959), and paroxysmal nocturnal hemoglobinuria (McKay, 1965).

The laboratory findings in acute or chronic ICF syndrome, whether severe or mild, are virtually the same, differing only in the degree of abnormality. The basic pattern is predictable from a knowledge of those factors which disappear when blood clots *in vitro*, namely, fibrinogen, prothrombin, factor V, factor VIII, and platelets. Not so easily explained is the occasional deficiency of some of the other factors which are not supposed to be coagulation-sensitive, such as factors VII and X. Because the prothrombin time depends on fibrinogen, prothrombin, and factor V, as well as on other factors, it is regularly found to be prolonged in this syndrome. The partial thromboplastin time, which is influenced in part by deficiency of factor VIII, and the plasma clot time test, which also requires an ample supply of platelets, both tend to be abnormal. Thrombocytopenia can be measured precisely by a platelet count or examination of a peripheral blood smear, but it can be suspected from inspection of lightly centrifuged blood. Hypofibrinogenemia is obvious if flimsy clots with indistinct end-points characterize all clotting tests.

Fibrinolysis may be detected by such a simple test as observation of a clot of the patient's whole blood. Much more sensitive is the euglobulin lysis time test or some measurement of fibrinogen–fibrin split-products in the patient's serum. If fibrinogen–fibrin intermediates exist in the patient's plasma, the thrombin clot time is prolonged and is imperfectly corrected by the addition of normal plasma. This latter step rules out a simple hypo-fibrinogenemic state.

ILLUSTRATIVE CASE: ABNORMALITIES OF ICF SYNDROME IN CASE OF OPERATIVE BLEEDING. A 35-year-old woman experienced profuse vaginal bleeding after curettage for removal of a fetus which had been dead for about 4 weeks. Her whole blood clot time was 16 minutes with an indistinct endpoint (normal, 6–9 minutes), prothrombin time 22 seconds (normal, 18 seconds), platelet count 50,000/mm³ (normal, 130,000–370,000/mm³), and fibrinogen 125 mg/100 ml (normal, 190–365 mg/100 ml). Tests for fibrinolysis were strongly positive: dissolution of a whole blood clot and very rapid euglobulin lysis. Fortunately, the patient recovered and several days later her coagulation tests all gave normal results.

B. Treatment

1. Acute ICF SYNDROME

In the acute syndrome with sudden, massive bleeding, the patient requires replacement of erythrocytes and of coagulation-sensitive clotting factors (fibrinogen, prothrombin, platelets, and factors V and VIII). Fresh whole blood supplies all these components, so whole-blood transfusion is the treatment of choice. Adequate replacement of blood loss will prevent shock which may initiate or perpetuate intravascular coagulation. Fresh-frozen plasma furnishes all the coagulation components except platelets, and it is usually available whereas fresh blood may not be. It is common practice to supplement the infused plasma or blood with fibrinogen (commercial preparations of Cohn's fraction I of human plasma), but each unit of blood (500 ml) or plasma (250–300 ml) contains about 1 gm of fibrinogen and is much less likely to transmit the hepatitis virus than is a fibrinogen concentrate. If fibrinogen replacement is desired, cryoprecipitate is preferable to the commercial preparations of Cohn fraction I because it is made from single units of plasma.

If transfusions of blood or plasma do not reverse the bleeding condition, serious consideration must be given to active interference with the intravascular clotting. Heparin is the only agent which can do this promptly and effectively. It is not easy to convince oneself to treat a bleeding diathesis with heparin, yet on occasion, cessation of bleeding promptly follows the administration of this agent. Accompanying clinical improvement is a significant increase in the platelet count and fibrinogen level.

When very active fibrinolysis is demonstrable during the acute ICF syndrome, EACA (Amicar) may be used along with the heparin to block the fibrinolysis as well as the coagulation. In such instances we give 50 mg of heparin sodium and 5 gm of EACA intravenously. We think that the temptation to give EACA alone should be suppressed; such a course is potentially dangerous because the fibrinolysis may be the body's only defense against the intravascular coagulation.

2. CHRONIC ICF SYNDROME

Direct treatment of the chronic ICF syndrome is difficult or impossible. If therapy of the primary disease (cancer, hemangioma) is effective, the bleeding tendency usually subsides. When treatment of the primary disease is not possible or is not accompanied by relief of bleeding, we administer heparin intravenously only when severe exacerbations of bleeding occur. Long-term therapy with heparin is impractical. In some instances it may be possible to use oral anticoagulants such as warfarin sodium.

XI. HYPOPLASIA OF BONE MARROW

A. Acquired Hypoplastic Anemia

Thrombocytopenia due to bone marrow failure forms part of the clinical picture of hypoplastic anemia. In rare instances an isolated neutropenia or thrombocytopenia has been described, but the majority of patients exhibit a decrease of all the peripheral blood elements. Hypoplasia of the bone marrow can be caused by a number of toxic substances although in at least half the patients no history of exposure to such an agent can be elicited. Exposure to hair dyes and insecticides may be injurious to the bone marrow but it should be emphasized that the evidence incriminating these substances, as well as many drugs, is purely circumstantial. The bone marrow can always be depressed by the use of oncolytic agents, including nitrogen mustard, busulfan, chlorambucil, cyclophosphamide, and antimetabolites. Ionizing radiation, administered acutely or chronically, will always cause thrombocytopenia if the dose is high enough. In view of the fact that the normal platelet has a life-span of 7–10 days, it will take this length of time after exposure to the radiation for thrombocytopenia to appear.

A large (and increasing) number of drugs may, on occasion, produce bone marrow aplasia. The effect of these drugs is unpredictable in a given patient and has been attributed to excessive dosage, prolonged use, intermittent use, and individual susceptibility. It seems quite likely that the affected person develops an idiosyncrasy for the drug and that the mechanism of action depends on the particular drug. No attempt will be made to give a complete list of drugs and chemicals that have been reported to produce bone marrow aplasia, but they include antibacterial agents (organic arsenicals and chloramphenicol) and anticonvulsants (mephenytoin and trimethadione). There have been isolated reports of bone marrow hypoplasia associated with the use of antithyroid drugs, antihistaminics, insecticides, hair dyes, chlorpromazine, and heavy metals (bismuth, mercury, gold, and silver).

Use of chloramphenicol frequently has been associated with a hypoplastic anemia with neutropenia and thrombocytopenia. Careful inquiries should be made regarding previous exposure to this drug, and it is a good idea to describe the capsule to the patient. There is convincing evidence that, if the drug is given in large enough doses, toxic changes, including vacuoles, appear in the erythrocyte precursors. In addition, there is evidence of bone marrow depression and, in patients being treated for pernicious anemia and iron-deficiency anemia, the reticulocyte response is delayed until the chloramphenicol administration is discontinued. Experiments *in vitro* suggest that chloramphenicol blocks the attachment of template RNA to ribosomal RNA (Saidi *et al.*, 1961; Ward, 1966).

1. CLINICAL AND HEMATOLOGIC PICTURE

In at least half the patients with hypoplastic anemia there is no recognizable cause. It must be emphasized, however, that we are continually being exposed to potentially etiologic agents, in our environment and in our food, and that many persons take drugs and chemicals without being aware of their exact nature. Although it would be dangerous to ascribe hypoplastic anemia to environmental agents without more evidence, the investigation of insecticides and food preservatives is certainly warranted. The unexpected effect of DDT on birds and fish is a good example of why we should always consider these agents suspect.

Hypoplastic anemia can occur at any age, and it affects both sexes equally. If the onset is acute and fulminating, abnormal bleeding is often the presenting manifestation. In most cases, however, the disease develops gradually and is slowly progressive. Abnormal bleeding is the result of thrombocytopenia, the increased susceptibility to infections is the result of neutropenia, and the other symptoms are attributable to anemia. Splenomegaly, hepatomegaly, and enlargement of lymph nodes are not part of the picture of this disease and, if present, should suggest some other diagnosis.

The blood picture is that of anemia, leukopenia, and thrombocytopenia. The morphology of the erythrocytes is normal, although many of the erythrocytes examined in the peripheral blood smear may have been provided by transfusions. The reticulocyte count is low and may be zero. Increased quantities of fetal hemoglobin may be present. There is no immaturity of the erythrocyte or leukocyte line in the peripheral blood. Thrombocytopenia may be severe. A representative area of bone marrow shows increased amounts of fat with decrease of all blood cell precursors. There is a relative increase in lymphocytes and occasionally in plasma cells. Mast cells also may be increased in number. The bone marrow involvement may affect some areas more than others, so it is possible to have a cellular specimen if the needle samples such an area fortuitously.

2. TREATMENT

Many patients will undergo spontaneous remission, so it is important to treat complications early and vigorously. If a drug or chemical is implicated, exposure to it should be stopped completely. Anemia should be treated with transfusions of packed erythrocytes. Hemosiderosis is a frequent occurrence in these patients after numerous transfusions. Intercurrent infections due to neutropenia and bleeding as the result of thrombocytopenia are the commonest causes of death. Transfusions of platelets are important in the therapy of these patients during a bleeding episode, and it may be desirable to give maintenance platelet transfusions on a regular basis. After numerous transfusions, the patient may become refractory because of the production of platelet antibodies. In such a situation, compatible platelets may be obtained from HL-A identical siblings (Yankee *et al.*, 1969) (the major antigenic system involved in tissue histocompatibility has been designated HL-A and several of the antigens are present on platelets). Antibiotics should be used to control infections, and leukocyte transfusions may be possible in the near future. In our opinion, corticosteroids are best avoided but may be used in certain patients who have thrombocytopenia with a marked bleeding tendency that is not being controlled by platelet transfusions. The use of androgens is advocated although the effects of their use in adults is not entirely certain. Improvement has been reported from the use of androgens in children (Shahidi and Diamond, 1959), although here again the evidence is conflicting (Heyn *et al.*, 1969).

B. Megakaryocytic Hypoplasias including Fanconi's Anemia

Fanconi (1927) described a fatal illness in three brothers, which he called "familial infantile pernicious-like anemia." The patients have a pancytopenia and bone marrow hypoplasia. Patchy brown pigmentation is common. A number of associated congenital disorders have been described, including dwarfism, microcephaly, hypogenitalism, anomalies of the thumbs, mental retardation, strabismus, and renal abnormalities (Dawson, 1955). The inheritance appears to be recessive and the pancytopenia usually develops between 4 and 12 years of age.

There have been occasional reports of congenital absence of megakaryocytes with resultant thrombocytopenia. Some of these patients may have an associated absence of the radii (Stefanini and Dameshek, 1962). The condition may be part of Fanconi's syndrome but differs in that thrombocytopenia arises in the first few months of life (Shaw and Oliver, 1959).

The bleeding manifestations should be treated with platelet transfusions. In Fanconi's anemia, splenectomy has yielded variable results; in general, it has not been helpful although an occasional good result has been reported (Dawson, 1955).

XII. INFILTRATION OF THE BONE MARROW

When the bone marrow begins to be replaced by foreign cells, a myelophthisic blood picture may result. The peripheral blood picture is characterized by the presence of immature erythrocyte and leukocyte precursors and, because the patient often is not anemic, it is better to use the term "leukoerythroblastic blood picture." Similar manifestations in the peripheral blood also can occur when the marrow is stimulated by acute hemolysis or acute blood loss.

The commonest cause of marrow replacement is metastatic cancer, particularly from the lung, breast, prostate, and thyroid and also from neuroblastomas. Multiple myeloma, Waldenström's macroglobulinemia, and lymphomas also may involve the bone marrow and produce a leukoerythroblastic blood picture. Agnogenic myeloid metaplasia is associated with leukoerythroblastosis, but this differs from the other conditions mentioned in that there are striking morphologic abnormalities of the erythrocytes. In agnogenic myeloid metaplasia the bone marrow is replaced by fibrous tissue. Occasionally, Gaucher's disease and Niemann-Pick disease may cause enough encroachment of the bone marrow to cause myelophthisis; in both these diseases, enlargement of the spleen may result in hypersplenism which may be an additional cause of thrombocytopenia.

The peripheral blood changes produced by the involvement of bone marrow by metastatic and other foreign cells are often attributed to the resultant replacement of the marrow. The involvement of the bone marrow is often patchy, however, and the degree of involvement seems to bear no definite relationship to the peripheral blood picture. Therefore, the exact explanation for a leukoerythroblastic blood picture is not entirely clear. It has been suggested that there is an "irritative" phenomenon—a suggestion that is more emotional than scientific.

The peripheral blood shows normochromic normocytic erythrocytes. Immature erythroid precursors and leukocyte precursors are seen, and in occasional patients the numbers of normoblasts may be extremely high. There may be leukopenia or leukocytosis. In most cases the platelet count is normal although, occasionally, thrombocytopenia occurs and there may be a platelet anisocytosis. Occasionally, megakaryocyte fragments and megakaryocytes themselves may be present in the peripheral blood. Because the bone marrow involvement may be spotty, it is necessary to examine very carefully all areas of the bone marrow aspirate. In these situations it is advisable to examine, in addition, serial sections of bone marrow tissue.

Thrombocytopenia occurs commonly in the acute leukemias. In these conditions the bone marrow may be practically replaced by sheets of immature granulocytes or lymphoblasts. Although it was thought at one time that these cells were rapidly dividing, it appears now that their maturation is actually delayed. In the entity known as myelomonocytic leukemia (Linman, 1966), all the cellular elements of the bone marrow are involved. The megakaryocytes often show striking abnormalities and it seems reasonable to suppose that this would result in defective platelet production.

The treatment of this diverse group of diseases is that of the primary disease.

XIII. INHERITED THROMBOCYTOPENIAS

A. Inherited Thrombocytopenia without Associated Abnormalities

This type of inherited thrombocytopenia is quite rare. The subject has been reviewed in detail (Bithell *et al.*, 1965; Seip and Kjaerheim, 1965; Woolley, 1956). Bithell and colleagues (1965) studied a large kindred and found mild thrombocytopenia in 11 members of three generations. Other hemostatic defects were excluded and the fact that the disease was inherited over three generations ruled out the possibility of ITP. The thrombocytopenia was inherited as an autosomal dominant trait. The disease is clearly distinct from Fanconi's syndrome (Fanconi, 1927) and the Aldrich syndrome (Aldrich *et al.*, 1954). Bone marrow examination showed normal numbers of megakaryocytes with little evidence of platelet formation; no other abnormality was found.

Four other families have been reported with a sex-linked type of inheritance (Canales and Mauer, 1967; Schaar, 1963; Vestermark and Vestermark, 1964). In another family there appeared to be a dominant type of inheritance with incomplete expression in females (Ata *et al.*, 1965). In these patients there was no other evidence of the Aldrich syndrome.

In general, the patients with the sex-linked type of inheritance have responded well to splenectomy. Corticosteroids have not been helpful. The decision as to therapy should be predicated on the severity of the hemorrhagic symptoms. If the hemorrhagic symptoms are mild, no treatment is indicated.

B. Hereditary Thrombopathic Thrombocytopenia

Quick and Hussey (1963) described this inherited type of thrombocytopenia in eight patients representing four generations of one family. In

addition to moderate thrombocytopenia there was evidence that the platelets were qualitatively abnormal because they exhibited decreased procoagulant activity. The symptoms were epistaxis, mucous membrane
bleeding, and menorrhagia. In the male members the hemorrhagic tendency lessened until about the fifth decade, at which time gastrointestinal
bleeding often developed.

The platelets are strikingly abnormal morphologically with many large
forms and resemble the platelets described by Bernard and Soulier (1948)
as "dystrophie thrombocytaire-hemorrhagipare." There are several other
reports of a similar syndrome and, in all of them, platelet anisocytosis is
increased and the platelets are large (Cullum *et al.*, 1967; Gröttum and
Solum, 1969; Hirsch *et al.*, 1950; Kurstjens *et al.*, 1968; Seip, 1963) although
not all of them are as big as lymphocytes (as they were in the disease described by Bernard and Soulier). In most families the disease has been
inherited as an autosomal dominant trait. With rare exception, platelet
survival appears to be short.

There is evidence that, despite the decreased life-span of the patients'
platelets, normal platelets survive normally (Gröttum and Solum, 1969;
Hirsch *et al.*, 1950), so platelet transfusions should be effective. Splenectomy
has not been a successful mode of therapy and, even if the platelet count
were to increase, the platelets would presumably still be thrombopathic.

C. May-Hegglin Anomaly

Döhle's inclusion bodies are found in the leukocytes of these patients in
association with large platelets, usually about $4\,\mu$ in diameter although
platelets up to $50\,\mu$ in diameter have been described. In some of the patients,
thrombocytopenia has developed; in the family described by Oski and colleagues (1962) only one of three members had thrombocytopenia. The
May-Hegglin anomaly is extremely rare and the patients are well clinically,
so no treatment is necessary. The cause of the disease remains obscure.

D. Aldrich Syndrome

Aldrich and colleagues (1954) described a patient who had thrombocytopenia, draining ears, eczematoid dermatitis, and bloody diarrhea. Nine
other members of the family had a similar syndrome although the presence
of thrombocytopenia in them could not be established with certainty. There
was a high mortality rate, and the pattern of inheritance was consistent

with a sex-linked recessive gene. No clear-cut deficiency of immune response has been shown, but isoagglutinins are absent; γ-globulin levels are normal or increased (Krivit and Good, 1959). The Aldrich syndrome probably represents an example of ineffective thrombocytopoiesis in that the platelet life-span is normal but the platelet count is decreased because the megakaryocytes in the bone marrow do not produce platelets adequately (Baldini, 1966; Krivit et al., 1966). Qualitative platelet abnormalities recently have been described, including absence of aggregation with ADP, epinephrine, and collagen. Epinephrine fails to produce the usual increase in the activity of the citric acid cycle in the platelet (Baldini et al., 1969).

E. Congenital Absence of "Thrombopoietin"

An interesting type of thrombocytopenia was reported by Schulman and colleagues (1960). The patient was an 8-year-old girl who had thrombocytopenia which responded to transfusions of blood or plasma. The thrombocytopenia was apparently due to the absence of a stimulating factor which appears to be responsible for megakaryocytic maturation and the production of platelets. It was found that the factor was stable in banked blood on storage. A similar case has been reported by Upshaw (1967).

XIV. MEGALOBLASTIC ANEMIAS

DNA synthesis is disturbed by a deficiency of vitamin B_{12} or folate, and this leads to megaloblastic changes in the bone marrow. The cellular changes do not affect the erythrocytes alone but are seen in all the cells of the marrow and indeed in all the cells of the body. Hypoprothrombinemia has been reported in pernicious anemia (Warner and Owen, 1942) and this perhaps is on the basis of hepatocellular involvement. The involvement of the bone marrow results in leukopenia and thrombocytopenia which are almost always found in advanced cases of megaloblastic anemia. Morphologic abnormalities of the platelet have been described in pernicious anemia and, in electron microscope studies, these changes in the platelets have been shown to persist despite adequate treatment with vitamin B_{12} (Rebuck et al., 1961). Even though there is thrombocytopenia, bleeding manifestations are rare. Bleeding times and tests of capillary function are often normal. It has been suggested that in this situation there may be a higher proportion of adhesive platelets than normal so that normal hemostasis occurs despite the thrombocytopenia.

XV. THROMBOCYTHEMIA

The level of circulating platelets may be increased in a number of circumstances including acute hemorrhage, acute hemolysis, cancer, iron deficiency, and splenectomy. The increase in platelet count associated with these conditions usually is called "thrombocytosis" to distinguish it from "thrombocythemia" which is a myeloproliferative disorder due to primary abnormality of the bone marrow.

Primary thrombocythemia forms part of the spectrum of the myeloproliferative syndromes which include myeloid metaplasia, polycythemia vera, and chronic myelogenous leukemia. Gunz (1960) published a critical review of the literature, outlining the clinical and hematologic features which he thought established the syndrome as a distinct entity. In the same year, Ozer and associates (1960) published a review including experience with six cases of the syndrome. More recently, Silverstein (1968) further delineated the syndrome by publishing experience with 15 cases. Although one would expect patients with such high platelet counts to have thromboembolic manifestations, it is intriguing and paradoxic that most of these patients have unusual bleeding instead.

A. Clinical Picture

The platelet counts usually are in excess of 1,000,000/mm^3 and may be two or three times higher. There is a report of one patient whose platelet count was 14,000,000/mm^3. On the peripheral blood smear the platelets often occur in large clumps or sheets and, because of hemorrhage, there may be a hypochromic microcytic anemia. There usually is a moderate leukocytosis with a slight degree of immaturity. The spleen is nearly always palpable. On bone marrow examination there usually is megakaryocytic hyperplasia and the smears of the marrow show numerous platelets. Silverstein's criteria for diagnosis are a history of recurrent hemorrhage or thrombosis, a platelet count in excess of 1,000,000/mm^3, absence of an increase in circulating erythrocytes, absence of leukemic features in peripheral blood and bone marrow, and absence of bone marrow fibrosis.

The hemorrhagic symptoms include ease of bruising, hematuria, and recurrent gastrointestinal hemorrhage. Thromboembolic phenomena also may occur, including hepatic and splenic vein thrombosis and painful priapism. In occasional patients the spleen is not enlarged and there may be Howell-Jolly bodies in the peripheral blood consistent with infarction atrophy of the spleen. In some patients, hemorrhage and thromboembolism occur concurrently.

Gastrointestinal bleeding is common in these patients. The gastrointestinal blood loss often is occult and a hypochromic anemia develops. A massive hemorrhage may lead to thrombocytosis and leukocytosis on its own account, but the presence of splenomegaly and a platelet count greater than 1,000,000/mm³ should suggest the possibility of primary thrombocythemia. In these situations a period of observation after the gastrointestinal bleeding has stopped may be helpful in making the diagnosis.

Death often is due to thromboembolic complications. Because of the rarity of the disease, accurate survival data are difficult to obtain. In Silverstein's series, six of eight patients were alive 2–5 years after the diagnosis was established.

B. Treatment

Although many patients have long periods without symptoms, it seems reasonable to advise myelosuppressive therapy in all patients whose platelet count is greater than 1,000,000/mm³. The goal of therapy is to decrease the platelet count in order to decrease the incidence of thrombosis and hemorrhage. There is no evidence that myelosuppressive therapy has any other influence on survival rate. Treatment with radioactive phosphorus (sodium ³²P-phosphate) or busulfan has been used most frequently, and there is some evidence that radiophosphorus may be preferable in that the length of remission is slightly greater (Silverstein, 1968).

If patients are having transient visual disturbances or other evidence of transient cerebral ischemic attacks, the situation should be regarded as an emergency and immediate steps should be taken to decrease the platelet count as rapidly as possible. The most effective way of doing this is to administer a full dose of nitrogen mustard intravenously and immediately follow this by "plateletpheresis" with the idea of rapidly removing as many as possible of the circulating platelets (Colman et al., 1966). Nitrogen mustard also can be used to decrease the platelet count before an urgent surgical procedure.

C. Pathophysiology of Bleeding

The occurrence of bleeding in these patients is paradoxic and has been the subject of a number of speculations. Our work, as well as that of others

(Bowie *et al.*, 1965a; Spaet, 1957), has shown that high concentrations of platelets have an inhibitory effect on the thromboplastin generation test. It has been suggested that this may be the mechanism of bleeding in these patients (Spaet, 1957). It seems more likely that the qualitative platelet abnormalities which have been demonstrated in patients with primary thrombocythemia (Didisheim and Bunting, 1966; McClure *et al.*, 1966) are more important causes of the hemostatic defects. Spaet and colleagues (1969) reported platelet aggregation studies in three patients with essential thrombocythemia. They found the aggregation response to epinephrine to be absent, that to ADP decreased, and that to collagen normal. There was no abnormality of platelet factor 3 availability.

Our own observations in this disease also have disclosed qualitative platelet defects. In one patient, ADP aggregation was abnormal but became normal when the platelet-rich plasma was diluted (with the patient's own plasma) to a platelet concentration of approximately 300,000/mm^3. In other patients, ADP aggregation remained abnormal despite dilution to a low platelet count. We also have found both normal and abnormal platelet factor 3 activity. There seems to be no question that qualitative platelet defects are common in patients with primary thrombocythemia and they may well be associated with abnormal bleeding.

There also is evidence that some of these patients have acute episodes of intravascular coagulation with depletion of coagulation factors, and it would seem possible that some patients may be found who have chronic intravascular coagulation, although such a patient has not yet been described. A plausible explanation for the recurrent episodes of gastrointestinal bleeding in these patients is the development of small hemorrhagic infarcts in the intestinal mucosa.

The situation is obviously complex and is far from being solved. It seems that bleeding may be due to a number of different causes but that qualitative platelet defects make an important contribution to the hemorrhagic diathesis.

XVI. QUALITATIVE PLATELET DEFECTS: GENERAL ASPECTS

Platelets have intense metabolic activity; at least 30 enzymes have been demonstrated, including a major glycolytic pathway which depends on ATP for energy. On exposure to certain stimuli, such as thrombin, epinephrine, and collagen, platelets release ATP and ADP. The freshly released ADP is a powerful agent for making platelets aggregate (as used herein in regard to platelets, "aggregate" means adhere to each other). When platelets aggregate, serotonin (Ashford and Freiman, 1967; Mustard *et al.*, 1967; Mustard and Packham, 1968), acid phosphatase, β-glucuronidase, and adenylate kinase are released and platelet factor 3 is activated (Zucker and Peterson, 1968).

At least 15 proteins are known to be present in platelets. These include various plasma proteins and plasma clotting factors and also some unique proteins such as thrombosthenin (Bettex-Galland and Lüscher, 1961; Nachman *et al.*, 1967a), which is remarkably similar to the protein of muscle cells, and a protein which inhibits the anticoagulant property of heparin (it is known as platelet factor 4).

The lipids of the platelet have been of particular interest because they are important in the coagulation of blood. Since phospholipids (Marcus, 1966; Marcus and Zucker, 1965; Marcus *et al.*, 1962) such as phosphatidyl serine and phosphatidyl ethanolamine (Marcus and Spaet, 1958; Marcus *et al.*, 1966) can substitute for platelets in the clotting reaction, the procoagulant action of platelets is often attributed to these two phosphatides. But other lipids also may be important. These lipids are found in the wall of the platelet (Hardisty, 1968; Marcus, 1966; Sixma and Nijessen, unpublished data), in internal granules (Marcus *et al.*, 1966, 1969; White, 1965), and in a nonsedimentable form (Horowitz and Papayoanou, 1967); it is difficult to know which group is primarily important in clotting. Furthermore, phospholipids within the cell are undoubtedly complexed with proteins. Whether or not this is the reason, platelet lipoprotein has greater coagulant power than have individual phospholipids (Marcus, 1966). Thus, the procoagulant property of platelets is described simply as "platelet factor 3" without attempts to assign the activity to any specific molecule or site within the platelet. The term will undoubtedly persist until considerably more is known about the biochemistry of platelet lipoproteins. A deficiency of this platelet factor 3 activity is known as "thrombocytopathy," "thrombocytopathia," or simply "thrombopathy."

Many platelet factors related to hemostasis have been described and several even have been assigned numbers (Seegers, 1961, 1962). Two of the numbered factors seem to be the same as plasmatic coagulation factors —platelet factor 1 = plasma factor V (Hjort *et al.*, 1955) and platelet factor 5 = plasma factor I or fibrinogen (Salmon *et al.*, 1957)—and another, platelet factor 7 (Lee *et al.*, 1957), has not been distinguished clearly from platelet factor 3.

We propose that the designations platelet factors 1, 5, and 7 be abandoned and, furthermore, that no additional platelet factor numbers be assigned until they have undergone the same scrutiny that has been given the plasmatic factors. In accord with this proposal, the platelet factors become: platelet factor 1, unassigned; platelet factor 2, that platelet activity which shortens the clotting time of purified thrombin and purified fibrinogen (Ware *et al.*, 1948); platelet factor 3, the procoagulant activity of the platelet necessary for intrinsic blood coagulation (Deutsch *et al.*, 1955; Van Creveld and Paulssen, 1952); platelet factor 4, the antiheparin activity of platelets (Conley *et al.*, 1948); platelet factor 5, unassigned, although the fibrinogen within the platelet is partially incoagulable (Nachman *et al.*, 1967b) and may be different from plasmatic fibrinogen; platelet factor 6, the antifibrinolytic activity of platelets (Johnson and Schneider, 1953); and platelet factor 7, unassigned.

Whether ADP, vasoactive amines (such as serotonin), and thrombosthenin should be numbered or not might be left until we have more definite knowledge about the role of these components.

Despite the steadily accumulating knowledge about platelet structure and function, most of the abnormalities of platelet function still cannot be explained. They have been discovered, for the most part, because patients presented with bleeding tendencies. The abnormalities may be lumped together as "qualitative platelet defects" because in these patients the platelet counts are within the range of normal yet one or another function is impaired. The platelet functions which are measured currently are as follows.

a. PLATELET ADHESIVENESS TO GLASS. Normal platelets easily become sticky and adhere readily to foreign surfaces. To quantitate this property, Wright (1941) measured the number of platelets adhering to a specific area of the glass surface in a rotating tube, Hellem (1960) increased the area of available glass surface by filling the tube with small glass beads, and Salzman (1963) drew the blood directly through the column of beads by vacuum. In our adaptation (Bowie *et al.*, 1969a), heparinized blood is forced through the column at a fixed rate. In Glanzmann's thrombasthenia, platelets are found not to be adhesive by any of these methods. Characteristically, in von Willebrand's disease, Salzman's test and our test give abnormal results but Wright's method gives normal results (Bowie *et al.*, 1967). A disease, "athrombia," has been described in which the only abnormality is in adhesiveness of platelets to glass (Inceman, 1955).

b. PLATELET ADHESIVENESS *in Vivo*. Borchgrevink (1961) found that the platelet count decreases rapidly in blood exuding from a puncture wound in a normal person. In von Willebrand's disease the platelet count decreases little or not at all, which may be related to the tendency of these patients to have long bleeding times. We use the Didisheim-Bunting adaptation of the Borchgrevink test to measure platelet adhesiveness *in vivo* (Didisheim and Bunting, 1966).

c. PLATELET AGGREGATION. The discovery that something in the erythrocyte (factor "R"), in association with one or more plasmatic substances in addition to calcium, induces platelets to aggregate has led to a flurry of activity in recent years. The erythrocytic constituent was found to be ADP (Gaarder *et al.*, 1961) and could be replaced by pure ADP. Thus, a test was developed in which platelet-rich plasma is mixed with ADP under standardized conditions of temperature and mixing speed (Born, 1962; O'Brien, 1962). As the platelets aggregate, less of a beam of light is absorbed by the platelet-rich plasma, and the amount of this change in absorbance of light reflects the amount of platelet aggregation. If the amount of ADP is carefully adjusted, the absorption of light decreases in two waves, one almost instantaneously and the second after about half a minute. The second wave is attributed to the release of the platelet's own ADP as a consequence of the initial aggregation (Mills *et al.*, 1968) and coincides with the release of serotonin and platelet factor 3 activity. In thrombocythemia, primary platelet aggregation on addition of ADP occasionally is decreased, and in thrombasthenia this aggregation is absent. If the patient has been taking one of several antiinflammatory drugs, notably aspirin, the release reaction, and consequently the second wave of ADP aggregation, is inhibited. A similar inhibition is found in some inherited platelet diseases.

Other substances such as epinephrine (O'Brien, 1963), norepinephrine, serotonin, thrombin, and collagen will induce platelet aggregation.

d. PLATELET–COLLAGEN INTERACTION. Because the adhesion of platelets to collagen is important in initiating hemostasis, this function will be considered separately. When an extract or suspension of collagen is added to stirred platelet-rich plasma, aggregation occurs after a delay and corresponds with the second wave (or release reaction) of ADP- or epinephrine-induced aggregation (Hovig, 1963). Divalent cations such as calcium are not required for platelets to adhere to collagen (Spaet and Zucker, 1964) although they are necessary for the release reaction (Hovig, 1964). Free amino acid groups, particularly the ε-amino groups of lysine, are critical for platelet aggregation with collagen, but carboxyl groups do not seem to be necessary (Wilner *et al.*, 1968b). Several patients have now been reported whose platelets aggregated ineffectively when collagen was added; if this function is hemostatically important (Baumgartner *et al.*, 1967; Branemark and Ekholm, 1968; Spaet and Cintron, 1964; Tranzer and

Baumgartner, 1967), it might explain their bleeding tendency. It seems clear that platelets adhere to connective tissue beneath damaged endothelium (Ashford and Freiman, 1967; French *et al.*, 1964; Mustard and Packham, 1968; Mustard *et al.*, 1967). It also has been suggested (Johnson *et al.*, 1969) that platelets may adhere directly to the damaged endothelial cell itself. Collagen also seems to activate factor XII (Niewiarowski *et al.*, 1965; Wilner *et al.*, 1968a).

e. CLOT RETRACTION. This is one of the oldest tests of platelet function. Clot retraction is characteristically absent in severe thrombocytopenia and in Glanzmann's thrombasthenia. Because the mechanism by which a clot retracts is incompletely understood and because the triggering mechanism in the platelet has not been discovered, this must remain an empiric test, albeit a simple and good one. The contractile protein of the platelet, thrombosthenin, apparently is normal in Glanzmann's disease. Although platelet fibrinogen is sharply decreased in this disease, no inferences can be made as to the importance of this finding in clot retraction.

f. PLATELET FACTOR 4 ACTIVITY. This is measured by the extent of inhibition of the effect of heparin in a plasma clotting system when platelets are added. No disease has been ascribed to abnormality of this factor. but the release of platelet factor 4 activity is inhibited by aspirin.

g. PLATELET FACTOR 3 ACTIVITY. Unlike "complete" thromboplastins or tissue juices, which induce clotting through the extrinsic pathway, platelet factor 3 is a "partial" thromboplastin and not until it has interacted in some way with factors XII (Iatridis and Ferguson, 1965), XI, IX, and VIII is an activity like that of tissue juices attained, although it has been reported that this activity is attained spontaneously if platelet-rich plasma is left at 37°C for at least 16 hours (Biggs *et al.*, 1968). Even so, unlike tissue juice thromboplastin, the generated thromboplastin apparently does not require factor VII to complete the formation of prothrombinase from factors V and X and phospholipid. Platelet factor 3 activity can be measured only by biologic tests. The following systems have been used.

i. *Plasma clot time.* If the platelet count of anticoagulated plasma is progressively decreased by centrifugation, the clot time of the plasma on recalcification increases steadily. The degree of correction of this clot time by addition of platelet-poor plasma has been used as a test of platelet factor 3 activity (Husom, 1961). Yet, in thrombocytopenic states or thrombopathic states, plasma clot times rarely are significantly prolonged. When the plasma clot time is abnormally long, the platelet is clearly involved if the partial thromboplastin time is normal because, in this test, a platelet substitute is added to the plasma before recalcification.

ii. *Prothrombin consumption test.* Although the mechanism is not understood, the prothrombin time of serum from patients with thrombocytopenia or thrombopathy is abnormally short. Quick and Geppert (1963) attribute the short serum prothrombin times to high levels of residual prothrombin in the serum. However, Johnson and co-workers (1957) found short serum prothrombin times, despite little residual prothrombin, in some sera from thrombocytopenic patients, suggesting that other coagulation activities may influence the "prothrombin consumption" test. Whatever the mechanism, a short serum prothrombin time is so characteristic of thrombopathy and thrombocytopenia that we have found it to be the best screening test for certain qualitative platelet disorders. Since other abnormalities also affect the prothrombin consumption test, we have modified the standard test of Quick by collecting two tubes of blood, to one of which is added a platelet substitute. If the serum prothrombin time is short in the unmodified test and is normal in the serum from the supplemented blood and if the platelet count is normal, we think that this is good evidence for a thrombopathic state.

iii. *Stypven test.* Rapid clotting of platelet-rich plasma is induced by the venom (Stypven) of the Russell viper if adequate amounts of platelet factor 3, factors V and X, prothrombin, and fibrinogen are present. The shortening of the Stypven clotting time after inducing platelet factor 3 release (for example, by the addition of kaolin) can be used as an index of platelet factor 3 activity (Hardisty, 1968; Spaet and Cintron, 1965).

iv. *Thromboplastin generation test.* This test, which actually measures the generation of prothrombinase rather than thromboplastin, consists of mixing serum, adsorbed plasma, platelets, and a solution of calcium chloride. At intervals the amount of prothrombinase is assayed by adding aliquots of the mixture to a solution containing prothrombin and fibrinogen (normal decalcified plasma). If the serum (containing factors XII, XI, IX, VII, and X) and the absorbed plasma (containing factors XII, XI, VIII, and V) are normal, all the plasmatic clotting factors but prothrombin are present in normal amounts. The rate of generation of prothrombinase from this mixture therefore is strictly dependent on the amount of platelet factor 3 added because little prothrombinase forms, and that slowly, if no platelets or substitutes are added. As we perform the test (Bowie *et al.*, 1965b), normal and patient's platelets are carefully harvested, washed, and suspended in buffered saline to a fixed concentration based on light transmittancy. The rate of generation of prothrombinase and the amount generated, from normal serum and absorbed plasma, are measured with the patient's platelets and compared with those with normal platelets. If platelet factor 3 activity is clearly impaired, both sets of platelets are fragmented by ultrasonic vibration for 3 seconds at 0°C and the thromboplastin generation test is repeated to see if platelet factor 3 activity is now demonstrable.

v. *Assay for platelet factor 3.* This has been based on the activation of purified prothrombin by platelet extract and diphenhydramine (Benadryl) (Alkjaersig *et al.,* 1955). The thrombin formed is measured quantitatively by clotting fibrinogen.

With these various tests, several abnormalities of platelet function have been described, including thrombopathy, Glanzmann's thrombasthenia, von Willebrand's disease, Portsmouth syndrome, and changes secondary to ingestion of various drugs.

The task of classifying the qualitative platelet diseases is formidable. The confusion is due to a number of things. In the first place, tests of platelet function have definite limitations. The techniques used for a given test may vary so much from laboratory to laboratory that the test actually may be measuring different functions in different laboratories. Furthermore, the interpretation and clinical significance of these tests are often uncertain.

Whereas at one time it was suggested (Braunsteiner, 1955; Braunsteiner and Pakesch, 1956) that platelet diseases could be divided into two clearcut groups, thrombocytopathy and thrombasthenia, it has become clear that qualitative platelet diseases often are much more complex, and often a number of abnormalities are combined. Thus, any classification based purely on isolated functional disturbances is difficult because there are a number of conditions, both inherited and acquired, in which several functional disturbances coexist. The situation is complicated by the lack of agreement on terminology. For example, the term "thrombopathy" has been used to mean a defect in platelet factor 3 activity (Bowie and Owen, 1968), a defect in platelet aggregation and ADP release (Weiss, 1967), and a defect in clot retraction (Pittman and Graham, 1964).

We think that, although the terms "thrombopathy" and "thrombasthenia" leave much to be desired, it would be best to retain these terms at the present time, using "thrombopathy" to mean abnormalities of platelet factor 3 activity and "thrombasthenia" to mean abnormalities of clot retraction. We would add another subgroup of qualitative platelet diseases, comprising abnormalities of platelet aggregation with normal clot retraction.

It is already clear that all these groups may be heterogeneous and their causes may be related to disorders of platelet membranes, granule membranes, platelet content of nucleotide and phospholipids, release (secretory) reaction, or platelet metabolism. Final classification can come only when further research clarifies the causes of the qualitative platelet disorders and makes an etiologic classification possible.

XVII. THROMBOPATHY (THROMBOCYTOPATHY)

The term "thrombopathy" is a misnomer because it implies a defective clot. Actually it is a shorter form of the term "thrombocytopathy," and we use it to parallel the term "thrombasthenia."

The thrombopathic states are those in which platelet factor 3 activity is abnormal (Bowie and Owen, 1968). In other words, coagulation tests give results consistent with thrombocytopenia but the platelet count is not decreased and even may be significantly increased (McClure *et al.*, 1966). Because standardized measurement of platelet factor 3 activity is difficult, there still is considerable skepticism about the very existence of thrombopathy. Marcus (1969) recently stated that the possibility of a hemorrhagic disorder developing solely on the basis of a primary platelet factor 3 deficiency or abnormality is slight. In our experience, serious bleeding is an uncommon complication of thrombopathy except when the condition is unsuspected and the patient is subjected to surgical or other traumatic procedures. However, in many patients whose only complaint is easy bruising we find a slightly abnormal prothrombin consumption test fully corrected by the addition of a platelet substitute. Such mild bleeders are by no means rare, but they are deserving of a correct diagnosis if an operation is contemplated. In some of these patients, results of other tests of platelet function, such as adhesiveness to glass and aggregation, may be abnormal, but in other patients no other abnormality except decreased procoagulant activity can be demonstrated.

We have divided the simple thrombopathic states into six classes (Table I) based on whether the disease is congenital (primary) (Marcus and Zucker, 1965; Ulutin, 1963, 1965, 1969) or acquired and whether the platelet lacks normal platelet factor 3 activity (deficit thrombopathy) or is simply unable to release it (functional thrombopathy) (Bowie and Owen, 1968; Johnson *et al.*, 1958, Ulutin and Karaca, 1959).

Functional thrombopathy, in its mildest forms, is so common that one perhaps cannot state that it is abnormal. If platelets from men are the reference standard, many platelets from women function less efficiently in the thromboplastin generation test. These women have as their main, and often only, complaint the tendency to develop black and blue spots without known cause. Except from the cosmetic point of view, this mild and common form of thrombopathy is probably unimportant. However, there are congenital and acquired forms of functional thrombopathy in which bleeding may be serious. Functional thrombopathy, like deficit thrombopathy, is characterized by an abnormal prothrombin consumption test which is fully corrected when a platelet substitute is added to the freshly drawn blood and by an abnormality in the thromboplastin generation test when intact platelets are used. It is distinguished from the deficit type by a normal thromboplastin generation test when the patient's platelets are first fragmented; in deficit thrombopathy, fragmented platelets remain ineffective.

It is tempting to attribute functional thrombopathic states to an inability of such platelets to release ADP and to aggregate because Weiss (1967) found such a correlation. This would be supported by the experience that in Glanzmann's disease and von Willebrand's disease the platelet tends to be thrombopathic. On the other hand, we have seen patients in whom there was defective release of platelet factor 3 but all other aspects of platelet function including aggregation were normal.

A. Congenital Deficit Thrombopathy

This diagnosis is warranted when there is a lifelong history of epistaxes, gingival bleeding, ecchymoses, and menorrhagia and the laboratory findings are those of deficit thrombopathy. The congenital nature of the disease is established if others in the family exhibit the same defect. Thrombopathy is diagnosed in our laboratory by two criteria: an abnormal prothrombin consumption test which is clearly corrected by the addition of platelet substitute; and ineffective generation of prothrombinase when the patient's platelets are tested in the thromboplastin generation test. Deficit thrombopathy is suggested when the patient's platelets are still ineffective after they have been disrupted by ultrasonic vibration.

ILLUSTRATIVE CASE: DEFICIT THROMBOPATHY. The patient, a 35-year-old man, had noticed ease of bruising and gingival bleeding since childhood. At age 21 he had hemorrhaged from a duodenal ulcer and was transfused with blood. He had had an episode of hemoptysis for which no cause was found, and at that time a diagnosis of pseudohemophilia was made elsewhere.

Studies of hemostasis were performed at this institution as part of the preparation for surgery for a protruded lumbar disk. The results were: platelet count, 265,000 and 287,000/mm³; bleeding time, Ivy, 3, 4, 4, 3½, 4, and 5 minutes; bleeding time, Duke, 3½ and 3½ minutes; clot retraction, normal; platelet adhesiveness to glass, 98% (normal, >70%); prothrombin consumption test, 20.3 seconds; prothrombin consumption test with Inosithin, 36.2 seconds; platelet thromboplastin generation test, decreased platelet factor 3 (Fig. 1); platelet aggregation with ADP, normal; platelet aggregation with collagen, normal. Whole blood clot time, plasma clot time, prothrombin time, and thrombin time were normal. Factor VIII level was 80%.

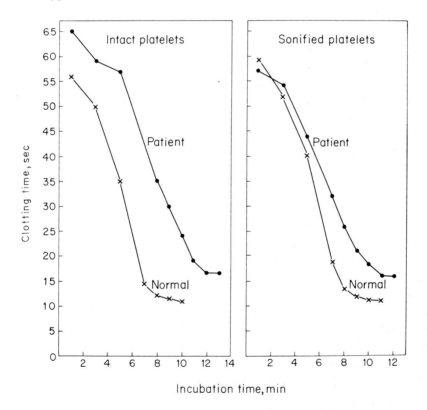

FIG. 1. Deficit thrombopathy. Equal concentrations of platelets from patient and normal subject are compared in thromboplastin generation test consisting of normal adsorbed plasma and normal serum. Patient's platelets cannot support normal thromboplastin generation. Abnormality is not corrected when platelet content of platelet factor 3 is released by destroying platelets with ultrasound, suggesting that patient's platelets have decreased content of platelet factor 3.

B. Acquired Deficit Thrombopathy

Most cases of true deficit thrombopathy are secondary to disease states such as renal failure (Altschuler *et al.*, 1960; Rabiner and Hrodek, 1968), liver disease (Ulutin, 1963, 1969), leukemia, and perhaps scurvy (Çetingil *et al.*, 1958). The clinical and laboratory findings are those of deficit thrombopathy, but there is no history of unusual bleeding before onset of the primary disease. Perhaps the most common form of deficit thrombopathy is that associated with renal failure. The exact agent which injures the platelet is not known, but guanidinosuccinic acid has been implicated (Horowitz *et al.*, 1967). The damage seems to be reversible because it is corrected by dialysis (Stewart and Castaldi, 1967).

C. Congenital Functional Thrombopathy

This is common, often familial, and may affect both sexes in consecutive generations.

D. Acquired Functional Thrombopathy

This is considerably less common than the congenital form. It has been recognized in several conditions characterized by the presence of abnormal plasma proteins which are thought to "coat" the platelet. If such coating rendered the platelet factor 3 phospholipoproteins in the surface ineffective, but not the granular or nonsedimentable ones, it would explain the impaired thromboplastin generation tests with intact platelets but a normal test with disintegrated ones. Whether this explanation is correct or not, these laboratory findings do characterize some patients with macroglobulinemia (Pachter *et al.*, 1959), multiple myeloma, monoclonal gammopathy, Waldenström's hypergammaglobulinemic purpura (Weiss *et al.*, 1963), and, most commonly, systemic lupus erythematosus (Bowie *et al.*, 1963).

The anticoagulants present in the blood of patients with lupus erythematosus have not received adequate attention. In some patients the primary laboratory abnormality is a prolonged prothrombin time which is poorly corrected by the addition of normal plasma. This characterizes coagulation inhibitors but, because the prothrombin time does not depend on the platelet, such an inhibitor must work in the plasmatic coagulation chain and there is evidence that in some cases the anticoagulant inhibits the interaction of activated factor X and factor V (Breckenridge and Ratnoff, 1963). In other patients the plasma clot time is prolonged, the partial thromboplastin time is normal, and the prothrombin consumption of blood is abnormal but is corrected by the addition of a platelet substitute. Both of these abnormalities, in the presence of a normal prothrombin time, clearly link the defect to the platelet. In a third group of patients with lupus, both platelet defect and plasmatic inhibition are evident. All this warrants the assumption that two inhibitors must exist in this disease, but these could equally well be two groups of inhibitors with many subspecies. When the properties of these inhibitors are better defined and clinical correlations are made, systemic lupus may be found to be a spectrum of abnormalities.

ILLUSTRATIVE CASE: FUNCTIONAL THROMBOPATHY WITH NORMAL PLATE-LET AGGREGATION BY COLLAGEN AND ADP. A 54-year-old woman had noted ease of bruising for 2 years. A diagnosis of giant follicular lymphoma had been made elsewhere 1 year previously and she had been treated with cyclophosphamide (Cytoxan) and radiotherapy to the neck. On examination she appeared myxedematous, and ecchymoses were present on her forearms. The hemoglobin concentration was 9.4 gm/100 ml, and a blood smear was suggestive of vitamin B_{12} or folate deficiency. The blood level of vitamin B_{12} was normal (269 pg/ml), and the folate level was low (1.2 ng/ml). The BMR was -10%, and the thyroxine level was decreased to 1.7 μg/100 ml. Other relevant laboratory data were: platelet count, 135,000 and 177,000/mm^3; bleeding time, Ivy, $7\frac{1}{2}$, 8, $9\frac{1}{2}$, 11, 14, and $14\frac{1}{2}$ minutes; bleeding time, Duke, 4 and $4\frac{1}{2}$ minutes; clot retraction, normal; platelet adhesiveness to glass, 96 and 98% (normal, $>70\%$); prothrombin consumption test, 14.8 seconds; prothrombin consumption test with Inosithin, 48.6 seconds; platelet thromboplastin generation test, ineffective release of platelet factor 3; platelet aggregation with ADP, normal; platelet aggregation with collagen, normal. The whole blood clot time, plasma clot time, and thrombin time were normal. Factor VIII level was 80%.

E. Plasmatic Thrombopathy

This type of thrombopathy is uncommon. The prothrombin consumption test is abnormal and is corrected by a partial thromboplastin equivalent to platelet factor 3, suggesting abnormal platelet function. However, the patient's platelets show normal procoagulant activity when tested in the thromboplastin generation test. Neither normal platelets nor the patient's platelets can support normal thromboplastin generation when tested in a thromboplastin generating system consisting of the patient's absorbed plasma and serum. One possible explanation for these findings is that there is an activity in normal plasma necessary for normal platelet function and that this activity is absent from the plasma of these patients (Bowie et al., 1964).

F. Macrothrombocytic Thrombopathy

Morphologic abnormalities have been described in thrombopathies, including an increase in platelet anisocytosis and an increase in intermediate and spread forms when platelets are examined under the electron microscope after being allowed to adhere to a collodion-covered glass slide. In some patients the morphologic abnormalities are striking, with the occurrence of giant forms as big as lymphocytes (Bernard and Soulier, 1948; Hirsch et al., 1950; Kanska et al., 1963; Quick and Hussey, 1963). These platelets may be 4–12 μ in diameter. The platelet count may be decreased or normal (Quick and Hussey, 1963). In some patients with giant platelets there may be a decreased content of platelet factor 3.

XVIII. THROMBASTHENIA

"Weak platelets" (thrombasthenia) is as unsatisfactory a term as "diseased platelets" (thrombopathy) in characterizing a clinical entity. But again, tradition has assigned the name "thrombasthenia" to the disease first described by the Swiss pediatrician, Glanzmann, in 1918. His patients had abnormal clot retraction, but it is interesting to note that several of them had thrombocytopenia. The patients usually have normal platelet counts, a prolonged bleeding time, no or defective clot retraction, and no platelet aggregation by ADP.

A. Clinical Findings

The disease is inherited autosomally and occurs approximately equally in males and females (Friedman et al., 1964). Although dominant inheritance has been suggested (Glanzmann, 1918; Stefanini and Dameshek, 1962), most of the reports suggest a recessive mode of inheritance which is supported by an incidence of consanguinity as high as 10% (Botto, 1950; Braunsteiner and Pakesch, 1956; Caen et al., 1966; Friedman et al., 1964;

Larrieu *et al.*, 1961; Pitman and Graham, 1964). The bleeding tendency is moderately severe and is of the mucous membrane and cutaneous type. The bleeding starts early in life and tends to ameliorate as the patient gets older. There may be severe hemorrhage at operation. One of the patients we have seen may have had hemarthrosis of the knee, and his sister was exsanguinated by a spontaneous gastrointestinal hemorrhage.

B. Laboratory Findings

The bleeding time is abnormal by the Duke and Ivy techniques and there is severely impaired clot retraction; the platelet count is normal. Platelet adhesiveness is decreased. The platelets do not aggregate on the addition of ADP, and aggregating agents that operate through the ADP mechanism also are ineffective. These agents include connective tissue particles, thrombin, norepinephrine, and serotonin (Cronberg *et al.*, 1967; Hardisty *et al.*, 1964; Nachman, 1966; Nachman and Marcus, 1968; Weiss and Kochwa, 1968). The plasma clot time, partial thromboplastin time, prothrombin time, Stypven time, and thrombin time are normal. In the thromboplastin generation test, one of our patients had an abnormal serum reagent. The prothrombin consumption test is abnormal but is corrected on the addition of Inosithin because these patients have abnormal platelet factor 3 release (functional thrombopathy).

On the peripheral blood smear, the platelets are isolated, in contrast to the normal clumped appearance; this may give the first clue to the diagnosis In some patients with thrombasthenia, a deficiency of two enzymes of the glycolytic cycle, pyruvate kinase and glyceraldehyde phosphate dehydrogenase, has been demonstrated in platelets as well as a diminished ATP content (R. Gross *et al.*, 1960). Studies of platelet proteins have produced some interesting and unexpected results. Although the contractile protein of platelets, thrombosthenin, appears to be implicated in clot retraction, it does not appear to be decreased in amount in thrombasthenic platelets (Nachman and Marcus, 1968; Weiss and Kochwa, 1968). On the other hand, platelet fibrinogen content is low; 27% of the fibrinogen is present in the granules in normal platelets, whereas only 10% is present in thrombasthenic platelets (Nachman and Marcus, 1968). Nachman (1966) suggested that the fibrinogen was qualitatively abnormal. No qualitative abnormality was found by Weiss and Kochwa (1968).

It seems quite likely that the primary defect in thrombasthenia lies in the platelet membrane. It has been shown that the protein pattern of thrombasthenic platelets is abnormal and that the constituents of the membrane of thrombasthenic platelets are different from those of the normal platelet (Nachman and Marcus, 1968). The failure of kaolin to produce an increase of thromboplastic activity (Hardisty *et al.*, 1964) also may reflect a membrane abnormality. Although connective tissue does not cause aggregation of thrombasthenic platelets, adherence to connective tissue does occur *in vivo*, and ADP and serotonin are released (Caen *et al.*, 1966; Hardisty *et al.*, 1964; Zucker *et al.*, 1966). Furthermore, thrombin also induces a release reaction. Thrombasthenic platelets, however, are unable to aggregate on exposure to the released ADP. The shape change from disk to spiny sphere occurs normally on exposure to ADP or after chilling (Zucker *et al.*, 1966).

Electron microscope studies have given variable results although increased vacuolation, abnormal granules, and abnormal Golgi vesicules have been described (Caen *et al.*, 1966; Friedman *et al.*, 1964).

C. Treatment

The treatment of these patients remains a matter of controversy. Cronberg and colleagues (1967) were unable to normalize the defect by transfusion of platelet concentrate, fraction 1–0, or fresh exercise-activated plasma. These authors found that cortisone shortened the bleeding time although no effect was found by Caen and associates (1966). A dental extraction was performed in one patient during treatment with EACA. Platelet transfusion in one patient (Hardisty *et al.*, 1964) gave disappointing results in that the infused platelets failed to circulate for more than an hour or two.

It is obvious that further therapeutic studies are needed in these patients but, in the meantime, we concur with Marcus (1969) that these patients should be treated with platelet concentrates or platelet-rich plasma.

XIX. ABNORMALITIES OF PLATELET AGGREGATION

Various drugs, notably aspirin but also chlorpromazine and imipramine (Mills and Roberts, 1967), inhibit release of ADP from platelets and hence inhibit the second wave of aggregation (Doery *et al.*, 1969; G. Evans *et al.*, 1968; Weiss and Aledort, 1967; Weiss *et al.*, 1968). Aspirin has demonstrable effects on normal subjects: ingestion of as little as 1.3 gm of aspirin lengthens the bleeding time (Quick, 1966a,b; Weiss *et al.*, 1968) and inhibits platelet aggregation by epinephrine (O'Brien, 1968a,b) and by collagen (Bowie and Owen, 1969; Zucker and Peterson, 1968) within 2 hours.

Aspirin also prevents release of platelet serotonin and inhibits platelet factor 3 activation (Zucker and Peterson, 1968), perhaps by inhibition of glucose transport across the platelet membrane (Doery *et al.*, 1969). However, the drug does not prevent platelet aggregation by thrombin or serotonin and does not alter adhesiveness of platelets to glass (O'Brien, 1968a).

Aspirin's inhibitory effect on ADP release from platelets can be detected indirectly. Various substances induce only the secondary wave of aggregation (ADP-release phenomenon), including collagen (G. Evans *et al.*, 1968; O'Brien, 1968a; Weiss and Aledort, 1967; Weiss *et al.*, 1968; Zucker and Peterson, 1968), triethyl tin (O'Brien, 1968b), antigen–antibody complexes (G. Evans *et al.*, 1968), and γ-globulin-coated particles (G. Evans *et al.*, 1968). The effect of these substances on platelet is inhibited by aspirin. The aggregation of platelets by thrombin is inhibited by aspirin if the concentration of thrombin is small (G. Evans *et al.*, 1968). Epinephrine, which induces two waves of platelet aggregation (Macmillan, 1966) in the same way that exogenous ADP does, cannot overcome the effect of aspirin (O' Brien, 1968a,b).

The deleterious effect of aspirin on platelets is said to last for virtually the entire life of the platelet (7–10 days) (O'Brien, 1968a,b; Weiss *et al.*, 1968). This suggests that the damage is permanent and normal function is regained only when a new generation of platelets emerges.

In view of the fact that salicylates have been shown to affect dehydrogenases, aminotransferases, and the enzyme systems responsible for oxidative phosphorylation, it has been suggested that aspirin affects some enzyme pathway in the platelet (O'Brien, 1968b) or alters membrane permeability (O'Brien, 1968b; Weiss *et al.*, 1968). It recently has been found (Doery *et al.*, 1969) that aspirin inhibits platelet glycolysis, perhaps as a result of inhibition of glucose transport across the platelet membrane, although it seems that the inhibition of ADP release on exposure to collagen is mediated by a different mechanism. Further evidence of a membrane effect is provided by experiments using ^{14}C-labeled aspirin. When the acetyl group was labeled, platelet radioactivity was detected in the membrane of granule subcellular fractions only; no radioactivity was detectable in the platelet when the carboxyl group of aspirin was labeled (Al-Mondhiry *et al.*, 1969).

It seems unlikely that the doses of aspirin taken by most persons is important hemostatically, although a number of instances of occult and massive gastrointestinal bleeding have been reported when excessive amounts were ingested (Alvarez and Summerskill, 1958; Douthwaite and Lintott, 1938; Holt, 1960). In contrast, even though aspirin's effect is subtle, it may be serious in a patient who already has a hemorrhagic diathesis (Beaumont *et al.*, 1955; Quick, 1966a,b; Zucker and Peterson, 1968). Quick (1966a,b) particularly emphasized the need for avoidance of aspirin by all hemophiliacs.

Inceman (1955) suggested that abnormalities of platelet adhesiveness and aggregation were associated with a bleeding disease. There now have been reported a small number of cases of bleeding tendency with impaired or absent aggregation of platelets by collagen (Caen *et al.*, 1968; Hardisty and Hutton, 1967; Hirsh *et al.*, 1967; O'Brien, 1967; Ulutin and Balkuv, 1967). Since O'Brien's patient was observed in Portsmouth, England, he suggested the term "Portsmouth syndrome." In these cases, the bleeding time was prolonged but the platelet counts were normal. The platelet aggregation was abnormal not only with collagen but also with other agents such as epinephrine or thrombin which cause aggregation by the release of ADP from platelets. The first wave of ADP aggregation was normal but, in some of the patients described, deaggregation was rapid (Hardisty and Hutton, 1967). Platelet adhesiveness to glass was normal in some patients and abnormal in others, being abnormal in most of the patients reported. Weiss (1967) described a group of six women who appear to have a similar type of abnormality. In addition, he demonstrated defective platelet factor 3 availability and defective release of aggregating activity from platelets when they were incubated with kaolin. It seems likely that the basic abnormality is a failure of platelets to release ADP in response to aggregating agents but, although the platelets can aggregate when ADP is added, in many instances deaggregation is rapid. These patients could be considered to have a type of functional thrombopathy.

Because aspirin induces the same phenomenon as seen in Portsmouth syndrome, it is important that collagen aggregation be studied at least 7–10 days after the last ingestion of aspirin. Whether it is aspirin-induced or innate, the collagen-platelet defect probably interferes with the adherence of platelets to subendothelial tissue at the site of vascular injury (Ashford and Freiman, 1967). This could explain prolonged bleeding times and a bleeding tendency in these patients and might also explain the prolonged survival of platelets in subjects taking aspirin (G. Evans *et al.*, 1968). If the adhesiveness of platelets to collagen diminishes with age (Bankowski *et al.*, 1969), a tendency toward Portsmouth syndrome with advanced age might be normal.

It has been suggested that these diseases be called essential idiopathic athrombia and that they be divided into types I, II, and III on the basis of ADP aggregation, collagen aggregation, and Salzman test results (Ulutin, 1969).

Illustrative Case: Absence of Collagen Aggregation

A 28-year-old woman had noted ease of bruising since early childhood and recurrent epistaxes since age 19. Bleeding had been considered excessive

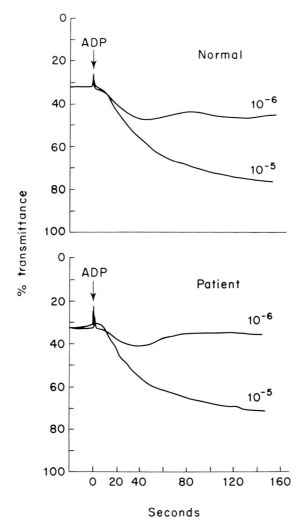

FIG. 2. Abnormal aggregation with ADP. ADP in a variety of final concentrations between 10^{-4} and 10^{-7} M is added to stirred platelet-rich plasma, and light transmission is recorded. Curves for the 10^{-5} and 10^{-6} M concentrations are illustrated. Plasma from normal subject shows two waves of aggregation; plasma from patient failed to show two waves of aggregation at any concentration of ADP but instead showed rapid deaggregation.

after a tonsillectomy, and she had bled for 10 days after the extraction of a third molar. She required four transfusions of blood because of post-partum hemorrhage after her first pregnancy. A large retroperitoneal hematoma developed after a cesarean section in her second pregnancy. Her third pregnancy was complicated by placenta accreta which resulted in massive hemorrhage requiring 14 transfusions of blood and a cesarean hysterectomy. Relevant laboratory data were: platelet count, 328,000 and 366,000/mm³; bleeding time, Ivy, 3½, 3½, and 4 minutes; bleeding time, Duke, 2½ minutes; clot retraction, normal; platelet adhesiveness to glass, 23, 37, and 38% (normal, >70%); prothrombin consumption test, 26.1 and 29.3 seconds (normal, >20 seconds); platelet aggregation with ADP, second wave not demonstrable (Fig. 2); platelet aggregation with collagen, absent (Fig. 3). Whole-blood clot time, plasma clot time, prothrombin time, and thrombin time were normal. The thromboplastin generation test showed the mild serum defect which occurs in normal females. Coagulation factor levels were: VIII, 115%; IX, 100%; XI, 110%; and XII, 50%.

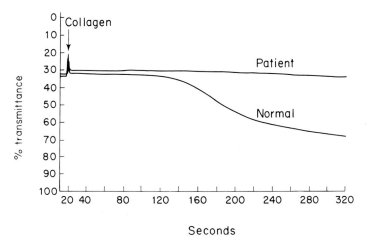

FIG. 3. Absence of platelet aggregation with collagen. Homogenized extract of collagen causes usual delayed single wave of aggregation of platelets from normal subject but no aggregation of platelets from patient.

XX. VON WILLEBRAND'S DISEASE

Shortly after von Willebrand (1926) first described the now-famous familial bleeding tendency among the inbred Åland islanders, he and Jür-gens (1933a) restudied the patients with a "capillary thrombometer."

This test consisted of driving freshly drawn blood back and forth through a temperature-controlled capillary tube. Normally, the tube became obstructed within 4 or 5 minutes but the thrombometer times in the islanders were much longer. The technique has been criticized as being simply a complicated whole-blood clotting time. However, this seems unlikely because the thrombometer times were said to be normal in hemophiliacs (Jürgens, 1937; von Willebrand and Jürgens, 1933b).

von Willebrand and Jürgens attributed the prolonged capillary thrombometer times to a platelet defect and thus seem to have anticipated the modern glass-adhesiveness tests by 30 years. With present-day adhesiveness tests, platelets adhere to glass beads very poorly in von Willebrand's disease (Bowie et al., 1969a; Salzman, 1963). However, there is no evidence that the defect actually resides in the platelet; it equally well could reflect a plasmatic defect. At least one plasmatic defect has been identified in von Willebrand's disease, a deficiency of factor VIII. It does not seem likely that this is responsible for the abnormal platelet adhesiveness because platelet adhesiveness is normal in classic hemophilia.

XXI. COMPOUND PLATELET DISEASES

Deficiencies of plasmatic coagulation factors may occur in association with thrombopathy (Bowie et al., 1965a; Owen and Thompson, 1960; Ulutin, 1963, 1969). Decreased level of factor VIII occurs most commonly, but factor IX deficiency occasionally is found. A combination of functional platelet abnormalities also may occur, such as abnormalities of clot retraction and of platelet factor 3 release. The term "thrombasthenic thrombopathy" or "thrombopathic thrombasthenia" has been proposed for this type of abnormality (Ulutin, 1963). However, it has been shown (Hardisty et al., 1964) that an abnormal release of platelet factor 3 is part of the picture of Glanzmann's thrombasthenia and it seems unnecessary to describe thrombopathic thrombasthenia as a separate disease entity.

The association of qualitative platelet abnormalities and factor VIII deficiency suggests that there may be some relationship to von Willebrand's disease. In one of our families with von Willebrand's disease (Bowie et al., 1967), thrombopathy was demonstrable, so it seems likely that thrombopathy with factor VIII deficiency (thrombopathic hemophilia) is part of the spectrum of von Willebrand's disease.

REFERENCES

Ackroyd, J. F. (194>). *Quart. J. Med.* **18**, 299.

Ackroyd, J. F. (1960). *In* "Lectures on Haematology" (F. G. J. Hayhoe, ed.), pp. 217–247. Cambridge Univ. Press, London and New York.

Aggeler, P. M., Perkins, H. A., and Watkins, H. B. (1967). *Transfusion (Philadelphia)* **7**, 35.

Aldrich, R. A., Steinberg, A. G., and Campbell, D. C. (1954). *Pediatrics* **13**, 133.

Alkjaersig, N., Abe, T., and Seegers, W. H. (1955). *Amer. J. Physiol.* **181**, 304.

Al-Mondhiry, H., Marcus, A., and Spaet, T. H. (1969). *Fed. Proc., Fed. Amer. Soc. Exp. Biol.* **28**, 576 (abstr.).

Altschuler, G., Marcus, A. J., and Ullman, H. L. (1960). *Blood* **16**, 1439.

Alvarez, A. S., and Summerskill, W. H. J. (1958). *Lancet* **2**, 920.

Amris, A., and Amris, C. J. (1964). *Thromb. Diath. Haemorrh.* **11**, 404.

Amundsen, M. A., Spittell, J. A., Jr., Thompson, J. H., Jr., and Owen, C. A., Jr. (1963). *Ann. Intern. Med.* **58**, 608.

Ashford, T. P., and Freiman, D. G. (1967). *Amer. J. Pathol.* **50**, 257.

Aster, R. H. (1964). *Clin. Res.* **12**, 219.

Aster, R. H. (1965). *Trans. Assoc. Amer. Physicians* **78**, 362.

Aster, R. H., and Keene, W. R. (1969). *Brit. J. Haematol.* **16**, 61.

Ata, M., Fisher, O. D., and Holman, C. A. (1965). *Lancet* **1**, 119.

Baehr, G., Klemperer, P., and Schifrin, A. (1936). *Trans. Assoc. Amer. Physicians* **51**, 43.

Baldini, M. (1966). *N. Engl. J. Med.* **274**, 1245, 1301, and 1360.

Baldini, M., Costea, N., and Ebbe, S. (1962). *Proc. 8th Congr. Eur. Soc. Haematol.*, 1961 Part II, p. 378.

Baldini, M., Kuramoto, A., and Steiner, M. (1969). *Blood* **34**, 852 (abstr.).

Bańkowski, E., Niewiarowski, S., and Rogowski, W. (1969). *Thromb. Diath. Haemorrh.* **21**, 441.

Baumgartner, H.-R., Tranzer, J.-P., and Stader, A. (1967). *Thromb. Diath. Haemorrh.* **18**, 592.

Beaumont, J.-L., Willie, A., and Lenègre, J. (1955). *Bull. Soc. Med. Hop. Paris* **2**, 1077.

Bedson, S. P. (1924). *Lancet* **2**, 1117.

Bernard, J., and Soulier, J.-P. (1948). *Sem. Hop.* **24**, 3217.

Bettex–Galland, M., and Lüscher, E. F. (1961). *Biochim. Biophys. Acta* **49**, 536.

Biggs, R., Denson, K. W. E., Reisenberg, D., and McIntyre, C. (1968). *Brit. J. Haematol.* **15**, 283.

Bithell, T. C., Didisheim, P., Cartwright, G. E., and Wintrobe, M. M. (1965). *Blood* **25**, 231.

Blix, S., and Aas, K. (1961). *Acta Med. Scand.* **169**, 63.

Bonnar, J., and Crawford, J. M. (1965). *Lancet* **1**, 241.

Bonnin, J. A. (1961). *Brit. J. Haematol.* **7**, 250.

Borchgrevink, C. F. (1961). *Acta Med. Scand.* **170**, 231.

Born, G. V. R. (1962). *Nature (London)* **194**, 927.

Botto, A. (1950). *Haematol. Lat.* **34**, 171.

Bouroncle, B. A., and Doan, C. A. (1969). *J. Amer. Med. Assoc.* **207**, 2049.

Bowie, E. J. W., and Owen, C. A., Jr. (1968). *Semin. Haematol.* **5**, 73.

Bowie, E. J. W., and Owen, C. A., Jr. (1969). *Circulation* **40**, 757.

Bowie, E. J. W., Thompson, J. H., Jr., Pascuzzi, C. A., and Owen, C. A., Jr. (1963). *J. Lab. Clin. Med.* **62**, 416.

Bowie, E. J. W., Thompson, J. H., Jr., and Owen, C. A., Jr. (1964). *Thromb. Diath. Haemorrh.* **11**, 195.

Bowie, E. J. W., Thompson, J. H., Jr., and Owen, C. A., Jr. (1965a). *Mayo Clin. Proc.* **40**, 625.

Bowie, E. J. W., Thompson, J. H., Jr., and Owen, C. A., Jr. (1965b). *Amer. J. Clin. Pathol.* **44**, 673.

Bowie, E. J. W., Didisheim, P., Thompson, J. H., Jr., and Owen, C. A., Jr. (1967). *Thromb. Diath. Haemorrh.* **18**, 40.

Bowie, E. J. W., Owen, C. A., Jr., Thompson, J. H., Jr., and Didisheim, P. (1969a). *Amer. J. Clin. Pathol.* **52**, 69.

Bowie, E. J. W., Maldonado, J. E., Brown, A. L., Didisheim, P., and Owen, C. A., Jr. (1969b). *Thromb. Diath. Haemorrh.* Suppl. **36**, 305.

Branemårk, P. I., and Ekholm, R. (1968). *Blut* **16**, 274.

Braunsteiner, H. (1955). *Wien. Z. Inn. Med. Ihre Grenzgeb.* **36**, 421.

Braunsteiner, H., and Pakesch, F. (1956). *Blood* **11**, 965.

Breckenridge, R. T., and Ratnoff, O. D. (1963). *Amer. J. Med.* **35**, 813.

Bridges, J. M., Baldini, M., Fichera, C., and Dameshek, W. (1963). *Nature (London)* **197**, 364.

Brittingham, T. E., III, and Chaplin, H., Jr. (1957). *Blood* **12**, 480.

Bull, B. S., Rubenberg, M. L., Dacie, J. V., and Brain, M. C. (1968). *Brit. J. Haematol.* **14**, 643.

Bunting, W. L., Kiely, J. M., and Campbell, D. C. (1961). *Arch. Intern. Med.* **108**, 733.

Caen, J. P., Castaldi, P. A., Leclerc, J. C., Inceman, S., Larrieu, M. J., Probst, M., and Bernard, J. (1966). *Amer. J. Med.* **41**, 4.

Caen, J. P., Sultan, Y., and Larrieu, M. J. (1968). *Lancet* **1**, 203.

Canales, L., and Mauer, A. M. (1967). *N. Engl. J. Med.* **277**, 899.

Carpenter, A. F., Wintrobe, M. M., Fuller, E. A., Haut, A., and Cartwright, G. E. (1959). *J. Amer. Med. Assoc.* **171**, 1911.

Cetingil, A. I., Ulutin, O. N., and Karaca, M. (1958). *Brit. J. Haematol.* **4**, 350.

Christensen, L. K. (1958). *Acta Med. Scand.* **162**, 407.

Cohen, P., and Gardner, F. H. (1961). *N. Engl. J. Med.* **265**, 611.

Cohen, P., Gardner, F. H., and Barnett, G. O. (1961). *N. Engl. J. Med.* **264**, 1294 and 1350.

Colman, R. W., Sievers, C. A., and Pugh, R. P. (1966). *J. Lab. Clin. Med.* **68**, 389.

Conley, C. L., Hartmann, R. C., and Lalley, J. S. (1948). *Proc. Soc. Exp. Biol. Med.* **69**, 284.

Cooper, T., Stickney, J. M., Pease, G. L., and Bennett, W. A. (1952). *Amer. J. Med.* **13**, 374.

Corn, M., and Upshaw, J. D., Jr. (1962). *Arch. Intern. Med.* **109**, 157.

Croizat, P., and Favre–Gilly, J. (1949). *Sang* **20**, 417.

Cronberg, S., Nilsson, I. M., and Zetterqvist, E. (1967). *Acta Paediat. Scand.* **56**, 189.

Cullum, C., Cooney, D. P., and Schrier, S. L. (1967). *Brit. J. Haematol.* **13**, 147.

Dameshek, W. (1960). *J. Amer. Med. Assoc.* **173**, 1025.

Dameshek, W. (1965). *Ser. Haematol.* **9**, 61.

Dameshek, W., and Estren, S. (1947). "The Spleen and Hypersplenism." Grune & Stratton, New York.

Dameshek, W., and Reeves, W. H. (1956). *Amer. J. Med.* **21**, 560.

Dameshek, W., and Schwartz, R. (1960). *Trans. Assoc. Amer. Physicians* **73**, 113.

Dameshek, W., Rubio, F., Jr., Mahoney, J. P., Reeves, W. H., and Burgin, L. A. (1958). *J. Amer. Med. Assoc.* **166**, 1805.

Dameshek, W., Ebbe, S., Greenberg, L., and Baldini, M. (1963). *N. Engl. J. Med.* **269**, 647.

Dawson, J. P. (1955). *Pediatrics* **15**, 325.

Delhaes, M. F. M., Van Dam, F. E., and Haanen, C. (1966). *Folia Med. Neer.* **9**, 131.

Denis, L. H., Stewart, J. L., and Conrad, M. E. (1967). *Lancet* **1**, 1088.

Deutsch, E., Johnson, S. A., and Seegers, W. H. (1955). *Circ. Res.* **3**, 110.

Didisheim, P., and Bunting, D. (1966). *Amer. J. Clin. Pathol.* **45**, 566.

Didisheim, P., Bowie, E. J. W., and Owen, C. A., Jr. (1969). *Thromb. Diath. Haemorrh.* Suppl. **36**, 215.

Diggs, L. W., and Hewlett, J. S. (1948). *Blood* **3**, 1090.

Doan, C. A., Bouroncle, B. A., and Wiseman, B. K. (1960). *Ann. Intern. Med.* **53**, 861.

Doery, J. C. G., Hirsh, J., and de Gruchy, G. C. (1969). *Science* **165**, 65.

Douthwaite, A. H., and Lintott, G. A. M. (1938). *Lancet* **2**, 1222.

Ebbe, S., Wittels, B., and Dameshek, W. (1962). *Blood* **19**, 23.

Epstein, R. D., Lozner, E. L., Cobbey, T. S., Jr., and Davidson, C. S. (1950). *Amer. J. Med.* **9**, 44.

Erickson, W. D., Burgert, E. O., and Lynn, H. B. (1968). *Amer. J. Dis. Child.* **116**, 1.

Evans, G., Packham, M. A., Nishizawa, E. E., Mustard, J. F., and Murphy, E. A. (1968). *J. Exp. Med.* **128**, 877.

Evans, R. S., and Duane, R. T. (1949). *Blood* **4**, 1196.

Fanconi, G. (1927). *Jahrb. Kinderheilk.* **117**, 257.

Fine, N. L., Applebaum, J., Elguezabal, A., and Castleman, L. (1967). *Arch. Intern. Med.* **119**, 522.

Fisher, J. A. (1947). *Quart. J. Med.* **16**, 245.

Frank, E. (1915). *Berlin. Klin. Wochenschr.* **52**, 454.

Freireich, E. J., Kliman, A., Gaydos, L. A., Mantel, N., and Frei, E., III. (1963). *Ann. Intern. Med.* **59**, 277.

French, J. E., Macfarlane, R. G., and Sanders, A. G. (1964). *Brit. J. Exp. Pathol.* **45**, 467.

Friedman, L. L., Bowie, E. J. W., Thompson, J. H., Jr., Brown, A. L., Jr., and Owen, C.A., Jr. (1964). *Mayo Clin. Proc.* **39**, 908.

Gaarder, A., Jonson, J., Laland, S., Hellem, A., and Owren, P. A. (1961). *Nature (London)* **192**, 531.

Ghitis, J., and Bonelli, V. (1963). *Ann. Intern. Med.* **59**, 737.

Gigon, J.-P., Thölen, H., Schmutzler, R., Scheidigger, S., Stamm, H., and Koller, F. (1964). *Deut. Med. Wochenschr.* **89**, 1881.

Glanzmann, E. (1918). *Jahrb. Kinderheilk.* **88**, 1.

Gollub, S., Ulin, A., Paxon, N. F., Winchell, H. S., O'Riordan, J., Back, N., and Ambrus, J. L. (1959). *J. Lab. Clin. Med.* **53**, 765.

Gross, P., and Benz, E. J. (1947). *Surg. Gynecol. Obstet.* **85**, 315.

Gross, R., Gerok, W., Löhr, G. W., Vogell, W., Waller, H. D., and Theopold, W. (1960). *Klin. Wochenschr.* **38**, 193.

Gröttum, K. A., and Solum, N. O. (1969). *Brit. J. Haematol.* **16**, 277.

Gunz, F. W. (1960). *Blood* **15**, 706.

Hagedorn, A. B., Thompson, J. H., Jr., Bowie, E. J. W., and Owen, C. A., Jr. (1969). *Thromb. Diath. Haemorrh.* Suppl. **36**, 233.

Hammond, J. D. S., and Verel, D. (1959). *Brit. J. Haematol.* **5**, 431.

Hardaway, R. M., Watson, H. E., and Weiss, F. H. (1960). *Arch. Surg.* (*Chicago*) **81**, 983.

Hardisty, R. M. (1968). *In* "Experimental Biology and Medicine: Platelets in Haemostasis" (E. Hagen, W. Wechsler, and F. Zilliken, eds.), Vol. 3, pp. 189–192. Karger, Basel.

Hardisty, R. M., and Hutton, R. A. (1967). *Lancet* **1**, 983.

Hardisty, R. M., Dormandy, K. M., and Hutton, R. A. (1964). *Brit. J. Haematol.* **10**, 371.

Harrington, W. J., Minnich, V., Hollingsworth, J. W., and Moore, C. V. (1951). *J. Lab. Clin. Med.* **38**, 1.

Harrington, W. J., Sprague, C. C., Minnich, V., Moore, C. V., Aulvin, R. C., and Dubach, R. (1953). *Ann. Intern. Med.* **38**, 433.

Harrington, W. J., Minnich, V., and Arimura, G. (1956). *Progr. Hematol.* **1**, 166.

Hellem, A. J. (1960). *Scand. J. Clin. Lab. Invest.* **12**, Suppl. 51, 1.

Heyn, R. M., Ertel, I. J., and Tubergen, D. G. (1969). *J. Amer. Med. Assoc.* **208**, 1372.

Hilgartner, M. W., Horowitz, H., Erlandson, M., Ferguson, A., and Smith, C. H. (1961). *Amer. J. Dis. Child.* **102**, 591 (abstr.).

Hill, J. B., and Cooper, W. M. (1968). *Arch. Intern. Med.* **122**, 353.

Hirsch, E. O., and Dameshek, W. (1951). *Arch. Intern. Med.* **88**, 701.

Hirsch, E. O., Favre–Gilly, J., and Dameshek, W. (1950). *Blood* **5**, 568.

Hirsh, J., Castellan, D. J., and Bronwen Loder, P. (1967). *Lancet* **2**, 18.

Hjort, P. F., and Rapaport, S. I. (1965). *Annu. Rev. Med.* **16**, 135.

Hjort, P., Rapaport, S. I., and Owren, P. A. (1955). *Blood* **10**, 1139.

Hollard, D., and Kolodié, L. (1968). *Nouv. Rev. Fr. Hematol.* **8**, 131.

Holt, P. R. (1960). *J. Lab. Clin. Med.* **56**, 717.

Horowitz, H. I., and Papayoanou, M. F. (1967). *J. Lab. Clin. Med.* **69**, 1003.

Horowitz, H. I., Des Prez, R. M., and Hook, E. W. (1962). *Blood* **20**, 760.

Horowitz, H. I., Cohen, B. D., Martinez, P., and Papayoanou, M. F. (1967). *Blood* **30**, 331.

Hovig, T. (1963). *Thromb. Diath. Haemorrh.* **9**, 264.

Hovig, T. (1964). *Thromb. Diath. Haemorrh.* **12**, 179.

Husom, O. (1961). *Scand. J. Clin. Lab. Invest.* **13**, 609.

Iatridis, P. G., and Ferguson, J. H. (1965). *Thromb. Diath. Haemorrh.* **13**, 114.

Inceman, S. (1955). *Sang* **26**, 190.

Innes, D., and Sevitt, S. (1964). *J. Clin. Pathol.* **17**, 1.

Jackson, D. P., Schmid, H. J., Zieve, P. D., Levin, J., and Conley, C. L. (1963). *J. Clin. Invest.* **42**, 383.

Johansson, S.-A. (1964). *Acta Med. Scand.* **175**, 177.

Johnson, S. A., and Schneider, C. L. (1953). *Science* **117**, 229.

Johnson, S. A., Caldwell, M. J., and Monto, R. W. (1957). *Thromb. Diath. Haemorrh.* **1**, 433.

Johnson, S. A., Monto, R. W., and Caldwell, M. J. (1958). *Thromb. Diath. Haemorrh.* **2**, 279.

Johnson, S. A., Wojcik, J. D., Webber, A. J., and Yun, J. (1969). *In* "Dynamics of Thrombus Formation and Dissolution" (S. A. Johnson and M. M. Guest, eds.), pp. 72–94. Lippincott, Philadelphia, Pennsylvania.

Jürgens, R. (1937). *Ergeb. Inn. Med. Kinderheilk.* **53**, 795.

Kańska, B., Niewiarowski, S., Ostrowski, L., Poplawski, A., and Prokopowicz, J. (1963). *Thromb. Diath. Haemorrh.* **10**, 88.

Karpatkin, S., and Siskind, G. W. (1969). *Clin. Res.* **17**, 330 (abstr.).

Kazmier, F. J., Didisheim, P., Fairbanks, V. F., Ludwig, J., Payne, W. S., and Bowie, E. J. W. (1969). *Thromb. Diath. Haemorrh.* Suppl. 36, 295.

Kaznelson, P. (1916). *Wien. Klin. Wochenschr.* **29**, 1451.

Kowalski, E., Budzyński, A. Z., Kopeć, M., Latallo, Z. S., Lipiński, B., and Wegrzynowicz, Z. (1965). *Thromb. Diath. Haemorrh.* **13**, 12.

Krevans, J. R., Jackson, D. P., Conley, C. L., and Hartmann, R. C. (1957). *Blood* **12**, 834.

Krivit, W., and Good, R. A. (1959). *Amer. J. Dis. Child.* **97**, 137.

Krivit, W., Yunis, E., and White, J. G. (1966). *Pediatrics* **37**, 339.

Kurstjens, R., Bolt, C., Vossen, M., and Haanen, C. (1968). *Brit. J. Haematol.* **15**, 305.

Larrieu, M.-J., Caen, J., Lelong, J.-C., and Bernard, J. (1961). *Nouv. Rev. Fr. Hematol.* **1**, 662.

Lasch, H. G., Krecke, H.-J., Rodriguez–Erdmann, F., Sessner, H. H., and Schütterle, G. (1961). *Folia Haematol. (Leipzig)* **6**, 325.

Lasch, H. G., Róka, L., and Heene, D. (1966). *Thromb. Diath. Haemorrh.* Suppl. 20, 97.

Ledingham, J. C. C., and Bedson, S. P. (1915). *Lancet* **1**, 311.

Lee, P.-H., Johnson, S. A., and Seegers, W. H. (1957). *Thromb. Diath. Haemorrh.* **1**, 16.

Lerner, R. G., Rapaport, S. I., and Meltzer, J. (1967). *Ann. Intern. Med.* **66**, 1180.

Linman, J. W. (1966). "Principles of Hematology." Macmillan, New York.

Loewy, F. E. (1934). *Lancet* **1**, 845.

McClure, P. D., Ingram, G. I. C., Stacey, R. S., Glass, U. H., and Matchett, M. O. (1966). *Brit. J. Haematol.* **12**, 478.

McKay, D. G. (1965). "Disseminated Intravascular Coagulation: An Intermediary Mechanism of Disease." Harper (Hoeber), New York.

McKay, G. F., Pisciotta, A. V., and Johnson, S. A. (1962). *Amer. J. Clin. Pathol.* **38**, 357.

McKenna, J. I., and Pisciotta, A. V. (1962). *Blood* **19**, 664.

Macmillan, D. C. (1966). *Nature (London)* **211**, 140.

Marcus, A. J. (1966). *Advan. Lipid Res.* **4**, 1.

Marcus, A. J. (1969). *N. Engl. J. Med.* **280**, 1213, 1278, and 1330.

Marcus, A. J., and Spaet, T. H. (1958). *J. Clin. Invest.* **37**, 1836.

Marcus, A. J., and Zucker, M. B. (1965). "The Physiology of Blood Platelets." Grune & Stratton, New York.

Marcus, A. J., Ullman, H. L., Safier, L. B., and Ballard, H. S. (1962). *J. Clin. Invest.* **41**, 2198.

Marcus, A. J., Zucker–Franklin, D., Safier, L. B., and Ullman, H. L. (1966). *J. Clin. Invest.* **45**, 14.

Marcus, A. J., Ullman, H. L., and Safier, L. B. (1969). *J. Lipid Res.* **10**, 108.

Meyers, M. C. (1961). *Amer. J. Med. Sci.* **242**, 295.

Mills, D. C., and Roberts, G. C. (1967). *Nature (London)* **213**, 35.

Mills, D. C. B., Robb, I. A., and Roberts, G. C. K. (1968). *J. Physiol. (London)* **195**, 715.

Moschcowitz, E. (1925). *Arch. Intern. Med.* **36**, 89.

Murphy, S., Oski, F. A., and Gardner, F. H. (1969a). *N. Engl. J. Med.* **281**, 857.

Murphy, S., Oski, F. A., and Gardner, F. H. (1969b). *Blood* **34**, 853 (abstr.).

Mustard, J. F., and Packham, M. A. (1968). *Plen. Sess. Pap., 12th Congr. Int. Soc. Hematol.*, 1968, pp. 306–314.

Mustard, J. F., Glynn, M. F., Hovig, T., Jorgenson, L., Packham, M. A., Nishizawa, E., and Rowsell, H. C. (1967). *In* "Physiology of Hemostasis and Thrombosis" (S. A. Johnson and W. H. Seegers, eds.), pp. 288–326. Thomas, Springfield, Illinois.

Nachman, R. L. (1966). *J. Lab. Clin. Med.* **67**, 411.

Nachman, R. L., and Engle, R. L. (1963). *Blood* **22**, 828 (abstr.).

Nachman, R. L., and Marcus, A. J. (1968). *Brit. J. Haematol.* **15**, 181.

Nachman, R. L., Marcus, A. J., and Safier, L. B. (1967a). *J. Clin. Invest.* **46**, 1380.

Nachman, R. L., Marcus, A. J., and Zucker–Franklin, D. (1967b). *J. Lab. Clin. Med.* **69**, 651.

Niewiarowski, S., Bańkowski, E., and Rogowicka, I. (1965). *Thromb. Diath. Haemorrh.* **14**, 387.

Nilsson, I. M., Skanse, B., and Gydell, K. (1957). *Acta Med. Scand.* **159**, 463.

O'Brien, J. R. (1962). *J. Clin. Pathol.* **15**, 452.

O'Brien, J. R. (1963). *Nature (London)* **200**, 763.

O'Brien, J. R. (1967). *Lancet* **2**, 258.

O'Brien, J. R. (1968a). *Lancet* **1**, 204.

O'Brien, J. R. (1968b). *Lancet* **1**, 779.

Oski, F. A., Naiman, J. L., Allen, D. M., and Diamond, L. K. (1962). *Blood* **20**, 657.

Oski, F. A., Naiman, J. L., and Diamond, L. K. (1963). *N. Engl. J. Med.* **268**, 1423.

Owen, C. A., Jr., and Thompson, J. H., Jr. (1960). *Amer. J. Clin. Pathol.* **33**, 197.

Owen, C. A., Jr., Bowie, E. J. W., Didisheim, P., and Thompson, J. H., Jr. (1969a). "The Diagnosis of Bleeding Disorders." Little, Brown, Boston, Massachusetts.

Owen, C. A., Jr., Oels, H. C., Bowie, E. J. W., Didisheim, P., and Thompson, J. H., Jr. (1969b). *Thromb. Diath. Haemorrh.* Suppl. **36**, 197.

Ozer, F. L., Traux, W. E., Miesch, D. C., and Levin, W. C. (1960). *Amer. J. Med.* **28**, 807.

Pachter, M. R., Johnson, S. A., Neblett, T. R., and Truant, J. P. (1959). *Amer. J. Clin. Pathol.* **31**, 467.

Pascuzzi, C. A., Spittell, J. A., Jr., Thompson, J. H., Jr., and Owen, C. A., Jr. (1961). *J. Clin. Invest.* **40**, 1006.

Pearson, H. A., Shulman, N. R., Marder, V. J., and Cone, T. E., Jr. (1964). *Blood* **23**, 154.

Penny, R., Rozenberg, M. C., and Firkin, B. G. (1966). *Blood* **27**, 1.

Pepper, H., Liebowitz, D., and Lindsay, S. (1956). *A.M.A. Arch. Pathol.* **61**, 1.

Peshkin, M. M., and Miller, J. A. (1934). *J. Amer. Med. Assoc.* **102**, 1737.

Pisciotta, A. V., Stefanini, M., and Dameshek, W. (1953). *Blood* **8**, 703.

Pittman, M. A., Jr., and Graham, J. B. (1964). *Amer. J. Med. Sci.* **247**, 293.

Pritchard, J. A., and Ratnoff, O. D. (1955). *Surg., Gynecol. Obstet.* **101**, 467.

Quick, A. J. (1966a). *Amer. J. Med. Sci.* **252**, 265.

Quick, A. J. (1966b). *Fed. Proc., Fed. Amer. Soc. Exp. Biol.* **25**, 498 (abstr.).

Quick, A. J., and Geppert, M. (1963). *Thromb. Diath. Haemorrh.* **9**, 113.

Quick, A. J., and Hussey, C. V. (1963). *Amer. J. Med. Sci.* **245**, 643.

Rabiner, S. F., and Hrodek, O. (1968). *J. Clin. Invest.* **47**, 901.

Rabinowitz, Y., and Dameshek, W. (1960). *Ann. Intern. Med.* **52**, 1.

Rapaport, S. I., and Chapman, C. G. (1959). *Amer. J. Med.* **27**, 144.

Ratnoff, O. D., Pritchard, J. A., and Colopy, J. E. (1955). *N. Engl. J. Med.* **253**, 63.

Rebuck, J. W., Riddle, J. M., Brown, M. G., Johnson, S. A., and Monto, R. W. (1961). *In* "Blood Platelets" (S. A. Johnson *et al.*, eds.), pp. 533–552. Little, Brown, Boston, Massachusetts.

Redleaf, P. D., Davis, R. B., Kucinski, C., Hoilund, L., and Gans, H. (1963). *Ann. Intern. Med.* **58**, 347.

Reid, H. A., Chan, K. E., and Thean, P. C. (1963). *Lancet* **1**, 621.

Risak, E. (1935). *Z. Klin. Med.* **128**, 605.

Robson, H. N. (1949). *Quart. J. Med.* **18**, 279.

Robson, H. N., and Davidson, L. S. P. (1950). *Lancet* **2**, 164.

Robson, H. N., and Duthie, J. J. R. (1950). *Brit. Med. J.* **2**, 971.

Rolovic, Z., Baldini, M., and Dameshek, W. (1966). *Fed. Proc., Fed. Amer. Soc. Exp. Biol.* **25**, 703 (abstr.).

Rubenberg, M. L., Regoeczi, E., Bull, B. S., Davie, J. V., and Brain, M. C. (1968). *Brit. J. Haematol.* **14**, 627.

Saidi, P., Wallerstein, R. O., and Aggeler, P. (1961). *J. Lab. Clin. Med.* **57**, 247.

Salmon, J., Verstraete, M., and Bounameaux, Y. (1957). *Arch. Intern. Physiol.* **65**, 632.

Salzman, E. W. (1963). *J. Lab. Clin. Med.* **62**, 724.

Schaar, F. E. (1963). *J. Pediat.* **62**, 546.

Schneider, C. L. (1951). *Surg., Gynecol. Obstet.* **92**, 27.

Schulman, I., Pierce, M., Lukens, A., and Currimbhoy, Z. (1960). *Blood* **16**, 943.

Seegers, W. H. (1961). *In* "Blood Platelets" (S. A. Johnson *et al.*, eds.), pp. 241–251. Little, Brown, Boston, Massachusetts.

Seegers, W. H. (1962). "Prothrombin," pp. 145–185. Harvard Univ. Press, Cambridge, Massachusetts.

Seip, M. (1963). *Acta Paediat. Scand.* **52**, 370.

Seip, M., and Kjaerheim, Å. (1965). *Scand. J. Clin. Lab. Invest.* **17**, Suppl. 84, 159.

Shahidi, N. T., and Diamond, L. K. (1959). *Amer. J. Dis. Child.* **98**, 293.

Shaw, S., and Oliver, R. A. M. (1959). *Blood* **14**, 374.

Shulman, N. R. (1963). *Trans. Assoc. Amer. Physicians* **76**, 72.

Shulman, N. R., Aster, R. H., Leitner, A., and Hiller, M. C. (1961). *J. Clin. Invest.* **40**, 1597.

Shulman, N. R., Marder, V. J., Hiller, M. C., and Collier, E. M. (1964). *Progr. Hematol.* **4**, 222.

Shulman, N. R., Marder, V. J., and Weinrach, R. S. (1965a). *Ann. N. Y. Acad. Sci.* **124**, 499.

Shulman, N. R., Weinrach, R. S., Libre, E. P., and Andrews, H. L. (1965b). *Trans. Assoc. Amer. Physicians* **78**, 374.

Silverstein, M. N. (1968). *Arch. Intern. Med.* **122**, 18.

Singer, K., Bornstein, F. P., and Wile, S. A. (1947). *Blood* **2**, 542.

Sixma, J. J., and Nijessen, J. G. Unpublished data.

Smith, C. H., Erlandson, M., Schulman, I., and Stern, G. (1957). *Amer. J. Med.* **22**, 390.

Soardi, F. (1959). *Haematologica* **44**, 789.

Soulier, J. P. (1958). *Nouv. Rev. Fr. Hematol.* **13**, 437.

Soulier, J. P., Petit, P., and LeBolloch, A. G. (1952). *Rev. Hematol.* **7**, 48.

Spaet, T. H. (1957). *J. Appl. Physiol.* **11**, 119.

Spaet, T. H., and Cintron, J. (1964). *Thromb. Diath. Haemorrh.* Suppl. **13**, 335.

Spaet, T. H., and Cintron, J. (1965). *Brit. J. Haematol.* **11**, 269.

Spaet, T. H., and Zucker, M. B. (1964). *Amer. J. Physiol.* **206**, 1267.

Spaet, T. H., Lejnieks, I., Gaynor, E., and Golstein, M. L. (1969). *Arch. Intern. Med.* **124**, 135.

Spittell, J. A., Jr., Pascuzzi, C. A., Thompson, J. H., Jr., and Owen, C. A., Jr. (1960). *Proc. Staff Meet. Mayo Clin.* **35**, 37.

Stefanini, M., and Chatterjea, J. B. (1952). *Proc. Soc. Exp. Biol. Med.* **79**, 623.

Stefanini, M., and Dameshek, W. (1962). "The Hemorrhagic Disorders: A Clinical and Therapeutic Approach," 2nd ed., Grune & Stratton, New York.

Stefanini, M., Plitman, G. I., Dameshek, W., Chatterjea, J. B., and Mednicoff, I. B. (1953). *J. Lab. Clin. Med.* **42**, 723.

Steinkamp, R., Moore, C. V., and Doubek, W. G. (1955). *J. Lab. Clin. Med.* **45**, 18.

Stewart, J. H., and Castaldi, P. A. (1967). *Quart. J. Med.* **36**, 409.

Takeda, Y. (1966). *J. Clin. Invest.* **45**, 103.

Tocantins, L. M. (1936). *A.M.A. Arch. Pathol.* **21**, 69.

Tranzer, J. P., and Baumgartner, H. R. (1967). *Nature (London)* **216**, 1126.

Trinkner, R. L., and Perkins, H. A. (1964). *J. Amer. Med. Assoc.* **189**, 158.

Tullis, J. L. (1962). *J. Amer. Med. Assoc.* **180**, 958.

Tytgat, G. N., Collen, D. J., and de Vreker, R. A. (1968). *Nouv. Rev. Fr. Hematol.* **8**, 123.

Ulin, A. W., and Gollub, S. S. (1966). "Surgical Bleeding: Handbook for Medicine, Surgery and Specialties." McGraw-Hill (Blakiston), New York.

Ulutin, O. N. (1963). *Turk. J. Pediat.* **5**, 237.

Ulutin, O. N. (1965). *Isr. J. Med. Sci.* **1**, 857.

Ulutin, O. N. (1969). *Proc. 5th Congr. Asian Pac. Soc. Hematol.*, 1969.

Ulutin, O. N., and Balkuv, S. (1967). *Lancet* **2**, 421.

Ulutin, O. N., and Karaca, M. (1959). *Brit. J. Haematol.* **5**, 302.

Upshaw, J. D. (1967). *3rd Conf. Blood Platelets*, 1967 Comment.

Van Creveld, S., and Paulssen, M. M. P. (1952). *Lancet* **1**, 23.

Vazquez, J. J., and Lewis, J. H. (1960). *Blood* **16**, 968.

Vestermark, B., and Vestermark, S. (1964). *Acta Paediat. Scand.* **53**, 365.

von Willebrand, E. A. (1926). *Finska Lakaresallsk. Handl.* **68**, 87.

von Willebrand, E. A., and Jürgens, R. (1933a). *Klin. Wochenschr.* **12**, 414.

von Willebrand, E. A., and Jürgens, R. (1933b). *Deut. Arch. Klin. Med.* **175**, 453.

Ward, H. P. (1966). *J. Lab. Clin. Med.* **68**, 400.

Ware, A. G., Fahey, J. L., and Seegers, W. H. (1948). *Amer. J. Physiol.* **154**, 140.

Warner, E. D., and Owen, C. A., Jr. (1942). *Amer. J. Med. Sci.* **203**, 187.

Weiss, H. J. (1967). *Amer. J. Med.* **43**, 570.

Weiss, H. J., and Aledort, L. M. (1967). *Lancet* **2**, 495.

Weiss, H. J., and Kochwa, S. (1968). *J. Lab. Clin. Med.* **71**, 153.

Weiss, H. J., Demis, D. J., Eegart, M. L., Brown, C. S., and Crosby, W. H. (1963). *N. Engl. J. Med.* **268**, 753.

Weiss, H. J., Aledort, L. M., and Kochwa, S. (1968). *J. Clin. Invest.* **47**, 2169.

Whitaker, A. N. (1967). *Fed. Proc., Fed. Amer. Soc. Exp. Biol.* **26**, 319 (abstr.).

White, J. G. (1965). *Thromb. Diath. Haemorrh.* **13**, 573 (abstr.).

Wilner, G. D., Nossel, H. L., and LeRoy, E. C. (1968a). *J. Clin. Invest.* **47**, 2608.

Wilner, G. D., Nossel, H. L., and LeRoy, E. C. (1968b). *J. Clin. Invest.* **47**, 2616.

Wiseman, B. K., Doan, C. A., and Wilson, S. J. (1940). *J. Amer. Med. Assoc.* **115**, 8.

Woolley, E. J. S. (1956). *Brit. Med. J.* **1**, 440.

Wright, H. P. (1941). *J. Pathol. Bacteriol.* **53**, 255.

Yankee, R. A., Grumet, F. C., and Rogentine, G. N. (1969). *N. Engl. J. Med.* **281**, 1208.

Zucker, M. B., and Peterson, J. (1968). *Proc. Soc. Exp. Biol. Med.* **127**, 547.

Zucker, M. B., Pert, J. H., and Hilgartner, M. W. (1966). *Blood* **28**, 524.

16

TRANSFUSION AND PRESERVATION

SEYMOUR PERRY and RONALD A. YANKEE

I. HISTORICAL REVIEW

Thrombocytopenia is one of the most common causes of abnormal bleeding and although the usefulness of replacement therapy was suggested years ago, it is only relatively recently that the value of platelet transfusions has been widely accepted. The role of platelets in coagulation was hypothesized during the last century (Bizzozero, 1882; Hayem, 1882) but Duke was the first to describe (1910) the relationship between thrombocytopenia and bleeding in a paper reporting three cases of bleeding associated with low platelet counts which responded to transfusions of fresh whole blood. Cessation of bleeding appeared to be related to increased platelet levels and the tendency to bleed resumed when the platelet counts fell. Duke confirmed this clinical impression by demonstrating in dogs rendered thrombocytopenic with benzol, that there was a relationship between low platelet counts and serious hemorrhage.

However, nearly half a century elapsed before the effectiveness of platelet replacement in thrombocytopenic hemorrhage was clearly demonstrated. Dillard *et al.* (1951) devised a procedure for separating and concentrating platelets from whole blood and showed that these could prevent bleeding in heavily irradiated dogs. The same group subsequently reported that thrombocytopenia could explain the defects in hemostasis in irradiated animals and that these defects were corrected by platelets both *in vivo* and *in vitro* (Cronkite *et al.*, 1952).

Since platelets contain potent thromboplastic materials (Alkjaersig *et al.*, 1955) and hemostasis of short duration can be achieved without intact platelets (Klein *et al.*, 1956a), attempts were made to utilize platelet extracts or platelet substitutes clinically (Klein *et al.*, 1956b; Djerassi *et al.*, 1962). However, this approach has not been particularly encouraging and has been abandoned. Animal studies (Jackson *et al.*, 1959) showed that lyophilized platelets, although improving prothrombin consumption, were of little value in correcting thrombocytopenic bleeding compared to fresh intact platelets. Firkin *et al.* (1960) demonstrated that lyophilized platelets, brain phospholipid extract, and soya bean extract failed to correct bleeding in thrombocytopenic rats and mice.

The use of platelet transfusions was given great impetus by several developments including the recognition of the importance of thrombocytopenic hemorrhage in acute leukemia and in whole-body irradiation, and the design of appropriate nontoxic containers for platelet collection. Hemorrhage, predominantly due to decreased circulating platelets, occurs at some time during the course of disease in approximately 75% of patients with untreated acute leukemia and in 30% of patients with chronic leukemia (Kirshbaum and Preuss, 1943). In addition, thrombocytopenia is the usual accompaniment of the modern treatment of acute leukemia and is frequently a limiting factor. There is a rough relationship between the height of the platelet count and the incidence of hemorrhage. Serious hemorrhage, such as melena, hematuria, and hematemesis, is infrequent in patients with platelet counts above 20,000–50,000/mm^3 (Freeman and Hyde, 1952; Freireich, 1966; Gaydos *et al.*, 1962). Gross hemorrhage occurred on 30% of hospital days of patients with acute leukemia when the platelet count was below 1000/mm^3 but on less than 1% of the days when the count was 20,000–50,000/mm^3. However, patients with counts as low as 10,000/mm^3 may be free of symptoms so that the absence of bleeding does not exclude severe thrombocytopenia. Previous to the use of platelets, hemorrhage was the cause of or a major factor in the death of patients of acute leukemia with an incidence as high as approximately 70% (Hersh *et al.*, 1965; Boggs *et al.*, 1962; Southam *et al.*, 1951). Although other abnormalities in the hemostatic mechanism also occur in patients with acute leukemia (Perry, 1957; Snyder *et al.*, 1967; Dameshek and Gunz, 1964) their incidence is relatively low compared to the incidence of quantitative platelet deficiencies.

At about the same time that the role of thrombocytopenia in the hemorrhagic diathesis of acute leukemia was being elucidated, its importance in bleeding associated with whole-body exposure to ionizing radiation was being reported (Cronkite *et al.*, 1952; Woods *et al.*, 1953). This was emphasized with the observation of purpuric bleeding in the Japanese population exposed to the atomic bomb explosions in World War II (Leroy, 1950).

Following the recognition that bleeding due to thrombocytopenia could be prevented or controlled with platelet replacement transfusions, widespread application of this procedure did not occur due to practical problems in the procurement of large quantities of platelets. With the appearance of silicone coated and plastic containers (Gardner *et al.*, 1954; Klein *et al.*, 1956c; Kissmeyer-Nielsen and Madsen, 1961b), it became possible to develop programs to improve platelet collection techniques and to provide platelet replacement therapy in thrombocytopenic patients.

Although no firm guidelines can be followed as indications for platelet transfusions there are situations where the decision is quite clear (National Academy of Sciences–National Research Council, and the Leukemia Task Force, 1966). Patients who are thrombocytopenic with significant bleeding manifestations or where these can be anticipated should be transfused. The relationship between the level of the platelet count and the incidence of bleeding has been discussed above and should be borne in mind in considering the risk of hemorrhage in an individual patient. The clinician, however, should not be guided solely by the platelet count since it is well recognized that in certain forms of thrombocytopenia, such as chronic idiopathic thrombocytopenia purpura, bleeding is less likely to occur at levels, where in other diseases, i.e., acute leukemia, it is quite frequent.

II. PLATELET PROCUREMENT

Acid-citrate-dextrose (ACD) is universally accepted as the anticoagulant of choice for blood transfusions and the same anticoagulant or some modification is now generally utilized to prepare platelet suspensions for the treatment of thrombocytopenic individuals. These modifications, which are important for the preparation of platelet concentrates, will be discussed. Ethylene diaminetetraacetate (EDTA) was used in the early experimental platelet transfusion studies in both animals (Dillard *et al.*, 1951) and man (Stefanini and Dameshek, 1953; Gardner *et al.*, 1954). However, it has largely been abandoned because of evidence suggesting that it causes morphologic changes in platelets and may be toxic. The platelets lose their usual disklike shape and become spherical (Zucker and Borrelli, 1954) and there are alterations in ultrastructure, particularly in the cell membrane (White and Krivit, 1968). In addition, there appear to be disturbances in phosphonucleotide synthesis (Rossi, 1964), in serotonin uptake *in vitro* (Ozge *et al.*, 1964) and in clot retraction (Zucker and Borrelli, 1958). There is also increased glucose utilization in platelets suspended in EDTA compared to citrate (Rossi, 1967). Studies of platelet kinetics in man utilizing ^{51}Cr have demonstrated that platelets prepared in EDTA result in relatively poor recoveries compared to platelets prepared in citrate (Aster, 1965) due to temporary sequestration in the liver (Davey and Lander, 1964; Aster and Jandl, 1964) followed by destruction in the spleen. This results in a loss of more than two-thirds of the transfused platelets (Aster and Jandl, 1964). However, it has been pointed out that differences between ACD and EDTA may not be real because of the elution of the chromium-51 from platelets prepared in EDTA (Gardner and Cohen, 1966). Platelet survival time with the two anticoagulants was approximately the same (Abrahamsen, 1965; Gardner and Cohen, 1966). Nevertheless, even if this is taken into account, ACD appears to be superior and the fact that EDTA cannot be used for red blood cell storage would make ACD the anticoagulant of choice for platelet transfusions.

Citrate-phosphate-dextrose (CPD) which has recently been approved as an anticoagulant has been reported to have some advantages compared to ACD for red cell transfusions (Kevy *et al.*, 1965). The preparation contains less citrate and hence, results in a smaller decrease in blood calcium; the pH of the blood containing citrate-phosphate-dextrose remains higher, less potassium is lost from the red cells on storage, and there is less hemolysis. Unfortunately, platelet concentrates (PC) prepared from blood anticoagulated with citrate-phosphate-dextrose show marked clumping and *in vivo* recovery following transfusion is less than 50% relative to ACD platelet concentrates (Pert *et al.*, 1967). The clumping is probably due to the higher pH of the blood when citrate-phosphate-dextrose is used for anticoagulation; ACD added to citrate-phosphate-dextrose platelet-rich plasma (PRP) allows the preparation of satisfactory platelet concentrates.

Heparin results in marked platelet clumping and even when combined with ACD does not permit the preparation of satisfactory platelet suspensions (Morrison and Baldini, 1967).

Platelets may be transfused as fresh whole blood, platelet-rich plasma, or platelet concentrates. Fresh whole blood, preferably from patients with polycythemia vera and thrombocytosis, was used commonly in the years prior to the development of platelet separation and concentration techniques. The blood must be carefully collected in ACD to assure satisfactory mixing of blood and anticoagulant so that platelet clumping is prevented. The blood must then be transfused within 6 hours of collection to obtain maximum platelet recovery (80–90%) in the recipient (Hirsch and Gardner, 1952). However, it has been reported that recovery may be quite satisfactory (45%) even after 24 hours at 4°C (Kissmeyer-Nielsen and Madsen, 1961a) although survival is compromised.

Fresh whole blood for platelet replacement should now be used only if the patient requires erythrocytes and plasma as well as platelets, but even in such circumstances, supplementation with additional platelets is often necessary. Platelet-rich plasma is easily prepared and when properly produced is as effective as whole blood. However, platelet concentrates are used more commonly because multiple transfusions are almost invariably necessary and large volumes of plasma as whole blood may result in overloading the cardiovascular system. Unfortunately, there are still large institutions in this country where neither platelet-rich plasma nor platelet concentrates are available; this should now be considered as a failure to keep up with the modern era of transfusion practices.

Platelet-rich plasma should be prepared from freshly drawn whole blood. In general, the interval between bleeding and transfusion should be as brief as possible, preferably less than 6 hours. Platelet-rich plasma which has been kept for longer than 6 hours results in lower *in vivo* recoveries so that at 24 hours the recovery may be only about 50% and the survival is markedly shortened. The blood flow should be rapid and uninterrupted into a closed double pack plastic bag system* which permits the collection of two units of platelet-rich plasma at each donation (Kliman *et al.*, 1961). The first unit is separated but the indwelling needle is kept patent by a slow drip of saline and the whole blood is then centrifuged in a swing bucket rotor at 1500 g for 3 minutes in a refrigerated centrifuge (PR-2[†]) at 10°–20°C (Freireich *et al.*, 1963). The supernatant platelet-rich plasma is expressed into the satellite bag taking care to exclude the buffy coat. The packed red cells diluted with 50–100 ml normal saline are returned to the donor. Following the infusion, the second unit of blood is collected and processed in

---

* Fenwal Cat. #JD-2.

† International Centrifuge, International Equipment Company, Boston, Massuchusetts.

the same way. A unit of platelet-rich plasma (approximately 250 ml plasma) prepared from a unit of fresh whole blood from a normal donor will contain approximately 10^{11} platelets. The platelet-rich plasma is transfused to an appropriate recipient directly from the satellite bag through a platelet recipient set including a filter chamber in order to trap macroscopic aggregates. Less than 3% of platelets are trapped in such a chamber and *in vivo* recovery and survival is unimpaired (Morrison, 1966). The same donor can be used repeatedly without ill effect as was demonstrated by Freireich *et al.* (1963) who subjected donors to plasmapheresis of 1000 ml per week and observed no significant changes in their hemograms. Only slight changes in plasma proteins were observed.

With the increasing appreciation of the utility of platelet replacement therapy and the need for multiple and repeated platelet transfusions, a great deal of work has gone into the preparation of satisfactory platelet concentrates. Although platelet concentrates are more difficult and more time consuming to prepare, the smaller resulting volume and salvaging of platelet-poor plasma present important advantages. In both children and adults large and frequent transfusions are usually required to effect hemostasis so that if platelet-rich plasma were to be used, the cardiovascular system would be quickly overloaded. Before elucidation of the mechanism of platelet aggregation and the role of ADP (Gaarder *et al.*, 1961), it was difficult to prepare smooth suspensions of platelet concentrates for transfusion. Platelet clumping can be induced by small amounts of ADP and it is quite probable that regardless of the agent initially involved, platelet aggregation is usually mediated by this nucleotide. Platelet aggregation precedes viscous metamorphosis and is considered to be important in the early stages of clotting (Sharp, 1958). ADP-induced clumping can be inhibited by a number of agents including thrombin, antihistamines, acidification, competitive inhibitors of ADP, chelating agents, and low calcium (Sharp, 1965; Greenwalt and Perry, 1969).

In platelet-rich plasma, clumping due to ADP can be reversed with little or no residual damage. However, in the preparation of platelet concentrates, persistent injury to the platelets occurs during centrifugation and concentration; consequently, the recovery of transfused platelets in the recipient was reduced to less than 25% as compared to platelet-rich plasma (Gardner *et al.*, 1954). That physical damage occurs during centrifugation is supported by the demonstration that ultrastructural damage develops during centrifugation (Arnaud *et al.*, 1963).

Freshly prepared platelet concentrates have been successfully used for replacement therapy in thrombocytopenic individuals with acute leukemia and other conditions (Djerassi *et al.*, 1963; Alvarado *et al.*, 1965), but the quantities required in order to achieve hemostasis were very large even in children (8–10 concentrates, each from 500 ml fresh blood) and the loss of platelets was presumably marked in these early studies.

Since clumping in platelet concentrates is usually irreversible and smooth suspensions cannot be obtained even after carefully kneading, the aggregated platelets are caught in the filter upon transfusion. However, even if clumping is prevented by using EDTA in the preparation of platelet concentrates, recovery in recipients is low approximating that obtained with ACD (Levin *et al.*, 1965). Thus, the advantage gained with EDTA is apparently lost because of the damaging effect of this anticoagulant. Similarly, the resuspending medium, whether plasma or saline, does not appear to be a factor particularly when platelet concentrates are transfused promptly after preparation. It appears, therefore, that the available evidence indicates that physical injury sustained by the platelet during centrifugation is responsible for the poor yields obtained with platelet concentrates prepared in ACD.

Although the transfusion of platelet concentrates results in a reduced recovery in the recipient compared to platelet-rich plasma, it should be pointed out that survival of the circulating platelets is relatively unimpaired (Levin *et al.*, 1965). Presumably, following the removal of the damaged platelets, the surviving fraction of cells has the same intravascular survival as the undamaged platelets in platelet-rich plasma.

The poor platelet recoveries with the clinical use of platelet concentrates led to numerous attempts to improve methods of preparation. Since the aggregation of platelets in platelet-rich plasma is usually a reversible process, Flatow *et al.* (1966) employed ADP-induced aggregations in an attempt to decrease the centrifugal force necessary for the preparation of platelet concentrates and hence reduce the physical injury to the platelet. With ADP at a concentration of 10 μg/ml and with centrifugation at 50 g, concentrates 80–90% as effective as platelet-rich plasma were observed. Unfortunately, the use of ADP for this purpose is associated with some practical problems and potential clinical hazards which prevent its general application.

The problem of platelet aggregation in platelet concentrates was not resolved until the important observation by Aster and Jandl that clumping with sequestration in the liver could be avoided if the pH of the suspending medium was lowered (Aster and Jandl, 1964). Viability of the platelets was preserved equally well with ACD as the anticoagulant at pH 7.4 or pH 6.5 when centrifugation was not performed. However, in the preparation of concentrates, ACD at pH 6.5 rather than at the usual pH 7.1 or 7.2 gave the best recoveries (Aster, 1965, 1969). At this lower pH, platelet survival and viability seem unimpaired. This has subsequently been substantiated by extensive clinical experience (Flatow and Freireich, 1966; Shively *et al.*, 1966). Platelet concentrates prepared in acidified plasma upon transfusion result in recoveries of 80–90%, and unimpaired intravascular survival compared to platelet-rich plasma (Flatow and Freireich, 1966). Acidification has been accomplished in a variety of ways including modification of the ACD (Aster and Jandl, 1964), the addition of excess ACD to platelet-rich plasma (Cohen *et al.*, 1965; Shively *et al.*, 1966), and the addition of excess citric acid to platelet-rich plasma (Flatow and Freireich, 1966).

However, there are objections to all these approaches but one practical technique is that of Chappell (1966) usually referred to as the "split-ACD" method. This procedure is schematically shown in Fig. 1. Standard ACD-A

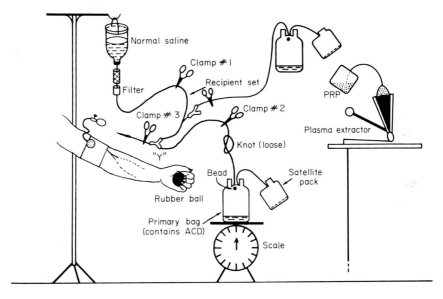

FIG. 1. Procedure for obtaining platelet-rich plasma (PRP) using the "split ACD" method (see text). The small satellite bags contain 15 ml of ACD-A.

contains approximately 16% more sodium citrate than is necessary for anticoagulation of a unit of whole blood. Using the standard double blood plastic bags,* 15 ml of the 75 ml ACD-A in the large bag is expressed into the satellite bag before use. 480 gm of blood may then be drawn into the

* Fenwal JD-2.

large bag without danger of clotting. The entire pack is centrifuged at 1500 g for 3 minutes in a PR-2 centrifuge at room temperature and the supernatant platelet-rich plasma is expressed into the satellite bag. Centrifugation is then carried out for 20 minutes at 1500 g and the platelet-poor plasma, except for 15–30 ml, is returned to the large bag for resuspension of the red cells. Such reconstituted blood has not been approved as of this writing by the Division of Biologic Standards. The platelet concentrate is resuspended in the residual plasma and should then be promptly infused usually through a small platelet filter* in order to remove large aggregates. Small aggregates do not appear to give rise to any clinical problems.

The need for acidification in the preparation of platelet concentrates is not universally accepted, however. Cavins et al. (1968a) and Djerassi et al. (1963, 1964) obtained satisfactory in vivo recoveries following the transfusion of platelet concentrates without lowering the pH. The procedure was essentially as above except that platelet-rich plasma was obtained by centrifuging whole blood for 4 minutes at 750 g in a refrigerated centrifuge (4°–10°C) and then the platelet-rich plasma was spun at 750 g for 30 minutes to yield the platelet concentrates. Persistent platelet clumps were minimal. In vivo recovery of platelets following the infusion of platelet concentrates prepared with this technique compared favorably with platelet concentrates prepared with the addition of excess ACD-A or citric acid (Cavins et al., 1968b).

The reasons for the different results obtained in various laboratories are not clear but temperature and the conditions of centrifugation may have been the most important factors. Most of the acidification studies were done at room temperature, whereas most of unmodified concentrates were prepared at 4°C. There were significant differences in the g forces employed, and it is felt that higher g forces enhance platelet aggregation. The role of ADP in this situation is not completely clear, although the reaction is temperature dependent. Aggregation appears to be maximum at room temperature but spontaneous reversal is optimal at 37°C (Salzman and Chambers, 1965; Hellem and Owren, 1964; Constantine, 1965). Platelet concentrates prepared at 4°–10°C contain aggregates; if these are kept at room temperature for one hour before resuspension, there appears to be no difference in aggregation between nonacidified and acidified suspensions. Pert et al. (1967) have recommended that platelet concentrates be prepared at 10°–14°C rather than 4°C since microscopic clumping appeared to be less frequent at the warmer temperature (Pert et al., 1967). Mourad (1968a)

* Fenwall #HE-92-D.

recommends centrifugation of whole blood at 2500 g for 100 seconds at 10°C to prepare platelet-rich plasma. The platelet-rich plasma is brought to 25°C by agitation at room temperature or in a water bath and the platelet concentrate is then prepared by centrifugation at 5100 g for 10 minutes at 25°C. Finally, the platelet concentrate is kept at room temperature for 30 minutes before resuspension. Aggregates were not detected macroscopically or microscopically and platelet integrity appeared intact since only 2% of platelet enzymes including nucleoside diphosphokinase, 3-phosphoglycerate kinase, and enolase were released. In contrast, at 0°C there were many aggregates, and enzyme release reached 10–20%. With centrifugation at 25°C followed by immediate resuspension, aggregation occurred and approximately 10% of the enzymes were released. This appears to be an important observation since platelet enzyme release is related to both aggregation and injury (Mourad, 1968b) strongly suggesting that platelet concentrates are best prepared at temperatures warmer than previously employed.

Although the present techniques of preparing platelet concentrates are relatively simple, they are tedious and time consuming. There have been many efforts to improve collection of blood components but the work begun by Cohn and his collaborators in 1949 is particularly noteworthy (Tullis *et al.*, 1956) and eventually led to the development of the Cohn-ADL centrifuge. A completely closed centrifugation system was utilized with the design of the bowls on a "falling film" principle. Recently, the bowls have been modified* and the operation simplified so that the device can be operated in commonly available refrigerated centrifuges by use of a special adapter (Tullis *et al.*, 1967). Bowls with various design configurations in clear plastic or stainless steel have been developed for different purposes. The operation is essentially a batch-type procedure in that for separation of the various blood components, blood flow must be interrupted at various intervals and the centrifugation decelerated. Recently, Tullis and his co-workers (1968) reported initial studies using the modified Cohn centrifuge to prepare platelet concentrates. Platelet recovery from normal donors was 60% (range, 36–82%) of the platelets theoretically available in an average volume of blood of approximately 2 liters per donor. Leukocyte contamination was 4–5% of the white blood cells passing through the machine. The procedure apparently was generally well tolerated by the donors and no important effects on donor erythrocytes, platelets, and calcium were detected. Red cell contamination was considered insignificant. When these

---

* Manufactured by A. D. Little Company, Acord Park, Cambridge, Massachusetts.

platelet concentrates were transfused into three thrombocytopenic non-bleeding recipients with an average pretransfusion platelet count of 3000/mm³, the average posttransfusion rise was 26000/mm³, representing 69% (range, 26–112%) recovery of the transfused platelets. After 24 hours, the average count was 20,000/mm³ indicating that survival was relatively intact. Viability seemed unimpaired as determined by various coagulation tests done before and after transfusion.

The modified Cohn centrifuge has recently been used successfully to prepare platelet concentrates from platelet-rich plasma (Miller *et al.*, 1969). The platelet-rich plasma was obtained from fresh whole blood utilizing the "split-ACD" technique described above. The platelet concentrate contained 80% of the platelets in the platelet-rich plasma and upon transfusion to thrombocytopenic individuals averaged about 30% (range, 15–45%). This compared favorably with conventional "split-ACD" platelet transfusions. Unfortunately, sterilization of the equipment was difficult since the plastic bowls could not be sterilized in conventional autoclaves and repeated exposure to ethylene oxide resulted in opacification of the plastic. However, with modification in the sterilization procedure, this is no longer a problem.

The recent development of the NCI-IBM Cell Separator* offers another approach for the rapid procurement of platelets (Buckner *et al.*, 1968, 1969; Graw *et al.*, 1970). In contrast to the Cohn-ADL centrifuge, the Cell Separator operates on a continuous flow basis at rates up to 200 ml/minute although *in vivo* processing is usually done at a blood flow of 40 ml/minute. The various components of the blood are isolated in a specially designed bowl and are drawn off separately. Most of the emphasis to date with this device has been on separation of white blood cells and only a few attempts at platelet procurement have been made. However, when patients with chronic myelocytic leukemia have been utilized as donors, as many as 2×10^{11} platelets have been obtained from a single donor in a 4-hour run (Graw and Eisel, 1969).

III. CLINICAL STUDIES IN THROMBOCYTOPENIC RECIPIENTS

Numerous clinical studies clearly document the effective control of hemostasis by platelet transfusion in patients with thrombocytopenia, particularly leukemia and aplastic anemia (Farber and Klein, 1957; Stefanini

* Now being marketed under the trade name "Celltrifuge Blood Cell Separator" by American Instrument Co., Inc., 8030 Georgia Avenue, Silver Spring, Maryland 20910.

and Dameshek, 1953; Cronkite and Jackson, 1959; Freireich *et al.*, 1963; Alvarado *et al.*, 1965; Maupin, 1969). It is significant that platelet trans-fusions have resulted in a marked reduction in the hemorrhagic complica-tions which in the past was the major contributor to the cause of death in patients with leukemia (Hersh *et al.*, 1965; Han *et al.*, 1966; Didisheim, 1967; Shively *et al.*, 1966).

A concept of prophylactic replacement therapy has evolved from clinical and experimental observations. In 1966, the National Cancer Institute and the National Academy of Sciences-National Research Council issued a statement entitled "Clinical Application of Platelet Transfusions" (Na-tional Academy of Sciences—National Research Council, and the Leukemia Task Force, 1966), and in 1968 the Platelet Transfusion Subcommittee of the Acute Leukemia Task Force outlined a number of the current techniques for platelet procurement and developed guidelines for the use of platelet transfusions in patients with leukemia and other diseases. Although there are diverse approaches to the practical aspects of platelet preparation and transfusion and patient selection, these reports are representative of current opinion and illustrate the magnitude of interest in this area of therapy.

In early studies, Duke (1910) emphasized that hemorrhage was un-common in patients with platelet counts of 30,000/mm³ or greater, whereas below this level bleeding manifestations were frequently observed. In the leukemic patients studied by Gaydos, Freireich, and Mantel (1962) bleeding occurred over a wide range of platelet values but a precise threshold for the appearance of hemorrhage could not be delineated. The most severe bleeding, however, was observed at platelet values which were in the range of 20,000/mm³ or below. Cronkite (1966) emphasized that an increased tendency to bleed at a higher level of platelets is observed in patients with rapidly falling platelet counts. In general, evidence of disturbed hemostasis is most often clinically apparent at circulating platelet levels below 50,000/mm³ (Freeman and Hyde, 1952; Boggs *et al.*, 1962).

As mentioned above, other coagulation defects may coexist with thrombo-cytopenia, particularly in patients with leukemia, and these may increase the likelihood of clinical hemorrhage. Qualitative platelet defects may also occur and result in hemorrhage at higher platelet levels (Friedman *et al.*, 1964; Zittuouin and Samama, 1968). The decision to use platelet transfusion therapy requires consideration of many factors and these have been em-phasized by the statement issued by the Leukemia Task Force in which a "probability or risk of hemorrhage" can be used as a guide to therapy (Platelet Transfusion Subcommittee of the Acute Leukemia Task Force, 1968).

Platelet transfusions are advised for most patients who develop overt hemorrhage in the presence of a platelet count below 50,000/mm³. Three categories were used to classify thrombocytopenia: (1) severe, when the platelet count is below 10,000/mm³; (2) moderate, if between 10,000 and 30,000/mm³; and (3) mild, if between 30,000 and 100,000/mm³. Prophylactic platelets should be given to maintain platelet counts above 10,000/mm³ if possible. In patients with moderate thrombocytopenia the presence of hemorrhage, fever, infection, or mucosal ulceration, is probably an indication for platelet transfusions depending on the "trend" of the platelet count determined at a minimum of 24-hour intervals.

The effectiveness of platelet transfusions is ultimately judged by the ability to correct the defect caused by thrombocytopenia, i.e., bleeding or the tendency to bleed. As previously mentioned, measurement of the red blood cell output in the thoracic duct lymph of animals made thrombocytopenic by irradiation (Dillard et al., 1951; Woods et al., 1953) is a valuable technique for determining the efficacy of transfused platelets but is obviously not useful in patients. The determination of the bleeding time, introduced by Duke in 1910, was considered a reflection of the level of circulating platelets. A number of tests have been evaluated (Raccuglia and Bethell, 1960; McGovern, 1957; Arnaud et al., 1963; Castaldi and Firkin, 1964) including prothrombin consumption, capillary fragility, platelet count, and clot retraction; it was concluded that the bleeding time was the most useful indicator of disturbed hemostasis and thus could be utilized to measure the effectiveness or "viability" of transfused normal platelets. Discomfort to the patient and variability in technique represent the major drawbacks to its application in routine transfusion therapy. It is of interest that lyophilized, disintegrated, or stored platelets when transfused may result in clot retraction and improve prothrombin consumption but will not raise the circulating platelet count nor result in significant hemostasis (Hjort et al., 1959; Raccuglia and Bethell, 1960; Estes et al., 1962).

Transfusions that fail to elevate the levels of circulating platelets do not appear to be effective in controlling hemorrhage (Cronkite and Jackson, 1959; Firkin et al., 1960; Baldini, 1960). A useful indication of platelet "viability" can thus be obtained by measuring the increment in platelet count and relating this to the dose of platelets infused and the recipients' weight, body surface area, or blood volume (Freireich, 1966; Murphy and Gardner, 1969; Alvarado et al., 1965). The platelet increment has been shown to be proportional to the dose of infused platelets (Cavins et al., 1968b; Freireich et al., 1963). Percent recovery or yield derives from measurement of the actual increase in total circulating platelets compared to a theoretical value based on simple dilution of the infused platelets within the blood volume of the recipient. Differences in methods of calculating results have made it difficult to compare results from different laboratories (Cavins et al., 1968b). Formulas for representative calculations are shown below:

	Posttransfusion	Pretransfusion

$$\text{Percent recovery} = \frac{\text{Platelet count} - \text{Platelet count}}{\text{Total number of platelets infused}} \times \text{Blood volume} \times 100 \qquad (1)$$

$$\text{Increment} \times \text{m}^2/10^{11} \text{ platelets} = \frac{\text{Platelet count} - \text{Platelet count}}{\text{Total number of platelets infused}} \times \text{m}^2 \qquad (2)$$

$$\text{Increment} \times \text{m}^2/\text{unit platelets} = \frac{\text{Platelet count} - \text{Platelet count}}{\text{Number of units of platelets infused}} \times \text{m}^2 \qquad (3)$$

Percent recovery and increment times m^2 per 10^{11} platelets are the most precise methods for comparison of a single preparation given to multiple individuals but increment times m^2 per unit is the most practical as it eliminates the necessity for counting the number of platelets infused. The average number of platelets obtained from a unit of blood can be determined and the figure used for the other calculations, i.e., 0.75×10 platelets/unit of platelet concentrate (Alvarado et al., 1965).

Current estimates of the recovery of ^{51}Cr-labeled autologous normal platelets, prepared with acidification at room temperature, average 68% (compiled by Aster, 1969). The normal survival of platelets in the blood ranges between 7 and 10 days (Aster and Jandl, 1964; Morrison and Baldini, 1967; Bosch et al., 1962; Cohen et al., 1961; Davey, 1966; Najean et al., 1969). Damage during processing (McGovern, 1957; Aster and Jandl, 1964), during storage (Murphy and Gardner, 1969; Baldini et al., 1960) or following transfusion (Shulman, 1966; Freireich, 1965; Salmon and Schwartz, 1960; Arnaud et al., 1963) may reduce platelet survival.

Although, wide variations in the recovery of transfused platelets given to thrombocytopenic patients have been observed, in large series the range of recovery of transfused platelet concentrates has varied between 25 and 39% (Davey and Lander, 1964; Levin et al., 1965; Cohen, 1962; Alvarado et al., 1965).

IV. ADVERSE REACTIONS

It is well recognized that alloimmunization may develop following the repeated use of platelets (Stefanini and Dameshek, 1953; Svejgaard, 1969; Shulman, 1966) and platelet antibodies are a frequent finding in most multitransfused patients receiving more than 100 transfusions (Aster, 1965; Shulman, 1966; Dausset et al., 1960). Antibodies may be directed either against specific platelet antigens (Shulman, 1966; Aster, 1965; Adner et al., 1969) or against antigens found both on leukocytes and platelets (Dausset et al., 1960; Shulman et al., 1964). Transfusion of platelets to sensitized individuals results in decreased platelet recovery and survival (Aster and Jandl, 1964; Baldini et al., 1962; Bosch et al., 1965; Shulman et al., 1964).

The spleen appears to be the primary site of platelet removal in patients with weak antibodies whereas the liver removes the bulk of transfused platelets in individuals with greater degrees of sensitization (Aster and Jandl, 1964; Shulman, 1965; Najean et al., 1969). Evidence that transfused platelets may transiently be effective in hemostasis despite sensitization has been reported (Cavins et al., 1968; Djerassi, 1966). Alloimmunization occurs less frequently in patients with leukemia (Djerassi et al., 1963; Aster et al., 1964b) than in nonimmunosuppressed patients receiving platelets (Bosch et al., 1965). It is likely that the dose and schedule of administration of platelets as well as immunosuppressive chemotherapy bears on the development of sensitization in these patients. The use of platelets obtained from relatives results in reduced sensitization (Freireich et al., 1963; Shulman, 1966; Bosch et al., 1965), probably due to lesser degrees of antigenic disparity. Long-term support with platelet transfusion in patients with bone marrow aplasia has been reported (Flatow and Freireich, 1966b; Baldini, 1964; Yankee et al., 1969). Flatow and Freireich transfused platelets regularly for 7 months in two patients and intermittently for over 2 years in another; all three patients eventually recovered. Splenectomy improved both the recovery and survival of the transfused platelets. Djerassi (1966) was also able to transfuse platelets repeatedly to a number of patients with one patient receiving 300 transfusions representing 1200 platelet concentrates during a 4-year period.

Platelet typing has not been practical in the routine use of platelet transfusions and selection of compatible platelets by identification of antibody specificity in the serum of recipients has been accomplished only rarely (Shulman et al., 1964; Adner et al., 1969). Bosch et al. (1965) were able to select "compatible" donors for a patient with aplastic anemia who had become refractory to platelets and whose serum contained a weak leukoagglutinin. Leukocyte groups were determined and platelets obtained from relatives having similar leukocyte antigens (mother, sister, and brother) were found to sustain circulating platelet levels in the patient. Recent studies indicate that lymphocyte genotyping may be used to determine platelet compatibility among family members of patients with aplastic anemia who are refractory to platelets (Yankee et al., 1969). In these patients, platelets from random donors disappeared from the circulation in less than 24 hours following transfusion. Platelets from each of the family members were also rapidly destroyed except for those obtained from siblings who were HL-A genotypically identical. The median recovery of transfused acidified platelet concentrates from the HL-A matched siblings ranged from 60 to 80% of the expected value. The median increment times m^2 per unit was $26,000/mm^3$ at 1 hour and $15,000/mm^3$ at 20 hours following transfusions. Four units of platelets obtained twice weekly by plasmapheresis of the compatible siblings, were transfused for 15, 18, and 24 months without decreases in response. These studies provide strong evidence that the genetic determinants of lymphocyte antigenicity are also primary determinants of platelet antigenicity. The complex nature of the HL-A system limits the direct application of these techniques at the present time to selection of compatible donors from among family members. Whereas the chance of finding an HL-A genotypic match among siblings is 1 in 4, a phenotypic match in the random population has been estimated at greater than 1 in 1000 (Bach, 1968). The presence of platelet specific antigens may further reduce the possibility of finding platelet compatibility among random and possibly even family donors. In the authors' opinion the use of platelets from single donors, preferably family members and preferably HL-A matched siblings, seems the most reasonable approach to the long-term platelet support required in patients with life-threatening thrombocytopenia.

ABO substances have been detected on the surface of platelet membranes by serologic techniques (Coombs and Bedford, 1955; Dausset and Maleward, 1954; Gurevitch and Nelken, 1954; Lewis et al., 1960). In comparative studies, Aster (1965) noted that the percent recovery of platelets transfused between ABO compatible individuals was 65%. When group A_1 donors were transfused to 0 recipients, the recovery was 19% and when group B donors were given to either A or O recipients the recovery was 57%. In group O recipients of A_1B platelets, recoveries approximated only 8%. Scanning data indicate that the liver is the primary organ of sequestration. Although platelet survival was shortened in two instances, the platelets remaining after the initial loss appeared to survive normally (8 days). An inverse relationship was observed between the height of the issoagglutinin titer and the percent recovery. Infusion of 0.25 ml of red blood cells from an A_1 donor concomitant with reinfusion of ^{51}Cr-labeled autologous platelets to an O individual did not result in decreased platelet recovery (58%), whereas infusion of A substance resulted in a significant decrease (25%). Pfisterer et al. (1966) using a modification of Aster's technique observed a platelet life-span of 9.69 days for compatible platelet infusion and 9.10 days (SD = 1.43 days) for transfusion of ABO incompatible platelets. A rising survival curve during the first 24 hours was seen in all compatible infusions and a falling curve with ABO incompatible platelets. The recovery at 20 to 24 hours was 46% for the compatible and 26% for the incompatible group. Recoveries were reduced by 40% for B donors given to A_1 recipients, 43% for A_1 donors to B recipients and 61% for A_1 donors to O recipients. Rh incompatibility did not significantly influence platelet recovery or survival. In studies of patients with leukemia, ABO incompatibility has not been associated with significant reduction in recovery or survival (Freireich, 1966; Clifford et al., 1965; Shulman et al., 1964). Red blood cell sensitization was also an infrequent finding in these patients.

It remains controversial whether specific immune destruction of platelets per se is responsible for the mild chills and transient fevers that occur with platelet transfusion (Harrington, 1953; Shulman, 1966; Aster and Jandl, 1964; Wierdt and Vander, 1965, as mentioned by Svejgaard, 1969). Available evidence suggests that most reactions following infusion of platelets are due to interaction of antibodies against contaminating leukocytes. Despite the rapid disappearance of transfused platelets from the circulation in the presence of antibody, reactions were not observed when highly purified platelet suspensions were given (Wierdt and Vander, 1965, as mentioned by Svejgaard, 1969).

Reactions to platelets usually consist of chills occurring within 20 minutes after transfusion followed by a fever lasting 1 to 4 hours. Occasionally dyspnea and cyanosis occur necessitating cessation of the infusion administration of epinephrine or corticosteroids.

V. PRESERVATION

There have been many reports of methods for platelet preservation and storage, but at present none appears completely satisfactory. Platelets stored at 4°C rapidly lose the ability to circulate when transfused (Jackson, 1956; Baldini et al., 1960; Levin et al., 1964; Morrison and Baldini, 1967) and the reduction in viability has been shown to have an almost logarithmic relationship with time (Baldini *et al.*, 1960). Viability as measured by a "viability index" was very low when platelets were stored for 24 hours at 4°C compared to fresh platelets. McGovern in 1957 noted that platelet concentrates prepared in ACD at room temperature are as effective as those prepared at 4°C and resuspend more readily when kept at room temperature (Mourad, 1968a). Recent studies indicate that the optimal temperature for retention of viability of platelets stored as acidified platelet-rich plasma is 22°C (Murphy and Gardner, 1969). Platelets stored at this temperature for 18 hours were reduced by only 14% compared with fresh platelets, whereas a 27% reduction in recovery occurred with storage at 4°C. The disappearance of transfused platelets was curvilinear with 4°C storage and linear at 22°C storage using ^{51}Cr. Although these results are of great practical importance, the risk of bacterial growth at the higher temperature must be more fully explored.

There have been numerous studies on cryopreservation of platelets. Early work suggesting that lyophilized platelets and platelets frozen in gelatin or plasma might be of value in the treatment of thrombocytopenia (Tullis, 1953; Stefanini and Dameshek, 1953; Klein *et al.*, 1956) was later subjected to more critical evaluation in irradiated animals where it was concluded that the platelets did not circulate and were of little benefit in controlling bleeding (Jackson *et al.*, 1959; Fliedner *et al.*, 1958; Firkin *et al.*, 1960; Baldini *et al.*, 1960). From the above studies as well as many others one must conclude that most of the *in vitro* tests that have been used to compare various preservation procedures have not been useful to predict *in vivo* platelet viability. Metabolic activity and effectiveness in tests of *in vitro* coagulation are generally better preserved than the ability of platelets to circulate after transfusion (Marcus and Zucker, 1966; Zucker and Lundberg, 1966; Morrison, 1968). Quantitation of radioactive serotonin uptake as well as the release of certain platelet enzymes, such as nucleoside phosphokinase, 3-phosphoglycerate kinase, and enolase, hold promise as parameters of platelet damage; however, further correlation of *in vivo* results is needed to determine their usefulness (Mourad and Pert, 1967; Lundberg *et al.*, 1967).

The most successful methods for the preservation of human platelets for transfusion currently in use include either dimethylsulfoxide (DMSO) or glycerol as additives. Cohen *et al.* (1961, 1965) studied the effect of glycerol in freezing canine platelets and human platelets. In the human studies platelets were frozen at 1°C per minute to −30°C and then 5°C per minute to −80°C. After rapid thawing the platelets were treated for 10 minutes with sodium citrate for dehydration, and deglycerolized and buffered by gradual addition of autologous plasma. The optimum protective concentration was found to be 10–12%. Recovery of transfused platelets measured at 1 hour by the ^{51}Cr technique in normal individuals was 23% and in thrombocytopenic recipients significant increments above baseline values were obtained. Djerassi et al. (1963) used rats to study the effect of various combinations of sugars and dimethylsulfoxide on platelets slowly frozen to −195°C. Optimum increments of 70–80% of controls were observed with the combination of 5% dimethylsulfoxide in 5% dextrose. Despite good recovery, the survival of the preserved platelets was approximately 50% of the controls. Dimethylsulfoxide used alone was consistently less effective than when combined with sugars. Clot retraction with platelets at −195°C is retained at slow rates of freezing in dimethylsulfoxide (Iossifides et al., 1962). With the addition of sugars to dimethylsulfoxide at higher rates of freezing (19.5°C/minute), both the capability to cause clot retraction and morphology are maintained (Djerassi et al., 1964). Platelets frozen at 1°C per minute in 5% dimethylsulfoxide and 5% dextrose have been transfused to patients with leukemia and aplastic anemia and recoveries approximating one-third of that observed with fresh platelets have been reported (Djerassi, 1966; Lundberg et al., 1967). Thus far no severe side effects have been reported with either dimethylsulfoxide or glycerol. Although local venospasm and pain are not uncommon, they can be ameliorated if the platelet suspension is diluted with small amounts of plasma just before use. Nausea and vomiting also occur with some frequency and the odor of dimethylsulfoxide is very objectionable to many patients. Intravenous glycerol has been shown to be readily cleared in large doses over prolonged periods (Haynes et al., 1960). Although cataracts have been reported in dogs receiving prolonged high levels of dimethylsulfoxide, no evidence of this has been observed in humans (Jacobs and Rosenbaum, 1966). However, patients should have careful eye examinations before receiving platelets preserved in dimethylsulfoxide and then reexamined approximately 1 month later.

Recent studies in animals suggest that hydroxyethyl starch may be useful as a cryopreservative for platelets (Spencer et al., 1969).

Under a contract from the National Cancer Institute, a standard Teflon container for platelet preservation has been developed and a controlled study is in progress comparing cryopreserved platelets with fresh platelets. As a result of this study, data should be forthcoming to define more clearly the use of preserved platelets for replacement therapy.

REFERENCES

Abrahamsen, A. F. (1965). *Scand. J. Haematol.* **2**, 52.

Adner, M. M., Fisch, G. R., Starobin, S. G., and Aster, R. H. (1969). *N. Engl. J. Med.* **280**, 244.

Alkjaersig, N., Abe, T., and Seegers, W. H. (1955). *Amer. J. Physiol.* **181**, 304.

Alvarado, J., Djerassi, I., and Farber, S. (1965). *J. Pediat.* **67**, 13.

Arnaud, S. R., Greenwalt, T. J., Pawlowski, J. M., and Johnson, S. A. (1963). *Transfusion (Philadelphia)* **3**, 8.

Aster, R. H. (1965). *Blood* **26**, 732.

Aster, R. H. (1969). *Vox Sang.* **17**, 23.

Aster, R. H., and Jandl, J. H. (1964a). *J. Clin. Invest.* **43**, 843.

Aster, R. H., Levin, R. H., Cooper, H. C., and Freireich, E. J. (1964b). *Transfusion* **4**, 428.

Bach, F. H. (1968). *Science* **159**, 1196.

Baldini, M., Costea, N., and Dameshek, W. (1960). *Blood* **16**, 1669.

Baldini, M., Costea, N., and Ebbe, S. (1962). *Proc. 8th Congr. Eur. Soc. Haematol.*, 1961 p. 378.

Bizzozero, G. (1882). *Virchows Arch. Pathol. Anat. Physiol.* **90**, 261 (cited in Tocantins, 1948).

Boggs, D. R., Wintrobe, M. M., and Cartwright, G. E. (1962). *Medicine (Baltimore)* **41**, 163.

Bosch, L. J., Jansz, A., Lammers, H. A., Van Leeuwen, A., and Van Rood, J. J. (1962). *Proc. 8th Congr. Eur. Soc. Haematol.*, 1961, p. 380.

Bosch, L. J., Eerrisse, J. G., Van Leeuwen, A., Loeliga, E. A., and Van Rood, J. J. (1965). *Rev. Belge Pathol. Med. Exp.* **31**, 139.

Buckner, D., Eisel, R., and Perry, S. (1968). *Blood* **31**, 653.

Buckner, D., Graw, R. G., Jr., Eisel, R. J., Henderson, E. S., and Perry, S. (1969). *Blood* **33**, 353.

Castaldi, P. A., and Firkin, B. G. (1964). *Med. J. Aust.* **51**, 861.

Cavins, J. A., Farber, S., and Roy, A. J. (1968a). *Transfusion (Philadelphia)* **8**, 24.

Cavins, J. A., Pirnar, A., Roy, A. J., and Farber, S. (1968b). *Transfusion (Philadelphia)* **8**, 289.

Chappell, W. (1966). *Transfusion (Philadelphia)* **6**, 308.

Clifford, G. O., Bettigale, R. E., and Glaser, I. (1965). *Transfusion (Philadelphia)* **5**, 378.

Cohen, P., Gardner, F. H., and Barnett, A. C. (1961). *N. Engl. J. Med.* **264**, 1294.

Cohen, P., Watrouse, P., and Gardner, F. H. (1965). *Blood* **25**, 608.

Constantine, J. W. (1965). *Nature (London)* **205**, 1075.

Coombs, R. R. A., and Bedford, P. (1955). *Vox Sang.* **5**, 111.

Cronkite, E. P. (1966). *Transfusion (Philadelphia)* **6**, 18.

Cronkite, E. P., and Jackson, D. P. (1959). Cited in Tocantins (1959).

Cronkite, E. P., Jacobs, G. J., Brecher, G., and Dillard, G. H. L. (1952). *Amer. J. Roentgenol., Radium Ther. Nucl. Med.* **67**, 796.

Dameshek, W., and Gunz, F. (1964). "Leukemia," 2nd ed., p. 331. Grune & Stratton, New York.

Dausset, J., and Maleward, G. (1954). *Vox Sang.* **4**, 204.

Dausset, J., Colin, M., and Colombani, J. (1960). *Vox Sang.* **5**, 4.

Davey, M. G. (1966). "The Survival and Destruction of Human Platelets," p. 137. Karger, Basel.

Davey, M. G., and Lander, H. (1964). *Brit. J. Haematol.* **10**, 94.

Didisheim, P. (1967). *Amer. J. Clin. Pathol.* **47**, 622.

Dillard, G. H. L., Brecher, G., and Cronkite, E. P. (1951). *Proc. Soc. Exp. Biol. Med.* **78**, 796.

Djerassi, I. (1966). *Transfusion* (*Philadelphia*) **6**, 55.

Djerassi, I. and Alvarado, J. (1964). *J. Ann. N. Y. Acad. Sci.* **115**, 366.

Djerassi, I., Farber, S., Roy, A. J., and Yoshimura, H. (1962). *J. Clin. Invest.* **41**, 770.

Djerassi, I., Farber, S., and Evans, A. E. (1963). *N. Engl. J. Med.* **268**, 221.

Djerassi, I., Roy, A., and Alvarado, J. (1964). *Thromb. et Diath. Haemat.* **11**, 222.

Duke, W. W. (1910). *J. Amer. Med. Ass.* **55**, 1185.

Estes, J. W., McGovern, J. J., Goldstein, R., and Rota, M. (1962). *J. Lab. Clin. Med.* **59**, 436.

Farber, S., and Klein, E. (1957). *Ann. Paediat. Fenn.* **3**, 348.

Firkin, B. G., Arimura, G., and Harrington, W. J. (1960). *Blood* **15**, 388.

Flatow, F. A., Jr., and Freireich, E. J. (1966a). *Blood* **27**, 449.

Flatow, F. A., Jr., and Freireich, E. J. (1966b). *New Eng. J. Med.* **274**, 242.

Flatow, F. A., Jr., Levin, R. H., and Freireich, E. J. (1966). *Transfusion* (*Philadelphia*) **6**, 205.

Fliedner, T. M., Sorenson, D. K., Bond, V. P., Cronkite, E. P., Jackson, D. P., and Adamik, E. (1958). *Proc. Soc. Exp. Biol. Med.* **99**, 731.

Freeman, G., and Hyde, J. S. (1952). *Blood* **7**, 311.

Freireich, E. J. (1966). *Transfusion* (*Philadelphia*) **6**, 50.

Freireich, E. J., Kliman, A., Gaydos, L. A., Mantel, N., and Frei, E., III (1963). *Ann. Intern. Med.* **59**, 277.

Friedman, I., Schwartz, S. O., and Leithold, S. L. (1964). *Arch. Intern. Med.* **113**, 177.

Gaarder, A., Jonsen, J., Laland, S., Hellem, A., and Woren, P. A. (1961). *Nature* (*London*) **192**, 531.

Gardner, F. H., and Cohen, P. (1966). *Transfusion* (*Philadelphia*) **6**, 23.

Gardner, F. H., Howell, D., and Hirsh, E. O. (1954). *J. Lab. Clin. Med.* **43**, 196.

Gaydos, L. A., Freireich, E. J., and Mantel, N. (1962). *N. Engl. J. Med.* **266**, 906.

Graw, R. G., Jr., and Eisel, R. (1969). Unpublished observations.

Graw, R. G., Jr., Henderson, E. S., and Perry, S. (1970). *Int. Symp. C.N.R.S. White Cell Transfusion*, 1969 (in press).

Greenwalt, T. J., and Perry, S. (1969). *Progr. Hematol.* **6**, 148.

Gurevitch, J., and Nelken, D. (1954). *J. Lab. Clin. Med.* **44**, 562.

Han, T., Shutzman, L., Cohen, E., and Kim, V. (1966). *Cancer* **19**, 1937.

Harrington, W. J. (1953). *Ann. Intern. Med.* **38**, 433.

Hayem, G. (1882). *C. R. Acad. Sci.* **94**, 200; **96**, 18 (cited in Tocantins, 1948).

Haynes, L., Tullis, J., Pyle, A., Sproul, M., and Wallach, S. (1960). *J. Amer. Med. Ass.* **173**, 1657.

Hellem, A., and Owren, P. A. (1964). *Acta Haematol.* **31**, 230.

Hersh, E. M., Bodey, G. P., Nies, B. A., and Freireich, E. J. (1965). *J. Amer. Med. Ass.* **193**, 105.

Hirsch, E. O., and Gardner, F. H. (1952). *J. Lab. Clin. Med.* **39**, 556.

Hjort, P. F., Perman, V., and Cronkite, E. P. (1959). *Proc. Soc. Exp. Biol. Med.* **102**, 31.

Iossifides, I. A., Glester, P., Eichman, M. F., and Tocantins, L. M. (1962). *Blood* **20**, 762.

Jackson, D. P., Sorensen, D. K., Cronkite, E. P., Bone, V. P., and Fliedner, T. M. (1959). *J. Clin. Invest.* **38**, 1689.

Jacobs, S., and Rosenbaum, E. (1966). *Headache* **6**, 127.

Kevy, S. V., Gibson, J. G., II, and Bartton, L. (1965). *Transfusion (Philadelphia)* **5**, 427.

Kirshbaum, J. D., and Preuss, F. S. (1943). *Arch. Intern. Med.* **71**, 777.

Kissmeyer–Nielsen, F., and Madsen, C. B. (1961a). *J. Clin. Pathol.* **14**, 630.

Kissmeyer–Nielsen, F., and Madsen, C. B. (1961b). *J. Clin. Pathol.* **14**, 626.

Klein, E., Arnold, P., Earl, R. T., and Wake, E. (1956c). *N. Engl. J. Med.* **254**, 1132.

Klein, E., Farber, S., Djerassi, I., Toch, R., Freeman, G., and Arnold, P. (1956b). *J. Pediat.* **49**, 517.

Klein, E., Toch, R., Farber, S., Freeman, G., and Fiorentino, R. (1956a). *Blood* **11**, 693.

Kliman, A., Gaydos, L. A., Schroeder, L. R., and Freireich, E. J. (1961). *Blood* **18**, 303.

Leroy, G. V. (1950). *Arch. Intern. Med.* **86**, 691.

Levin, R. H., Freireich, E. J., and Chappell, W. C. (1964). *Transfusion* **4**, 251.

Levin, R. H., Pert, J. H., and Freireich, E. J. (1965). *Transfusion (Philadelphia)* **5**, 54.

Lewis, J., Draude, J., and Kuhns, W. (1960). *Vox Sang.* **5**, 434.

Lundberg, A., Yankee, R. A., Henderson, E. S., and Pert, J. H. (1967). *Transfusion (Philadelphia)* **7**, 380.

McGovern, J. J. (1957). *N. Engl. J. Med.* **256**, 922.

Marcus, A. J., and Zucker, M. B. (1966). "The Physiology of Blood Platelets," p. 103. Grune & Stratton, New York.

Maupin, B. (1969). "Blood Platelets," Vol. I, Pergamon, New York.

Miller, W. V., Gillem, H. G., Yankee, R. A., and Schmidt, P. J. (1969). *Transfusion (Philadelphia)* **9**, 251.

Morrison, F. S. (1968). *Cryobiology* **5**, 29.

Morrison, F. S. (1966). *Transfusion (Philadelphia)* **6**, 493.

Morrison, F. S. and Baldini, M. (1967). *Vox Sang.* **12**, 90.

Mourad, N. (1968a). *Transfusion (Philadelphia)* **8**, 48.

Mourad, N. (1968b). *Transfusion (Philadelphia)* **8**, 363.

Mourad, N., and Pert, J. H. (1967). *Proc. Soc. Exp. Biol. Med.* **125**, 643.

Murphy, S. and Gardner, F. H. (1969). *N. Engl. J. Med.* **280**, 1094.

Najean, Y., Ardaillou, N., and Dresch, C. (1969). *Annu. Rev. Med.* **20**, 47.

National Academy of Sciences–National Research Council, and the Leukemia Task Force, National Cancer Institute. (1966); *Transfusion (Philadelphia)* **6**, 62.

Ozge, A., Baldini, M., and Goldstein, R. (1964); *J. Lab. Clin. Med.* **63**, 378.

Perry, S. (1957). *J. Lab. Clin. Med.* **50**, 229.

Pert, J. H., Zucker, M. B., Lundberg, A., Yankee, R., and Henderson, E. S. (1967). *Vox Sang.* **13**, 119.

Pfisterer, H., Thierfelder, S., Thiede, C., and Stich, W. (1966). *Klin. Wochenschr.* **44**, 613.

Platelet Transfusion Subcommittee of the Acute Leukemia Task Force. (1968). *Can. Chem. Rep.* **1**, 1.

Raccuglia, G., and Bethell, F. H. (1960). *Amer. J. Clin. Pathol.* **34**, 505.

Rossi, E. C. (1964). *J. Lab. Clin. Med.* **64**, 100.

Rossi, E. C. (1967). *J. Lab. Clin. Med.* **69**, 204.

Salmon, C., and Schwartz, D. (1960). *Rev. Hematol.* **15**, 162.

Salzman, E. W., and Chambers, D. A. (1965). *Nature (London)* **206**, 727.

Sharp, A. A. (1958). *Brit. J. Haematol.* **4**, 28.

Sharp, A. A. (1965). *N. Engl. J. Med.* **272**, 89.

Shively, J. A., Sullivan, M. P., and Chiu, J. S. (1966). *Transfusion (Philadelphia)* **6**, 302.

Shulman, N. R. (1966). *Transfusion (Philadelphia)* **6**, 39.

Shulman, N. R., Marder, V. J., Hiller, M. C., and Collie, E. M. (1964). *Progr. Haematol.* **4**, 222.

Snyder, J., Brakman, P., Henderson, E. S., and Astrup, J. (1967). *Proc. Amer. Ass. Cancer Res.* **8**, 62.

Southam, C. M., Craver, L. F., Dargeon, H. W., and Burchenal, J. H. (1951). *Cancer* **4**, 39.

Spencer, H. H., Starkweather, W. H., and Knorpp, C. T. (1969). *Clin. Res.* **17**, 344.

Stefanini, M., and Dameshek, W. (1953). *N. Engl. J. Med.* **248**, 797.

Svejgaard, A. (1969). *Ser. Haematol.* **2**, 4.

Tocantins, L. M. (1948). *Blood* **3**, 1073.

Tocantins, L. M. (1959). *Progr. Hematol.* **2**, 239.

Tullis, J. L. (1953). *Am. J. Med. Sciences* **226**, 191.

Tullis, J. L., Surgenor, D. M., Tinch, R. J., D'Hont, M., Gilchrist, F. L., Driscoll, S., and Batchelor, W. H. (1956). *Science* **124**, 792.

Tullis, J. L., Tinch, R. J., Gibson, J. G., II, and Baudanza, P. (1967). *Transfusion (Philadelphia)* **7**, 232.

Tullis, J. L., Eberle, W. G., II, Baudanza, P., and Tinch, R. (1968). *Transfusion (Philadelphia)* **8**, 154.

White, J. G., and Krivit, W. (1968). *Scand. J. Haematol.* **5**, 241.

Woods, M. C., Gamble, F. N., Furth, J., and Bigelow, R. R. (1953). *Blood* **8**, 545.

Yankee, R. A., Grumet, F. C., and Rogentine, G. N. (1969). *N. Engl. J. Med.* **281**, 1208.

Zittuouin, A. B. and Samama, M. (1968). *Sem. Hop.* **44**, 183.

Zucker, M. B. and Borrelli, J. (1954). *Blood* **9**, 602.

Zucker, M. B. and Borrelli, J. (1958). *J. Appl. Physiol.* **12**, 453.

Zucker, M. B. and Lundberg, A. (1966). *Anesthesiology* **27**, 385.

AUTHOR INDEX

Numbers in italics refer to the pages on which the complete references are listed.

A

Aas, K. A., 28, 31, *39*, 500, *532*
Abe, T., 337, 343, 344, *349*, 518, *532*, 542, *560*
Abildgaard, C. F., 27, *39*
Abood, L. G., 151, *179*
Abrahamsen, A. F., 32, *39*, 96, *118*, 544, *560*
Achard, C., 6, *14*, 417, *416*
Ackroyd, J. F., 455, *467*, 482, 493, *532*
Adam, A., 140, *185*
Adamik, E. R., 12, *15*, 22, 27, *40*, 558, *561*
Adams, W. S., 25, 26, *40*
Addison, W., 2, *14*
Adelson, E., 31, 33, *39*, 208, *223*
Adler, A., 193, *204*
Adner, M. M., 460, *467*, 555, *560*
Afrelius, B. A., 177, *184*
Aggeler, P. M., 328, *349*, 494, 504, *532*, *538*
Ahmed, K., 152, *179*
Akazaki, K., 13, *14*
Albers, R. W., 152, 165, 166, 167, 170, *179*
Albrechtsen, O. K., 397, *411*
Alder, A., 9, *14*
Aldrich, R. A., 507, 508, *532*
Aledort, L. M., 76, 109, *117*, *119*, 164, *179*, 232, *239*, 261, 264, 265, 266, 268, 273, 274, 276, *278*, *281*, 526, 527, *539*
Alexander, B., 192, *203*
Alkjaersig, N., 200. *204*. 306, 307, 327, 337, 340, 343, 344, *349*, *353*, 396, 398, 399, 406, 409, *411*, *412*, 518, *532*, 542, *560*

Allen, D. M., 508, *537*
Allen, R. D., 106, *117*
Al-Mondhiry, H., 527, *532*
Alpers, H. S., 270, 271, *280*, 423, 434, 435, *470*
Alton, H. G., 329, 344, *349*
Altschul, R., 378, *391*
Altschuler, G., 522, *532*
Alvarado, J., 547, 549, 552, 553, 554, 559, *560*, *561*
Alvarez, A. S., 527, *532*
Ambrus, J. L. 500, *534*
Ames, S. B., 260, *279*, 361, *392*
Amorosi, E. L., 463, *467*
Amris, A., 498, *532*
Amris, C. J., 498, *532*
Amundsen, M. A., 499, *532*
Anderson, B., 34, *42*, 196, *203*, *205*
Andrews, H. L., 461, *471*, 486, 488, *538*
Angrist, A. A., 54, *119*, 194, *200*
Aoki, N., 308, 322, 323, 323, *349*, *353*
Apitz, K., 309, *349*
Applebaum, J., 500, *534*
Ardaillou, N., 34, *41*, 554, 555, *562*
Ardlie, N. G., 262, 277, *278*
Arimura, G. K., 143, 144, *187*, 486, 488, 535, 542, 553, 558, *561*
Arnaud, S. B., 285, *298*, 546, 553, 554, *560*
Arnold, P., 542, 543, 558, *562*
Asano, M., 25, 26, *42*
Ascari, E., 324, *350*
Ash, B. J., 314, *351*
Ashford, S. P., 357, *391*

565

Nelson, R. A., Jr., 421, 437, 438, 439, *470,* *471*

Nemerson, Y., 30, *41,* 145, 147, 155, 159, 161, *184, 185,* 344, *352*

Neri, L. L., 31, 32, *42,* 145, 148, 149, 151, 153, 154, 160, 161, *179, 180, 186,* 222, *224,* 227, 234, 235, *238, 239,* 264, 265, 268, 275, 277, *278, 280*

Neumeister, E., 171, *184*

Newcomb, T. F., 131, 135, 136, 140, 155, 157, 162, 168, *183*

Newsholme, E. A., 130, *182*

Niemetz, J., 109, *117,* 164, *179,* 261, 268, 273, *278,* 454, *470*

Niemeyer, G., 138, 145, 151, 157, 158, 159, 161, 168, 175, *184, 185, 186*

Nies, B. A., 542, 552, *561*

Niewiarowski, S., 7, *16,* 47, *119,* 132, 153, *184,* 191, *204,* 216, *224,* 274, 275, *280,* 302, 343, 346, *351, 352,* 381, 385, *393,* 409, *412,* 516, 524, 528, 532, *536, 537*

Nigam, V. N., 135, *185*

Nijessen, J. G., 513, *538*

Nilsson, I. M., 525, 526, 527, 528, *533, 537*

Nishizawa, E. E., 270, *280,* 371, 381, *393,* 441, 443, *470,* 513, 516, 526, 527, 528, *534, 537*

Norden, A., 142, *185,* 196, *205*

Nordland, M., 12, *15*

Nordling, S., 191, *205*

Nordøy, A., 132, *185,* 377, *391*

Norman, P. S., 398, *412*

Nosal, R., 201, *204*

Nossel, H. L., 272, *281,* 315, *352,* 382, *393,* 515, 516, *539*

Novak, L. V., 138, *183*

Nunnari, A., 190, *205*

O

O'Brien, J. R., 132, 152, *185,* 261, 262, 266, 268, 276, *280,* 328, 346, *349, 352,* 365, *393,* 515, 526, 527, 528, *537*

Odartchenko, N., 20, 22, *40*

Ødegaard, A. E., 132, *185,* 264, 266, *280, 281*

Odell, T. T., Jr., 12, *16,* 23, 24, 25, 26, 27, 29, 34, *40, 41, 42,* 145, 146, 173, *181,* 196, *203, 205*

Odense, P. H., 7, *17*

Odland, G. F., 285, *299*

Oelhafen, H., 12, *16*

Oels, H. C., 498, *537*

O'Grady, L. F., 21, *41*

Ohi, Y., 169, *187*

Ohler, W. G. A., 127, 140, 179, *185*

Ohnashi, T., 108, *119*

Ohnishi, Tomoko, 178, *185*

Ohnishi, Tsuyoshi, 178, *185*

Okuma, M., 30, *42*

Olbromski, J., 346, *349*

Oldfield, R., 160, *182*

Oliveira, B., 444, *471*

Oliver, R. A. M., 505, *538*

Ollegaard, E., 5, *16*

Olsson, I., 142, *185,* 196, 197, *205*

Olwin, J. H., 138, *183,* 335, *351*

O'Neill, J., 160, *182*

Onoue, K., 443, 451, *470*

Opie, E. L., 401, *412*

Orbison, J. L., 463, *470*

Org, L., 268, *278*

O'Riordan, J., 500, *534*

Oski, F. A., 484, 493, 494, 508, *536, 537*

Osler, A. G., 420, 422, 423, 424, 426, 430, 431, 437, 443, *468, 469, 671*

Osler, W., 2, *17,* 46, *119*

Ostrowski, L., 524, *536*

Otto, P., 171, *184*

Overcash, J., 11, *15,* 25, 26, 27, *40*

Owen, C. A., Jr., 7, *14,* 474, 477, 478, 491, 498, 499, 500, 509, 512, 514, 515, 517, 518, 519, 522, 524, 526, 531, *532, 533,* *535, 537, 539*

Owren, P. A., 5, *15,* 260, 263, 266, *279,* 342, *350,* 361, *391,* 549, *561*

Ozer, F. L., 510, *537*

Ozge, A., 33, *41, 185,* 544, *562*

P

Pachter, M. R., 522, *537*

Packham, M. A., 270, *279, 280,* 371, 381, *393,* 441, 443, *470,* 513, 516, 526, 527, 528, *534, 536, 537*

Paetkau, V., 170, 173, *183*

SUBJECT INDEX

A